Methods
in Pharmacology

Volume 2

METHODS IN PHARMACOLOGY

a series of monographs
edited by Arnold Schwartz

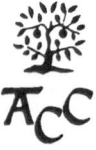

APPLETON-CENTURY-CROFTS
Educational Division
MEREDITH CORPORATION
New York

METHODS IN PHARMACOLOGY

Volume 2
Physical Methods

edited by COLIN F. CHIGNELL

Laboratory of Chemical Pharmacology
National Heart and Lung Institute
National Institutes of Health
Bethesda, Maryland

ISBN 978-1-4757-0198-2   ISBN 978-1-4757-0196-8 (eBook)
DOI 10.1007/978-1-4757-0196-8

Copyright © 1972 by MEREDITH CORPORATION

Softcover reprint of the hardcover 1st edition 1972

72 73 74 75 76/10 9 8 7 6 5 4 3 2

Library of Congress Catalog Card Number: 70-92660

390-19055-1

to Anke

Contributors

JEFFREY BARON
Department of Biochemistry, University of Texas (Southwestern) Medical School at Dallas, Dallas, Texas

THEODOR H. BENZINGER
National Bureau of Standards, Gaithersburg, Maryland

RAYMOND F. CHEN
Laboratory of Technical Development, National Heart and Lung Institute, National Institutes of Health, Bethesda, Maryland

COLIN F. CHIGNELL
Laboratory of Chemical Pharmacology, National Heart and Lung Institute, National Institutes of Health, Bethesda, Maryland

DEREK A. CHIGNELL
Department of Biological Chemistry, University of California School of Medicine, Los Angeles, California

B. L. VAN DUUREN
Laboratory of Organic Chemistry and Carcinogenesis, Institute of Environmental Medicine, New York University Medical Center, New York, New York

RONALD W. ESTABROOK
Department of Biochemistry, University of Texas (Southwestern) Medical School at Dallas, Dallas, Texas

CATHERINE FENSELAU
Department of Pharmacology and Experimental Therapeutics, The Johns Hopkins University School of Medicine, Baltimore, Maryland

RAYMOND J. GAJAN
Division of Chemistry and Physics, Food and Drug Administration, Department of Health, Education, and Welfare, Washington, D.C.

O. HAYES GRIFFITH
Institute of Molecular Biology and Department of Chemistry, University of Oregon, Eugene, Oregon

ALFRED HILDEBRANDT
Department of Biochemistry, University of Texas (Southwestern) Medical School at Dallas, Dallas, Texas

DONALD P. HOLLIS
Department of Physiological Chemistry, The Johns Hopkins University, School of Medicine, Baltimore, Maryland

JORDAN L. HOLTZMAN
Clinical Pharmacology Division, Minneapolis Veterans Administration Hospital, Minneapolis, Minnesota, and Department of Pharmacology, University of Minnesota, Minneapolis, Minnesota

PATRICIA JOST
Institute of Molecular Biology and Department of Chemistry, University of Oregon, Eugene, Oregon

S. H. KIM
Department of Biology, Massachusetts Institute of Technology, Cambridge, Massachusetts

JULIAN PETERSON
Department of Biochemistry, University of Texas (Southwestern) Medical School at Dallas, Dallas, Texas

PALMER W. TAYLOR
Division of Pharmacology, Department of Medicine, University of California, San Diego, La Jolla, California

DAVID N. TELLER
Associate Research Scientist, Biochemistry, New York State Research Institute for Neurochemistry and Drug Addiction, Wards Island, New York, New York

G. WITZ
Laboratory of Organic Chemistry and Carcinogenesis, Institute of Environmental Medicine, New York University Medical Center, New York, New York

Preface

This volume, the second in the Methods in Pharmacology series, contains some of the physical methods which either have been or could be applied to pharmacological problems. A major emphasis has been placed on spectroscopic techniques, particularly those, such as optical rotatory dispersion and circular dichroism, fluorescence spectroscopy, magnetic resonance spectroscopy, ultraviolet absorption spectroscopy, stopped flow and relaxation spectrometry, Mössbauer spectroscopy, light scatter and x-ray crystallography, that can be used to study drug interactions with biological systems at a molecular level. Although phosphorescence spectroscopy and oscillographic polarography can also be used to study drug interactions, their main usefulness is in the detection and estimation of drugs and their metabolities in body tissues and fluids. Mass spectrometry is a powerful tool for studying the metabolism of drugs as well as for detecting abnormal endogenous metabolites in the body. Finally, heatburst microcalorimetry is a nonspectroscopic technique that can be used to study how drugs and other ligands interact with biological macromolecules.

Each chapter contains a brief introduction to the theoretical basis for each technique as well as a description of the instrumentation involved. This is followed by a section describing the application of the technique to pharmacological problems. Where these are not available, examples have been drawn from the other life sciences. In a final section, some further applications of each technique to problems in pharmacology are suggested. After a research worker has read any given chapter, it should be possible for him to decide whether the technique described could be applied in his own research. Since most of these techniques require extensive training in the operation of expensive equipment, it is unlikely that the reader will carry out the experiments himself. For this reason, this volume does not contain the kind of detailed instructions found in the first volume. Rather, we have attempted to provide the research worker with sufficient background so that he can seek out a specialist in one or more of these techniques and be able to discuss intelligently with him the application of the methodology to his own particular problem. While no attempt has been made to make each chapter comprehensive, the authors have been encouraged to include sufficient material so that this book can serve as a reference for those already working in the fields described. Although this volume is primarily aimed at the needs of the pharmacologist, its contents are equally suitable for physiologists, biological and medicinal chemists, organic and other chemists, and researchers in many other disciplines concerned with analytic techniques.

Finally, it should be emphasized that the selection of subjects for this volume reflects the personal prejudices of the editor. There are no doubt many other techniques that could have been included in a book such as this. Hopefully these can appear in succeeding volumes in this series.

I should like to thank Mrs. B. J. Chambers and Mrs. D. M. Sherwood for typing several of the chapters, and Mrs. D. K. Starkweather and Miss D. DiMasi for help in proofreading the manuscripts. I am also greatly indebted to Dr. Elwood O. Titus for advice and encouragement given during the preparation of this volume.

Colin F. Chignell

Contents

Chapter **1**

Fluorescence Spectroscopy— Theory and Measurement

Raymond F. Chen

Laboratory of Technical Development, National Heart and Lung Institute, National Institutes of Health, Bethesda, Maryland

BACKGROUND AND THEORY

Introduction

Pharmacologists have long been interested in fluorometry, a technique naturally suited to the detection and study of drugs. The specificity and sensitivity of fluorometric assays are indispensible in many areas of pharmacology; conversely, pharmacologists have contributed in many ways to the development of fluorescence spectroscopy. Many of the most interesting fluorescent compounds such as quinine, carcinogenic hydrocarbons, the coumarins, heterocyclic antibiotics, and certain psychoactive drugs have been brought to the attention of the fluorescence spectroscopist as a result of their physiological importance. The need to develop fluorometric apparatus for pharmacologic uses has provided a significant part of the commercial incentive to develop instrumentation which can be purchased also by the theoretical chemist interested in fluorescence processes.

At the outset, one should distinguish between the use of fluorometric methods to assay a drug, and the use of more sophisticated fluorescence spectroscopic techniques to study other phenomena such as molecular interactions. As Udenfriend (1962) has pointed out, the former usage requires simple instrumentation and little understanding of the underlying phenomena. In contrast, a greater appreciation of the potential of fluorescence spectroscopy can be rewarding and may suggest practical approaches to the solution of difficult problems. This chapter will

1

review briefly the basic nature of the light-emission process and methods of measurement involved in fluorescence spectroscopy. This discipline is now well established in the biomedical field and cannot be neglected.

Historical

Although it is not exactly clear when the first accounts of fluorescence appeared, E. N. Harvey (1957) has written a history of luminescence including references to light phenomena in ancient times. Since concepts about the nature of luminescence are intimately connected with scientific theories about the nature of matter and energy, it is obvious in retrospect that in earlier times there was no adequate framework for distinguishing between different forms of light phenomena such as fluorescence, light scattering, reflection, phosphorescence, and even phosphenes—the light one "sees" when pressing on the eyeball. Modern ideas about fluorescence depended on the development of electromagnetic theory in the late nineteenth century.

The visible blue emission of quinine held in sunlight was recognized by Herschel (1845) to be different from scattered white light. This and many other observations were sorted and classified by Stokes (1852) in a classic, lengthy (112 pages) paper. Stokes is often considered the father of fluorescence not only because he coined the term, but also because he clearly understood that the process involved actual absorption and subsequent emission of energy.

Both fluorescence and phosphorescence arise from molecules which have been excited to a higher state by the absorption of light. Therefore, the phenomena should more properly be considered to be forms of *photoluminescence*. Light emission may also arise from excited states reached by different routes; hence we have chemiluminescence, electroluminescence, biochemiluminescence, and the like. Fluorescence differs from phosphorescence in that the former seems to disappear upon extinguishing the exciting light, while the latter persists for a perceptible time afterwards.

The term phosphorescence is derived from Greek roots meaning "light bearing." The etymology of "fluorescence" is less obvious. The term derives from fluorspar, a mineral which is used as a flux in the refinement of ores and exhibits fluorescence. "Fluorspar" in turn is derived from the Latin *fluere*, to flow; i.e., fluorspar is a "flow stone" (Shipley, 1945).

Measurements of fluorescence with commercially produced instruments were performed largely with filter fluorometers until the mid–1950's. Apparatus for recording spectra was not available except to physicists or other specialists who built their own instruments. In the late 1940's, marked developments were made in photomultiplier tubes; and sensitive and quantitative fluorometric measurements became possible. Commercially produced spectrofluorometers became available in the late 1950's. Workers were also measuring fluorescence polarization about the same time by modifying commercially available light scattering instruments. In recent years there have been improvements in spectrofluorometers, offerings of automatic "corrected" spectrofluorometers, and even apparatus for determining fluorescence lifetimes. The current intense interest in fluorescence is due both to the availability of instrumentation and to realization of the potential of the technique.

Basis of Photoluminescence

When a molecule absorbs a photon, a quantum of light energy, it is said to be in an excited state. The normal, or ground, state is reached again when the excited molecule emits fluorescence or loses the excess energy by some other mechanism. Whether a molecule is in a ground or excited state is determined by the potential energy of electrons in the molecular orbitals. Light absorption and light emission (fluorescence) involve movement of electrons from one orbital to another; hence optical spectra are considered to be due to these "electronic transitions." The total energy of a molecule is, of course, made up of many other factors including rotational and vibrational energy. Thus, while quantum theory indicates that there are discrete electronic states for each molecule, in practice there are almost an infinite number of energetic states due to the many possible substates involving different vibrational energy levels. In atomic spectra, fewer energy levels are available, and the absorption and emission spectra are typically simple lines. In contrast, the absorption spectra of organic molecules in solution are typically broad bands which represent electronic transitions from the ground state to many vibrational levels of higher states.

The only quantum theory equation we need to concern ourselves with here is Planck's equation, which describes the dual nature (both particulate and wave-like) of light:

$$e = h\nu \tag{1}$$

Here e is the energy of a quantum of energy, h is Planck's constant, and ν is the frequency of the radiation. Spectra are often expressed in terms of wavelength λ which is related to the frequency ν, by the equation $\nu = c/\lambda$, where c is the speed of light. From this one can see that light of short wavelength has higher energy than light of longer wavelength; or, put another way, blue photons are more energetic than red ones. Stokes (1852) noted that in true fluorescence the emitted light was always of longer wavelength than that of the exciting light. This observation, known as Stokes' Law, merely states that the emitted photon cannot have higher energy than that of the absorbed photon.

The abscissa in an optical spectrum is usually presented in terms of wavelength, λ, in most publications in biology and chemistry. However, physicists prefer to use either the frequency, ν, or the wave-number, which is the reciprocal of wavelength, $1/\lambda$, since these quantities are directly related to the energy of a photon (equation 1). The units of wavelength most often used are angstroms (1 Å $= 10^{-8}$ cm), millimicrons, or nanometers (1 mμ $= 1$ nm $= 10^{-7}$ cm). In this chapter, nm will be used except for some figures taken from other publications.

Our discussion of the quantum jumps called electronic transitions may be illustrated by Figure 1, which will also serve to introduce some common spectroscopic terminology. The ground state and higher states have the symbols S_0, S_1, S_2,

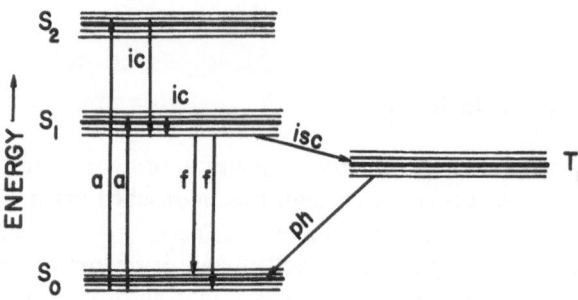

FIG. 1. Energy diagram showing the types of electronic transitions involved in photoluminescence. For definition of abbreviations, see text.

. . . , S_n. The S stands for singlet state, a quantum mechanical term for a structure
where the molecular orbitals contain paired electrons with opposing spin. T_1 represents the lowest triplet state, which differs from singlet states in that one electron
has undergone a reversal of spin, so that the molecule as a whole is now paramagnetic. (Not shown in Figure 1 are higher triplet states, T_2, T_3, . . . , T_n.) As
shown in Figure 1, fluorescence arises from S_1 and phosphorescence arises from T_1.
The symbols used represent the various types of electronic transitions: a, absorption; f, fluorescence; ic, internal conversion; isc, intersystem crossing; and ph,
phosphorescence. Internal conversion is the process whereby energy is lost by heat,
and an excited molecule passes from one singlet state to another. Intersystem crossing is the process of going from a singlet to a triplet state, or vice versa.

Optical spectra are frequently referred to as "electronic spectra" since, as
shown in Figure 1, the energy changes which are involved are due to electrons
changing their orbitals. In absorption spectra, the longest wavelength band (lowest
in energy) usually represents the $S_0 \rightarrow S_1$ transition, the next longest wavelength
band the $S_0 \rightarrow S_2$ transition, and so forth. However, note that fluorescence is simply
the $S_1 \rightarrow S_0$ transition, so that the fluorescence spectrum is always much simpler
than the complete absorption spectrum. In fact, for many compounds in aqueous
solution, the fluorescence emission spectrum is a single, structureless band. At low
temperatures, some structure may be evident in fluorescence spectra due to resolution of vibrational levels rather than due to additional electronic transitions.

Figure 1 does not show the radiationless transitions from S_1 and T_1 to S_0.
These radiationless transitions are modes of energy loss involving dissipation of
heat and can be considered to compete with fluorescence and phosphorescence.
Radiationless processes can be considered to have rates, just as fluorescence does.
Strongly fluorescent compounds, then, have fluorescence rate constants which are
much faster than those for radiationless processes, and the reverse is true for weakly
fluorescent compounds.

Since an absorbed photon does not split into more photons, the number of
emitted photons is never greater than that absorbed. The quantum yield, in other
words, cannot exceed unity. For most compounds, in addition, it is thought that the
process of internal conversion from higher states down to the lowest level of S_1
occurs with 100% quantum efficiency. Thus, the quantum yield will be identical

whether the absorbed photon represents the transition $S_0 \rightarrow S_1$ or $S_0 \rightarrow S_n$. Practically speaking, this means that excitation at any wavelength will produce fluorescence in proportion to the strength of absorption; i.e., the absorption and excitation spectra should coincide.

A more precise definition of fluorescence and phosphorescence can be made in view of the discussion of Figure 1. Fluorescence can be thought of as luminescence arising from a singlet state, while phosphorescence arises from a triplet state. This definition is generally true for molecules whose ground states are singlet in character, but there are rare exceptions such as stable free radicals, which may have unpaired electrons in the ground state. Actually, the original definition of Lewis and Kasha (1944, 1945) stated that fluorescence involved an electronic transition between the same type of state while phosphorescence involved a transition between different spin states.

We may consider further some of the times involved in the electronic transitions discussed above. The absorption of light is essentially an instantaneous process depending only on the width of the molecule and the speed of light. Thus absorption is said to take place in the order of 10^{-15} to 10^{-18} sec. Also very rapid are the internal conversions from higher states to the lowest excited state S_1; these occur in perhaps 10^{-12} sec or so. Fluorescence, radiationless transitions, and intersystem crossing are slower and may be of the same order of magnitude, taking place in 10^{-10} to 10^{-7} sec. Phosphorescence is slow, because the probability of the necessary electron spin reversal is low; the process occurs in time ranges from 10^{-4} to 10^{+3} seconds.

For more detailed description of the basis of luminescence processes, the reader is referred to texts by Reid (1957), Pringsheim (1949), Calvert and Pitts (1966), Seliger and McElroy (1965), and Parker (1969). Useful multiauthored volumes expanding on the above material are the works edited by Hercules (1966) and Guilbault (1967). Elementary exposition of this material will also be found in the widely used texts of Udenfriend (1962, 1969).

Fluorescence and Chemical Structure

Almost all fluorescent compounds which will be encountered by the pharmacologist are aromatic or heteroaromatic ring compounds. A common feature of these substances is a system of conjugated pi electrons such as in benzene. Apparently the electrons in unsaturated bonds are held "loosely" enough that they may be raised to other quantum mechanically allowed states by ultraviolet and visible light. In contrast, saturated hydrocarbons in which the bonding electrons are of the sigma type are nonfluorescent. These compounds do not absorb light above 200 nm unless they have some other chromophoric group. To excite the sigma electrons, higher energy photons are needed (wavelengths of under 150 nm) and this can result in bond scission.

An empirical observation is that the more extensive the pi electron system, the longer is the wavelength at which the fluorescence peaks. Thus, benzene, naphthalene, anthracene, and other acenes are highly fluorescent and emit at successively longer wavelengths. In cyclohexane, the approximate peak wavelengths of emission are 280 nm for benzene, 390 nm for naphthalene, and 450 nm for anthracene.

Due to the involvement of pi electrons in fluorescence, one sometimes sees the term "$\pi^* \to \pi$" fluorescence, indicating that emission is due to an excited pi electron. Another type of fluorescence is encountered occasionally, namely "$\pi^* \to n$" fluorescence, which arises from "$n \to \pi^*$" absorption. The terminology refers to absorption and fluorescence due to an electronic transition between a ground state nonbonding electronic orbital and an excited state pi orbital. Such fluorescence is exhibited by aromatic carbonyl and nitrogen heterocyclic compounds and is usually weaker than $\pi^* \to \pi$ fluorescence.

When an aromatic compound is substituted in the ring system by halogen atoms, the fluorescence may be markedly affected. Fluorine may enhance fluorescence yield, as in the fluorophenylalanines, which are more fluorescent than phenylalanine itself (Chen, 1967a). Chlorine may not have much of an influence, but bromine and iodine generally quench fluorescence. In fact, there are few iodinated compounds which are fluorescent. Ring substitution by $-NO_2$ usually results in a nonfluorescent product. On the other hand, other radicals such as -OH, -COOH, $-SO_3H$, $-OCH_3$, $-CH_3$, $-(CH_2)_nCH_3$ and $-\phi$ are all compatible with fluorescence. Ionization of a phenolic hydroxyl group may cause loss of fluorescence; this is true of phenol and tyrosine, but may cause only a shift in emission wavelength as in the case of naphthols.

The mechanism by which these radicals affect fluorescence is not known in every case. However, in some instances such as iodine substitution, the resulting compound may have no fluorescence, but the phosphorescence is markedly enhanced over that of the parent compound. This suggests that the substituent increases the rate of intersystem crossing to the triplet state; i.e., the strong electric field of the substituent atom or radical is conducive to spin reversal in one of the pi electrons of the parent molecule.

It should be emphasized that the preceding discussion attempts to correlate fluorescence with chemical structure alone, but actually the presence or absence of fluorescence is always dependent on many other factors as well, such as temperature, solvent, pH, and sensitivity to quenching agents such as the omnipresent O_2. Caffeine is a notable example of a compound which is "nonfluorescent" at room temperature but at liquid N_2 temperature (77°K) has intense fluorescence (Longworth, 1962).

Events Occurring in the Excited State

Although fluorescence appears to be "instantaneous," there is actually a finite interval between absorption and emission. During the excited state lifetime, denoted by the symbol τ, which has a magnitude of the order of 10^{-8} sec (or 10 nsec, where nsec $= 10^{-9}$ sec) for organic molecules, a number of events may occur which will be reflected in the character of the fluorescence. The following is a listing of events which may occur after a molecule A has been excited to the S_1 singlet state, becoming A^*:

1. $A^* \rightarrow A + h\nu$ (fluorescence)
2. $A^* \rightarrow A + h\nu'$ (phosphorescence)
3. $trans\text{-}A^* \rightarrow cis\text{-}A^*$ (cis-trans isomerization)
4. $A^* + B \rightarrow C$ (photochemical reaction)
5. $A^* \rightarrow A'^*$ (rotation)
6. $A^* + H^+ \rightarrow AH^+$ (excited state protonation)
7. $A^* \rightarrow A^{-*} + H^+$ (photoionization)
8. $A^* \rightarrow A$ (quenching)
9. $A^* \rightarrow A''^*$ (solvent reorientation, configurational changes)
10. $A^* + B \rightarrow B^* + A$ (energy transfer)

Some of the above reactions are self-explanatory. An example of *cis-trans* isomerization is the isomerization of *trans*-stilbene to *cis*-stilbene by light, or isomerization of all-*trans*-retinene to Δ^{11}-*cis*-retinene. Such isomerizations usually are slower than fluorescence, so that fluorescence is usually unaffected except that continued exposure of the solution will result in a change or loss of fluorescence due to a change in the compound.

Event 5, above, is of interest because it is possible to study the rotations undergone by molecules due to their Brownian motion by means of *fluorescence polarization* methods. The basic principle is simple: If a fluorescent molecule is excited with polarized light, the resulting fluorescence will be polarized provided that the molecule does not rotate during the interval between the absorption and emission of light. In some cases the fluorescence is only partially polarized, and here it is possible to say how much rotation has taken place provided one can accurately measure the polarization and the fluorescence lifetime, τ. The relevant equations and examples of the use of fluorescence polarization are given on p. 10, below.

Events 6 and 7 (above) refer to the acid-base properties of fluorescent molecules. The protonation or ionization constants of an excited molecule A^* may be completely different from those of the ground-state molecule A. The pK_a of naphthols typically changes from about 9 to near 3 in the excited state (Weller, 1961). A general rule is that phenols and naphthols become stronger acids by about 6 pK_a units in the excited state, and bases become stronger bases (Wehry and Rogers, 1966). An interesting example of event 6, excited-state protonation, occurs with acid solutions of 5-hydroxytryptamine (serotonin). This substance has an absorption peak at about 274 nm and in neutral solution emits at about 340 nm (Figure 2). However, in acid solution, a bright green fluorescence develops even though the absorption spectrum is unchanged. The green fluorescence is the basis of the well-known fluorometric assay of serotonin (Bogdanski et al., 1956). It has been shown that the green fluorescence is due to an excited-state protonated form of serotonin and that the protonation is probably at position 6, where serotonin in the ground state has no tendency to accept a proton (Chen, 1968).

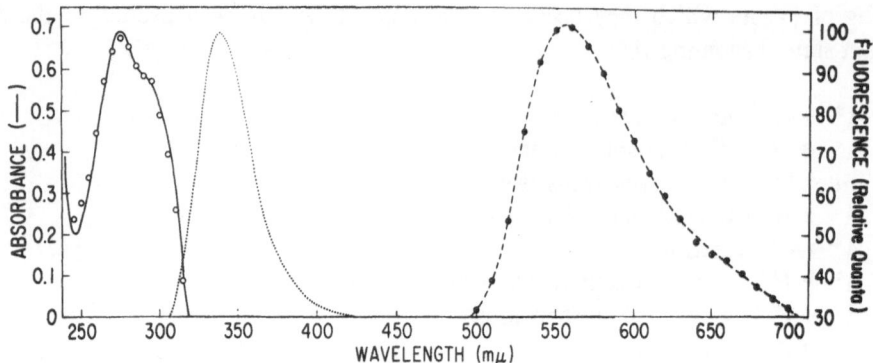

FIG. 2. Spectra of serotonin. The curves represent absorption (—), ultraviolet fluorescence (- - -), visible fluorescence (-●-), and excitation (-o-). UV fluorescence was obtained in 0.01 M Tris-Cl⁻ buffer, pH 7; while visible fluorescence was measured in 3 M HCl. The absorption and excitation spectra were identical in the two solvents. (From Chen. 1968. *Proc. Nat. Acad. Sci. U.S.A.*, 60:598.)

Event 9, the change in molecule shape or solvation which may occur after a molecule is excited but before it emits a photon, is the basis of many fluorescence spectral shifts. The change in orientation of solvent molecules has been particularly well studied by Lippert (1957). When a molecule is placed in different solvents, the fluorescence spectrum may shift markedly; this effect is illustrated by dansyl[1] tryptophan in Figure 3. It is now known that the excited states responsible for $\pi^* \to \pi$ fluorescence involve molecules whose dipole moments are much higher than they were in the ground state. Since the solvent molecules, like H_2O, are also dipoles, there is an increased attraction between the solvent and excited state fluorescer. This attraction causes the solvent molecules to reorient themselves, a process which uses up energy, so that when the fluorescent photon is finally emitted, it has less energy than it would have had without the solvent interaction. This means that the average emitted photon is of a longer wavelength (or lower frequency) in polar solvents than in nonpolar solvents which would interact less strongly with the excited state solute molecule. The position of the emission spectral peak is related to the dielectric constant of the solvent; this was quantitated by Lippert (1957) in a number of equations whose validation was strong evidence for the dipole-dipole interaction theory as the basis of such fluorescence spectral shifts. It should also be noted that Figure 3 shows that the strength of fluorescence also seems to increase, the less the spectrum is shifted towards higher wavelengths. This perhaps indicates that collisional encounters with polar molecules are more frequent, resulting in more energy dissipation.

Energy transfer, event 10 above, is a process which is most often studied by fluorescence spectroscopy since few other techniques are applicable. The basic principle may be likened to setting one tuning fork into vibration by vibrating another tuning fork that has the same frequency nearby. Resonance is *induced* in

---

[1] Abbreviation used: dansyl, 1-dimethylamino-5-sulfonyl

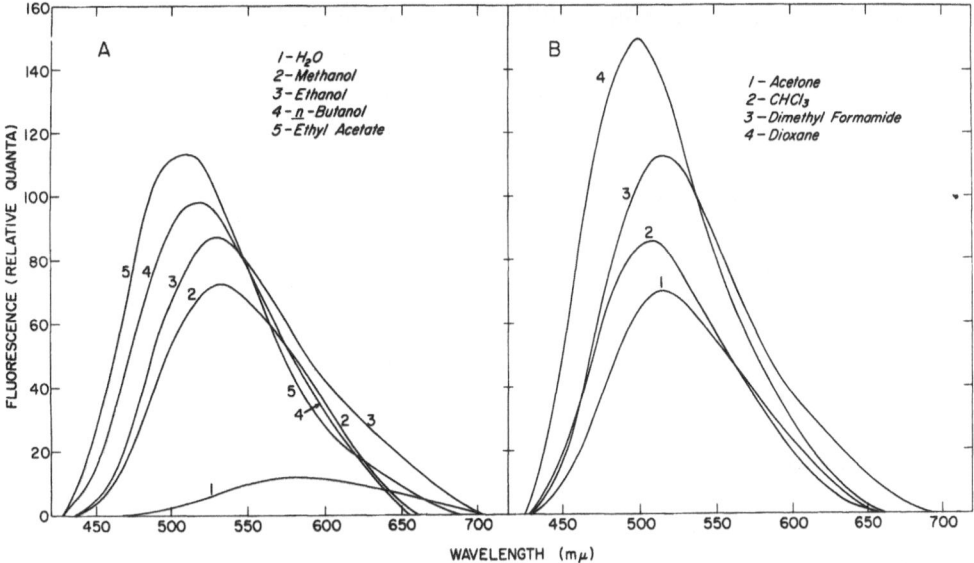

FIG. 3. Emission spectra of dansyl DL-tryptophan in water and organic solvents, excited at 332 nm. The areas beneath the curves are directly related to the fluorescence quantum yields. (From Chen. 1967b. *Arch. Biochem. Biophys.*, 120:609.)

the first tuning fork. Similarly, energy transfer may occur between organic molecules provided that they share the same light frequencies for fluorescence and absorption. The process is often called "induced resonance," or energy transfer by the Förster mechanism, so called because of the investigator who was instrumental in elucidating the process. In terms of spectra, in the case of the energy transfer process $A^* + B \rightarrow B^* + A$, the emission spectrum of A must overlap the absorption spectrum of B. In this way, if the two molecules are close to one another, excitation of A may give rise to fluorescence from B, while at the same time the fluorescence from A is quenched. If B is nonfluorescent, the only evidence of energy transfer will be the quenching of fluorescence of A.

The reason for the importance of energy transfer resides in the ability of this phenomenon to impart knowledge about the distances between donor and acceptor molecules. Using an equation developed by Förster (1951) it is possible to calculate R_0, the distance between A and B where the probability of energy transfer is equal to the probability of fluorescence. Knowing R_0, one can measure the actual degree of energy transfer either by the degree of quenching of fluorescence from A, or by the amount of sensitized fluorescence elicited from B by excitation of A. If the energy transfer is 50%, the two molecules are separated by the distance R_0. If the fraction of absorbed photons which is transferred is X, the separation distance is given by (Chen and Kernohan, 1967):

$$1 - X = \frac{1}{(R_0/R)^6 + 1} \qquad (2)$$

The Förster equation (Förster, 1951) for calculating R_0 is:

$$R_0 = \sqrt[6]{\frac{1.66 \times 10^{-33} \times \tau J}{n^2 \, X \, \bar{v}_0^2}} \tag{3}$$

where $\bar{v}_0$ is the mean of the peak positions of the donor emission and lowest energy absorption bands, J is the "overlap integral," and n the refractive index. J is defined as $\int \varepsilon(v) f(v) \, dv$, a quantity which can be evaluated graphically by plotting out the corrected emission spectrum of the donor and the absorption spectrum of the acceptor in terms of the frequency v. The probability of energy transfer is clearly enhanced by a long fluorescence lifetime, a strong overlap of fluorescence and absorption bands, and a high extinction coefficient of the acceptor.

Actual examples of the use of energy transfer calculations in studying intermolecular distances will be cited in Chapter 2.

Fluorescence Polarization

Fluorescent molecules may be viewed as having linear arrays of absorbing or emitting oscillators. When one excites a solution with linearly polarized light, only those molecules whose absorbing dipole vectors are parallel to the direction of polarization will absorb light energy. Fluorescence will also be polarized to a degree depending on how much Brownian motion has randomized the orientation of these molecules during the excited state lifetime. For most small molecules like the dye fluorescein, in nonviscous solvents such as water, so much Brownian motion can occur that the fluorescence is practically completely unpolarized. However, if a more viscous solvent like glycerol is used, or if low temperatures are employed, one can see polarization even of small molecules. Large molecules like nucleic acids and proteins show marked fluorescence polarization, and from this the amount of Brownian motion may be quantitated to give information on the size and shape of the molecule.

Perrin (1925, 1926) and Levshin (1925) worked out the basic theory relating the polarization P[1], lifetime τ, and molecular size:

$$1/P - 1/3 = (1/P_0 - 1/3)(1 + \frac{RT\tau}{\eta V}) \tag{4}$$

Here R is the gas constant, P_0 is the maximum polarization, which would be observed at infinite viscosity, η is the viscosity, V is the molecular volume with the assumption that the shape is a sphere, and T is the absolute temperature. The above

---

[1] Details of the definition and measurement of P will be given under the section on Fluorescence Methods. The equations given here assume that the fluorescence is excited with polarized light. P can then have a maximum value of 0.5, although the polarization will be near 0 for most small molecules in nonviscous solvents.

relation, called the Perrin equation, refers to spheres only, but since many small dye molecules are approximately spherical when considered with their solvent shells, the measurement of polarization can be used as an indirect method for determining τ. The other quantities in equation 4 are easily measured, except for V, which can be estimated from the chemical structure. The quantity P_0 is usually obtained by extrapolation of a plot of $1/P - 1/3$ vs. T/η obtained by measuring P at different temperatures. Such a "Perrin plot" extrapolated to $T/\eta = 0$ gives the limiting polarization.

If one knows the fluorescence lifetime, τ, one can use equation 4 to calculate the molecular volume. This has been done by Singleterry and Weinberger (1951), who adsorbed the dye rhodamine B onto soap micelles and studied the micellar size by polarization of fluorescence.

An important use of fluorescence polarization is the detection of binding of small fluorescent molecules onto larger, relatively stationary macromolecules such as proteins. Upon binding, the polarization increases from a value near zero to a very high level. Such binding studies have been carried out for adsorption of dyes onto serum albumin (Ainsworth and Flanagan, 1969), antigen-antibody interactions (Haber and Bennett, 1962; Dandliker and Feigen, 1961; Dandliker et al., 1965), and dye absorption to enzymes (Deranleau and Neurath, 1966).

The Perrin equation also applies to proteins which have been labeled with fluorescent dyes. Weber (1952) showed that the mean harmonic rotational relaxation time, ρ_h, which is a measure of a protein's Brownian rotation, may be estimated from a modification of the Perrin equation:

$$1/P - 1/2 = (1/P_0 - 1/3)\,(1 + \frac{3\tau}{\rho_h}) \tag{5}$$

The great usefulness of this relation is due to the fact that information on macromolecular size and shape is obtained even though it is the fluorescence of the small, attached dye molecules which is being measured. However, the equation is true only if the protein is approximately ellipsoidal, the dyes are rigidly bound, the protein rotates as a rigid entity, and the dyes are randomly oriented with respect to the protein axes. Equation 5 has been widely used to obtain relaxation times for proteins and to study changes in conformation due to denaturants or other factors. Although the basic assumptions such as rigid dye binding and absence of segmental rotations have not always been true (for review, see Chen, 1967c), the polarization method is still one of the most convenient and powerful tools for observing *changes* in structure.

Examples of Perrin plots of a dye-labeled protein are given in Figure 4. Most serum albumins are known to undergo molecular unfolding at about *p*H 4. Figure 4 shows the changes in Perrin plots obtained at different *p*H values with a dansyl rabbit albumin preparation. The increased slope of the plots at lower *p*H indicates faster Brownian rotation of the dyes, probably due to a relaxation of the macromolecular structure.

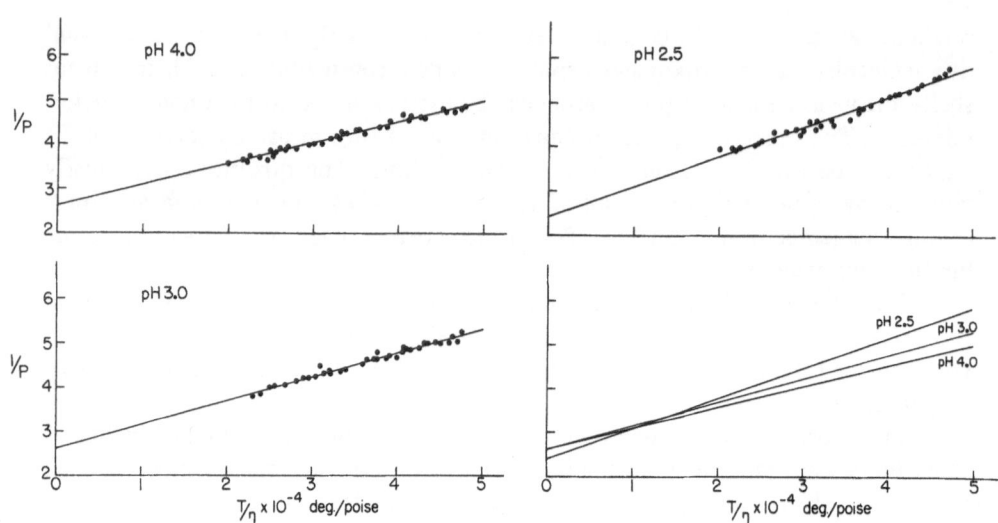

FIG. 4. Examples of Perrin plots. Data were obtained with a dansyl conjugate of rabbit serum albumin, which was dissolved in water. The pH of the resultant solutions was changed by addition of HCl to the values shown. Excitation was at 360 nm and emission was monitored at 500 nm. The greater slopes at lower pH indicate faster rotational movement of the dyes possibly due to increased flexibility due to unfolding of the albumin.

MEASUREMENT OF FLUORESCENCE

Fluorescence Parameters

There are various aspects to the fluorescence of an organic compound, but not all of these parameters are always relevant or necessary to measure in a given study. The parameters which may be measured are: (a) Fluorescence "intensity." (b) Spectra (absorption, excitation and emission). (c) Quantum yield. (d) Polarization. (e) Fluorescence lifetime.

(a). FLUORESCENCE INTENSITY. In analytical methods using fluorescence, the important numbers to obtain are the relative fluorescence intensities of the unknown samples and those of the standards. The comparative measurements may be carried out in a *filter fluorometer*. This type of instrument consists basically of a light source, a sample compartment, a photodetector system, and filters to provide some selectivity in the spectrum of light reaching the sample and detector. Instead of being in line with the light source and the sample, the detector is placed to the side, so that light emitted at right angles to the direction of excitation is actually observed. This orthogonal geometry is utilized in order to avoid contamination of the fluorescence signal by exciting light. The primary and secondary filters are placed between the lamp and cell, and between cell and detector, respectively. The primary filter ideally transmits those wavelengths which are effective in exciting the sample, while the secondary filter passes the emitted light but not the exciting wavelength. Any scattered exciting radiation will, therefore, be prevented from reaching the detector in the ideal situation. In practice, there is almost always a "background" signal due to scattered light, and this must be corrected for by suitable blanks.

While such measurements of fluorescence "intensity" have practical utility, there are serious limitations to the usefulness of filter fluorometers in more sophisticated experiments. The detector response is dependent on the spectrum of the sample, the filters used, and the wavelength sensitivity of the phototube. Thus comparisons of solutions containing the same fluorescent substance are valid, but comparisons of readings of different types of solutions are largely meaningless. The situation is analogous to the use of filter colorimeters to measure percentage of transmission. It is for this reason that the word "intensity" is in quotation marks. The units of measurement are arbitrary; the photodetector response is usually just a meter reading or a recorder pen deflection.

Filter fluorometers have the advantage of low cost and high sensitivity. There are at least a dozen American manufacturers of filter fluorometers, and some makers have more than one model. It is beyond the scope of this article to mention all the companies, but one can find these listed each year in either the *Guide to Scientific Instrumentation* published by *Science,* or in the *ACS Laboratory Guide,* published by *Analytical Chemistry.* The various fluorometers differ in numerous ways. Some may be equipped for automated sample reading, for solid samples, or for scanning thin-layer chromatograms. Others have devices for compensating for lamp fluctuations. A large variety of different ultraviolet- and visible-light emitting lamps are available, and the same is true of photomultiplier tubes. In addition to instruments designed specifically for fluorometry, some spectrophotometers may be modified for fluorometry.

(b). SPECTRA. The measurement of spectra requires a monochromator instrument. If the primary filter of a filter fluorometer is replaced by a prism or grating monochromator, the fluorescence intensity may be measured as a function of the exciting wavelength to give an *excitation spectrum*, sometimes also called an *activation* spectrum. Conversely, if the secondary filter of a simple fluorometer is replaced by a monochromator, one may measure fluorescence intensity as a function of emission wavelength to obtain an *emission spectrum*.

Some spectrophotometers may be fitted with fluorescence accessories which permit determination of either excitation or emission spectra, but sometimes a given instrument may not be adaptable to determination of both. Instruments designed for fluorescence spectral work which have both excitation and emission monochromators are called *spectrofluorometers*. Such an instrument was first described by Bowman et al. (1955), and subsequently commercially available models came on the scene. The development of this type of instrument and its widespread dissemination have greatly influenced the development of fluorescence theory and practice.

A slight digression may be appropriate here in order to appreciate the significance of the spectrofluorometer, whose short history coincides with the period of dynamic growth of fluorescence spectroscopy. The idea of a spectrofluorometer was suggested to Dr. R. L. Bowman by a pharmacologist, Dr. B. B. Brodie, with a view towards surveying compounds to see if they could be excited to give fluorescence either in the ultraviolet or visible regions. At that time, it was difficult to make such a survey with the filter fluorometers then available, because the lamps used did not emit a continuum of wavelengths. While a tungsten lamp would emit at all wavelengths in the visible and near red regions, there would be no ultraviolet light available. If a mercury arc lamp was used, one was limited to excitation with the specific lines characteristic of the mercury spectrum, namely, the strong lines at 254, 297, 303, 313, 366, 404, 436, 546, and 579 nm. With such a lamp, it was not possible to obtain an excitation spectrum. Bowman therefore introduced the high pressure xenon arc lamp as a source in fluorometry, the paper by Bowman et al. (1955) being the first reference to such use of the xenon arc. This type of lamp initially had some serious problems with stability, but there have been great improvements in power supplies as well as lamp construction since that time. The xenon arc is now universally used in spectrofluorometers because it has a continuous emission spectrum from 200 to 800 nm. The output of the xenon arc combines the

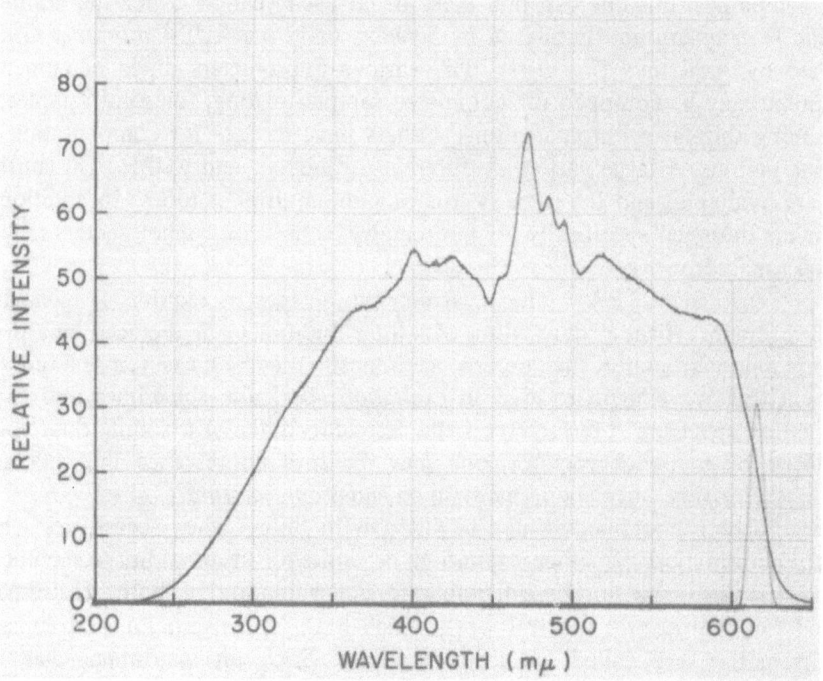

FIG. 5. Relative intensity of the excitation source of a spectrofluorometer at different wavelengths. This calibration of the xenon arc lamp source was obtained simply by measuring the fluorescence from the front surface of a concentrated rhodamine B solution (3 g/liter in ethylene glycol), which was excited at different wavelengths. The fluorescence was monitored at 615 nm; the scatter peak at that wavelength was obtained by replacing the dye solution with water. The measured fluorescence is proportional to the relative photon output of the light source up to about 580 nm. (From Chen. 1967d. *Anal. Biochem.*, 20:339.)

energy continuum of an incandescent source with a few lines characteristic of the xenon emission spectrum; Figure 5 shows the output as found in a modern spectrofluorometer. Aside from the xenon arc, the other major development which permitted development of an instrument having two monochromators was the sensitive photomultiplier tube. In contrast to filter fluorometers where the photo-detector may be placed quite close to the sample, there are greater light losses in a spectrofluorometer. With the instrument of Bowman et al. (1955), Duggan et al. (1957) were able to survey many compounds including drugs and in a very short time were able to discover that quite a few of them could be excited to fluorescence.

Block diagrams of two models of a commercial spectrofluorometer, the Aminco-Bowman instrument, are shown in Figure 6. This type of apparatus is also sometimes called a spectrophotofluorometer, or SPF, in order to indicate that a photomultiplier is employed. The two models shown in Figure 6 differ only in that SPF #2 has variable slits and a mirror condensing system for the lamp, while SPF #1 has fixed but interchangeable slits and has the xenon arc directly in front of the first monochromator with no entrance slit or mirror condenser. While the Aminco-Bowman instrument is the most widely used spectrofluorometer, there are other essentially similar instruments offered by Farrand Optical Co., Turner Associates, Baird-Atomic, Hitachi, Perkin-Elmer, Zeiss, and others. The different instruments differ in detals which may or may not be important to particular investigators; choosing between them is often difficult and ultimately is governed by considerations of cost, options available, accessibility to good service, as well as optical, electronic, and mechanical specifications. In this regard, it should be noted that Figure 6 does not show several necessary items: a power supply for the xenon arc lamp, a current source to operate the photomultiplier tube, an amplifier and metering system to read the detector response, and an X-Y recorder or oscilloscope to record spectra.

Spectrofluorometers may be used like filter fluorometers to measure fluorescence intensity for chemical assays. Excitation spectra are obtained usually by

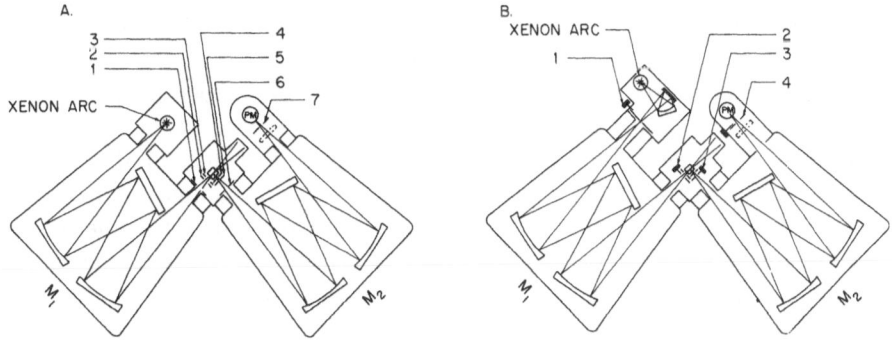

FIG. 6. Diagrams of different models of the Aminco-Bowman spectrofluorometer. *A.* Standard instrument. *B.* Instrument with mirror condensing system and variable slits in the numbered positions. The standard instrument has interchangeable but fixed slits in the positions shown. M_1 and M_2 are monochromators, and PM is the photomultiplier. (From Chen. 1967d. *Anal. Biochem.* 20:239.)

setting the emission monochromator to the wavelength of peak fluorescence and recording the intensity as a function of the exciting wavelength. Conversely, setting the first monochromator at a peak for excitation permits recording the emission spectrum.

It should be pointed out that spectrofluorometers such as that of Figure 6 have the disadvantage of measuring only "apparent" or "uncorrected" spectra. Both the emission of the xenon arc as well as the detector sensitivity are dependent on wavelength, thus distorting the spectra which are recorded. For instance, Figure 5 shows the way the xenon arc output differs with wavelength. An ideal source would put out exactly the same number of photons per second at each wavelength. Since such a source is unknown, the "true" spectrum of excitation can be obtained by correcting the apparent spectrum. This is usually done by measuring the xenon output to obtain a curve such as shown in Figure 5. Knowing exactly how the lamp output varies, one can make point-by-point corrections of the apparent spectra at, say, 5 or 10 nm intervals. The correction of excitation spectra has been discussed in detail by Parker and Rees (1960) and Chen (1967d) in relation to various spectrofluorometers.

Figure 5, a calibration curve for the xenon arc source, was obtained by the so-called "fluorescent screen" method. An adapter is used to permit fluorescence to be read from the front surface of a cell which is filled with a concentrated dye solution. With such a solution of rhodamine B, for instance, light of any wavelength up to about 580 nm will be essentially completely absorbed and converted into fluorescence. The fluorescence intensity depends only on the number of photons reaching the solution; hence the solution acts as a photon counter. The method relies on the assumption that the quantum yield of the rhodamine B is independent of exciting wavelength, and there is evidence that this is true (Melhuish, 1955). Aside from the fluorescent screen method of calibrating a light source, other methods include the use of thermopiles or other energy sensing devices as well as chemical actinometers, which are solutions undergoing photochemical changes in proportion to the amount of radiation received.

Emission spectra can be corrected by obtaining calibration curves for the photodetector response. This calibration is most often done by comparing the detector response with the known output of a standard lamp. Such lamps are available from the U.S. National Bureau of Standards or from several commercial firms. The light from the lamp is directed into the detector system, and the recorded intensity as a function of wavelength setting is all the information required. Most standard lamps are tungsten filament sources, which have little ultraviolet output. For calibration in the ultraviolet, one may use the xenon arc source in the spectrofluorometer since that source can be easily calibrated by the fluorescent screen method. Examples of detector response calibration curves are given in Figure 7. The open circles represent data obtained with the xenon arc as a standard, while the filled points were obtained with a U.S. National Bureau of Standards tungsten lamp. The curves of Figure 7 were obtained with various phototubes and gratings; both of these components are important in determining the overall detector response. $S(\lambda)$ of Figure 7 is the reciprocal of the sensitivity, so that the multiplication of

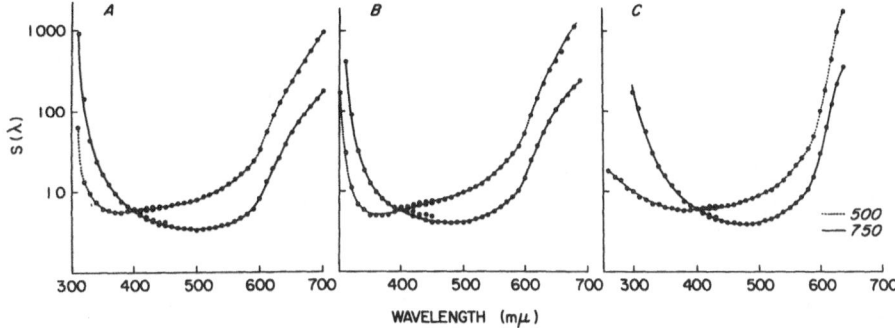

FIG. 7. Photodetector calibration curves for a spectrofluorometer. The correction factor S(λ) is used to convert uncorrected spectra into "true" emission spectra and is the reciprocal of the sensitivity. The different curves represent different combinations of phototube and grating types in the emission monochromator: the photomultiplier tubes used were: A, RCA 4472; B, RCA 1P21; C, RCA 1P28. Gratings were used whose wavelengths (in nm) of maximal efficiency are as shown in panel C. (From Chen. 1967d. *Anal. Biochem.*, 20:339.)

each point in the uncorrected emission spectrum by $S(\lambda)$ gives the corrected spectrum in terms of the relative number of photons emitted at each wavelength. The units for corrected excitation and emission spectra are frequently given simply as "relative quanta" or "$dq/d\lambda$" vs. wavelength, λ.

Before bothering to calibrate light source and detector systems, one may justifiably ask how often corrected excitation and emission spectra are needed. Actually, many investigators never bother to make the corrections, and many journals publish uncorrected spectra. In the days when the spectrofluorometer began to be popular, there were experts in the field who felt that only corrected spectra should be published, mainly to facilitate meaningful comparisons of results in different laboratories (Chapman et al., 1963). However, in practice everyone uses a xenon lamp, so that the distortions of the excitation spectrum are similar from one instrument to another, and most fluorometers are equipped with photomultipliers of the RCA 1P21 or 1P28 type so that emission spectra are distorted in similar ways in most instruments. In analytical articles the uncorrected spectra are satisfactory for showing the approximate peak wavelengths of excitation and emission. Furthermore, the use of fluorescence excitation and emission spectra as an index for the identification of compounds has been rather disappointing, so that corrected spectra are required for only certain special applications. Corrected emission spectra are needed when dealing quantitatively with spectral shifts, quantum yields, or with fluorescence which is in the red end of the spectrum, where the distortions of the photodetector system become very large. Corrected excitation spectra are of use in studies on energy transfer where it might be necessary to see whether the excitation and absorption spectra coincide. An experienced spectroscopist can imagine what the corrected spectra should look like if he knows the type of lamp and detector used. For practical analytical work, it turns out that comparisons of *uncorrected* spectra between different laboratories can be made if commercial instruments are used. However, in publishing uncorrected spectra, one

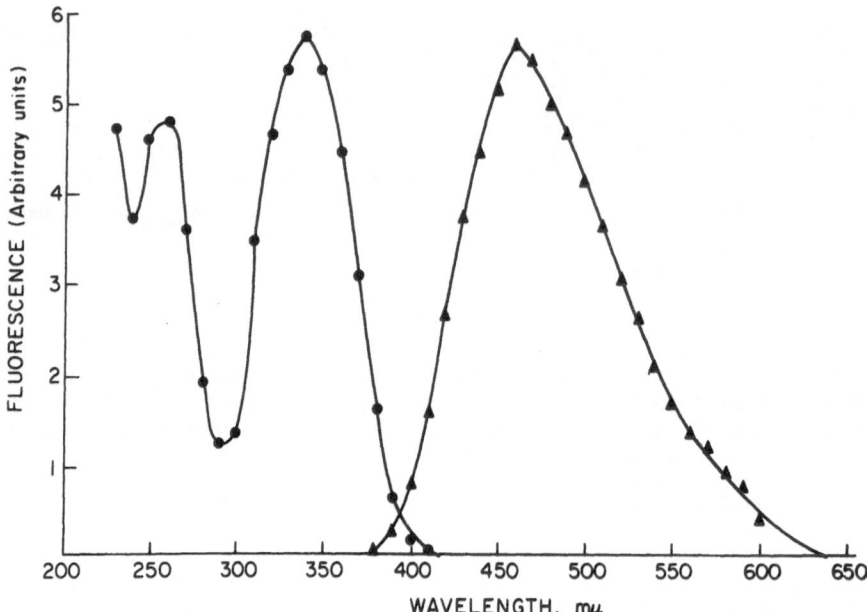

FIG. 8. Corrected spectra of excitation (-●-) and emission (-▲-) for NADH in 0.1 *M* NaHCO₃ at 10°C. (From Chen and Hayes. 1965. *Anal. Biochem.* 13:523.)

should specify the make and number of the phototube, and the type of grating used if that is known. An alternative is to include spectra of well-known standard compounds such as quinine and fluorescein.

Because of the need for corrected spectra in specialized work, in recent years instrumentation for automatic recording of corrected excitation and emission spectra has become available commercially. The Turner Model 210 spectrofluorometer (Turner, 1964) accomplishes the corrections automatically by cams and a lamp monitoring system. The Farrand Optical Co. has built an automatic instrument on special order (Cravitt and Van Duuren, 1968). The American Instrument Co. has attachments for its Aminco-Bowman spectrofluorometer which are said to give corrected spectra.

Examples of corrected excitation and emission spectra are given in Figures 8 and 9.

(c). QUANTUM YIELDS.   The efficiency of luminescence is expressed as the quantum yield Q. Q is defined as the ratio of the number of photons emitted to the number of photons absorbed, and may refer to either fluorescence or phosphorescence. For theoretical reasons, Q may not exceed 1 under normal circumstances and is 0 for nonfluorescent substances. The quantum yield of alkaline fluorescein in water was the first value of Q obtained for a solution (Vavilow, 1924). The value obtained, 0.85, was a surprise to many people in those days since it was generally assumed that only a very small fraction of the absorbed energy came back as fluorescence.

There are two general classes of quantum yield methods: the absolute (or

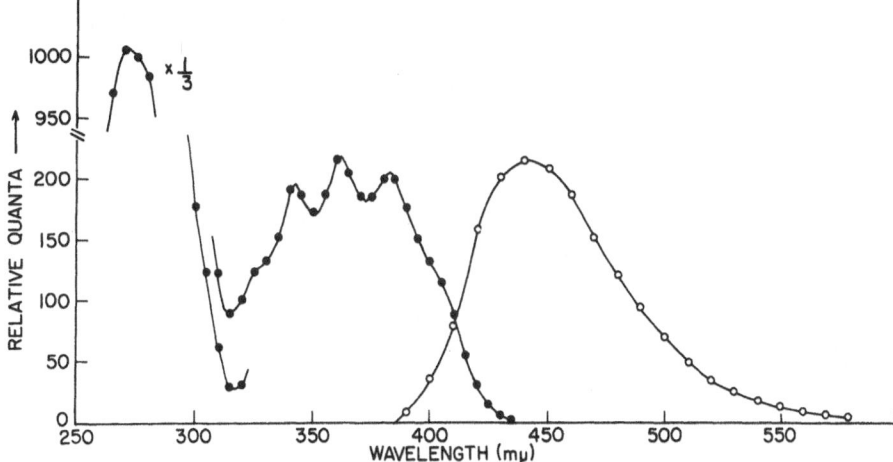

FIG. 9. Corrected spectra of a protein-dye conjugate, glutamate dehydrogenase labeled by reaction with anthracene-β-isocyanate. The dye-emission spectrum (-o-) was obtained by excitation at 362 nm, and the excitation spectrum (-•-) was obtained with the emission monochromator set at 450 nm. (From Chen. 1967c. *In* Guilbault, ed. *Fluorescence: Theory, Instrumentation, and Practice*. Courtesy of Marcel Dekker.)

direct) and the comparative methods. In the former, one actually measures or calculates the numbers of photons absorbed and emitted. This is no mean task, and is best left to the specialist in optics. Because there are now a number of compounds whose quantum yields are well established, determination of quantum yields by comparison with these standards is now the method of choice.

The quantum yield may be determined with a spectrofluorometer from the relation

$$\frac{Q_x}{Q_{st}} = \frac{F_x}{F_{st}} \qquad (6)$$

where x and st stand for the unknown and standard solutions, and Γ is the area under the corrected emission spectra. Here, it is necessary to excite both standard and unknown at the same wavelength and to have adjusted the concentrations so that the solutions have the same absorbance at that wavelength. If these two conditions are not met, a more general formula may be used:

$$\frac{Q_x}{Q_{st}} = \frac{F_x}{F_{st}} \cdot \frac{A_{st}}{A_x} \cdot \frac{\Phi_{st}}{\Phi_x} \qquad (7)$$

This relation takes into account the absorbance A and the relative photon output Φ of the exciting source at the wavelengths for exciting standard and unknown. Experience has shown that quantum yields can be more reliably obtained by exciting standard and unknown at their absorption peaks rather than at some wavelength where the solutions have equal absorbance. This is especially true when the standard and unknown have very different absorption spectra; at no single wavelength will the spectra of both solutions have a slope of 0, in most cases. Thus, any slight error in the wavelength setting of the excitation monochromator will result in large errors in the absorbance term.

The choice of fluorescence standard is usually made on the basis of similarity of the emission spectrum to that of the unknown. Errors in the calibration of the detector system for correction of the emission spectrum are thus minimized. Useful standards are fluorescein in 0.1 M NaOH, $Q=0.85$ (Parker and Rees, 1960; Vavilow, 1924; Umberger and La Mer, 1945) with an emission peak at 525 nm; quinine in 0.1 N H_2SO_4, $Q=0.54$ (Melhuish, 1955; Eastman, 1967; Dawson and Windsor, 1968) with emission peak at 458 nm; and tryptophan in 0.01 M Tris-Cl$^-$ buffer, pH 7, $Q=0.13$ (Chen, 1967a) with emission peak at 348 nm. All values refer to room temperature (23°C).

What is the need for quantum yield data? For most analytical purposes, quantum yield figures are an embellishment rather than a necessity. However, for development of analytical methods, it is often desirable to have an approximate knowledge of Q. If Q is very low, there is hope of improving the fluorescence by measuring the sample at lower temperatures or in different solvents; while, if Q is high, there is little possibility of significant improvement by these means. Quantum yields are of interest in binding studies involving proteins. When the value of Q is near unity, one can practically assume that the fluorescent compound is in a very shielded environment, protected from collisional encounters with solvent molecules which may lead to quenching. Also, in theoretical studies on the dissipation of excited state energy, including energy transfer processes, the quantum yield is of great importance.

(d). POLARIZATION. The degree of fluorescence polarization P is defined as the ratio

$$P = \frac{I_V - I_H}{I_V + I_H} \tag{8}$$

The intensities I_V and I_H are obtained by observing the fluorescence through an analyzing polarizer which is oriented vertically and then horizontally, as shown in Figure 10. Generally, the sample is illuminated with vertically polarized light, and the emission measured at right angles to the direction of propagation of the excitation. (Correctly, "vertically oriented" refers to alignment of a polarizer such that it passes light with its electric vector perpendicular to the plane defined by the axes of illumination and observation.)

Accurate measurements of P require reasonably well collimated excitation, in order that the directions of illumination and observation be well defined. Light scattering apparatus and spectrofluorometers have been adapted for polarization measurements with success (Singleterry and Weinberger, 1951; Steiner and Edelhoch, 1961; Chen and Bowman, 1965). However, filter fluorometers have generally proved unsatisfactory because of the close placement of sample to lamp and phototube.

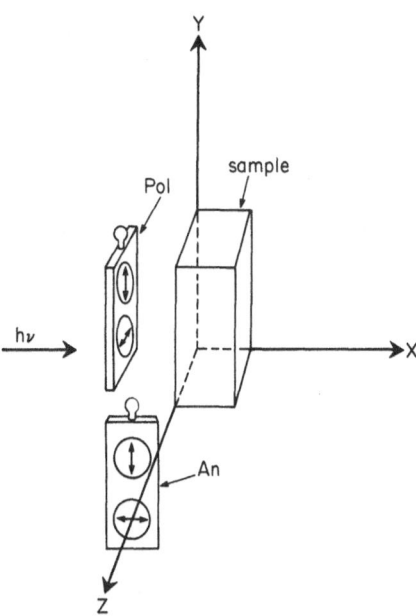

FIG. 10. Diagram of optical arrangement for measuring fluorescence polarization using filters. Light ($h\nu$) travels along the x-axis through the polarizer (Pol). Emission is observed through an analyzer (An). Y is the direction in which light is vertically polarized. (From Chen and Bowman. 1965. *Science*, 147:729.)

Figure 10 shows the filter arrangement used in the Aminco-Bowman spectro-fluorometer in the author's laboratory. Four filters are used as shown. In the polarizing position (Pol), light-fast filters (Polacoat Corp., Blue Ash, Ohio) are used; in the analyzing position (An) any polarizing material such as Polaroid film may be used since the light intensities encountered are not high enough to cause bleaching. Although normally one would use vertically polarized excitation only for measurements of P, the arrangement shown in Figure 10 allows use of horizontally polarized excitation as well. The latter would be expected to result in P-values of zero, but in practice the gratings introduce a polarization artifact. Excitation with horizontally polarized light allows for calculation of the correction factor needed to overcome this artifact, as follows (Azumi and McGlynn, 1962):

$$P = \frac{I_{VV} - GI_{VH}}{I_{VV} + GI_{VH}} \tag{9}$$

where $G = I_{HV}/I_{HH}$, and the first and second subscripts refer to vertical or horizontal orientation of the polarizer and analyzer.

Polarization can also be measured using unpolarized exciting light, provided that the emission is observed at right angles to the excitation. The maximum polarization with unpolarized excitation is $+\frac{1}{3}$, while with polarized light, P, can theoretically reach $+\frac{1}{2}$. If P_n and P_p are the polarizations observed for the same solution for natural and vertically polarized excitation, the general equation relating the quantities is

$$P_p = 2P_n/(1 + P_n) \tag{10}$$

The main advantage of unpolarized excitation is increased light level, but the loss in degree of polarization usually outweighs this consideration. Moreover, with spectrofluorometers, it may not be possible to obtain truly unpolarized light if gratings are present.

Instead of filters, more conventional materials may be used to polarize and analyze the light. Included in this classification are dichroic prisms such as Glan, Glan-Thompson, Nichol, and Rochon types. Some of these are available as accessories for various spectrofluorometers or they can be adapted to fit a particular instrument. Prisms generally have much better polarizing ability than filter materials, which may actually pass a significant amount of unpolarized light. However, the incompleteness of polarization in filtered light does not appear to seriously hinder the use of polarizing filters in fluorescence. Prisms involve considerable initial expense, and their alignment is quite critical.

(e). FLUORESCENCE LIFETIME.   The lifetime of fluorescence τ is the fluorescence parameter that is least often measured directly. Assuming that one had an ideal light source which could be extinguished instantaneously, the fluorescence would decay exponentially, and τ is the time required for the emission to decline to a value of $1/e$ of the initial intensity (where e is the base of natural logarithms). Fluorescent solutions have lifetimes, typically, in the range of 10 nsec (1 nsec $= 10^{-9}$ sec); therefore, measurement requires sophisticated electronic instrumentation.

In a recent review of fluorescence decay time measurements and applications Birks and Munro (1967) have divided the methods of determining τ into two classes: indirect and direct. An example of an indirect method is the use of the Perrin relations (equations 4 and 5), which requires only the measurement of fluorescence depolarization, from which τ is calculated. Other indirect methods are based on the fact that the lifetime is directly proportional to the quantum yield; i.e.,

$$\frac{Q_1}{Q_2} = \frac{\tau_1}{\tau_2} \tag{11}$$

where the subscripts refer to measurements at different conditions. For instance, a solution at different temperatures or in different solvents will normally have different values of Q, and it can be assumed that τ is changed proportionately. For the case of $Q = 1$, the limiting lifetime τ_0, which is also often called the "natural lifetime," obtains and is a measure of the inherent probability of a molecule to undergo an emissive transition from the excited singlet state. There are various approximate formulas based on quantum mechanical theory with which τ_0 may be calculated; the only data required are the absorption and corrected emission spectra. If one measures Q and has calculated τ_0, equation 11 may be used to determine τ. This indirect method is subject to serious limitations, including the approximate nature of the equations used to calculate the natural lifetime and the assumption that equation 11 is true for a given system.

Direct methods of measurement of lifetime are more reliable than the indirect. The *phase shift* method depends upon exciting the sample with light which fluctuates regularly at very high frequencies, usually in the range of 10^7 times per second. If this modulation of the exciting light is sinusoidal, the fluorescence is also sinusoidally modulated. However, the fluorescence lags behind the excitation by an amount determined by the decay time. The lag is expressed as an electrical phase shift in the detecting system used, and since such phase shifts can be measured very accurately, fluorescence lifetimes can be quite precisely measured. Phase shift apparatuses have been claimed to have been built which can measure lifetimes to within a few hundredths of a nanosecond (Müller et al., 1965; Spencer and Weber, 1969).

The *nanosecond flash* methods utilize special lamps designed to produce intense flashes lasting only a few nanoseconds. Ideally, such flashes should be infinitely short, and the resulting fluorescence decay rate will be given directly. In practice, such ideal lamps do not exist, although the flashes may be negligible in length compared with the duration of fluorescence. Most lamps described have an intensity-vs.-time profile which is roughly triangular with a width at half maximum of from 1 to 20 nsec. If $Y(t)$ is the resulting fluorescence signal, the true fluorescence decay function $f(t)$ usually cannot be seen directly but must be calculated from the following convolution integral (Steingraber and Berlman, 1963):

$$Y(t) = \int i(t) f(t) \, dt \qquad (12)$$

where $i(t)$ is the shape of the lamp pulse. The many pulse methods which have been described in the literature differ in the light sources, detector systems, and ways to deconvolute equation 12 to obtain $f(t)$, as well as other electronic details. The only complete lifetime apparatus that is commercially available is that manufactured by TRW Instruments (El Segundo, California), which has a small analog computer which solves equation 12 to give the decay time directly. The apparatus is of moderate sensitivity and quite convenient for fairly accurate work (Chen et al., 1967). In recent years, specialists in lifetime measurements have turned to photon counting methods (Birks and Munro, 1967) to obtain very high sensitivity and time resolution using the basic nanosecond flash technique. The principles and electronics of this method are complex and beyond the scope of this article. At present, both the phase shift and nanosecond flash techniques are being used by fluorescence spectroscopists.

Although lifetimes are not technically accessible to many laboratories interested in fluorescence, τ values are quite important especially in studies of fluorescence polarization. Lifetime measurements have many uses for the theoretical chemist and photochemist, since it represents a direct measurement of a kinetic process

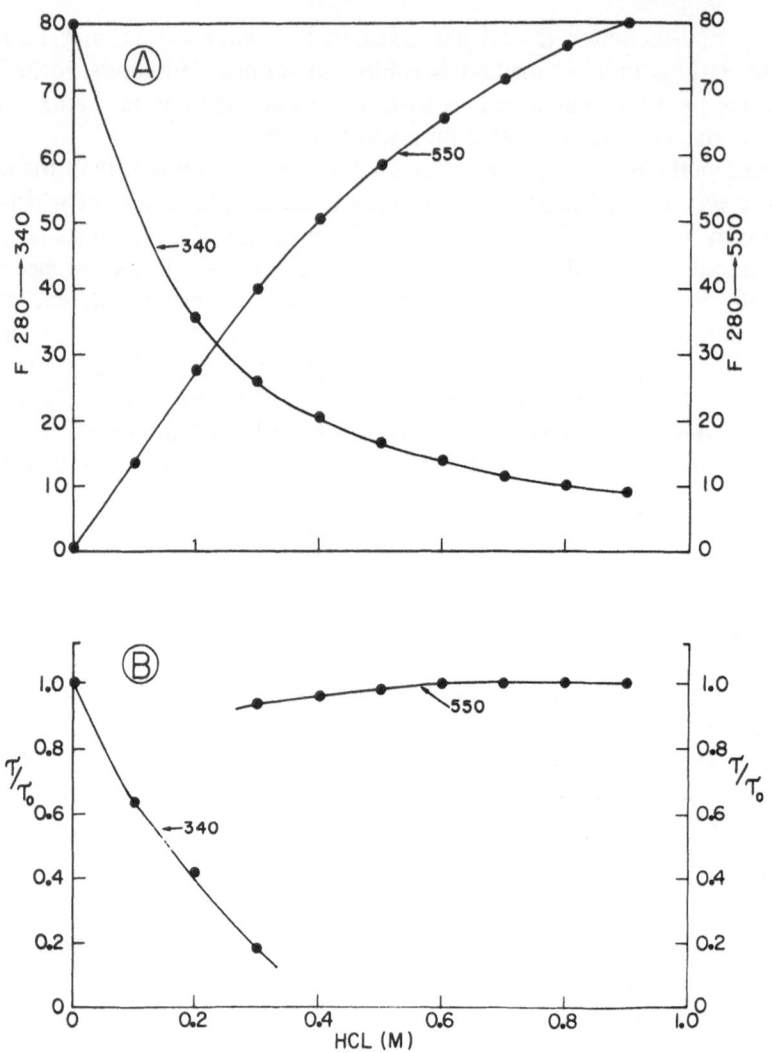

FIG. 11. Relation of quantum yield and lifetime of serotonin. A. Relative intensities of the normal ultraviolet fluorescence (monitored at 340 nm) and the green fluorescence (observed at 550 nm) upon addition of acid. B. Effect of acid on the fluorescence lifetime τ measured at 340 and 550 nm. τ_0 is the fluorescence lifetime of the solution where the intensity reading is 80 in panel A. Cf. Figure 2.

involving the first excited singlet state. Another interesting application of lifetime measurements is for the elucidation of quenching mechanisms. Quenching is defined simply as reduction of the quantum yield, and may be due to either "static" or "dynamic" mechanisms. A static quencher acts upon the fluorescent molecules in the ground state, effectively reducing the concentration of potentially fluorescent excited states; an example would be protonation of fluorescein, which is much more fluorescent in alkaline solution, or ionization of phenol, which fluoresces only in the nonionized state. In contrast, dynamic quenching occurs only in the excited state. Quenching by collisions with O_2 or I^- can be demonstrated for many molecules (Pringsheim, 1949). Lifetime measurements can distinguish between static and dynamic quenching; the former is not accompanied by a change in τ, while in dynamic quenching the decrease in quantum yield is proportional to a decrease in τ.

An example is shown in Figure 11, which shows the effect of acid on the two types of fluorescence (ultraviolet and visible) exhibited by 5-hydroxytrypta-mine, serotonin (cf. Figure 2). Acid quenches the normal ultraviolet fluorescence, and concomitantly, a visible fluorescence peaking at about 520 nm appears (Chen, 1968). At first glance, one might assume that H^+ protonates serotonin to give a species having only the visible fluorescence. However, if that were so, the mean lifetime of the remaining unprotonated serotonin molecules should be unchanged. If on the other hand the H^+ ions were dynamically quenching the serotonin by protonating only the excited molecules, the mean lifetime would be shortened. Figure 11 shows the latter to be the case, thus indicating the quenching to be of the dynamic type. Lifetime measurements thus provide direct evidence for excited state protonation, a process also suggested by the absence of pK_a of serotonin in the pH range of the acid quenching region, and by other evidence (Chen, 1968).

(f). COMMON PITFALLS IN THE MEASUREMENT OF FLUORES-CENCE. One of the commonest artifacts in fluorometry is the so-called *inner filter effect,* which refers to the reduction in intensity of either the exciting light or the fluorescence due to optical absorption by the sample under investigation. Usually one expects the intensity of fluorescence to be directly proportional to the concentration of the fluorescing substance. Actually, it is found that fluorescence is proportional to concentration only for dilute solutions. At higher concentrations, light is absorbed so strongly that the excitation does not penetrate to the center of the cuvette very well, and most of the fluorescence is given off from the solution near the illuminated face of the cuvette. Since the detector is usually focussed on the center of the cell, the filtering of incoming light by the solution itself reduces the signal, and at very high concentrations the fluorescence signal may actually be less than at lower concentrations. The same type of artifact may occur if the fluorescent solutions have high optical density at the wavelength used for monitoring the fluorescence.

The inner filter effect can be avoided or corrected for. Consider Figure 12, which shows the cross-sections of a 1×1 cm cuvette compared with a microcuvette with internal dimensions of 0.29×0.29 cm. The paths of excitation and observation are shown in cross-hatched areas, while the doubly cross-hatched regions in the center of the cells are actually those responsible for the signal. The shorter path length of the microcuvette means that there is less chance of encountering inner filter effects. At the same time, there is no loss in sensitivity, since the volume which is both illuminated and observed is identical in the two types of cells. It can be shown (Chen et al., 1969) that 5% of the exciting light is absorbed by the time the ray reaches the center of the 1×1 cm cell when the OD^{1cm} is 0.044; this amount of self-absorption is usually about the maximum permissible in analytical

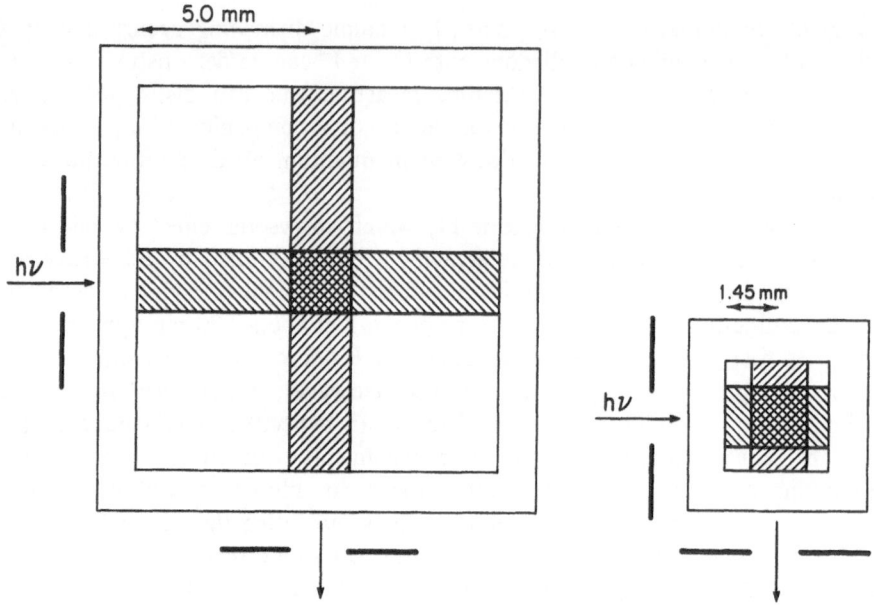

FIG. 12. Cross-sections of cuvettes used in the author's laboratory. The walls are 1.0 mm thick, and the slits which are shown are 1/16 inch wide. The hatched areas represent solution which is excited and/or observed by the detector. Only the central portion is both excited and observed; the area is the same for regular and microcuvettes. (From Chen. 1964. *Biochem. Biophys. Res. Comm.*, 17:141.)

tests. In contrast, the smaller path length of the microcuvette permits use of solutions with an OD^{1cm} of up to 0.152 before the effective excitation is reduced by 5%. Most laboratories use the large cells due to their easier handling, but there is normally no advantage in sensitivity and there may be disadvantages with regard to the inner filter effect. In terms of sensitivity, the large cells may be advantageous if dilute solutions and very large slits (3 to 4 mm) are employed; such large slits cannot be used in conjunction with the microcuvette since light would scatter off the corners of the cell and reduce the purity of the fluorescence signal.

If the absorbance of the solution is known, a correction can be made for the inner filter effect. The correction factor by which the reading must be multiplied is the antilogarithm of the effective optical density, which in turn is the absorbance measured in a 1 cm cuvette times half the width of the fluorescence cuvette (Weill and Calvin, 1963).

Light scatter may interfere with fluorescence measurements. When part of the exciting light reaches the photodetector, there is an increase in the blank reading and a corresponding decrease in the signal-to-noise ratio. Indeed, the sensitivity of some fluorometric methods is limited by the blank signal, which is largely scatter. Scatter appears in the signal in spite of monochromators and filters. In scanning to make spectra, a scatter peak is always encountered which has the same wavelength as the exciting light. *Second order* scatter peaks are sometimes encountered in spectrofluorometers that employ grating monochromators. When such a monochromator is set for a given wavelength λ, it will also pass light of wavelength $\lambda/2$. In exciting a sample at 280 nm, it should be recognized that the peaks in the emission spectrum at 280 nm and 560 nm are the same scattered light.

There are three main types of scatter. *Tyndall* scattering arises from dust or other relatively large particles in solution. Even with perfectly clear solutions, however, there is interaction between light and the solvent molecules giving rise to *Rayleigh* scatter. Tyndall and Rayleigh scattering occur at the wavelength of excitation. In making fluorescence measurements on very dilute solutions, one may encounter *Raman* scatter, which is due to molecular stretching vibrations of the solvent molecules. Raman scatter peaks occur at wavelengths which are shifted from the excitation wavelength; the amount of shift depends on the solvent. For example, in water excitation at 350 nm results in a Raman line at 395 nm, because the Raman water line is represented by a shift of 3300 cm^{-1} (on the wavenumber scale).

A rather simple trick is routinely used in the author's laboratory to minimize scatter (Chen, 1966). This is simply to excite the sample with horizontally polarized light, using no polarizer on the emission side. Typical results are shown in Figure 13. The scatter is almost eliminated by using the polarizer, because scattered light now has a high degree of polarization, but in the direction of observation, so that no signal is produced in the detector. Fluorescence is usually

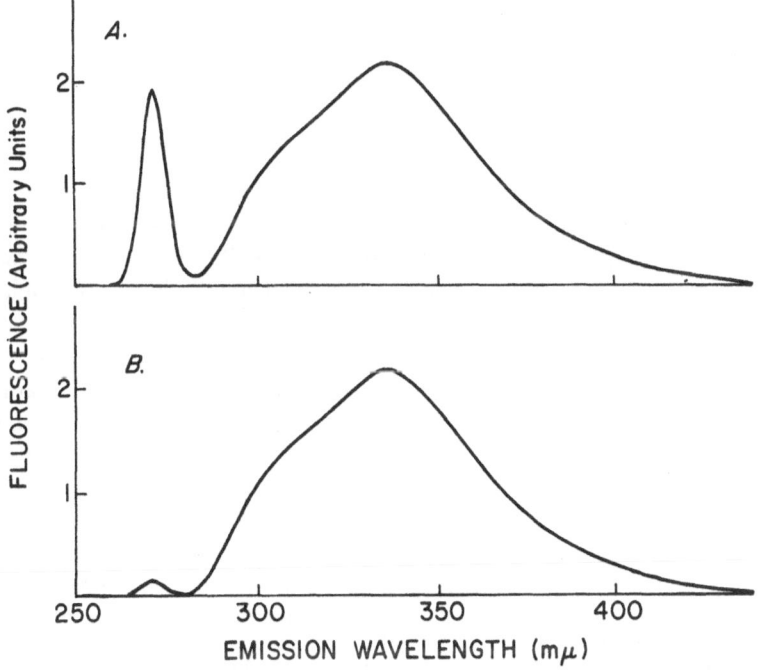

FIG. 13. Fluorescence spectrum of human serum albumin at pH 5.42 excited at 270 nm in a microcuvette (see Fig. 12). A. No polarizers present. B. Excited through a horizontally oriented Polacoat 105 UV filter. The phototube amplifier gain was increased to compensate for light loss through the filter. Note the marked diminution of the scatter peak relative to the fluorescence spectrum. (From Chen. 1966. *Anal. Biochem.*, 14:497.)

unpolarized or has considerably less polarization than does scatter; so that an improvement in signal-to-noise is effected. As shown in Figure 13, the improvement may be of the order of tenfold.

The simple device of a single, horizontally oriented polarizer in the exciting beam has the additional advantage of reducing the intensity of radiation and therefore the amount of *photodegradation* encountered. The high intensity lamps which most fluorometers are equipped with often cause sample destruction which is evidenced by slow loss of fluorescence signal. This change is sometimes erroneously attributed to poor instrumental stability, but, since the direction of change is always the same, one should suspect photochemical events. Another common cause of decreasing signal is *heating* of the sample in the compartment, which may be warmed by the powerful lamp. Fluorescence is much more temperature sensitive than absorption, so that temperature-controlled sample cells are desirable.

The use of horizontal polarizer in the exciting beam allows recording of the emission spectrum with reduced interference from scatter. Conversely, if a single horizontal polarizer is used in the emission side, scatter will be reduced when recording an excitation spectrum.

Turbid solutions should be avoided wherever possible. The scatter from the suspended particles acts to increase the effective illumination of the sample. This can increase the fluorescence signal. However, marked turbidity can also block penetration of the light into the sample as well as producing objectionable amounts of scatter.

CONCLUDING REMARKS

Fluorescence spectroscopy is a dynamic technique for studying many aspects of molecular interaction and structure in the biomedical fields. The last 15 years or so have seen the appearance of a variety of useful fluorometric instruments on the market, and the commercial availability of instrumentation is paralleled by a remarkable growth in interest in fluorescence. While in the past it was necessary for the individual investigator to be mechanically gifted, at present it is possible to purchase instruments to determine all the most useful fluorescence parameters. The years to come will undoubtedly see even more spectacular advances in this area.

REFERENCES

Ainsworth, S., and M. T. Flanagan. 1969. The effects that the environment exerts on the spectroscopic properties of certain dyes that are bound by bovine serum albumin. Biochim. Biophys. Acta, 194:213-221.

Azumi, T., and S. P. McGlynn. 1962. Polarization of the luminescence of phenanthrene. J. Chem. Phys., 37:2413-2420.

Birks, J. B., and I. H. Munro. 1967. The fluorescence lifetimes of aromatic molecules. Progress in Reaction Kinetics, 4:239-303.

Bogdanski, D. F., A. Pletscher, B. B. Brodie, and S. Udenfriend. 1956. Identification and assay of serotonin in brain. J. Pharmacol. Exp. Ther., 117:82-88.

Bowman, R. L., P. A. Caulfield, and S. Udenfriend. 1955. Spectrophotofluorometric assay in the visible and ultraviolet. Science, 122:32-33.

Calvert, J. G., and J. N. Pitts, Jr. 1966. Photochemistry. New York, John Wiley & Sons.

Chapman, J. H., Th. Forster, G. Kortum, C. A. Parker, E. Lippert, W. H. Melhuish, and G. Nebbia. 1963. Proposal for standardization of methods of reporting fluorescence emission spectra. Appl. Spectroscopy, 17:171.

Chen, R. F. 1964. Photoinactivation of L-glutamate dehydrogenase in a spectrophotofluorometer. Biochem. Biophys. Res. Commun., 17:141-145.

———— 1966. Reduction of scattered light in fluorometry by the use of horizontally polarized excitation. Anal. Biochem., 14:497-499.

———— 1967a. Fluorescence quantum yields of tryptophan and tyrosine. Anal. Lett., 1:35-42.

———— 1967b. Fluorescence of dansyl amino acids in organic solvents and protein solutions. Arch. Biochem. Biophys., 120:609-620.

———— 1967c. Extrinsic and intrinsic fluorescence in the study of protein structure: A review. In Guilbault, C. G., ed., Fluorescence: Theory Instrumentation and Practice, pp. 443-509. New York, Marcel Dekker.

———— 1967d. Practical aspects of the calibration and use of the Aminco-Bowman spectrophotofluorometer. Anal. Biochem., 20:339-357.

———— 1968. Fluorescence of protonated excited state forms of 5-hydroxytryptamine (serotonin) and related indoles. Proc. Nat. Acad. Sci. U.S.A., 60:598-605.

———— and R. L. Bowman. 1965. Fluorescence polarization: Measurement with ultra-violet-polarizing filters in a spectrophotofluorometer. Science, 147:729-732.

———— H. Edelhoch, and R. F. Steiner. 1969. Fluorescence of proteins. In Leach, S. J., ed., Physical Principles and Techniques of Protein Chemistry, Part A, pp. 171-244. New York, Academic Press.

———— and J. E. Hayes, Jr. 1965. Fluorometric assay of high concentrations of NADH and NADPH in a spectrophotofluorometer. Anal. Biochem., 13:523-529.

———— and J. Kernohan. 1967. Combination of bovine carbonic anhydrase with a fluorescent sulfonamide. J. Biol. Chem., 25:5813-5823.

———— G. G. Vurek, and N. Alexander. 1967. Fluorescence decay times: Proteins, coenzymes, and other compounds in water. Science, 156:949-951.

Cravitt, S., and B. L. Van Duuren. 1968. The design and performance of a new multi-purpose luminescence spectrophotometer. Chemical Instrumentation, 1:71-93.

Dandliker, W. B., and G. Feigen. 1961. Quantification of the antigen-antibody reaction by the polarization of fluorescence. Biochem. Biophys. Res. Commun., 5:299-304.

———— S. P. Halbert, M. C. Florin, R. Alonso, and H. C. Schapiro. 1965. Study of penicillin antibodies by fluorescence polarization and immunodiffusion. J. Exp. Med., 122:1029-1048.

Dawson, W. R., and M. W. Windsor. 1968. Fluorescence yields of aromatic compounds. J. Phys. Chem., 72:3251-3260.

Deranleau, D. A., and H. Neurath. 1966. The combination of chymotrypsin and chymotrypsinogen with fluorescent substrates and inhibitors for chymotrypsin. Biochemistry (Washington), 5:1413-1425.

Duggan, D. E., S. Udenfriend, R. L. Bowman, and B. B. Brodie. 1957. A spectrophotofluorometric investigation of compounds of biological interest. Arch. Biochem. Biophys., 68:1-14.

Eastman, J. W. 1967. Quantitative spectrofluorimetry. The fluorescence quantum yield of quinine sulfate. Photochem. Photobiol., 6:55-72.

Förster, T. 1951. Fluoreszenz organischer Verbindungen. p. 85. Göttingen, Vandenhoeck and Ruprecht.

Guilbault, G. G., ed. 1967. Fluorescence: Theory, Instrumentation and Practice. New York, Marcel Dekker.

Haber, E., and C. S. Bennett. 1962. Polarization of fluorescence as a measure of antigen-antibody interaction. Proc. Nat. Acad. Sci. U.S.A., 48:1935-1942.

Harvey, E. N. 1957. A History of Luminescence. Philadelphia, American Philosophical Library.

Hercules, D. M., ed. 1966. Fluorescence and Phosphorescence Analysis. New York, Wiley/Interscience.

Herschel, J. 1845. Philos. Trans. Roy. Soc. (London), 142:463 (cited by Harvey, 1957).

Levshin, V. L. 1925. Polarisierte Fluoreszenz und Phosphoreszenz der Farbstofflösungen. Z. Physik, 32:307-310.

Lewis, G. N., and M. Kasha. 1944. Phosphorescence and the triplet state. J. Amer. Chem. Soc., 66:2100-2116.

_____ and M. Kasha. 1945. Phosphorescence in fluid media and the reverse process of singlet-triplet absorption. J. Amer. Chem. Soc., 67:994-1003.

Lippert, E. 1957. Spektroskopische Bestimmung des Dipolmomentes aromatischer Verbindungen im ersten angeregten Singulettzustand. Z. Elektrochem., 61:962-975.

Longworth, J. W. 1962. The luminescence of purines and pyrimidines. Biochem. J., 84: 104P.

Melhuish, W. H. 1955. The measurement of the absolute quantum efficiencies of fluorescence. N. Zealand J. Sci. and Technology, B37: 142-149.

Müller, A., R. Lumry, and H. Kokubun. 1965. High performance phase fluorometer constructed from commercial subunits. Rev. Sci. Instrum., 36:1214-1226.

Parker, C. A. 1969. Photoluminescence of Solutions. New York, Elsevier.

_____ and W. T. Rees. 1960. Correction of fluorescence spectra and measurement of fluorescence quantum efficiency. Analyst, 85:587-600.

Perrin, F. 1925. Sur le mouvement brownien de rotation. C. R. Acad. Sci. (Paris), 181:514-516.

_____ 1926. Polarisation de la lumière de fluorescence. Vie moyenne des molécules dans l'état excité. J. Phys. Radium, 7:930-933.

Pringsheim, P. 1949. Fluorescence and Phosphorescence. New York, Interscience.

Reid, C. 1957. Excited States in Chemistry and Biology. New York, Academic Press.

Seliger, H. H., and W. D. McElroy. 1965. Light: Physical and Biological Action. New York, Academic Press.

Shipley, J. T. 1945. Dictionary of Word Origins. New York, Philosophical Library.

Singleterry, C. R., and L. A. Weinberger. 1951. The size of soap micelles in benzene from osmotic pressure and from the depolarization of fluorescence. J. Amer. Chem. Soc., 73:4574-4579.

Spencer, R. D., and G. Weber. 1969. Measurement of subnanosecond fluorescence lifetimes with a cross-correlation phase fluorometer. Ann. N. Y. Acad. Sci., 158:361-376.

Steiner, R. F., and H. Edelhoch. 1961. The properties of thyroglobulin. VI. The internal rigidity of native and denatured thyroglobulin. J. Amer. Chem. Soc., 83:1435-1444.

Steingraber, O. J., and I. B. Berlman. 1963. Versatile technique for measuring fluorescence decay times in the nanosecond region. Rev. Sci. Instrum., 34:524-529.

Stokes, G. Q. 1852. On the refrangibility of light. Philos. Trans. Roy. Soc. (London), 142:463-574.

Turner, G. K. 1964. An absolute spectrofluorometer. Science, 146:183-189.

Udenfriend, S. 1962. Fluorescence Assay in Biology and Medicine, Vol I. New York, Academic Press.

_____ 1969. Fluorescence Assay in Biology and Medicine, Vol. II. New York, Academic Press.

Umberger, J., and V. La Mer. 1945. Kinetics of diffusion controlled molecular and ionic reactions in solution as determined by measurements of the quenching of fluorescence. J. Amer. Chem. Soc., 67:1099-1109.

Vavilow, S. I. 1924. Die Fluoreszenzausbeute von Farbstofflösungen. Z. Physik, 22:266-272.

Weber, G. 1952. Polarization of the fluorescence of macromolecules. 2. Fluorescent conjugates of ovalbumin and bovine serum albumin. Biochem. J., 51:155-167.

Wehry, E. L., and L. B. Rogers. 1966. Fluorescence and phosphorescence of organic molecules. *In* Hercules, D. M., ed., Fluorescence and Phosphorescence Analysis. New York, Wiley/Interscience.

Weill, G., and M. Calvin. 1963. Optical properties of chromophore-macromolecule complexes: Absorption and fluorescence of acridine dyes bound to polyphosphates and DNA. Biopolymers, 1:401-417.

Weller, A. 1961. Fast reactions of excited molecules. Progr. Reaction Kinetics, 1:187-214.

Chapter **2**

Fluorescence Spectroscopy— a Tool for Studying Drug Interactions with Biological Systems

Colin F. Chignell

Laboratory of Chemical Pharmacology, National Heart and Lung Institute,
National Institutes of Health, Bethesda, Maryland

INTRODUCTION

By far the major use of fluorescence spectroscopy in pharmacology has been in the measurement of tissue drug levels as well as the estimation of biogenic amines such as norepinephrine and epinephrine in the brain and other organs. Since this particular application has been adequately covered elsewhere (Udenfriend, 1962, 1969) it will not be further discussed in this section. Instead, emphasis will be placed on the use of fluorescence spectroscopy to study how drugs interact with biological systems.

It may be seen from the previous chapter that the fluorescence of a given molecule may be characterized by several parameters including the wavelengths of maximal activation and emission, quantum yield, fluorescence lifetime, and degree of polarization. Since these parameters are often very sensitive to changes in the environment of the fluorophore it is not surprising that the fluorescence of a drug can be drastically altered when the drug interacts with a macromolecule. Similarly, the fluorescence characteristics of a macromolecule can be modified by the binding of a drug. When such changes in fluorescence occur it is often possible to gain valuable information about the nature of the drug-macromolecule interaction. If neither the drug nor the macromolecule possesses suitable fluorescence characteristics, the interaction can often still be examined by complexing (covalently or otherwise) the macromolecule with a fluorescent label.

APPLICATION OF FLUORESCENCE SPECTROSCOPY TO THE STUDY OF DRUG-MACROMOLECULE INTERACTIONS

Changes in Drug Fluorescence on Binding to Macromolecules

DRUG INTERACTIONS WITH NUCLEIC ACIDS. Ethidium bromide (I) (2,7-diamino-9-phenylanthridium-10-ethylbromide) is a trypanocidal drug

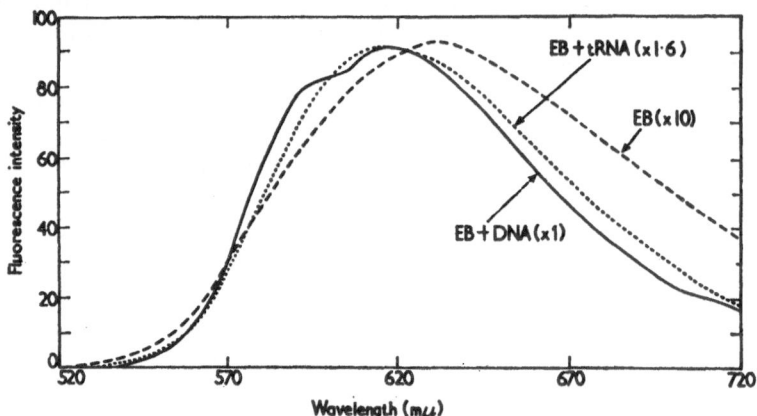

I

which also has antibacterial and antiviral properties. In cell-free systems ethidium bromide (EB) inhibits both DNA polymerase and DNA-dependent RNA polymerase probably by binding to the template DNA (Hawking, 1963; Newton, 1964). In 1964, LePecq et al. reported that the quantum yield of EB increased markedly when the drug bound to nucleic acids (Figure 1). For excitation in the region of the EB-nucleic acid absorption spectrum where there was no polynucleotide absorption, the ratio between the quantum efficiency of bound and free EB was 21 for DNA, and 26 for RNA (LePecq and Paoletti, 1967). When the EB-DNA complex was activated in the spectral range where the polynucleotides

FIG. 1. Corrected emission spectra of EB, and EB in the presence of tRNA and calf thymus DNA. The wavelength of excitation was 436.1 nm. Solutions were made in 0.1 M sodium phosphate buffer (pH 7.0) and contained 5×10^{-4} M EB. (From Bittmann. 1969. $J.$ $Molec.$ $Biol.$, 46: 251. Courtesy of Academic Press, Inc.)

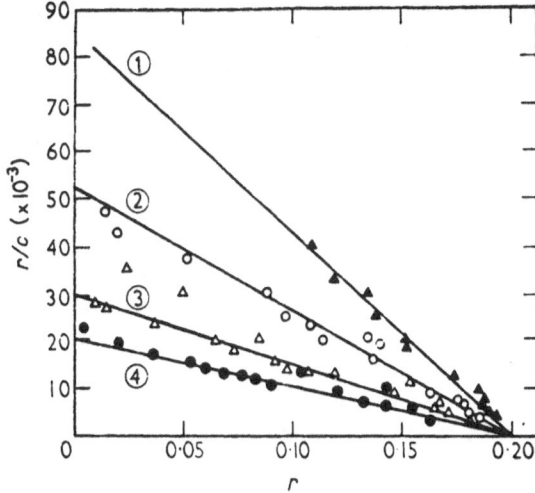

FIG. 2. Competition between quinacrine and ethidium bromide for the binding sites of DNA: r = Number of moles of ethidium bromide bound per mole of DNA nucleotide. c = Molar concentration of free ethidium bromide. Curve 1 shows the binding of ethidium bromide to DNA alone (4 μg/ml). Curves 2, 3, and 4 contain 3.2 μg, 9.6 μg, and 15 μg quinacrine/ml, respectively (corresponding to molar ratios, quinacrine/nucleotide, of 5.1, 15.3, and 24). Solutions contained 0.12 M sodium chloride, 0.08 M Tris-HCl (pH 7.5). (From LePecq and Paoletti. 1967. *J. Molec. Biol.*, 27:87. Courtesy of Academic Press, Inc.)

also absorbed light there was good evidence for energy transfer from the nucleic acid to EB. Quantum measurements showed that, at a P/D ratio (i.e., the ratio of nucleic acid phosphate groups to bound dye molecules) of 14, about half the energy absorbed by the DNA was transferred to the dye and re-emitted as fluorescence (LePecq and Paoletti, 1967).

Spectrofluorometric titration (see Appendix) revealed that at high salt concentration the RNA and DNA binding sites for EB were homogeneous and could therefore be described by a single association constant. There was about one EB binding site per five nucleotides for DNA (Figure 2) and one per ten nucleotides for RNA. Scatchard plots for several DNA's were very similar, suggesting that there was no base composition selectivity in EB binding. Spectrofluorometric titration of DNA by EB in the presence of quinacrine (Figure 2) or actinomycin C indicated that binding was competitive for the former but noncompetitive for the latter.

At high salt concentration EB bound almost exclusively to double-stranded hydrogen-bonded nucleotides or, in the case of denatured DNA and RNA, to short double-stranded hydrogen-bonded regions. However, at low salt concentrations (<0.01 M) fluorescence binding studies indicated the presence of two kinds of sites: (a) the same double-stranded (primary) site as at high salt concentrations, which was characterized by enhanced fluorescence, and (b) a second binding site (secondary site) at which the fluorescence was low. At the primary site both electrostatic and short range (van der Waals) forces were in operation, while at the secondary site only electrostatic interactions were important (LePecq and Paoletti, 1967).

In a later study Burns (1969) found that the decay time of EB was the same when the EB-DNA complex was excited with violet light (absorbed directly by the bound dye) as it was when ultraviolet light (absorbed mainly by the nucleic acid then transferred to the bound dye) was used for excitation. He concluded that energy transfer from DNA to EB occurred in an average time interval too short to be measured or less than 1 nanosecond. When EB was excited directly, Burns (1969) found that the fluorescence lifetime of the drug was 23 nanoseconds when bound to DNA, and 19.5 nanoseconds when bound to RNA. In contrast, the fluorescence lifetime of free EB was about 1 nanosecond. Since fluorescence lifetime is directly proportional to quantum yield it follows that the fluorescence yield of EB increased 23-fold on binding to DNA and 19.5-fold on binding to RNA. The large increase in the decay time and quantum yield of EB bound to DNA or RNA was attributed by Burns (1969) to a change in the conformation of the dye such that a forbidden transition became allowable. Förster (1946) has proposed that a change from a nonplanar to a planar conformation in certain dyes may permit fluorescence. However, LePecq and Paoletti (1967) have suggested that the increase in quantum fluorescence yield when EB binds to RNA or DNA is due to immersion of the drug in a hydrophobic region of the nucleic acid.

Burns (1969) has reported that when the EB-DNA complex is excited with violet light the polarization of the dye is 0.1, whereas excitation with ultraviolet light yields a value of 0.07. When the viscosity of the solution was increased by the addition of glycerol, the polarization of EB measured with violet light increased to 0.22, while polarization measured with ultraviolet light was unchanged. Since an increase in viscosity did not increase the polarization of light absorbed by DNA

TABLE 1

Drugs and Dyes That Change Their Fluorescence
on Interaction with Nucleic Acids

Drug	Nucleic Acid	Reference
Ethidium bromide	DNA, RNA	LePecq and Paoletti (1967)
Ethidium bromide	DNA, RNA	Burns (1969)
Ethidium bromide	tRNA, DNA	Bittman (1969)
Ethidium bromide	RNA, DNA	Sela (1969)
Acridine orange	DNA	Yamabe (1969)
Acridine orange	DNA	Borisova and Tumerman (1965)
Acridine orange	DNA	Boyle et al. (1962)
Acridine orange	DNA	Lerman (1961, 1963, 1964)
Acridine orange	DNA	MacInnes and Uretz (1966)
Acridine orange Proflavine Thionine Methylene blue	DNA, RNA	Tomita (1968)
Acridine orange Proflavine	DNA	Weill and Calvin (1963)
Proflavine	DNA	Thomes et al. (1969)
Proflavine	DNA	Ellerton and Isenberg (1969)
Acriflavine	DNA	Tubbs et al. (1964)
Berberine	DNA, RNA	Yamagishi (1962)

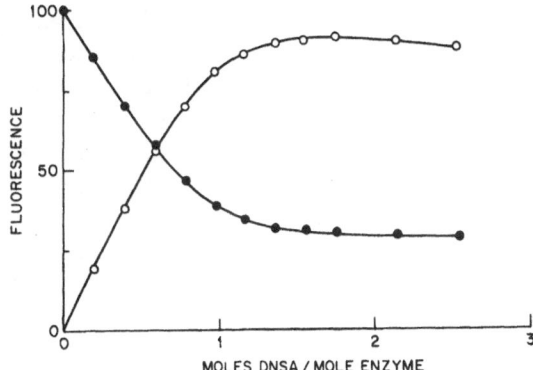

FIG. 3. Fluorometric titration of carbonic anhydrase at high concentration (8.2×10^{-6} *M*) with DNSA. The intensity of tryptophan fluorescence (-●—●-) was followed by excitation at 280 nm with the emission monochromator set at 336 nm; the corresponding wavelengths for ligand fluorescence (-o—o-) were 320 and 470 nm. The emission of free DNSA at 470 nm was negligible. Bandwidths of excitation and emission were 12 nm. (From Chen and Kernohan. 1967. *J. Biol. Chem.*, 242:5813. Courtesy of the editors of the *Journal of Biological Chemistry.*)

then re-emitted by bound EB, Burns concluded that energy transfer occurred only between DNA and intercalated dye molecules.

The fluorescence of many other drugs and dyes is also modified when they interact with DNA or RNA, and other examples will be found listed in Table 1.

DRUG INTERACTIONS WITH PROTEINS.   Erythrocyte carbonic anhydrase is a zinc-containing enzyme, which is inhibited by sulfonamides (Mann and Keilin, 1940) having the general formula $ArSO_2NH_2$, where Ar is an aromatic nucleus (homocyclic or heterocyclic) (Maren, 1967). Chen and Kernohan (1967) reported that 5-dimethylaminonaphthalene-1-sulfonamide (II) (DNSA) formed a

$N(CH_3)_2$

SO_2NH_2

II

highly fluorescent complex with bovine erythrocyte carbonic anhydrase. They found that while the fluorescence of free DNSA in water had a peak emission at 580 nm and a quantum yield of 0.055, when bound to carbonic anhydrase, DNSA had an emission maximum at 468 nm and a quantum yield of 0.84. The binding of DNSA to carbonic anhydrase also quenched the native tryptophan fluorescence of the enzyme. The protein fluorescence quenching curve and the DNSA fluorescence enhancement curve both indicated (Figure 3) that only 1 mole of inhibitor was bound per mole of enzyme; the dissociation constant at *p*H 7.4 was calculated (see Appendix) to be 2.5×10^{-7} *M*.

When the DNSA-carbonic anhydrase complex was activated at 290 nm some of the energy absorbed by the seven tryptophans in the enzyme was transferred to the bound inhibitor which then re-emitted it as fluorescence. The quantum yield for this transfer was 0.71. However, when the DNSA complex was activated at 320 nm (a wavelength where only the bound DNSA absorbs light) the quantum yield was 0.84. It is therefore obvious that the quanta of light absorbed by the tryptophan residues of carbonic anhydrase were transferred to the bound DNSA with a yield of 85% ($0.71/0.84 \times 100$). This transfer efficiency was much higher than any previously reported for a protein having one dimethylaminonaphthalene group. Although the diameter of the carbonic anhydrase molecule is roughly 50Å, the bound DNSA group was probably within the critical transfer distance of 21.3Å. This permitted Chen and Kernohan (1967) to calculate that the effective average transfer distance between DNSA and tryptophan was 16Å.

Chen and Kernohan (1967) calculated from a Perrin-Weber plot of $1/P$ vs T/η for the DNSA-carbonic anhydrase enzyme that the rotational relaxation time (ρ) for the complex was 28.9 nanoseconds at 25°C. The relaxation time (ρ_0) for an anhydrous sphere of equivalent molecular weight (30,000) would be 24.3 nanoseconds. This gave a value of 1.19 for ρ/ρ_0. Since for most proteins rotating as ellipsoids the relaxation time ratio ρ/ρ_0 is between 1.7 and 2.0, the investigators concluded that the carbonic anhydrase molecule had a low degree of asymmetry.

The very high quantum yield and the blue shift in the fluorescence emission maximum of DNSA on binding to carbonic anhydrase strongly suggested that the binding site was hydrophobic (Edelman and McClure, 1968). However, Chen and Kernohan (1967) pointed out that the blue shift in the fluorescence emission maximum of DNSA bound to carbonic anhydrase was much greater than that observed when DNSA bound to bovine serum albumin, a protein known to have a very hydrophobic binding site. They suggested that this was due to the loss of a proton by DNSA, i.e., the process $ArSO_2NH_2 \rightleftarrows ArSO_2NH^- + H^+$. Some experiments suggested that evidence for this postulation was obtained by demonstrating that when the pH of an aqueous solution of DNSA was raised by the addition of KOH the fluorescence emission spectrum shifted from 580 mμ to 540 mμ, while the quantum yield increased from 0.055 to 0.085.

Chignell (1970a) has recently reported that the binding of the anticoagulant drug warfarin to human serum albumin (HSA) results in a sixfold increase in the fluorescence yield of the drug and a small shift in its fluorescence emission maximum to shorter wavelengths. These fluorescence changes also suggest that the warfarin binding site is located in a hydrophobic region of the protein. Similar fluorescence changes were observed (Chignell, 1970b) when warfarin was bound to serum albumin from other species with rat, bovine, and canine serum albumins, causing the largest (20 nm) blue shifts in the fluorescence emission maximum of the drug (Table 2). Rat serum albumin also induced the largest (13-fold) increase in the quantum yield of warfarin. These results suggest that rat serum albumin has the most hydrophobic warfarin binding site and illustrate well the use of a drug molecule as a fluorescent probe for its own binding sites.

The increase in fluorescence polarization of a drug on binding to a macromolecule has been used to study the interaction of chlorpromazine with human

TABLE 2

The Quantum Yield and Fluorescence Emission Maximum of
Warfarin Bound to Different Serum Albumins[a]

Serum Albumin	Fluorescence Quantum Yield	Fluorescence Emission Maximum[b] (nm)
None	0.012	400
Human	0.070	390
Bovine	0.069	380
Rat	0.153	380
Porcine	0.080	385
Canine	0.083	380
Ovine	0.076	385
Equine	0.088	390
Rabbit	0.047	390

[a]From Chignell. 1970. *Fluorescence News*, 5:1-5. Courtesy of American Instrument Company.
[b]Activation wavelength was 320 nm using 12 nm bandwidth.

serum albumin (Teller et al., 1968) as well as the binding of chlorpromazine and thioproperazine to crab myosin B (Levine et al., 1968). This particular technique should find much wider application since it can be applied to any drug that is highly fluorescent both before and after binding to a macromolecule. A theoretical treatment of fluorescence polarization data and its relationship to binding has been given by Deranleau and Neurath (1966). A list of drugs that change their fluorescence characteristics on binding to proteins may be found in Table 3.

TABLE 3

Drugs and Other Ligands That Change Their
Fluorescence on Interaction with Proteins

Drug	Protein	Reference
Dansylsulfonamide	Carbonic anhydrase	Chen and Kernohan (1967)
Warfarin	Serum albumin	Chignell (1970a)
Hapten	Antibody	Berns and Singer (1964)
Chlorpromazine Thioproperazine	Myosin B	Levine et al. (1968)
Chlorpromazine	Serum albumin	Teller et al. (1968)

Changes in the Fluorescence of Macromolecules When They Bind Drugs

The fluorescence of proteins may be divided into two types: (a) intrinsic fluorescence which is due to the aromatic amino acids (phenylalanine, tyrosine and tryptophan), and (b) extrinsic fluorescence which originates from bound fluorescent molecules such as NADH, NADPH, and other coenzymes. In this section we will be concerned solely with the effect of drug binding on the intrinsic fluorescence of proteins. Weber (1960) divided proteins into two classes according to their native fluorescence. Class A proteins were those containing phenylalanine and tyrosine but no tryptophan. In these proteins phenylalanine fluorescence was absent, the fluorescence spectrum being characteristic of tyrosine with a maximum emission at 303 nm. However, the quantum yield of fluorescence in class A proteins such as insulin, ribonuclease, and zein, was found to be only one fifth to one seventh that of free tyrosine. Class B proteins were those containing tryptophan as well as tyrosine and alanine. In all these proteins the fluorescence of tryptophan dominated the emission spectrum. The quantum yield of fluorescence for class B proteins varied widely from 0.04 to 0.3, as compared with 0.2 for free tryptophan. For a more comprehensive discussion of the native fluorescence of proteins the reader is referred to reviews by Weber and Teale (1965) and Chen et al. (1969).

In 1958, Velick reported that the binding of either NAD or NADH to glyceraldehyde-3-phosphate dehydrogenase or lactate dehydrogenase quenched the native tryptophan fluorescence of these enzymes. Later, Velick and coworkers (1960) used this same technique to study the interaction of ε-N-2,4-dinitrophenyl-lysine with a rabbit antibody directed against the 2,4-dinitrophenyl group. Subsequently, fluorescence quenching has also been used to study the binding of thyroxine, steroids, bilirubin, and certain anionic drugs to serum albumin as well as the interaction of sulfonamide inhibitors with carbonic anhydrase (for references see Table 4).

TABLE 4

*Proteins That Show Fluorescence Changes
on Interaction with Drugs and Other Ligands*

Drug	Protein	Reference
Dansylsulfonamide	Carbonic anhydrase	Chen and Kernohan (1967)
Sulfonamides	Carbonic anhydrase	Taylor et al. (1970)
Warfarin, dicoumarol	Serum albumin	Chignell (1970a)
Flufenamic acid	Serum albumin	Chignell (unpublished)
Thyroxine	Serum albumin	Steiner et al. (1966)
Steroids	Serum albumin	Attalah and Lata (1968)
Bilirubin	Serum albumin	Chen (1971)
Chlorpromazine	Myosin	Levine et al. (1968)
Haptens	Acetylcholine antibody	Marlow et al. (1969)

The quenching of protein tryptophan fluorescence by the binding of a ligand is due to energy transfer from excited-state tryptophan residues to the bound ligand. Förster (1951) has shown that a general prerequisite for energy transfer to occur by the dipole resonance mechanism is that the emission band of the donor overlap the absorption band of the acceptor. Figure 4 shows, for example, that the tryptophan fluorescence emission band of human serum albumin is overlapped completely by the absorption spectrum of bilirubin. When bilirubin binds to either human or bovine serum albumin the native tryptophan fluorescence

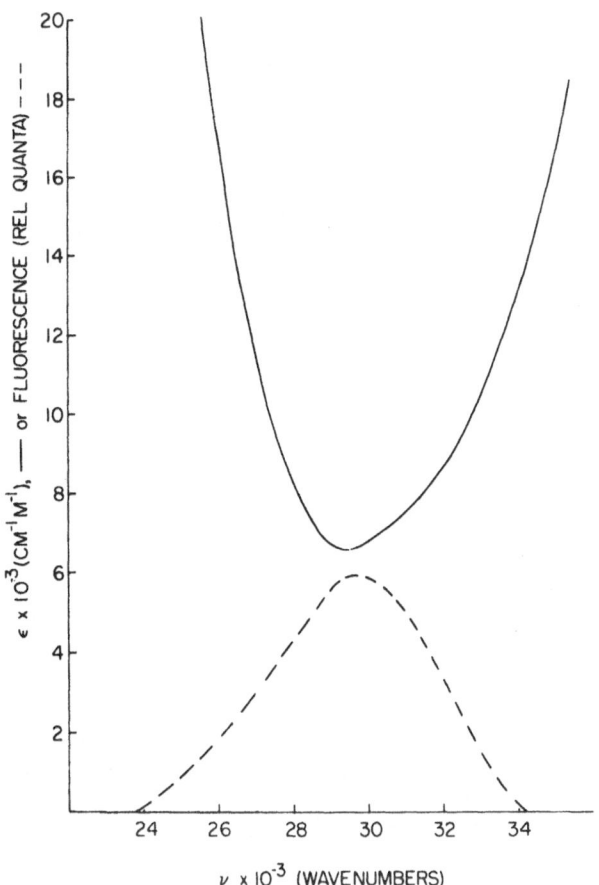

FIG. 4. Spectrum of human serum albumin fluorescence (- - - -) and part of the bilirubin-human serum albumin absorption spectrum (—) showing the spectral overlap necessary for energy transfer to occur. The solutions contained 0.1 M potassium phosphate buffer, pH 7.3; human serum albumin was excited at 290 nm. (Reproduced from Chen [unpublished results] with the permission of the author.)

of the protein is quenched (Figure 5). Scatchard plots derived from the fluorescence quenching curves (see Appendix) indicated that the association constants for the first two binding sites were 2×10^7 M^{-1} and 2×10^6 M^{-1} for bovine serum albumin and 7×10^7 M^{-1} and 6×10^6 M^{-1} for HSA (Chen, personal communication).

Chen and Kernohan (1967) have shown that the binding of DNSA to bovine erythrocyte carbonic anhydrase quenches the tryptophan fluorescence of the protein. Since the energy which was nonradiatively transferred from the tryptophans to the bound DNSA was re-emitted by the ligand as fluorescence, Chen and Kernohan (1967) were able to estimate the average transfer distance between the tryptophans and the DNSA (*vide supra*). Recently, Taylor and coworkers (1970) have used fluorescence quenching to study the binding of 24 aromatic sulfonamides to human carbonic anhydrases B and C. With 4-[(5,7-disulfonic acid naphth-2-ol)-

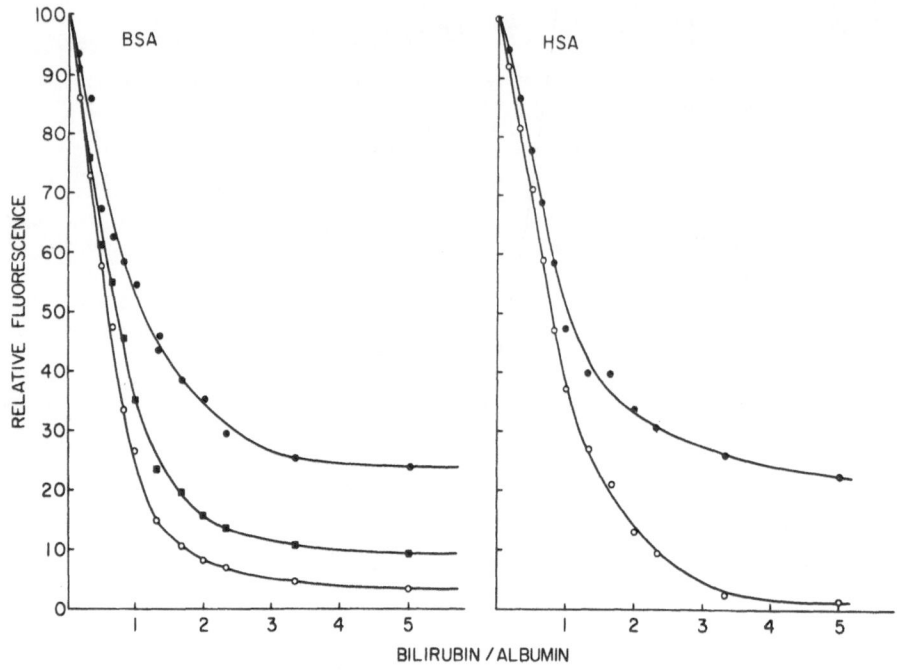

FIG. 5. Quenching of albumin fluorescence by bilirubin. The intensity of fluorescence excited at 290 nm and monitored at 340 nm is plotted against the ratio of the total concentrations of bilirubin and albumin. BSA = bovine serum albumin; HSA = human serum albumin. The titrations were carried out in the presence of albumin at 10^{-5} M (o), 10^{-6} M (■) and 10^{-7} M (●). The solutions were at 23°C and contained potassium phosphate buffer, pH 7.3. (Reproduced from Chen [unpublished results] with the permission of the author.)

1-azo] benzene sulfonamide (DNABS) (III), 90% of the enzyme fluorescence

III

was quenched at complete saturation. The affinity of sulfonamides that did not quench carbonic anhydrase fluorescence was estimated by measuring their ability to competitively displace DNABS from the enzyme (see Appendix). Taylor and coworkers (1970) were also able to use fluorescence quenching measurements in conjunction with stopped-flow techniques to study the kinetics of the reaction between sulfonamides and carbonic anhydrase. Their results indicated that the association rate was not diffusion controlled but that the formation of the complex required a distinct activation energy.

Solutions of the commonly occurring purines, pyrimidines, and their nucleotides and nucleosides do not emit fluorescence in the physiological range of pH

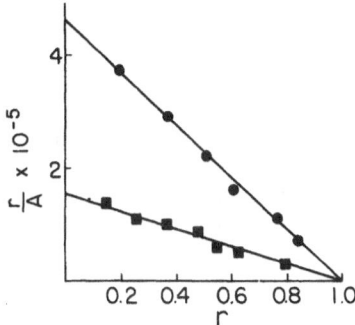

FIG. 6. Scatchard plot of the binding of dansylglycine to human serum albumin. A=molar concentration of free dansylglycine, n=number of moles of dansylglycine bound per mole of albumin. Binding was measured by monitoring the increase in dansylglycine fluorescence at 480 nm while activating at 350 nm. Human serum albumin alone (1×10^{-5} M) (-■—■-); human serum albumin (1×10^{-5} M)+phenylbutazone (2.5×10^{-5} M) (-●—●). (From Chignell. 1969a. *Molec. Pharmacol.*, 5:244. Courtesy of Academic Press, Inc.)

at room temperature. It is not, therefore, surprising that none of the nucleic acids examined by Udenfriend and Zaltzman (1962) exhibited any fluorescence at neutral pH and room temperature. Fluorescence can, however, be used to monitor drug interactions with nucleic acids by labeling them with fluorescent molecules such as acriflavine. This approach is discussed in the section on fluorescent labels.

Changes in the Fluorescence of Fluorescent Labels Attached to the Macromolecule

PROTEINS CONTAINING FLUORESCENT LABELS. Fluorescent labels are small molecules of known chemical structure, which, after attachment (covalently or noncovalently) to a macromolecule, can be used to detect changes in the various structural parameters of the macromolecule. The most commonly used labels for noncovalent attachment to proteins are 1-anilinonaphthalene-8-sulfonic acid (ANS) (IV), 2-p-toluidinylnaphthalene-6-sulfonic acid (TNS), and

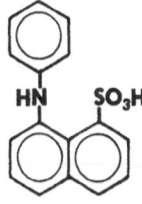

IV

5-dimethylaminonaphthalene-1-sulfonyl (dansyl) derivatives of amino acids such as glycine. These compounds all show a marked increase in their fluorescence quantum yields and a blue shift in their fluorescence emission maxima on going from a nonpolar to a polar environment (see review by Edelman and McClure, 1968). Similar fluorescence changes are also observed when ANS, TNS, or the dansyl

amino acids bind to certain proteins such as serum albumin. It has therefore been
suggested that the dye binding sites on these proteins are nonpolar and that ANS,
TNS, and the dansyl amino acids can be used as probes for the polarity of protein
binding sites (Edelman and McClure, 1968; Stryer, 1968).

When dansylglycine (V) binds to human serum albumin the quantum yield

V

of the ligand increases fivefold while its fluorescence emission maximum moves
from 580 nm to 480 nm (Chignell, 1970a). Fluorescence titration indicates that
binding occurs at a single site for which dansylglycine has an association constant
of $4.6 \times 10^5 \ M^{-1}$ (Figure 6). Chignell (1969a,b, 1970a) has shown that several
anionic drugs such as phenylbutazone (Figure 6), flufenamic acid and dicoumarol
(Figure 7) competitively displace dansylglycine from its binding site on human
serum albumin. These results not only indicate that these drugs have at least one
hydrophobic binding site on human serum albumin but also permit calculation of
their association constants for that site from their corresponding Scatchard or Hill
plots (see Appendix). Similarly, Chen and Kernohan (1967) have studied the
binding of ethoxzolamide, a nonfluorescent sulfonamide, to carbonic anhydrase
by measuring its ability to competitively displace DNSA.

Many studies of the antigen-antibody reaction have been made using antigens
and/or antibodies labeled with fluorescent dyes. For example, Dandliker and
Feigen (1961) have prepared antibodies to ovalbumin and fluorescein labeled
ovalbumin (F-ovalbumin) and carried out titrations of each with F-ovalbumin.
An increase in fluorescence quantum yield of F-ovalbumin was observed on titration
with anti-F-ovalbumin but not with anti-ovalbumin. Subsequently, Haber and
Bennett (1962) used fluorescence polarization techniques to follow titrations of
fluorescein-labeled ribonuclease, bovine serum albumin, and insulin B chain with
their corresponding antibodies. They observed an initial increase in polarization
in all instances, consistent with the expected increase in rotational relaxation times
of the antigen-antibody complex. An excellent review of the application of fluorescence polarization to antigen-antibody reactions has been published by Dandliker
et al. (1964). A list of complexes between fluorescent labels and macromolecules
that show fluorescence changes on interaction with drugs and other ligands may be
found in Table 5.

NUCLEIC   ACIDS   CONTAINING   FLUORESCENT   LABELS.
Nucleic acids, which show little or no fluorescence under normal physiological
conditions, have been labeled by fluorescent dyes such as acriflavine. For example,
Millar and Steiner (1965) have followed the helix→ coil transitions of polyadenylic
acid by measuring changes in the fluorescence polarization of acriflavine covalently

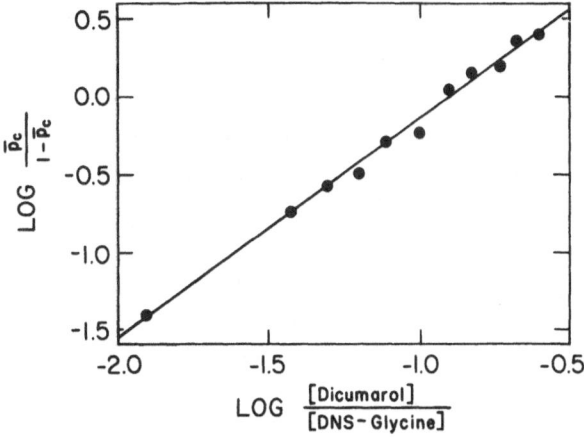

FIG. 7. Hill plot of the displacement dansylglycine from its binding sites on human serum albumin by the addition of dicoumarol. The concentrations were: HSA, 1×10^{-5} M; dansylglycine, 2×10^{-4} M; sodium phosphate buffer (pH 7.4), 0.1 M. Activation and emission wavelengths were 350 nm and 480 nm, respectively. Bandwidths for excitation and emission were 12 nm. $\bar{p}_c =$ Fractional occupation of dansylglycine-binding sites by dicoumarol. (From Chignell. 1970a. *Molec. Pharmacol.*, 6:1. Courtesy of Academic Press, Inc.)

TABLE 5

Complexes of Macromolecules with Fluorescent Labels That Show
Fluorescence Changes on Interaction with Drugs and Other Ligands

Fluorescent label	Ligand	Macromolecule	Reference
DNSA	Ethoxzolamide	Carbonic anhydrase	Chen and Kernohan (1967)
Dansylglycine	Dicoumarol	Serum albumin	Chignell (1970a)
Dansylglycine	Phenylbutazone	Serum albumin	Chignell (1969a)
Dansylglycine	Fenamic acids	Serum albumin	Chignell (1969b)
Fluorescein	Ovalbumin	Antibody	Dandliker and Feigen (1961)
Fluorescein	Ribonuclease	Antibody	Haber and Bennett (1962)
	Bovine serum albumin		
	Insulin (β-chain)		
Dye	Antigen	Antibody	Dandliker et al. (1964)
Acriflavine	—	RNA	Churchich[a] (1963)
Acriflavine	—	Poly A	Millar and Steiner[b] (1965)
Acriflavine	—	tRNA	Millar and MacKenzie[b] (1966)

[a]Measured the relaxation time of the acriflavine-RNA complex.
[b]Studied the helix → transition of the nucleic acid by measuring changes in the fluorescence polarization of the dye.

attached to the polymer. Similar studies have also been made by Millar and MacKenzie (1966) of an acriflavine conjugate with *Escherichia coli* tRNA. This technique could also be used to study changes in nucleic acid conformation on interaction with drug molecules.

TABLE 6

*Fluorescent Labels for Studying Drug Interactions
with Membrane Systems*

Fluorescent label	Ligand	Membrane system	Reference
ANS	Butacaine Aliphatic alcohols	Erythrocyte membranes	Feinstein et al. (1970)
ANS	Aliphatic alcohols	Erythrocyte membranes	Spero and Roth (1970)
ANS	Warfarin and other drugs	Liver microsomes	DiAugustine et al. (1970)
ANS	Flaxedil, *d*-tubocurarine	Electric eel organ membranes	Kasai et al. (1969)
ANS	CA^{++}butacaine, ATP, oligomycin, PCP	Mitochondria Mitochondrial membranes	Chance et al. (1969) Azzi et al. (1969) Chance and Lee (1969)
ANS	Various substrates	Mitochondria	Packer et al. (1969)
ANS	Various substrates	Mitochondria	Brocklehurst et al. (1970)
ANS	Cations, polymyxin B	Sarcoplasmic reticulum	Vanderkooi and Martonosi (1969)
ANS	Cations, ATP	Brain microsomes	Mayer and Avi-Dor (1969)
ANS	Cations, ATP, ouabain	Brain microsomes	Nagai et al. (1970)
Acridine orange	—	Crab nerve[a]	Tasaki et al. (1969)
ANS	—	Crab nerve[a]	Tasaki et al. (1969)

[a]Fluorescence changes observed after electrical stimulation of the nerve.

MEMBRANE PREPARATIONS CONTAINING FLUORESCENT LABELS. The binding of ANS to intact mitochondria or isolated mitochondrial membranes is accompanied by a marked shift in the fluorescence emission maximum of the dye to shorter wavelengths and an increase in dye fluorescence yield (Azzi et al., 1969; Chance and Lee, 1969; Chance et al., 1969; Packer et al., 1969). The addition of oligomycin, succinate, uncouplers of oxidative phosphorylation, or ATP produces changes in the fluorescence of membrane-bound ANS, which suggests that conformational changes precede the utilization of the intermediates of energy production by the mitochondrion. The addition of either butacaine (a local anesthetic) or Ca^{++} to ANS-labeled rat liver mitochondria caused an increase in the fluorescence yield of the dye but negligible changes in its fluorescence polarization (Chance et al., 1969). Chance and coworkers suggested that butacaine rendered the environment of membrane-bound ANS less polar by causing the extrusion of water from the membrane.

Other workers have found that the fluorescence of ANS bound to erythrocyte membranes is markedly affected by cations, such as Na$^+$ or Ca^{++}, or by local anesthetic drugs, such as butacaine or certain aliphatic alcohols (Wallach et al., 1970; Rubalcava et al., 1969; Feinstein et al., 1970; Spero and Roth, 1970). DiAugustine and coworkers (1970) have studied the interaction of ANS with liver microsomes and found that neither phenobarbital pretreatment nor reduction with $Na_2S_2O_4$ altered the fluorescence of bound ANS. While warfarin competitively displaced ANS from the microsomes, most of the other drugs tested increased the fluorescence of ANS.

Kasai et al. (1969) have found that the binding of ANS to membranes from the electric organ of the electric eel greatly enhanced the fluorescence intensity and polarization of the dye. The affinity of ANS for the membranes increased significantly in the presence of calcium ions, and in the presence of either d-tubocurarine or flaxedil, two drugs which are inhibitors of neuromuscular transmission. While it is at present unclear whether these fluorescence changes are directly related to the pharmacological effects of these agents, it does appear that the use of more specific fluorescence probes may permit the monitoring of the molecular events occurring during the transmission of impulses at the neuromuscular junction. In Table 6 will be found a list of fluorescent labels which have been used to study drug-membrane interactions.

One of the difficulties in interpreting data from membrane systems containing ANS is that the precise location of the fluorescent label is unknown. Several groups have suggested, however, that ANS is bound to membrane phospholipids (Feinstein et al., 1970; Spero and Roth, 1970; DiAugustine et al., 1970). Thus it appears probable that changes in ANS fluorescence may represent alterations not only in the conformation of membrane protein but also in the phospholipid environment of the dye. This problem has been overcome by Waggoner and Stryer (1970), who have synthesized several probes specifically for membrane studies. Three of these compounds, anthroyl stearic acid (VI), dansyl phosphatidyl

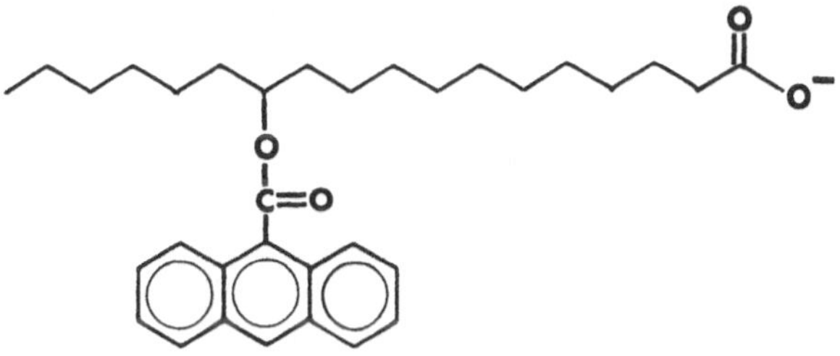

VI

ethanolamine (VII), and octadecyl naphthylamine sulfonic acid (VIII), were

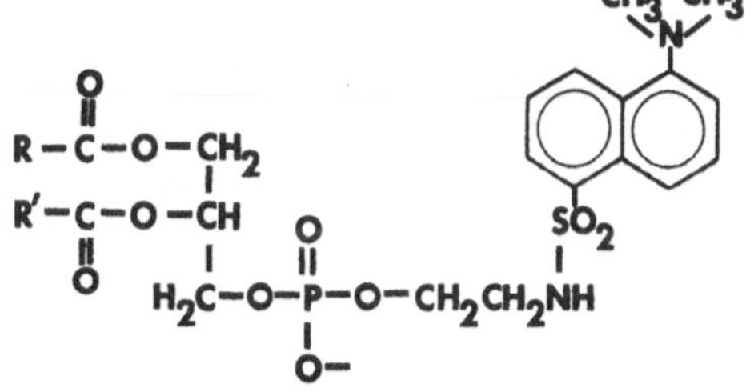

VII

VIII

found to be specifically incorporated into phospholipid bilayer vesicles. The emission spectra of these probes indicated that the chromophore of VI was located in the hydrocarbon region, that of VII was located in the glycerol layer, and that of VIII was located at the aqueous interface of the bilayer. When such specific fluorescent labels are incorporated into membranes, it will become easier to interpret the fluorescence changes that occur when drugs and other molecules perturb these systems.

APPENDIX — FLUORESCENCE TITRATIONS

SOME PRACTICAL CONSIDERATIONS

Fluorescence titrations may be carried out in a 1 cm^2 cuvette containing an accurately measured volume (2 to 4 ml) of solution. The cell compartment should be kept at a constant temperature throughout the titration since fluorescence intensity is temperature dependent. The titrant solution may be added from a microsyringe, while stirring can best be achieved with a small magnetic stirrer. Since fluorescence titration involves the making of multiple readings on a single sample, photodecomposition may become a problem. It is therefore important that the solution be exposed to light at the activating wavelength only during the actual measurement of fluorescence. At all other times the activating light should be screened from the sample. The problem of photodecomposition may also be overcome by preparing individual samples containing increasing amounts of the titrant. This approach has the advantage that it permits the use of microsample cells, which may in turn make the "inner filter" effect small enough to be neglected.

The observed fluorescent intensities must be corrected for the "inner filter" effect unless the optical density of the solution is less than 0.04 for a 1-cm pathlength. This may be done by carrying out a second titration in either the same cuvette used for the fluorescence measurements, or in another cuvette having the same pathlength. The optical density of the solution during titration is then determined at both the activating and emitting wavelengths. If the volume of titrant is small so that dilution factors are negligible, it is often possible to measure the optical density at the beginning and end of a titration and to obtain the intermediate values by calculation or graphically. The correction factor, X, by which each fluorescence intensity must be multiplied is given by

$$X = \text{antilog}\left(\frac{d_A + d_E}{2}\right)$$

where d_A = optical density at the activating wavelength, and d_E = optical density at the emitting wavelength.

The fluorescence values also must be corrected by the appropriate dilution factor. This correction may be avoided by adding small amounts of a concentrated solution of the titrant. Corrections for dilution are not generally necessary if the volume increase during titration is less than 5%. Another solution to this problem is to add the macromolecule to the titrant in the same concentration as it is present in the cuvette. Under these conditions the concentration of macromolecule does not change during the titration.

CALCULATION OF ASSOCIATION CONSTANTS FROM FLUORESCENCE TITRATION EXPERIMENTS

If, when a drug binds to a macromolecule, the intrinsic fluorescence of the drug increases or the intrinsic fluorescence of the macromolecule decreases, it is possible to calculate from fluorescence titration data an association constant for the interaction. In situations where the drug is nonfluorescent on binding it is often possible to calculate an association constant by measuring its ability to competitively displace from the macromolecule another drug or other ligand whose fluorescence is enhanced by binding. Similarly, if the binding of a drug does not quench the intrinsic fluorescence of a macromolecule, an association constant can be calculated if the drug competitively displaces a drug or other ligand that does quench the fluorescence of the macromolecule.

Drugs that Increase Their Fluorescence Yield on Binding to a Macromolecule

MACROMOLECULES WITH SINGLE DRUG-BINDING SITES. The interaction of a drug molecule (D) with a macromolecule (M) having a single binding site may be expressed as follows

$$D + M \rightleftarrows DM \tag{1}$$

The association constant (K_a) for this reaction is then given by

$$K_a = \frac{[DM]}{[D][M]} \tag{2}$$

where $[DM]$, $[D]$, and $[M]$ are the concentrations of the drug-macromolecule complex, free drug, and free macromolecule, respectively.

If the unbound drug shows no fluorescence at the wavelength where the bound drug fluoresces, the titration curve obtained by adding increments of the

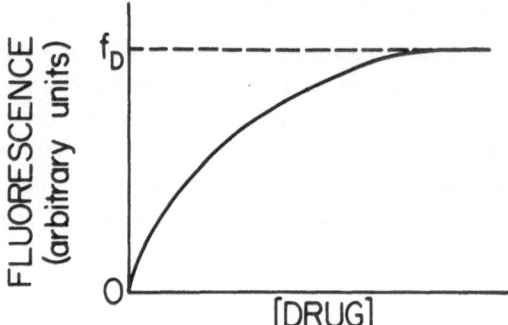

FIG. 8. The fluorescence titration curve of a drug that becomes fluorescent on binding to a macromolecule. Increments of drug have been added to a constant amount of the macromolecule. The drug is nonfluorescent when unbound.

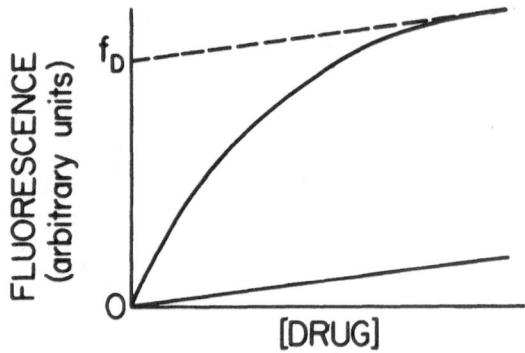

FIG. 9. The fluorescence titration curve (upper curve) of a drug that exhibits an increase in fluorescence yield on binding to a macromolecule. Increments of the drug have been added to a constant amount of the macromolecule. The intrinsic fluorescence of the drug in the absence of the macromolecule is shown in the lower curve.

drug to a fixed amount of macromolecule will have the form shown in Figure 8. However, if the unbound drug is also fluorescent, the titration curve will have the form shown in Figure 9. In order to correct the curve in Figure 9 a second titration must be performed in the absence of the macromolecule and the fluorescence of the drug alone must be subtracted from the fluorescence observed in the presence of the macromolecule. Throughout the rest of this section the term "drug fluorescence" when applied to a drug-macromolecule mixture will refer to the increase in the intrinsic fluorescence of the drug observed in the presence of the macromolecule.

If f is the fluorescence of a mixture containing the drug and the macromolecule, then the concentration of the complex will be given by

$$[DM] = Q \cdot M_t \tag{3}$$

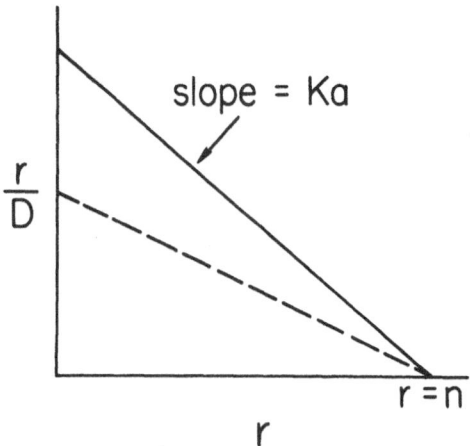

FIG. 10. A Scatchard plot of binding data: r=Number of moles of drug bound per mole of macromolecule, K_a=association constant for the interaction, n=total number of drug binding sites per macromolecule, D=concentration of free drug.

where $Q=f/f_D$, and f_D is the fluorescence observed when all the binding sites are completely saturated; and M_t is the total concentration of the macromolecule. The concentration of free drug, $[D]$, and the concentration of free macromolecule, $[M]$, are then given by

$$[D]=[D_t]-Q \cdot M_t \qquad (4)$$

$$[M]=M_t(1-Q) \qquad (5)$$

where $[D_t]$ is the total concentration of drug added.
    Combining equations (3), (4), and (5) with equation (2), we have

$$K_a=\frac{QM_b}{([D_t]-QM_t)M_t(1-Q)} \qquad (6)$$

The association constant can also be determined graphically by means of a Scatchard plot (Scatchard, 1949) based on the relationship

$$\frac{r}{D}=K_an-K_ar \qquad (7)$$

where r=number of moles of drug bound per mole of macromolecule, D=molar concentration of free drug, K_a=association constant (M^{-1}) for the interaction, and n=number of drug binding sites per macromolecule. The association constant is calculated from the slope of the line obtained by plotting r/D against r (Figure

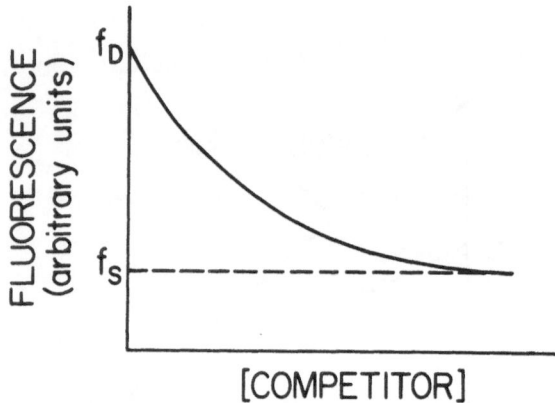

FIG. 11. The displacement of a fluorescent drug from a macromolecule by a nonfluorescent competitor. In this back titration a large excess of the fluorescent dye has been added to the macromolecule to ensure that all the binding sites were occupied before addition of the competitor.

10). A good example of this kind of approach is the binding of ethidium bromide to nucleic acids (LePecq and Paoletti, 1967) (Figure 2).

The association constant of a drug that is nonfluorescent on binding to a macromolecule can often be calculated by measuring its ability to competitively displace a fluorescent drug or other fluorescent ligand.

Let us assume that in the absence of the fluorescent drug (D) the interaction of a nonfluorescent competitor (C) with the macromolecule is given by

$$C + M \rightleftarrows CM \qquad (8)$$

The association constant (K_a') for this interaction would then be

$$K_a' = \frac{[CM]}{[C][CM]} \qquad (9)$$

The value of K_a' may be determined by adding increments of the fluorescent drug (D) to a mixture containing a fixed amount of the competitor (C) and macromolecule (M). The concentration of free and bound drug can be calculated as before from equations (3) and (4). The association constant (K_a') can then be determined from a Scatchard plot (Klotz et al., 1948). An example of this type of titration is the displacement of dansylglycine from HSA by phenylbutazone (Figure 6) (Chignell, 1969a).

The association constant (K_a') for a competitor can also be determined by back titration. In this approach an excess of drug (D) is added to the macromolecule (M) so that all the binding sites are occupied. The mixture will then have a fluorescence value f_D (Figure 11). Increments of the competitor are then added until there is no further decrease in fluorescence, which will reach a new value f_s (Figure 11). Since the competitor (C) is nonfluorescent, f_s will represent the fluorescence of the displaced drug (D). If the displaced drug is nonfluorescent, f_s will of course be zero.

The fluorescence (f) of the mixture at any point during the back titration is given by the expression

$$f = f_s + \frac{(f_D - f_s)\,[DM]}{[DM] + [CM]} \tag{10}$$

Equation (10) can be rearranged to give

$$f = \frac{f_s\,[CM] + f_D\,[DM]}{[CM] + [DM]} \tag{11}$$

Substituting for $[CM]$ and $[DM]$ the values derived from equations (2) and (9), we obtain

$$f = \frac{f_s K_a'\,[C] + f_D K_a\,[D]}{K_a'\,[C] + K_a\,[D]} \tag{12}$$

Equation 12 may then be rearranged to give

$$K_a' = \frac{f_D - f}{f - f_s} \cdot \frac{[D]}{[C]} \cdot K_a \tag{13}$$

Since it can be shown that

$$[D] = [D_t] - \frac{f - f_s}{f_D - f_s}\,[M_t] \tag{14}$$

and that

$$[C] = [C_t] - \frac{f_D - f}{f_D - f_s}\,[M_t] \tag{15}$$

equation (13) becomes

$$K_a' = \frac{f_D - f}{f - f_s} \cdot \frac{[D_t] - \left(\dfrac{f - f_s}{f_D - f_s}\right)[M_t]}{[C_t] - \dfrac{f_D - f}{f_D - f_s}\,[M_t]} \cdot K_a \tag{16}$$

A graphical solution is possible by rearranging equation (13) to the form

$$\frac{f_D-f}{f-f_s}=\frac{[C]}{[D]}\cdot\frac{K_a{}'}{K_a}\qquad\qquad(17)$$

and plotting $(f_D-f)/(f-f_s)$ against $[C]/[D]$. The slope of the resultant straight line will then be $K_a{}'/K_a$.

MACROMOLECULES WITH MULTIPLE DRUG-BINDING SITES. If a macromolecule is known to have more than one drug-binding site or if the number of drug-binding sites is unknown, a slightly different approach must be employed. First, a fixed amount of the drug D_b is titrated with increments of the macromolecule until there is no further increase in fluorescence. It is then assumed that all the drug is bound and that the observed fluorescence, f_B, is related to the concentration of bound drug, $[D_b]$, by the expression

$$[D_b]=P\cdot f_B\qquad\qquad(18)$$

where P is a constant of proportionality. A second fluorescence titration is then carried out in which increments of the drug are added to a fixed amount of the macromolecule. If the increase in the fluorescence quantum yield of the drug is the same at all binding sites, then at any given point during the titration when the mixture has a fluorescence value f, the concentration of bound drug will be given by $P\cdot f$. Since the total concentration of drug is known, it is possible to calculate how much is still unbound. Results may then be expressed in terms of a Scatchard plot (Figure 10) from which the association constant(s) for the interaction can be calculated.

The association constant of a nonfluorescent competitor can be determined by titrating a mixture of macromolecule and competitor with the fluorescent drug. Since the concentration of free and bound drug can still be calculated with the aid of equation (18), the association constant for the competitor can be obtained from the Scatchard plot (Klotz et al., 1948). Using this technique LePecq and Paoletti (1967) have studied the competitive displacement of ethidium bromide from DNA by quinacrine (Figure 2).

Flanagan and Ainsworth (1968) have shown that if the macromolecule has multiple binding sites that are heterogeneous, then association constants for some of these sites can be obtained by modifying equation (17) to give

$$\log\frac{f_D-f}{f-f_s}=\log\frac{[C]}{[D]}+\log\frac{K_a{}'}{K_a}\qquad\qquad(19)$$

and then plotting $\log (f_D-f)/(f-f_s)$ against $\log [C]/[D]$. For heterogeneous sites the slope of the line approaches unity only at the beginning and end of the titration. Extrapolation of the linear portions of the curve to the abscissa permits an estimation of the association constants for the first and last sites from which the drug is displaced. This kind of approach has been used by Chignell (1970a), who determined the affinity of dicoumarol for human serum albumin by the ability of the drug to competitively displace the fluorescent probe dansylglycine (Figure 7).

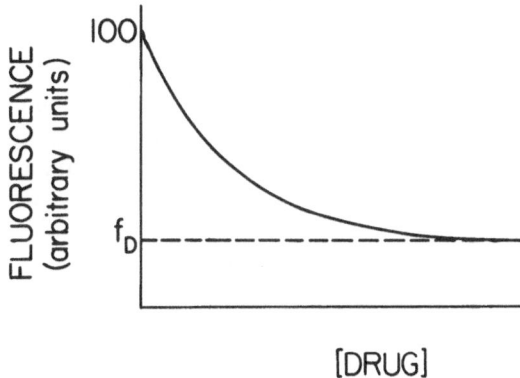

FIG. 12. The fluorescence titration curve of a macromolecule whose intrinsic fluorescence is quenched by the binding of a drug.

Nonfluorescent Drugs That Quench the Intrinsic Fluorescence of a Macromolecule on Binding

MACROMOLECULES WITH A SINGLE DRUG-BINDING SITE.   If the intrinsic fluorescence of a macromolecule is quenched by the binding of a drug molecule, the resultant titration curve will generally have the form shown in Figure 12. The concentration of free and bound drug can be calculated from equations (3) and (4) using a value of $Q = (100-f) / (100-f_D)$, where f = fluorescence of the macromolecule at a given point during the titration, and f_D = fluorescence of the macromolecule when all sites are occupied.

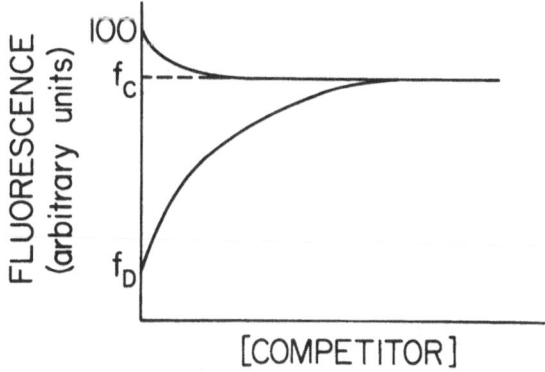

FIG. 13. The effect of competitor binding on the intrinsic fluorescence of a macromolecule measured in the absence (upper curve) and in the presence (lower curve) of a large excess of drug that quenches on binding.

The association constant K_a may be calculated from equation (6) or may be obtained from a Scatchard plot (Figure 10).

The association constant (K_a') of a competitor (C) that can displace the drug (D) but which does not itself quench the fluorescence of the macromolecule can also be determined by fluorescence titration. A mixture containing a fixed amount of the macromolecule and competitor is titrated with the drug. The concentration of free and bound drug is calculated as described above and a Scatchard plot is obtained. The association constant of the competitor can be calculated by the method of Klotz et al. (1948).

The association constant of the competitor can also be obtained by a back titration procedure. In this method a large excess of drug (D) is added to a solution containing the macromolecule (M) so that all drug binding sites are occupied and the fluorescence of the macromolecule has a value f_D (Figure 12). If increasing amounts of competitor (C) are now added to the system, the drug (D) will be displaced from the macromolecule. The intrinsic fluorescence of the macromolecule will therefore increase until it has reached the initial intensity observed before the addition of drug (D) (Figure 12). If, however, the binding of the competitor (C) quenches the fluorescence of the macromolecule to any significant extent, the fluorescence of the macromolecule will return instead to a new value f_C (Figure 13). The fluorescence, f, at any given point during such a titration can be expressed as follows

$$f = 100 - \frac{(100 - f_c)[CM]}{[CM] + [DM]} - \frac{(100 - f_D)[DM]}{[CM] + [DM]} \tag{20}$$

Equation (20) can be rearranged to give

$$f = \frac{f_c [CM] + f_D [DM]}{[CM] + [DM]} \tag{21}$$

Substituting for $[CM]$ and $[DM]$ the values derived from equations (2) and (9), we obtain

$$f = \frac{f_c K_a' [C] + f_D K_a [D]}{K_a' [C] + K_a [D]} \tag{22}$$

Equation (22) may then be rearranged to give

$$K_a' = \frac{f - f_D}{f_c - f} \cdot \frac{[D]}{[C]} \cdot K_a \tag{23}$$

Since it can be shown that

$$[D] = [D_t] - \frac{f_c - f}{f_c - f_D}[M_t] \tag{24}$$

and that

$$[C] = [C_t] - \frac{f - f_D}{f_c - f_D}[M_t] \tag{25}$$

equation (23) becomes

$$K_a' = \frac{f - f_D}{f_0 - f} \cdot \frac{[D_t] - \frac{f_0 - f}{f_0 - f_D} \cdot [M_t]}{[C_t] - \frac{f - f_D}{f_0 - f_D} \cdot [M_t]} \cdot K_a \tag{26}$$

A graphical solution is possible by rearranging equation (23) to give

$$\frac{f - f_D}{f_0 - f} = \frac{[C]}{[D]} \cdot \frac{K_a'}{K_a} \tag{27}$$

and plotting $(f - f_D)/(f_0 - f)$ against $[C]/[D]$. The slope of the line will then be K_a'/K_a. If the binding of the competitor (C) does not quench the intrinsic fluorescence of the macromolecule, then $f_C = 100$ can be substituted in equation (26).

A good example of this kind of approach is the work of Taylor et al. (1970), who studied the binding of various sulfonamides to carbonic anhydrase by measuring their ability to displace a sulfonamide (DNABS, III) that quenched the native fluorescence of the protein on binding.

MACROMOLECULES WITH MULTIPLE DRUG-BINDING SITES. Although fluorescence quenching may be employed to study the interaction of drugs with macromolecules containing multiple binding sites, the method of calculating association constants is somewhat different from that described in the previous section. Let us consider the case of a protein molecule, such as human serum albumin, which contains a single tryptophan group. If human serum albumin has several drug-binding sites each of which is located at a distance equal to the average transfer distance from the tryptophan group, then the binding of a single drug molecule to the protein will result in a 50% decrease in the intensity of tryptophan fluorescence. However, a 50% decrease in the fluorescence quantum yield of tryptophan must mean that the fluorescence lifetime of the amino acid has also been shortened by 50%. Since the probability of energy transfer from the tryptophan to the drug is dependent on the fluorescence lifetime of the amino acid, it follows that when a second drug molecule binds to the protein the efficiency of transfer will be less than 50%. Thus the observed quenching of tryptophan fluorescence will not be proportional to the number of drug molecules bound.

In order to calculate the association constant of a drug for multiple binding sites on a macromolecule by fluorescence quenching, titrations must be made over a range of macromolecule concentrations. The fluorescence intensities, expressed as a percentage of the initial fluorescence of the macromolecule, are then plotted as a function of the drug-macromolecule ratio (Figure 14). It will be found that above a certain critical concentration of macromolecule the titration curves are superimposable (Figure 14, curve C) since all the drug is bound. The concentration of bound drug in mixtures containing the macromolecule below this critical concentration can be calculated with the aid of this curve as shown in Figure 14. Results can then be expressed as a Scatchard plot. A good example of this kind of approach has been provided by Chen (personal communication), who has used fluorescence

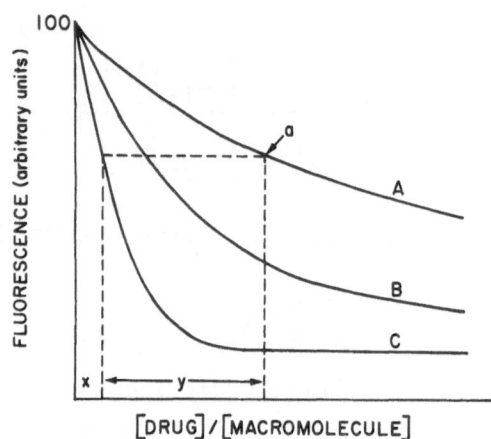

FIG. 14. The fluorescence titration curve of a macromolecule whose intrinsic fluorescence is quenched by drug binding to multiple sites. Curves A, B, and C represent experiments performed with increasing concentrations of macromolecule. The fraction of drug bound at point "a" is given by $x/(x+y)$.

quenching to study the binding of bilirubin to multiple sites on human and bovine serum albumins (Figure 5).

It should also be possible to use this technique to estimate the association constant of a competitor that does not quench the intrinsic fluorescence of the macromolecule by measuring its ability to displace a drug molecule that does quench on binding. Results are best expressed as a Scatchard plot, from which an association constant could be calculated by the method of Klotz et al. (1948).

REFERENCES

Attalah, N. A., and G. F. Lata. 1968. Steroid-protein interactions studied by fluorescence quenching. Biochim. Biophys. Acta, 168:321-333.

Azzi, A., B. Chance, G. K. Radda, and C. P. Lee. 1969. A fluorescence probe of energy dependent structural changes in fragmented membranes. Proc. Nat. Acad. Sci. U.S.A., 62:612-619.

Berns, D. S., and S. J. Singer. 1964. A fluorescence study of specific and non-specific dye-protein interactions. Immunochemistry, 1:209-217.

Bittmann, R. 1969. Studies of the binding of ethidium bromide to transfer RNA: Absorption, fluorescence, ultracentrifugation and kinetic investigations. J. Molec. Biol., 46:251-268.

Borisova, O. F., and L. A. Tumerman. 1965. Application of acridine orange luminescence to the study of secondary structure of nucleic acids. Biofizika, 10:32-36.

Boyle, R. E., S. S. Nelson, F. R. Dollish, and M. J. Olsen. 1962. The interaction of deoxyribonucleic acid and acridine orange. Arch. Biochem. Biophys., 96:47-50.

Brocklehurst, J. R., R. B. Freedman, D. J. Hancock, and G. K. Radda. 1970. Membrane studies with polarity-dependent and excimer-forming fluorescent probes. Biochem. J., 116:721-731.

Burns, V. W. F. 1969. Fluorescence decay time characteristics of the complex between ethidium bromide and nucleic acids. Arch. Biochem. Biophys., 133:420-424.

Chance, B., A. Azzi, L. Mela, G. Radda, and H. Vainio. 1969. Local anesthetic induced changes of a membrane-bound fluorochrome. A link between ion uptake and membrane structure. Fed. Eur. Biochem. Soc. Letters, 3:10-13.

———— and C. Lee. 1969. Comparison of fluorescence probe and light-scattering readout of structural states of mitochondrial membrane fragments. Fed. Eur. Biochem. Soc. Letters, 4:181-184.

Chen, R. F., H. Edelhoch, and R. F. Steiner. 1969. The fluorescence of proteins. In Leach, S. J., ed., Physical Principles and Techniques of Protein Chemistry, Vol. 1, pp. 171-244. New York, Academic Press.

———— and J. C. Kernohan. 1967. Combination of bovine carbonic anhydrase with a fluorescent sulfonamide. J. Biol. Chem., 242:5813-5823.

Chignell, C. F. 1969a. Optical studies of drug-protein complexes. II. The interaction of phenylbutazone and its analogs with serum albumin. Molec. Pharmacol., 5:244-252.

———— 1969b. Optical studies of drug-protein complexes. III. The interaction of flufenamic acid and other N-arylanthranilates with serum albumin. Molec. Pharmacol., 5:455-462.

———— 1970a. Optical studies of drug-protein complexes. IV. The interaction of warfarin and dicoumarol with human serum albumin. Molec. Pharmacol., 6:1-11.

———— 1970b. Fluorescence studies of drug interactions with biological systems—a review. Fluorescence News, 5:1-5.

Churchich, J. E. 1963. Fluorescence studies on soluble ribonucleic acid labelled with acriflavine. Biochim. Biophys. Acta, 75:274-276.

Dandliker, W. B., and G. A. Feigen. 1961. Quantification of the antigen-antibody reaction by the polarization of fluorescence. Biochem. Biophys. Res. Commun., 5:299-308.

———— H. C. Schapiro, J. W. Meduski, R. Alonso, G. A. Feigen, and J. R. Hamrick. 1964. Application of fluorescence polarization to the antigen-antibody reaction. Immunochemistry, 1:165-191.

Deranleau, D. A., and H. Neurath. 1966. The combination of chymotrypsin and chymotrypsinogen with fluorescent substrates and inhibitors for chymotrypsin. Biochemistry (Washington), 5:1413-1425.

DiAugustine, R. P., T. E. Eling, and J. R. Fouts. 1970. The interaction of a fluorescent probe with rat hepatic microsomes. Fed. Proc., 29:738.

Edelman, G. M., and W. O. McClure. 1968. Fluorescent probes and the conformation of proteins. Accounts Chem. Res., 1:65-70.

Ellerton, N. F., and I. Isenberg. 1969. Fluorescence polarization study of DNA-proflavine complexes. Biopolymers, 8:767-786.

Feinstein, M. B., L. Spero, and H. Felsenfield. 1970. Interactions of a fluorescent probe with erythrocyte membrane and lipids: Effects of local anesthetics and calcium. Fed. Eur. Biochem. Soc. Letters, 6:245-248.

Flanagan, M. T., and S. Ainsworth. 1968. The binding of aromatic sulfonic acids to bovine serum albumin. Biochim. Biophys. Acta, 168:16-26.

Förster, T. 1946. Das Fluoreszensvermögen organischer Farbstoffe. Naturwissenschaften, 33:220-221.

———— 1951. Fluoreszenz organischer Verbindungen. Göttingen, Vandenoeck and Ruprecht.

Gitler, C., B. Rubalcava, and A. Caswell. 1969. Fluorescence changes of ethidium bromide on binding to erythrocyte and mitochondrial membranes. Biochim. Biophys. Acta, 193:479-481.

Haber, E., and J. C. Bennett. 1962. Polarization of fluorescence as a measure of antigen-antibody interaction. Proc. Nat. Acad. Sci. U.S.A., 48:1935-1942.

Hawking, F. 1963. Chemotherapy of trypanosomiasis. In Schnitzer, R. J., and F. J. Hawking, eds., Experimental Chemotherapy, Vol. 1, pp. 129-256. New York, Academic Press.

Kasai, M., J. P. Changeux, and L. Monnerie. 1969. *In vitro* interaction of 1-anilino-8-naphthalene sulfonate with excitable membranes isolated from the electric organ of *Electrophorus electricus*. Biochem. Biophys. Res. Commun., 36:420-427.

Klotz, I. M., H. Triwush, and F. M. Walker. 1948. The binding of organic ions by proteins. Competition phenomena and denaturation effects. J. Amer. Chem. Soc., 70:2935-2941.

LePecq, J. B., and C. Paoletti. 1967. A fluorescent complex between ethidium bromide and nucleic acids. J. Molec. Biol., 27:87-106.

———— P. Yot, and C. Paoletti. 1964. Interaction du bromhydrate d'ethidium (BET) avec les nucléïques (A.N.). Etude spectrofluorimétrique. C. R. Acad. Sci. (Paris), 259:1786-1789.

Lerman, L. S. 1961. Structural considerations in the interaction of DNA and acridines. J. Molec. Biol., 3:18-30.

———— 1963. The structure of the DNA-acridine complex. Proc. Nat. Acad. Sci. U.S.A., 49:94-102.

———— 1964. Amino group reactivity in DNA-aminoacridine complexes. J. Molec. Biol., 10:367-380.

Levine, R. J. C., D. N. Teller, and H. C. B. Denber. 1968. Binding of chlorpromazine and thioproperazine *in vitro*. III. Fluorometric measurement of changes in *Limulus polyphemus* (horseshoe crab) myosin B structure and enzyme activity after treatment with phenothiazine drugs. Molec. Pharmacol., 4:435-442.

MacInnes, J. W., and R. B. Uretz. 1966. Organization of DNA in dipteron polytene chromosomes as indicated by polarized fluorescence microscopy. Science, 151:689-691.

Mann, T., and D. Keilin. 1940. Sulphanilamide as a specific inhibitor of carbonic anhydrase. Nature (London), 146:164-165.

Maren, T. H. 1967. Carbonic anhydrase: Chemistry, physiology and inhibition. Physiol. Rev., 47:595-781.

Marlow, H. F., J. C. Metcalfe, and A. S. V. Burgen. 1969. The specificity of drug receptors. An immunochemical model for cholinergic receptors. Molec. Pharmacol., 5:156-165.

Mayer, M., and Y. Avi-Dor. 1969. Fluorescence properties of anilino-naphthalene-sulfonate bound to microsomal particles. Israel J. Chem., 7:149 P.

Millar, D. B. S., and M. MacKenzie. 1966. The helix-coil transition of *E. coli* s-RNA as measured by fluorescence polarization. Biochem. Biophys. Res. Commun., 23:724-729.

———— and R. F. Steiner. 1965. Fluorescent conjugates of biosynthetic polyribonucleotides. Biochim. Biophys. Acta, 102:571-589.

Nagai, K., G. E. Lindenmayer, and A. Schwartz. 1970. Direct evidence for the conformational nature of the (Na^+, K^+)-ATPase system: Fluorescence and circular dichroism studies. Arch. Biochem. Biophys., 139:252-254.

Newton, B. A. 1964. Mechanisms of action of phenanthridine and aminoquinaldine trypanocides. Advances Chemother., 1:35-83.

Packer, L., M. P. Donovan, and J. M. Wrigglesworth. 1969. Oscillations of 8-anilinonaphthalene-1-sulfonic acid fluorescence in mitochondria. Biochem. Biophys. Res. Commun., 35:832-837.

Rubalcava, B., D. M. Munoz, and C. Gitler. 1969. Interaction of fluorescent probes with membranes. I. Effect of ions on erythrocyte membranes. Biochemistry (Washington), 8:2742-2747.

Scatchard, G. 1949. The attraction of proteins for small molecules and ions. Ann. New York Acad. Sci., 51:660-672.

Sela, I. 1969. Fluorescence of nucleic acids with ethidium bromide: An indication of the configurative state of nucleic acids. Biochim. Biophys. Acta, 190:216-219.

Spero, L., and S. Roth. 1970. Fluorescent hydrophobic probe study of the interaction between local anesthetics and red cell ghosts. Fed. Proc., 29:474.

Steiner, R. F., J. Roth, and J. Robbins. 1966. The binding of thyroxine by serum albumin as measured by fluorescence quenching. J. Biol. Chem., 241:560-567.

Stryer, L. 1968. Fluorescence spectroscopy of proteins. Science, 162: 526-533.

Tasaki, I., L. Carnay, and A. Watanabe. 1969. Transient changes in extrinsic fluorescence of nerve produced by electric stimulation. Proc. Nat. Acad. Sci. U.S.A., 64:1362-1368.

_____ L. Carnay, R. Sandlin, and A. Watanabe. 1969. Fluorescence changes during conduction in nerves stained with acridine orange. Science, 163:683-685.

Taylor, P. W., R. W. King and A. S. V. Burgen. 1970. Kinetics of complex formation between human carbonic anhydrases and aromatic sulfonamides. Biochemistry (Washington), 9:2638-2645.

Teller, D. N., R. J. C. Levine, and H. C. B. Denber. 1968. Binding of chlorpromazine and thioproperazine *in vitro*. II. Fluorometric measurement of stoichiometry. Agressologie, 9:1-20.

Thomes, J. C., G. Weill, and M. Daune. 1969. Fluorescence of proflavine-DNA:complexes: Heterogeneity of binding sites. Biopolymers, 8:647-659.

Tomita, G. 1968. Absorption and fluorescence of some basic dyes complexing with nucleic acids. Z. Naturforsch., 23:922-925.

Tubbs, R. K., W. E. Ditmars, and Q. Van Winkle. 1964. Heterogeneity of the interaction of DNA with acriflavine. J. Molec. Biol., 9:545-557.

Udenfriend, S. 1962. Fluorescence Assay in Biology and Medicine, Vol. I. New York, Academic Press.

_____ 1969. Fluorescence Assay in Biology and Medicine, Vol. II. New York, Academic Press.

_____ and P. Zaltzman. 1962. Fluorescence characteristics of purines, pyrimidines and their derivatives: Measurement of guanine in nucleic acid hydrolysates. Anal. Biochem., 3:49-59.

Vanderkooi, J., and A. Martonosi. 1969. Sarcoplasmic reticulum. VIII. Use of 8-anilino-1-naphthalene sulfonate as a conformational probe on biological membranes. Arch. Biochem. Biophys., 133:153-163.

Velick, S. F. 1958. Fluorescence spectra and polarization of glyceraldehyde-3-phosphate and lactic dehydrogenase coenzyme complexes. J. Biol. Chem., 233:1455-1467.

_____ C. W. Parker, and H. N. Eisen. 1960. Excitation energy transfer and the quantitative study of the antibody-hapten reaction. Proc. Nat. Acad. Sci. U.S.A., 46:1470-1482.

Waggoner, A. S., and L. Stryer. 1970. Fluorescent probes of biological membranes. Proc. Nat. Acad. Sci. U.S.A., 67:579-589.

Wallach, D. F. H., E. Ferber, D. Selin, E. Weidekamm, and H. Fischer. 1970. The study of lipid-protein interactions in membranes by fluorescent probes. Biochim. Biophys. Acta, 203:67-76.

Weber, G. 1960. Fluorescence-polarization spectrum and electronic energy transfer in proteins. Biochem. J., 75:345-352.

_____ and F. W. J. Teale. 1965. Interaction of proteins with radiation. *In* Neurath, H., ed., The Proteins, Vol. 3:445-475. New York, Academic Press.

Weill, G., and M. Calvin. 1963. Optical properties of chromophore-macromolecule complexes: Absorption and fluorescence of acridine dyes bound to polyphosphates and DNA. Biopolymers, 1:401-417.

Yamabe, S. 1969. A fluorospectrophotometric study on the binding of acridine orange with DNA and its bases. Arch. Biochem. Biophys., 130:145-155.

Yamagishi, H. 1962. Interaction between nucleic acids and berberine sulfate. J. Cell Biol., 15:589-592.

Chapter **3**

Phosphorescence Spectroscopy

B. L. Van Duuren and G. Witz

Laboratory of Organic Chemistry and Carcinogenesis, Institute of Environmental Medicine, New York University Medical Center, New York, New York

INTRODUCTION

The phenomena of phosphorescence, fluorescence, and delayed fluorescence are closely related aspects of what is termed luminescence or photoluminescence, as distinguished from chemiluminescence. Because of the close relationship between these manifestations of photoluminescence, the theory and definitions applicable to each should be, and are, in this volume, presented together in a preceding chapter on fluorescence spectroscopy. This chapter will be concerned primarily with the instrumentation and some applications of phosphorescence spectroscopy.

As with fluorescence, the use of phosphorescence as an analytical tool has only relatively recently become more widely used. This is somewhat surprising since luminescence of organic and inorganic compounds has been studied for over a century. An early version of a phosphoroscope was made in the mid-nineteenth century by E. Becquerel (1871). However, the advent of commercial instruments for phosphorescence measurements has made possible wider application of this mode of spectroscopy in organic chemical structural studies, in agricultural chemistry, petrochemistry, biochemistry, pharmacological chemistry, and lately in biomedical research.

Instrumentation

Instrumentation for phosphorescence varies in its degree of sophistication, depending on the requirements, from simple filter phosphoroscopes to complex

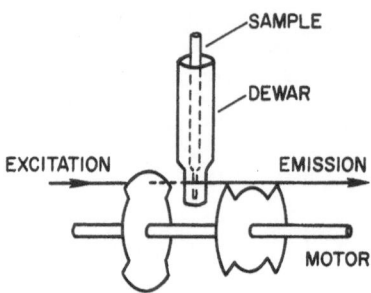

FIG. 1. Becquerel phosphoroscope.

spectrophosphorimeters, and it is frequently possible to measure both fluorescence and phosphorescence on the same instrument. The basic difference between measurement of fluorescence and phosphorescence is that in the former measurements are made while the sample is irradiated; in phosphorescence, however, the incident light does not impinge on the sample while the measurement is being made. In addition, phosphorescence is in most instances measured at low temperature, usually liquid nitrogen temperature, and this necessitates special sample chambers and solvent systems or solid matrices. For the rest the instrumentation required for measurement of phosphorescence is very similar to that required for fluorescence.

Phosphorescence provides additional luminescence information about a given material, namely, its phosphorescence emission spectrum, a phosphorescence decay curve or half-life, and a measure of the quantum efficiency of phosphorescence.

An essential part for the measurement of phosphorescence is the phosphoroscope, which is usually a mechanical device which allows for alternate irradiation of the sample and measurement of emitted phosphorescence. There are two basic designs for phosphoroscopes: one is a modified Becquerel phosphoroscope, shown schematically in Figure 1. This is also called a rotating disc phosphoroscope. This diagram indicates that excitation occurs out-of-phase with measurement of phosphorescence. A second type of phosphoroscope is the rotating hollow cylinder type shown in Figure 2. This design was developed by Lewis and Kasha (1944) and consists of a motor-driven hollow cylinder with equally spaced slits around the circumference. The slits are so spaced that, as the motor-driven cylinder rotates around the sample, excitation of the sample and measurement of phosphorescence emitted occur alternately. This type of phosphoroscope has been incorporated in a commercial phosphorescence spectrophotometer. The efficiency of these two types of phosphoroscopes has been compared based on an expression called the "observation efficiency factor." This factor is the ratio of the observed phosphorescence signal given by a phosphoroscope to the signal obtained by using continuous excitation and emission. The intensity of the phosphorescence signal when using a phosphoroscope will depend on the duration of excitation, the time interval between the end of excitation and the beginning of measurement, and the phosphorescence decay time. It was concluded that the Becquerel phosphoroscope is more versatile than the rotating cylinder version; with the latter, which has a maximum speed of

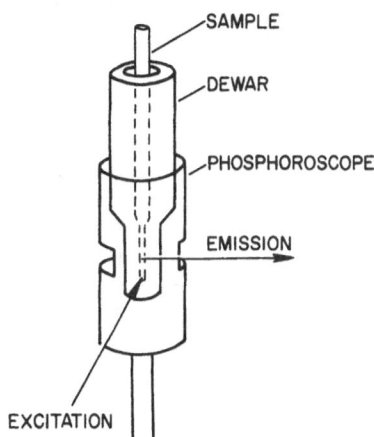

SAMPLE

DEWAR

PHOSPHOROSCOPE

EMISSION

EXCITATION

FIG. 2. Rotating cylinder phosphoroscope.

15,000 r.p.m. (O'Haver and Winefordner, 1966), phosphorescence decay times can be obtained effectively for compounds that have a decay time greater than 1 millisecond. It is less useful for compounds with a faster phosphorescence decay time. A recently described multipurpose luminescence spectrophotometer (Cravitt and Van Duuren, 1968) uses an optical chopper in the excitation beam for phosphorescence measurements. This instrument can be operated in either fluorescence or phosphorescence modes. The optical chopper consists of a tuning fork with flags attached to the ends. The on-to-off time of the chopper is ~1 msec, i.e., it allows for phosphorescence measurements when the decay time is 1 msec or longer. When the chopper is locked in the open position the instrument is in the fluorescence mode.

Parker (1968a) devised a phosphorescence spectrophotometer which uses neither the Becquerel nor Lewis and Kasha phosphoroscopes. In this instrument two chopper discs are used, driven by two separate synchronous motors. One chopper is placed at the exit slit of the excitation monochromator and the second at the entrance slit of the analyzing monochromator. In this manner the two choppers can readily be put in or out of phase so that either phosphorescence or total luminescence can be measured. When the choppers are run in phase the instrument is operating as a spectrofluorimeter. Parker (1968a) has also considered in detail the "phosphorimeter factor," called the "observation efficiency factor" by McCarthy and Winefordner (1967). Thus, if the lifetime of phosphorescence emission is of the same order of magnitude as the periods of illumination and darkness, the phosphorescence will decay appreciably during the dark period before observation by the photomultiplier. In Parker's terminology, the phosphorimeter factor is the ratio of the observed phosphorescence intensity, i.e., with the choppers out of phase, to the total emission. The magnitude of the correction which has to be made can be calculated and depends upon the mechanical and optical arrangement of the choppers or phosphoroscope used. This aspect has been discussed by Parker (1968a). Therefore, when quantitative analyses are being made by phosphores-

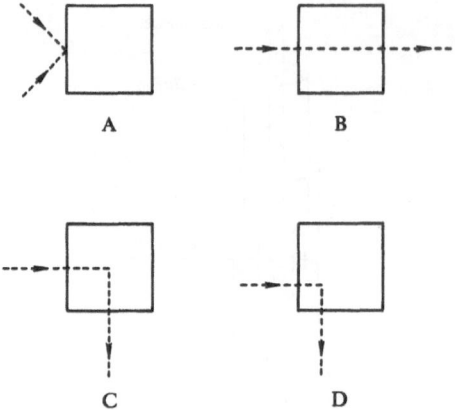

FIG. 3. Sample area geometry for phosphorescence.

cence, it is important to have some knowledge of the phosphorescence decay time of the material under investigation. This can be obtained by examining the effect of increasing the chopper or phosphoroscope speed on phosphorescence intensity.

The light sources, monochromators and/or filters, detectors, and read-out devices for the measurement of phosphorescence spectra are the same as those used for fluorescence as described elsewhere in this volume.

In addition to the phosphoroscope the only other major difference between fluorescence and phosphorescence measurements is the nature of the sample area. As in the case of fluorescence, various modes can be used for sample area geometry as depicted in Figure 3. The most commonly used mode is that with a 90° angle between the exciting beam and the angle of measurement, Figure 3c; the end-on mode, Figure 3b, is rarely used because of interference by scattered excitation energy and reabsorption problems. Since most compounds phosphoresce only in rigid media, phosphorescence measurements are usually made at liquid nitrogen temperature. This necessitates an optically clear Dewar flask for liquid nitrogen and a special quartz container for the frozen sample. Light passes through two unsilvered ports in the Dewar flask. In order to avoid frosting of the surfaces in the light path, it is desirable to have an airtight sample area which can be flushed with dry air or nitrogen. Various types of Dewar flasks and quartz sample cells have been described in the literature (Cravitt and Van Duuren, 1968; McCarthy and Winefordner, 1967).

The introduction of the phosphoroscope and cooling system into a luminescence spectrophotometer makes phosphorescence measurements more complicated than those of fluorescence. The additional quartz surfaces in the sample area, bubbles in the surrounding liquid nitrogen, and frosting of surfaces all enhance light scattering and, hence, decrease luminescence energy. Since excitation and emission energy pass through the cooling liquid, it is important that the latter not absorb light and also be free of fluorescent material. Liquid nitrogen fulfills these requirements, since it is transparent from 200 to 800 mμ; also it is safe and inexpensive to use. Conduction cooling systems have been devised in order to overcome the difficulties encountered in the use of a Dewar (Hoerman and Mancewicz, 1964). However, these systems also have some disadvantages, and the immersion cooling method is still the most commonly used.

MEDIA

The choice of a solvent matrix for measurement of phosphorescence at liquid nitrogen temperature is of great importance. In addition to the usual criteria required of solvents for fluorescence, i.e., purity and solubilizing properties, it is necessary that the solvent give a clear glass, free of cracks, at 77°K. Very few pure solvents show this property and hence solvent mixtures are usually employed. Extensive studies on suitable solvent mixtures of varying polarity have been made (Scott and Allison, 1962; Smith et al., 1962; Winefordner and St. John, 1963) and some of these are listed in Table 1. The most commonly used solvent mixture, EPA,

TABLE 1

Low Temperature Rigid Glass Systems

System	Composition (vol:vol)
Hydrocarbons	
3-Methylpentane	—
Isopentane:methylcyclohexane	1:4
Pentene-2(*cis*):pentene-2(*trans*)	—
Alcohols	
Methanol:ethanol	1:4
Ethanol	—
Isopropyl alcohol	—
1-Propanol	—
1-Butanol	—
Ether	
n-Butyl ether:isopropyl ether:diethyl ether	3:5:12
2-Methyltetrahydrofuran	—
Alcohol:Ethers	
Ethanol:diethyl ether	1:1
Propanol:diethyl ether	2:5
Butanol:diethyl ether	2:5
Alcohol:Hydrocarbon:Ether	
Ethanol:isopentane:diethyl ether	2:5:5
Isorpopyl alcohol:isopentane:diethyl ether	2:5:5
Ethers:Hydrocarbons	
Diethyl ether:isopentane	1:1
Diethyl ether:pentene-2(*cis*):pentene-2(*trans*)	2:1

consists of ether-isopentane-ethyl alcohol, 5:5:2, v/v. A convenient type of matrix that has also been used for phosphorescence analysis is provided by polymers that are rigid at room temperature. A number of polymers have been used for this purpose including polystyrene, polymethylmethacrylate, polyvinylacetate, etc. (Geacintov et al., 1968). These polymers offer certain advantages over frozen solvent mixtures, e.g., they can be made in a variety of sizes and shapes ranging from thin films to rods or blocks which are readily machined. On the other hand, some of the polymers influence the wavelength and intensity of phosphorescence because of solute-solvent interactions. Samples have to be degassed during preparation in order to minimize oxygen quenching. A potassium bromide pellet technique developed earlier for fluorescence measurements and found eminently suitable for that purpose (Van Duuren and Bardi, 1963) can also be used for phosphorescence measurements with the use of a Teflon pellet holder. Thus, spectra of solid solutions, as well as crystal dispersions in the potassium bromide matrix, can be measured. This technique has been used for the study of phosphorescence of aflatoxins B_1 and G_1 (Van Duuren et al., 1968). The phosphorescence of organic compounds has also been observed on paper chromatograms cooled to liquid nitrogen temperature and this procedure has been used for the examination of aromatic hydrocarbon air pollutants

PHOSPHORESCENCE LIFETIME

The rate of phosphorescence decay or phosphorescence lifetime depends on temperature, medium, etc., and is an important physical constant of the compound under examination. The decay rate can be measured in one of several ways depending on the length of the lifetime. Thus, long lifetimes, 5 seconds or more, may be determined by recording the decrease in the photomultiplier signal, when the excit-

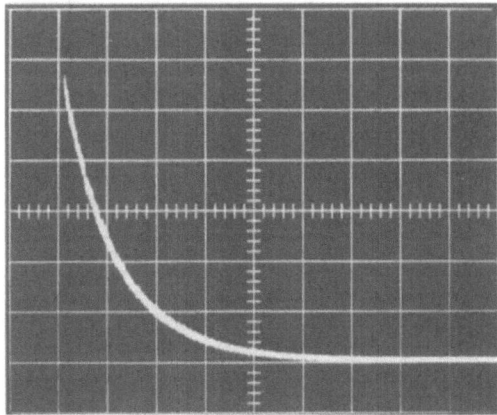

FIG. 4. Phosphorescence decay curve for aflatoxin B_1: excitation and emission wavelengths at 365 and 498 mμ, respectively; 5.0 mμ excitation and emission bandwidths. Solvent: ethanol-methanol (4:1), 2.5×10^{-5} M. Each box on the abscissa represents 1 second. (Adapted from Cravitt and Van Duuren. 1968. *J. Chem. Soc.*, Part 3:3893.)

ing light is shut off with a rapid mechanical shutter. The decay can thus be measured with a fast pen recorder. When the lifetime is between 0.1 and 5 sec, the decay rate can be determined from a photograph of an oscilloscope tracing, as is shown in Figure 4 for aflatoxin B_1 and Figure 5 for 1-indanone. Both of these decay curves were measured with a custom-built luminescence spectrophotometer (Cravitt and Van Duuren, 1968). The decay is obtained by using a capping shutter to block the excitation. The shutter keeps the light off the sample while the decay is measured and an on-to-off time of about 2 msec is realized. The shutter has a D'Arsonval-type meter movement with a blackened flag cemented to the needle. High-energy short-duration electrical pulses are applied to cause fast action of the shutter. The oscilloscope is simultaneously triggered to portray the decay curve. A swing-away Polaroid camera attachment is used to photograph the curves. With this arrangement, accurate decay curves of rates approaching 1 msec and as slow as

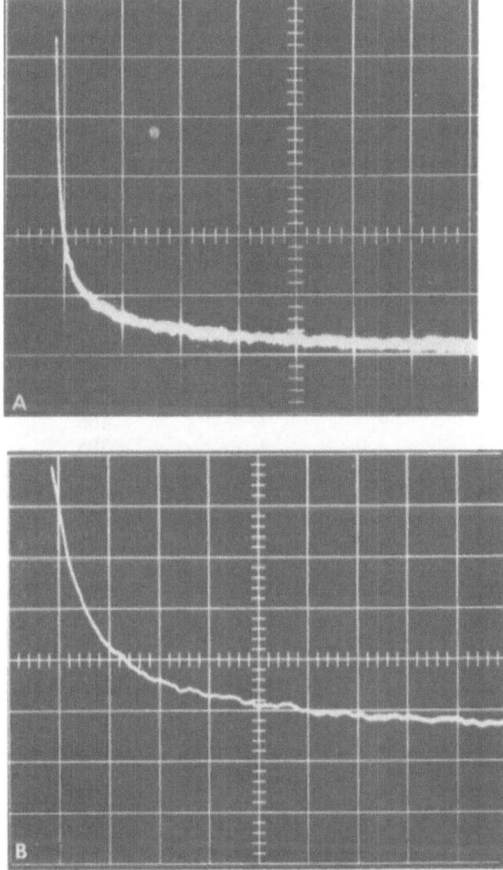

FIG. 5. Phosphorescence decay curves of 1-indanone, 2.5×10^{-5} M in EPA at 77°K, excitation at 292 mμ, emission at 403 mμ, excitation and emission bandwidth 5 mμ. A. Sweep time 50 msec/box; B. sweep time 5 msec/box. (Adapted from Cravitt and Van Duuren. 1968. *J. Chem. Soc.*, Part 3:3893.)

TABLE 2

Phosphorescence of Organic Compounds

Compound	Solvent[a]	Major Emission Maximum (mμ)	Excitation Wavelength (mμ)	Decay Time (sec)
Acenaphthene[c]	E	515	300	—
Acetaldehyde-4-nitro-phenylhydrazone[d]	EPA	525	395	0.50
Acetone-4-nitrophenylhydrazone[d]	EPA	525	392	0.48
p-Aminobenzoic Acid[e]	E	430	310	3.2
2-Amino-5-nitrobiphenyl[d]	—	520	380	0.56
2-Amino-6-nitrobenzothiazole[d]	EPA	515	375	0.41
2-Amino-7-nitrofluorene[d]	EPA	520	340	0.38
Anthracene[c]	E	462	300	—
Apomorphine[b,f]	E	470	320	3.1
Aramite[g]	E	400	285	3.3
Azosulfamide[h]	E	440	290	0.9
Benz(a)anthracene[c]	E	510	310	2.2
1,2-Benzfluorene[c]	E	502	315	—
2,3-Benzfluorene[c]	E	502	325	—
Benzocaine[e]	E	430	310	3.4
Benzoic acid[e]	E	400	240	2.4
Benzophenone-4-nitro-phenylhydrazone[d]	EPA	515	365	—
4-Benzoylbiphenyl-4-nitro phenylhydrazone[d]	EPA	520	370	0.38
Benzo(a)pyrene[c]	E	508	325	—
Biphenyl[i]	E	385	270	1.0
Brucine[f]	E	435	305	0.9
Butacaine sulfate[e]	E	430	310	5.7
Caffeine[e]	E	440	285	2.0
Chlorobenzilate[g]	E	415	275	< 0.2
p-Chlorophenol[g]	E	505	290	—
Chloretetracycline[e]	E	410	280	2.7
Cincophen[e]	E	520	350	0.8
Cocaine[b,e]	E	400	240	2.7
Codeine[f]	E	505	275	0.3
Cyclaine[b,e]	E	400	240	2.4
Diacetylsulfanilamide[h]	E	405	280	1.3
Diazinon[g]	E	395	275	5.0
Dibenz-(a,h)-anthracene[c]	E	550	340	1.3
2,6-Dichloro-4-nitroaniline[d]	EPA	525	368	0.47
2,4-Dichlorophenoxy acetic acid[g]	E	495	290	< 0.2
2,6-Diethyl-4-nitroaniline[d]	EPA	525	388	0.66
Dicoumarol[j]	E	475	305	0.6
N,N-Dimethyl-4-nitroaniline[d]	EPA	525	398	0.54
Diphenadione[j]	E	440	260	0.6
Ephedrine[e]	E	390	225	3.6
Guthion[g]	—	420	325	0.6
Lidocaine[e]	E	400	265	1.1
Mebaral[e]	E	380	240	2.2
Methoxychlor[g]	E	380	275	0.7
N-Methyl-4-nitroaniline[d]	EPA	522	390	0.5
Methycaine[b,e]	E	400	240	2.7
Morphine[f]	E	500	285	0.3
Morphine sulfate[f]	E	460	265	0.8
Naphthacene[c]	E	518	300	—
Naphthalene[k]	EPA	475	310	1.8
α-Naphthol[g]	E	475	320	1.2
Narceine[f]	E	440	290	0.5
5-Nitroacenaphthene[d]	EPA	540	380	—
4-Nitroaniline[d]	EPA	510	380	0.6

Compound	Solvent			
9-Nitroanthracene[d]	EPA	488	248	—
1-Nitroanthraquinone[d]	EPA	490	250	0.28
4-Nitrobiphenyl[d]	EPA	480	330	—
2-Nitrofluorene[d]	EPA	517	340	0.40
6-Nitroindole[d]	EPA	520	372	0.41
1-Nitronaphthalene[d]	EPA	520	340	—
2-Nitronaphthalene[d]	EPA	500	260	0.36
4-Nitro-1-naphthylamine[d]	EPA	578	400	—
3-Nitro-N-ethylcarbazole[d]	EPA	475	315	0.37
2-Nitro-N-methylcarbazole[d]	EPA	530	345	—
3-Nitro-N-methylcarbazole[d]	EPA	540	385	0.39
4-Nitro-o-toluidine[d]	EPA	520	375	0.53
4-Nitrophenylhydrazine[d]	EPA	520	390	0.48
p-Nitrophenol[g]	E	520	355	< 0.2
Orthotran[g]	E	395	260	< 0.2
Papaverine[b,f]	E	480	260	1.5
Phenanthrene[k]	EPA	465	340	2.6
Phenindione[j]	E	395	235	< 0.2
phenobarbital[e]	—	380	240	1.8
Phenylephrine[b,e]	E	390	290	2.4
Phthalylsulfacetamide[h]	E	415	290	0.6
Phthalylsulfathiazole[h]	E	405	305	0.9
Procaine[b,e]	E	430	310	3.5
Propionaldehyde-4-nitro-phenylhydrazone[d]	EPA	525	395	0.50
Quinidine Sulfate[e]	E	500	340	1.3
Quinine[b,e]	E	500	340	1.3
Retene[c]	—	510	265	—
Rutonal[e]	E	380	240	2.5
Strychnine phosphate[f]	E	440	290	1.2
Sodium sulfathiazole[h]	E	410	315	1.4
Succinyl sulfathiazole[h]	E	420	310	1.3
Sulfabenzamide[h]	E	405	305	0.7
Sulfacetamide[h]	E	410	280	1.3
Sulfadiazine[h]	E	410	275	0.7
Sulfaguanidine[h]	E	405	305	0.7
Sulfamerazine[h]	E	405	280	0.7
Sulfamethazine[h]	E	410	280	0.8
Sulfanilamide[h]	E	405	270	1.3
Sulfapyridine[h]	E	440	310	1.4
Sulfathiazole[h]	E	420	310	0.9
Sulfenone[g]	E	391	275	< 0.2
1,2,4,5-Tetramethylbenzene[k]	EPA	392	275	4.5
Thebaine[f]	E	500	315	1.0
Triphenylene[c]	E	461	291	15
2,4,5-Trichlorophenoxyacetic acid[g]	E	480	300	< 0.2
2,4,5-Trichlorophenol[g]	E	485	305	< 0.2
Tromexan[j]	E	460	295	0.6
Tronothane[b,e]	E	410	300	1.2
N-Acetyl-L-tyrosine ethyl ester[l]	H	395	250	—
Yohimbine[b,f]	E	410	290	7.4

[a]Solvent: E, ethanol; EPA, ether:isopentane:ethanol (5:5:2); H, water:methanol:ethanol (5:4:4); O, octane.
[b]Analyzed as hydrochloride.
[c]Hood and Winefordner (1966).
[d]Sawicki and Pfaff (1967).
[e]Winefordner and Tin (1964).
[f]Hollifield and Winefordner (1965).
[g]Moye and Winefordner (1965).
[h]Hollifield and Winefordner (1966).
[i]McCarthy and Winefordner (1965).
[j]Hollifield and Winefordner (1967).
[k]McGlynn, Neely, and Neely (1963).
[l]Freed and Vise (1963).

10 sec can be obtained. Lifetimes covering a whole range of values can be measured
with the use of a flash-excitation arrangement much the same as that used for measuring fluorescence lifetimes. This is particularly useful for phosphorescence lifetimes of less than 0.1 msec (Bäckström and Sandros, 1958). To determine the
phosphorescence lifetime (τ_0), the intensity of phosphorescence is plotted against
time after excitation energy has been shut off. The phosphorescence lifetimes for a
series of organic compounds are shown in Table 2.

QUANTUM EFFICIENCY OF PHOSPHORESCENCE

The quantum efficiency of phosphorescence is determined in the same way as
that of fluorescence, i.e., by comparison of the integrated area under the corrected
emission spectrum with that of a known standard. Depending upon the chopper
arrangement or phosphoroscope, a correction factor may have to be applied in
order to obtain reliable quantum efficiency data. Because of light scattering due to
cracking in rigid glasses and bubbles in the surrounding liquid nitrogen, determinations of phosphorescence quantum efficiencies are usually less accurate than those
of fluorescence quantum efficiencies obtained at room temperature. The method
used for the measurement of fluorescence efficiency is described in detail in the
chapter on fluorescence spectroscopy (p. 18). Of interest to luminescence spectroscopists is the ratio of the quantum efficiencies of phosphorescence and fluorescence, Φ_p/Φ_f, and how this ratio is affected by chemical structure, wavelength of
excitation, and environmental factors. The Φ_p and Φ_p/Φ_f are compared in Table
3 for a series of compounds at 77°K. In calculating these values it was assumed

TABLE 3

Fluorescence and Phosphorescence Efficiencies at 77° K[a]

Compound	τ(sec)	Φ_p/Φ_f	Φ_p	Φ_f
Benzene	8.0	0.89	0.19	0.21
Naphthalene	2.8	0.02	0.008	0.39
Phenanthrene	4.3	0.80	0.11	0.14
Fluorene	7.1	0.14	0.07	[0.5]
Diphenyl	5.1	1.4	0.25	0.17
Triphenylene	17.1	5.1	0.28	0.06
Phenol	2.6	0.93	0.37	0.40
Benzoic acid	2.0	> 10	0.27	—[b]
Acetanilide	3.6	> 10	0.05	—[b]
4-Nitro-N-ethylaniline	0.4	> 10	0.12	—[b]
N-Phenyl-2-naphthylamine	1.3	1.7	0.44	0.26
Acetophenone	0.008	> 10	1.0	—[b]
Benzophenone	0.005	> 10	0.71	—[b]
Benzoin	0.018	> 10	0.54	—[b]
Benzil	0.005	> 10	0.67	—[b]
Anthraquinone	0.004	> 10	0.41	—[b]

[a]From Parker and Hatchard. 1962. *Analyst*, 87:644-676. Courtesy of the Society for Analytical
Chemistry.
[b]Very low.

that the optical densities of all solutions were the same at 77°K as at 293°K. Usually Φ_p/Φ_f is independent of exciting wavelength; however, for some compounds such as fluorescein, chrysene, and hexahelicene, Φ_p/Φ_f increases with decreasing excitation wavelength. It is possible that in such cases intersystem crossing from the higher excited singlet states occurs with greater frequency than from the lowest excited singlet state.

PHOSPHORESCENCE SENSITIVITY

Luminescence sensitivity both for fluorescence and phosphorescence can be defined in one of several ways and it is important that those factors which determine sensitivity be clarified. Thus, it is frequently difficult to determine from published reports what terminology or definitions are used in discussions on sensitivity of instruments or methods. The various types of sensitivity that can be considered have been clearly defined and discussed by various authors. The sensitivity of the instrumentation used in a particular study or for an analytical procedure is of prime importance, and the various instrumental parameters used in a particular study should be clearly specified. These are: light source and its intensity; filter or monochromator characteristics; band width or slit width; wavelength settings on excitation and emission monochromators; characteristics of the photomultiplier, i.e., wavelength-response characteristics; time constant; sample size; concentration; and sample area geometry. Instrumental sensitivity has been defined as that concentration of a substance which is required to produce a recorder deflection equal to the overall dark-current fluctuation when the time constant of the detection system is one second (Parker, 1968b). This definition must be amplified by inclusion of data on the other parameters of the instrumentation used as described above. In addition to these rather specific instrumental parameters, there is a series of extraneous, but nevertheless important, factors which limit sensitivity. These factors can best be described as the instrument blank, i.e., light reaching the detector from sources other than the phosphorescence of the sample under investigation. The most important factors contributing to an instrument blank are scattered light, Raman bands from the medium, phosphorescence from impurities in the solute or medium and, finally, phosphorescence from the sample cell and surrounding cooling system. Thus, the sensitivity of a particular measurement will be limited by the magnitude of this "background" phosphorescence. The careful investigator in phosphorescence analysis will be likely to eliminate as much of this background as possible by choice of medium, phosphorescence-free cells and Dewars, and by maintaining the highest possible purity of solute or medium. The third and also very important aspect determining sensitivity concerns the intrinsic phosphorescence of a compound under a given set of experimental conditions of solvent, temperature, excitation wavelength, etc. For most substances, the quantum efficiency is independent of wavelength and hence the maximum sensitivity is obtained at the most intense peak in the excitation spectrum taking into consideration also source intensity and photomultiplier response at that wavelength.

It is worthwhile at this point to consider phosphorescence sensitivity compared to that attained by other spectroscopic and analytical methods. For inorganics, there are frequently other more sensitive tools, e.g., flame absorption spectrometry. However, certain elements in particular forms are still measured by luminescence methods. Luminescence measurements of organic compounds which are capable of photoluminescence are usually more sensitive than those by other spectroscopic methods, such as infrared-, ultraviolet-, visible-, or nuclear magnetic resonance spectrometry. However, luminescence spectra have the drawback that they are usually structurally less informative than other spectroscopic data. Furthermore, only absorbing compounds show luminescence, although nonluminescent materials can frequently be converted to luminescent ones.

ENVIRONMENTAL FACTORS IN PHOSPHORESCENCE

Photoluminescence is in many instances markedly influenced by environmental factors such as temperature, solvent viscosity, concentration, etc. These effects are at times a hindrance in phosphorescence studies, and by the same token they can, with proper prior knowledge, be used to advantage for a particular study. Some of these effects are discussed here. Effects on fluorescence are discussed in another chapter.

Temperature

The efficiency of fluorescence is usually decreased somewhat with increasing temperature; the phosphorescence efficiency, on the other hand, is frequently drastically decreased with increase in temperature. This is in part due to the fact that phosphorescence is critically dependent on solvent viscosity and is usually observed only at very low temperature. The temperature effect on phosphorescence is ascribed to the long radiative lifetime of the triplet state and hence the greater likelihood of intersystem crossing and quenching effects. The effect of temperature on phosphorescence is complicated by an additional factor, *the triplet formation efficiency*, Φ_t, which refers to the number of triplet molecules formed per quantum of exciting light absorbed. For many compounds Φ_t varies only slightly with temperature and it is possible to calculate the effect of temperature on phosphorescence quantum efficiency, Φ_p, by use of the formula:

$$\Phi_p/\Phi_t = \tau/\tau_R$$

where:

Φ_p = quantum efficiency of phosphorescence
Φ_t = triplet formation efficiency
τ = *actual* lifetime of triplet
τ_R = radiative lifetime of triplet.

Calculations of this nature have been made for eosin and for a series of aromatic hydrocarbons. Thus for hydrocarbons the radiative lifetime of triplets, τ_R, are of the order of 1 to 10 sec, and the phosphorescence efficiency in fluid solution at room temperature is expected to be lower than that at 77°K by a factor of approximately 1000. The phosphorescence efficiency of aromatic hydrocarbons at room temperature (in fluid solutions) has been measured. Thus, for phenanthrene, Φ_p at 295°K is less than 1/1000th of that at 77°K. Quantitative studies, including measurements of Φ_p and τ, have also been carried out concerning the effect of temperature on various radiative and radiationless processes for coronene and benzcoronene (Dawson and Kropp, 1969). The rate constants for radiationless and radiative deactivation of the lowest excited singlet and triplet states, S_1 and T_1 are constant between $-196°$ and 23°C for both compounds. The rate of intersystem crossing from S_1 to T_1 is also not affected in this temperature range. Radiationless deactivation of S_1 to the ground state does not occur for coronene between $-196°$ and 23°C, but for benzcoronene direct radiationless deactivation of S_1 to the ground state occurs at 23°, but not at $-196°C$. This latter finding is attributed to a decrease in quantum efficiency of fluorescence of benzcoronene with increasing temperature (Dawson and Kropp, 1969).

The phosphorescence of the carcinogen dibenz (a,h) anthracene was measured in a number of polymers over a wide temperature range (Geacintov et al., 1968) and it was found that in a rigid polymer such as a polycarbonate film, the phosphorescence was not affected in any significant way by changing the temperature in stages from 77°K to 298°K. Above 298°K phosphorescence intensity decreased sharply and the emission maximum became broad and diffuse.

Solvent Effects

The nature of the solvent markedly affects fluorescence, phosphorescence, and absorption spectra, and because of a frequent interplay of a variety of solvent effects they are at present incompletely understood. Solvent effects are due to three main factors; i.e., the solvent viscosity and polarity and the opportunities for hydrogen bonding and other interactions with the solvent. Photochemical reactions in or with the solvent are not considered here although they have to be borne in mind in the design of phosphorescence experiments. The heavy atom effect, discussed below, may be considered a special case of a solvent effect. Of these effects the most critical is viscosity since most compounds phosphoresce only in solid matrices. The range of solvent mixtures available for this purpose was discussed above. The viscosity of the medium is important since it determines the rate of diffusion controlled reactions according to the equation:

$$k_c = 8\,RT/3000\,n$$

where:

k_c = diffusion-controlled bimolecular rate constant

n = viscosity of the solvent in poises
R = gas constant
T = absolute temperature.

Hence, the phosphorescence of most organic molecules is measured in rigid glasses at 77°K, in polymers at 77°K to room temperature, and in pure crystals in the same temperature range.

It is known that the lifetime of triplet molecules in fluid solution is frequently seriously affected by traces of impurities in the solvent, and, for solvents of equal purity, the one with the higher viscosity usually gives the longest phosphorescence lifetime and the greatest phosphorescence intensity of the solute at the same concentration. This will be the case if there are no other complicating factors such as hydrogen bonding. It is not clear whether increased phosphorescence observed on lowering the temperature is due only to increased viscosity of the solvent, although this is probably a major contributing factor. It is not at present possible to differentiate completely between the effects of viscosity on diffusion-controlled quenching and its effect on intersystem crossing from the triplet to the ground state. A well-known example of the effect of viscosity on diffusion-controlled quenching is the quenching effect of oxygen on phosphorescence. At room temperature, phosphorescence is largely quenched by the presence of oxygen and, therefore, deaerated solvents have to be used. Phosphorescence spectra run at 77°K are rarely affected by oxygen. Other data suggest that viscosity also affects intersystem crossing. Thus, the phosphorescence efficiency of eosin in glycerol increases sharply at −60°C (Parker and Hatchard, 1961), at which temperature there is a sharp increase in the rigidity of the solvent. There is no increase in the phosphorescence efficiency in ethanol, which does not show markable viscosity changes at −60°C. These experiments suggest that in glycerol at −60°C the vibrational modes of triplet eosin molecules are restricted, resulting in a decrease or inhibition of radiationless intersystem crossing to the ground state.

The phosphorescence spectra of condensed rigid structures such as unsubstituted polynuclear aromatic hydrocarbons in n-paraffins at 77°K show a surprisingly large number of sharp peaks. These spectra, referred to as Shpol'skii spectra and observed by Shpol'skii and coworkers (Shpol'skii and Klimova, 1956), are characteristic also for the fluorescence of these compounds at 77°K. In these situations, the hydrocarbon molecule is incorporated into the crystal lattice of the solvent; i.e., it is molecularly dispersed rather than in the form of microcrystals; crystals of the hydrocarbons show at 77°K diffuse spectra with little fine structure. Coronene, for example, shows some 50 sharp bands in its phosphorescence spectrum in n-heptane at 77°K. When vitrification occurs the fine structure disappears. The degree of splitting of bands observed for a given polycyclic hydrocarbon is dependent upon the size of the n-alkane used as solvent.

Shpol'skii phosphorescence and fluorescence spectra are useful in analytical chemistry (Shpol'skii and Klimova, 1956); they are also of theoretical interest in measuring molecular vibrational frequencies of ground states of certain compounds. This is because in the condensed medium all radiative transitions take place from the lowest vibrational level from the first excited triplet (or singlet) state. Such vibrational analyses have been made for phenanthrene (Teplyakov, 1963) and for dibenz(a, h)anthracene (Geacintov et al., 1968).

Effect of pH

The phosphorescence characteristics of emitting species are often profoundly affected by the pH of the surrounding medium. The effect of pH on the phosphorescence intensity and emission maxima of purines, pyrimidines, their nucleosides, and nucleotides, DNA, and of tryptophan, tyrosine, and proteins is discussed in detail in another section of this chapter (pp. 85, 95, 100). These effects can be traced to partial or complete loss of a proton from the aromatic ring of the emitting species. In other molecules, the state of ionization of acidic or basic functional groups directly attached to the emitting moiety is responsible for changes of phosphorescence characteristics with changes in pH.

Concentration

The relationship between phosphorescence intensity and concentration is of considerable importance in quantitative analysis, especially in areas which involve determination of drug levels in biological fluids and tissues. Analytical calibration curves are constructed by plotting luminescence intensity of the emitting species at the maximum wavelength of emission versus concentration of standard solutions of the same species using the same instrument settings for the standard and the unknown. The concentration of the unknown is read from the calibration curve. Such plots are always corrected for background phosphorescence, which in some cases, e.g., serum or urine analysis, can be considerable.

Analytical phosphorescence curves are usually linear over a 10^4-fold or greater concentration range. In the linear range, the phosphorescence intensity is directly proportional to concentration, and therefore analyses which give drug concentrations within this region are reasonably accurate. At high concentrations, the curve reaches a plateau and with further increase in concentration phosphorescence intensity decreases due to self-absorption, formation of aggregates, and concentration quenching.

Oxygen Quenching

The presence of oxygen in solution may quench the fluorescence as well as the phosphorescence of an emitting species, resulting in a decrease of the observed emission intensity. Oxygen quenching has been studied in much greater detail for fluorescence than for phosphorescence. In the case of fluorescence it is not possible to predict whether the emission intensity will be decreased; some compounds, such as aromatic hydrocarbons, are sensitive to oxygen quenching, whereas others are not. However, most organic compounds which fluoresce, do not phosphoresce at room temperature in liquid media unless special precautions concerning the removal of oxygen are taken. One method for removing oxygen from solutions, especially when using hydroxylic solvents, consists of repeated freeze-thaw cycles. Another method is to bubble nitrogen or another inert gas through the solution.

Since oxygen quenching is a diffusion-controlled process, the presence of oxygen in liquid media results in efficient quenching. It follows then that increasing the viscosity of the medium results in a decrease of oxygen quenching, and the use of rigid glasses for phosphorescence measurements further reduces the likelihood of oxygen quenching.

Several mechanisms for oxygen quenching have been advanced. One such mechanism involves intermolecular energy transfer from the excited species to oxygen, resulting in excited singlet state oxygen (Kautsky, 1939; Kawaoka et al., 1967). Another mechanism, advanced by Porter and Wright (1959), is based on the fact that oxygen in the ground state is a diradical, and therefore paramagnetic. The presence of paramagnetic ions, such as Cu^{++}, Mn^{++}, and Co^{++}, has been shown to decrease sharply the phosphorescence of deoxyribonucleic acid, as described elsewhere in this chapter. Nitrogen monoxide, another paramagnetic ground state triplet species, can also cause effective excited-state quenching (Wehry, 1967).

Oxygen quenching, which makes proper determination of phosphorescence yields and lifetimes difficult, has, on the other hand, been used as a tool for oxygen analysis in liquid solutions (Tolmach, 1951).

Heavy Atom Effect

Atoms of high atomic number, or "heavy" atoms, often have a pronounced effect on the emission characteristics of a luminescent substance. This effect is caused by the interaction of the inhomogeneous electric fields, present in heavy atoms, with solute molecules in the excited state. The distinction is usually made between "internal" and "external" heavy atom or coupling effects, the former term being applied to situations where the heavy atom is a constituent of the luminescent molecule, and the latter when the heavy atom is part of the solvent molecules or present in solution as a third constituent.

The presence of inhomogeneous electric fields in heavy atoms results in an increase in spin-orbit coupling—i.e., a coupling of the orbital and spin motions between individual atoms. An increase in spin-orbit coupling may be reflected in the fluorescence and phosphorescence behavior of a substance due to an increase in one or more of the following processes:

(a) $S_1 \rightarrow T_1$ (intersystem crossing)
(b) $T_1 \rightarrow S_0 + h\nu$ (phosphorescence)
(c) $T_1 \rightarrow S_0$ (radiationless deactivation).

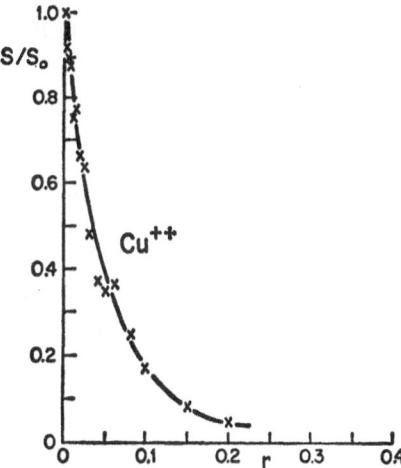

FIG. 6. Quenching of DNA phosphorescence by Cu^{++}. Relative amplitude of phosphorescence plotted against the ratio of cation added to DNA phosphate. (From Isenberg et al. 1965. *Science*, 150:1180. Copyright © 1965 by the American Association for the Advancement of Science. Reproduced by permission.)

If process (a) is affected by the presence of a heavy atom, the ratio Φ_p/Φ_f becomes larger since the singlet excited state is depopulated in favor of the triplet excited state. However, simultaneous increase of process (c) could mask the increase in intersystem crossing rates. Increase of spin-orbit coupling between the triplet excited state and the singlet ground state, process (b), results not only in an increase of the Φ_p/Φ_f ratio but also in a reduced lifetime of the triplet state. Perturbation of process (c)—radiationless deactivation of the triplet state—leads to a decrease in Φ_p and τ_b. The extent to which each process is affected by the presence of a heavy atom is often very difficult to assess.

An internal heavy atom effect was investigated in a series of 1-halonaphthalenes by McClure (1949). A steady decrease in τ_d and increase in Φ_p/Φ_f was observed with an increase in the atomic number of the halogen. 1-Fluoronaphthalene, the lightest halonaphthalene, and 1-iodonaphthalene, the heaviest halonaphthalene, had decay times of 1.5 and 0.0025 sec, respectively, compared to 2.6 sec for unsubstituted naphthalene.

An external heavy atom effect has been demonstrated for salmon sperm deoxyribonucleic acid (DNA) by Isenberg et al. (1965). These authors examined purified DNA in 1:1 mixtures of glycerol and water at 77°K at various ratios of paramagnetic cations, such as Cu^{++} and Ni^{++} to DNA. The results obtained for quenching by copper are shown in Figure 6, where S/S_0 represents the ratio of the phosphorescence intensity with and without added cation, and r represents the ratio of added cation to DNA phosphate. Similar curves were obtained for Ni^{++}, Co^{++}, and Mn^{++} added to DNA. The quenching efficiency decreased in the order $Cu^{++} > Ni^{++} > Co^{++} > Mn^{++}$. All the curves indicate strong quenching even at low values of r; i.e., addition of a small amount of paramagnetic cation causes a sharp decrease in phosphorescence intensity, and further addition produces a relatively smaller decrease. Rahn, Shulman, and Longworth (1966) confirmed the results obtained for DNA phosphorescence quenching by Mn^{++}.

A detailed study of the external heavy atom effect on naphthalene in alcohol solutions containing propyl chloride, propyl bromide, and propyl iodide was undertaken by McGlynn, Daigre, and Smith (1963). These authors measured relative phosphorescence to fluorescence quantum yields and phosphorescence lifetimes and calculated from these results and other published data the following first-order rate constants: k_f, fluorescence rate constant; kq_f, the rate constant for internal fluorescence quenching; k_p, the phosphorescence rate constant; kq_p, the rate constant for internal quenching of phosphorescence; and k_{Is}, the rate constant for intersystem crossing, i.e., $S^1 \rightarrow T^1$. Some of McGlynn's results are summarized in Table 4. As the

TABLE 4

Relative Fluorescence Yields, Rates of Intersystem Crossing,
and Phosphorescence Quenching of Naphthalene in Various Media at 77°K[a]

Medium	Fluorescence yield	k_{qp}	$k_{Is} \times 10^{-6}$
EM[b]	—	1.0	1.0
PCl[c]	1.0	1.1	3.7
PBr[c]	0.33	1.5	33
PI[c]	0.09	2.0	89

[a]Adapted from McGlynn, Daigre, and Smith. 1963. J. Chem. Phys., 39:675-679. Courtesy of the American Institute of Physics.

[b]EM refers to 4 parts ethanol and 1 part methanol, by volume.

[c]Ethanol:methanol:propyl halide (16:4:5 by volume).

atomic number of the heavy atom increases, the fluorescence yield of naphthalene decreases drastically and the intersystem crossing rate constant increases, up to a factor of 89 in propyl iodide, compared to that of naphthalene in an ethanol-methanol glass without any added propyl halide. Phosphorescence quenching also increases with an increase in the atomic number of the heavy atom, but the increase is very slight compared to that found for the $S^1 \rightarrow T^1$ intersystem crossing rates. Thus, the authors concluded that the presence of an external heavy atom mainly increases the probability of intersystem crossing, and affects the following processes in decreasing order of sensitivity: $S^1 \rightarrow T^1$ (intersystem crossing from first excited singlet to lowest excited triplet) $> T^1 \rightarrow S_0$ (radiationless phosphorescence quenching) $> T^1 \rightarrow S_0 + h\upsilon$ (phosphorescence emission).

Since addition of an external heavy atom frequently results in an increase of the phosphorescence quantum yield, McGlynn, Daigre, and Smith (1963) suggested that the heavy atom effect could be of analytical use. Hood and Winefordner (1966) investigated the heavy atom effect as a means of improving the sensitivity of analysis by phosphorimetry. These authors examined the phosphorescence intensity of polynuclear hydrocarbons in ethanol-ethyl iodide mixtures at 77°K. Among the compounds investigated were benzo(a)pyrene, dibenz(a,h)anthracene, and benz(a)anthracene, compounds which are of biological interest because they are known to be carcinogenic. The effect of ethyl iodide on the phosphorescence

TABLE 5

Effect of a Heavy Atom Solvent on Phosphorescence Intensity
of Polynuclear Aromatic Hydrocarbons at 77° K[a]

Hydrocarbons	Concentration	(P/P_o)[b]		
		Ethanol:ethyl iodide (vol:vol)		
	μg/ml	*19/1*	*9/1*	*5/1*
Naphthalene	13.0	0.3	0.2	0.1
Anthracene	18.0	0.6	0.7	0.9
Phenanthrene	1.8	0.6	0.4	0.2
Triphenylene	2.3	0.2	0.1	0.05
Retene	6.0	1.1	1.1	0.8
Naphthacene	6.0	2.4	3.1	4.6
Dibenz(a,h)anthracene	2.8	1.2	1.2	1.3
Benz(a)anthracene	23.0	1.2	1.3	1.4
Benzo(a)pyrene	25.0	1.5	2.2	3.5
Acenaphthene	15.0	0.9	0.9	0.7
11-H-Benzo(a)fluorene	22.0	6.4	9.8	13.0
11-H-Benzo(b)fluorene	22.0	8.7	15.0	25.0

[a]From Hood and Winefordner. 1966. *Anal. Chem.*, 38:1922-1924. Courtesy of the American Chemical Society.

[b]Ratio of phosphorescence intensity in ethanol:ethyl iodide mixture(P) to phosphorescence intensity in ethanol (P_o).

intensity for these and other hydrocarbons is summarized in Table 5. The results indicate that addition of ethyl iodide causes an increase of the phosphorescence intensity of the two benzfluorenes listed and a less marked increase for the carcinogenic hydrocarbons dibenz(a,h)anthracene, benz(a)anthracene, and benzo(a)-pyrene. Other compounds, such as naphthalene and anthracene, actually exhibit quenched phosphorescence in the presence of ethyl iodide. A further increase in the amount of ethyl iodide in the solvent sometimes causes additional intensification of the phosphorescence emission, as in the case of the carcinogenic hydrocarbons and the benzfluorenes. Other compounds, such as phenanthrene and naphthalene, show phosphorescence quenching upon further increase in the amount of ethyl iodide in the solvent mixture. The range of linear response of phosphorescence intensity with respect to concentration becomes larger when determined in 9:1 ethanol-ethyl iodide than in ethanol alone. Furthermore, those compounds which show enhanced phosphorescence have correspondingly lower limits of detection in the presence of a heavy atom solvent.

PHOSPHORESCENCE AND
MOLECULAR STRUCTURE

Phosphorescence emission always occurs at longer wavelengths than fluorescence emission because the excited state of a molecule of lowest energy is always the triplet state. This follows from theoretical considerations which indicate that the state of highest multiplicity among states with the same orbital distribution of electrons is the most stable state and therefore of lowest energy (Streitwieser, 1961). The lowest excited triplet state may be due to either a π-π^* or an n-π^* transition. Criteria for distinguishing between π-π^* and n-π^* phosphorescence can be found in a discussion by Kasha (1960). Most aromatic hydrocarbons, heterocyclics, and their derivatives exhibit π-π^* phosphorescence. However, some types of compounds, such as quinones, ketones, nitro-compounds, and some heterocyclics such as pyrimidine and pyrazine show the less frequently observed n-π^* phosphorescence.

The O,O band, i.e., the band of shortest wavelength of a phosphorescence spectrum, represents the energy of the lowest vibrational level of the triplet state, and frequently the band of maximum phosphorescence emission is the O,O band. However, if the molecular configuration of the triplet state is significantly different from that of the ground state, the O,O-band intensity may be quite low. In such cases, assignment of the O,O band and determination of the energy between the lowest triplet and the ground state is difficult. Since the O,O band represents the lowest vibrational level of the triplet state, all other bands at wavelengths longer than that of the O,O band correspond to the various vibrational levels of the ground state. Therefore, analysis of the fine structure emission peaks of phosphorescence spectra is useful in the determination of the energy distribution of ground-state vibrational levels. A number of vibrational analyses of phosphorescence spectra have appeared in the literature, among them the vibrational analysis of benzene (Shull, 1949; Lewis and Kasha, 1944) and naphthalene (Ferguson et al., 1954). Many compounds have phosphorescence spectra that are broad and show few structural details. However, by employing hydrocarbon matrices, such as cyclohexane at 77°K, spectra with increased fine structure and higher O,O-band intensity may be obtained (Sponer et al., 1960). The increase in fine structure in the phosphorescence spectrum of benzene in going from an EPA matrix to a cyclohexane matrix is shown in Figure 7.

Ethylene, the simplest organic molecule capable of π-π^* electron promotion,

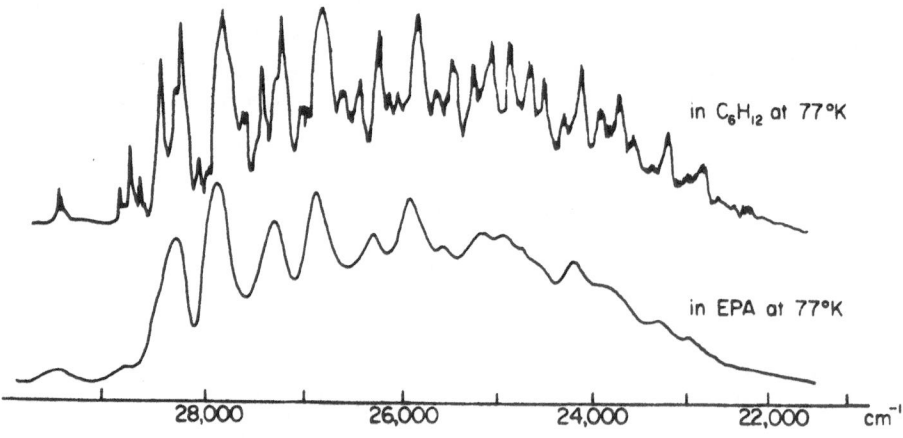

FIG. 7. Phosphorescence spectra of benzene in cyclohexane and EPA at 77°K. (From Sponer et al. 1960. *Spectrochimica Acta,* 16:1135.)

does not phosphoresce. Data on conjugated alkenes containing two or more double bonds are sparse. The long-chain polyene lycopene, $C_{40}H_{56}$, does not phosphoresce when all the double bonds are in the *trans* configuration. However, isomerization to *cis* groupings results in phosphorescence, with no observable fluorescence (Lewis and Kasha, 1944). Beer (1956) investigated the luminescence behavior of poly-acetylenes containing up to four conjugated triple bonds. All of the polyacetylenes examined by Beer phosphoresce; however, with the exception of diphenylacetylene, none of the compounds examined by Beer with less than four triple bonds exhibited fluorescence. Of the aliphatic aldehydes, the simplest aldehyde, formaldehyde, fluoresces, but does not phosphoresce (Brand, 1956). Glyoxal (CHOCHO) exhibits weak phosphorescence (Brand, 1954), and biacetyl ($CH_3COCOCH_3$) phosphoresces intensely, not only in solid matrices and liquid solutions, but also in the vapor state (Sidman and McClure, 1955a, b; Bäckström and Sandros, 1960). Phosphorescence has also been observed for the aliphatic ketones acetone, methyl ethyl ketone, and diethyl ketone (McClure, 1949).

Benzene, naphthalene, anthracene, and higher linear homologs all phosphoresce. In this series, the O,O-phosphorescence band is displaced progressively towards longer wavelengths (Lewis and Kasha, 1944; McGlynn et al., 1955). Increasing linear annulation in the phenanthrene, benz(a)anthracene, and pentaphene series also results in a red shift of the O,O band. A red shift of the O,O band is also observed upon introduction of a halogen, hydroxyl, sulfhydryl, or amino substituent into aromatic hydrocarbons. The phosphorescence O,O bands for a number of unsubstituted and substituted aromatic hydrocarbons are shown in Table 6.

TABLE 6

O,O-Band Phosphorescence Wavelengths of Aromatic Hydrocarbons and Substituted Derivatives

Compound	O,O-Band Wavelength (mμ)
Benzene[a]	339.0
Naphthalene[a]	470.7
Anthracene[a,b]	669.9
Tetracene[b]	975.6
1-Fluoronaphthalene[c]	474.8
1-Chloronaphthalene[c]	484.4
1-Bromonaphthalene[c]	484.2
Phenol[a]	350.9
1-Naphthol[a]	487.8
Nitrobenzene[a]	473.9
4-Nitroaniline[e]	515.5
1-Nitronaphthalene[d]	531.9
4-Nitro-1-naphthylamine[d]	574.7
Thio-2-naphthol[a]	480.8

[a]Lewis and Kasha (1944).
[b]McGlynn et al. (1955).
[c]Ferguson et al. (1954).
[d]Corkill and Graham-Bryce (1961).
[e]Foster et al. (1956).

Aromatic nitro-compounds exhibit n-π^* phosphorescence (Zudin, 1959), and show no fluorescence. The phosphorescence of various aromatic nitro-compounds has been investigated by Lewis and Kasha (1944), and the ten isomeric dinitronaphthalenes were examined by Corkill and Graham-Bryce (1961). The luminescence behavior of nitroanilines and nitronaphthylamines, reported by Foster et al. (1956) and Corkill and Graham-Bryce (1961), respectively, is unique in that either phosphorescence or fluorescence, but never both, is observed. Among the nitroanilines, 4-nitroaniline phosphoresces, whereas 3-nitroaniline and 2-nitroaniline fluoresce. Of the 14 isomeric nitronaphthylamines, 1-nitro-2-naphthylamine, 4-nitro-1-naphthylamine, and 5-nitro-1-naphthylamine phosphoresce exclusively, while all the remaining isomers fluoresce. Conjugation between the amino and nitro substituents in these compounds seems to be a necessary, but not sufficient, requirement for phosphorescence. Eleven of the twelve possible isomers with either steric inhibition of resonance or unfavorable resonance interaction between the nitro and amino substituent exhibit fluorescence only.

Aromatic carbonyl compounds, such as aromatic aldehydes, ketones, carboxylic acids, etc., like aromatic nitro-compounds, phosphoresce from the n-π^*-excited state (Kasha, 1960). These compounds, as a rule, show only phosphorescence, and no fluorescence. Phosphorescence O,O bands for benzaldehyde, 1-naphthaldehyde, acetophenone, benzophenone, anthrone, benzoic acid, and 2-naphthoic acid have been measured by Lewis and Kasha (1944). The luminescence behavior of quinones was investigated by Zander (1967). Para-benzoquinone, naphtho-1, 4-quinone, anthra-1,4-quinone, tetracene-5,12-quinone, and pentacene-6,13-quinone exhibit well-defined, intense n-π^* phosphorescence emission, and no fluorescence. Hexacene-6,15-quinone and heptacene-7,12-quinone, on the other hand, fluoresce intensely at room temperature, but do not phosphoresce under any conditions.

The aromatic heterocycles pyridine (Evans, 1957), furan, pyrrole, and thiophene (Heckman, 1958) do not phosphoresce, and the last three also do not fluoresce. Pyrimidine and pyrazine hydrochloride (Krishna and Goodman, 1961) show intense n-π^* phosphorescence. Pyridazine, however, does not phosphoresce (Kasha, 1950). Quinoline phosphoresces, but does not fluoresce, in nonpolar solvents. However, both triplet and singlet emission is observed for quinoline in polar solvents (Kasha, 1960).

As mentioned in the beginning of this section, phosphorescence spectra are extremely useful in the determination of triplet state energies. A large number of compounds exhibit sensitized phosphorescence, or phosphorescence of a species which is excited to the triplet state by way of energy transfer from another species in the triplet state. Such transfer can take place only from a species that has a triplet energy level higher than that of the species that is excited by the energy transfer. Sensitized phosphorescence was first observed by Terenin and Ermolaev (1956) upon irradiation of an ethanolic solution of naphthalene and benzaldehyde at 77°K. Irradiation at 366 mμ of a solution containing equal concentrations of naphthalene and benzaldehyde resulted in intense naphthalene phosphorescence. Under the same conditions, naphthalene alone did not luminesce, for naphthalene does not absorb at 366 mμ. Therefore, the excitation energy is absorbed by benzaldehyde and the energy transferred to naphthalene. Singlet-singlet energy transfer was ruled out because benzaldehyde has a lower singlet state than naphthalene. Terenin and Ermolaev (1956) proposed the following scheme for sensitized phosphorescence:

$$S \xrightarrow{h\nu} {}^1S*$$
$${}^1S* \rightarrow {}^3S* \text{ (intersystem crossing)}$$
$${}^3S* + {}^1A \rightarrow S + {}^3A* \text{ (triplet energy transfer)}$$
$${}^3A* \rightarrow A + h\nu \text{ (sensitized phosphorescence)}$$

In this scheme, S is the donor of the transferred triplet energy, or the sensitizer, which promotes the acceptor of the transferred energy, A, to the triplet excited state. Triplet energy transfer from a donor to an acceptor is a spin-allowed process which is much more efficient in solution than singlet energy transfer (Terenin and Ermolaev, 1956). Theoretically, sensitized phosphorescence may occur in a solution containing two solutes with different triplet energy levels. Acetophenone, benzaldehyde, and benzophenone, for example, may act as triplet energy donors for diphenyl and naphthalene (Terenin and Ermolaev, 1956). Heckstroeter et al. (1964) have published triplet excitation energies for a large number of compounds. These energy values were obtained from the O,O bands of phosphorescence spectra of compounds in polar and nonpolar solvents at 77°K.

Photochemical reactions, or reactions initiated by irradiation with light, are extremely complex in terms of mechanism and often result in a multitude of products. These products arise not only from excited state reactants, but also from secondary reactions involving photosensitive, and therefore unstable, intermediates. The proper choice of a sensitizer often facilitates the formation of desired products (Hammond et al., 1964; Hammond and Liu, 1963) and may lead to information concerning the elucidation of photochemical mechanisms (Wilkinson, 1962).

PHOSPHORESCENCE IN BIOCHEMISTRY AND PHARMACOLOGY

Pyrimidines, Purines, and Derivatives

An investigation of the phosphorescence of adenine compounds was first undertaken by Steele and Szent-Györgyi (1957), and intensive phosphorescence studies on purines, pyrimidines, their nucleoside and nucleotide derivatives, DNA, and model polynucleotides followed in the late 1960's. In these studies, the purity of the compound in question is of extreme importance, and the first fact to be established is the correspondence between the excitation spectrum of the compound in question and its absorption spectrum. Thus, only those emission spectra are valid which are recorded with wavelengths of excitation lying within the regions of absorption of the compound studied, a precaution not always followed by early investigators.

Shulman and his group (Longworth et al., 1966) examined in detail the

phosphorescence behavior of purines, pyrimidines, and their nucleoside and nucleotide derivatives in 1:1 mixtures of ethylene or propylene glycol and water at 77°K
at various pH values. The phosphorescence emission of all bases and derivatives
examined was found to be extremely sensitive to pH; i.e., luminescence is strongly
dependent on the nature of the various tautomeric structures.

Thymine, cytosine, and uracil fluoresce at all pH values at 77°K, but phosphorescence occurs only in strong alkaline solutions where the N_1 proton is lost by
thymine and uracil, and the N_3 proton is lost by cytosine. The phosphorescence
emission spectra of these bases, upon excitation at 270 mμ, are broad and structureless, with maxima at 430, 400, and 410 mμ, respectively, for thymine, cytosine, and
uracil. Phosphorescence quantum yields are very low, the highest being 0.03,
observed for cytosine. The excited state protolytic equilibrium pK_a^* of each pyrimidine differs by less than one pH unit from the value of the corresponding ground
state species, compared to the singlet state ionization constants, which show changes
from 2.4 to 7.5 pH units from the ground state values. Excited state pK_a^*'s between
two species A^- and HA may be determined by the method of Weller (1961) from
the equation:

$$pK^* = pK - (0.625/T)\,\Delta\nu$$

where

pK = ground state equilibrium constant,
$\Delta\nu = \nu_{HA} - \nu_{A^-}$, in cm^{-1} (defined as the arithmetic
mean of the spectral shifts in absorption and
phosphorescence upon ionization).

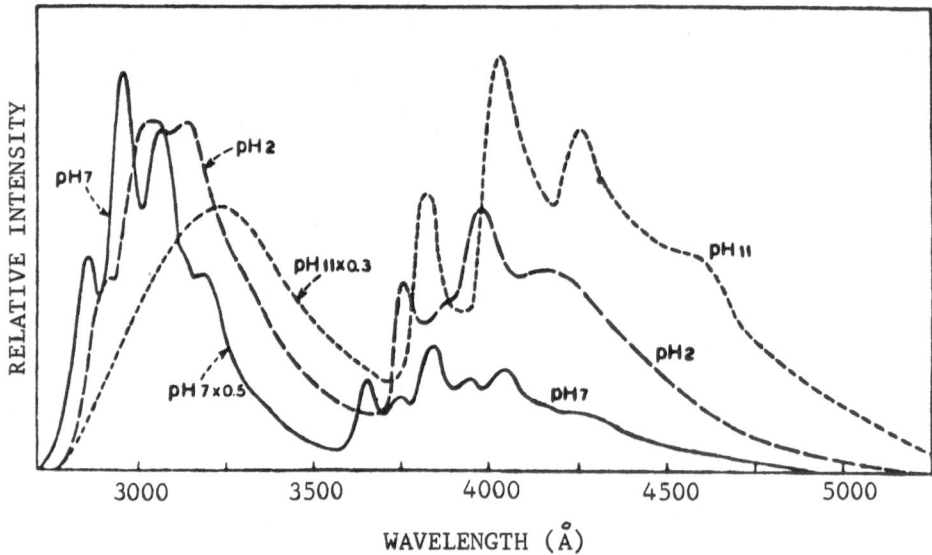

FIG. 8. Luminescence of adenine at pH 2.0, 7.0, and 11.0. Concentrations were 1×10^{-3} M
in ethylene glycol and water at 77°K. Amplifier gain was 1.0, 0.5, and 0.3, as indicated. (From
Longworth et al. 1966. *J. Chem. Phys.*, 45:2936. Courtesy of the American Institute of Physics.)

The phosphorescence emission behavior of the nucleoside and nucleotide derivatives is very similar to that of the parent pyrimidines. With the exception of cytidine, which does not phosphoresce since the N_3 proton is replaced by ribose, the nucleosides phosphoresce only in strong alkaline solution. Their emission spectra are structureless, the maxima are slightly displaced (5 and 10 mμ red-shifted for thymidine and uridine, respectively), and the quantum yields are again low. Thymidine, upon titration with base, gives a 30-fold increase in phosphorescence intensity upon going from pH 7 to pH 12 (loss of N_1 proton). Uridine, in a similar titration, shows a 6-fold enhancement. The pK_a* of phosphorescence activation of thymidine is ~10.6, as compared to the pK_a of 9.8 of the ground state species, corresponding to the loss of the N_1 proton.

In contrast to the pyrimidines, which phosphoresce only in strong alkaline solution, the purines adenine and guanine phosphoresce in alkaline, neutral, or acidic solutions. The phosphorescence emission spectra of these compounds and their corresponding nucleoside and nucleotide derivatives show considerable fine structure, each spectrum being characteristic of the pH-dependent tautomer and the specific derivative in question. Adenine, however, exhibits a more extensive fine structure than guanine, and much more variation in spectral emission is observed between adenine, its riboside and ribonucleotide than that observed for the corresponding guanine compounds. The total luminescence spectra of adenine at various pH values are shown in Figure 8. The phosphorescence quantum yields are again

TABLE 7

Phosphorescence Characteristics of Purines,
Nucleosides, and Nucleotides at 77°K[a]

Compound	pH	Emission maxima (mμ)	τ_d (sec)	Quantum yield
Adenine	1	375,398,418	3.35	0.03
	7	365,384,404,425	2.2	0.035
	11	381,402.5,425	2.8	0.095
Adenosine	1	405,535	—	0.003
	7	380,401,424,448	2.5	0.008
5'-Adenylic acid	1	420	—	0.0008
	7	381,402.5,427.5, 459	2.45	0.004
Guanine	1	385,405,425	(40%) 0.42±0.05 (60%) 1.6±0.1	0.04
	7	360,380,409,417	1.42	0.07
	11	408	1.35	0.06
Guanosine	1	435	(63%) 0.77±0.2 (37%) 0.17±0.1	0.002
	7	380,403,422	1.3	0.03
	11	418	1.3	0.04
5'-Guanylic acid	1	435	(60%) 0.64±0.1 (40%) 0.17±0.1	0.002
	7	380,405,422	1.25	0.04
	11	418	1.25	0.02

[a]From Longworth, Rahn, and Shulman. 1966. *J. Chem. Phys.*, 45:2930-2939. Courtesy of the American Institute of Physics.

generally low, and vary with the nature of the tautomeric form and the specific derivative. The emission maxima, quantum yields, and decay times of purines and their derivatives at various pH values are given in Table 7.

Phosphorescence decay measurements, performed with a Sanborn recorder with a 0.01 sec response time, are generally characteristic of π-π* states, which, at 77°K, are usually of the order of 1 sec, in contrast to n-π* states of triplets, which are usually several orders of magnitude lower. The appearance of two components in the triplet decay of guanine at pH 1 is not well understood, since only one guanine species is expected to exist at that pH. Decay times obtained by electron spin resonance (ESR) measurements (Shulman and Rahn, 1966) are generally in agreement with those found by phosphorescence techniques. According to ESR measurements, 5'-guanylic acid at pH 7 and pH 1 has decay times of 1.26 and 0.37 sec, respectively.

Polynucleotides

The phosphorescence behavior of polynucleotides is complicated by several factors: (a) hydrogen bonding between bases, which may lead to proton transfer in the excited state; (b) energy transfer between bases; (c) conformation, which in turn affects hydrogen bonding and energy transfer; (d) changes in intersystem crossing and nonradiative transition rates. These factors complicate the luminescence behavior of polynucleotides; however, the characterization of the phosphorescence behavior of the individual purines, pyrimidines, and their derivatives does provide a starting point for the interpretation of the often unexpected luminescence behavior of polynucleotides, specifically that of DNA.

The influence of conformation on phosphorescence emission was investigated for the homopolymer polyadenylic acid (poly-A) (Rahn, Yamane, et al., 1966). At neutral pH, room temperature, and in aqueous solution, optical rotatory dispersion, optical absorption, and viscosity measurements indicate that poly-A is in the form of a flexible single strand; at low pH, poly-A consists of a double-stranded helix (Holcomb and Tinoco, 1965). At 25°C in 1:1 ethylene glycol and water at neutral pH, Rahn, Shulman, and Longworth (1966), performing similar measurements, found poly-A to be completely disordered. However, lowering the temperature to 77°K results in the formation of a single-stranded helix, comparable to the one formed in water at neutral pH and room temperature. At 77°K, pH 7, in an ethylene glycol and water glass, poly-A has a structured phosphorescence emission spectrum very similar to that of adenosine monophosphate (AMP) under the same conditions, except that it is shifted to the red by $\sim$10 mμ relative to that of AMP, as shown in Figure 9. The triplet decay time of poly-A is 2.4 sec, i.e., identical with that of AMP. Thus, incorporation of AMP into a polynucleotide, with stacking of the bases, does not greatly alter the phosphorescence characteristics.

Double-stranded poly-A is formed upon protonation of the N_1 proton of adenine, and less than 50% protonation results in a completely ordered, double-stranded helix. Protonation of $\sim$60% of poly-A results in almost total quenching of the poly-A phosphorescence, in contrast to AMP, where quenching increases

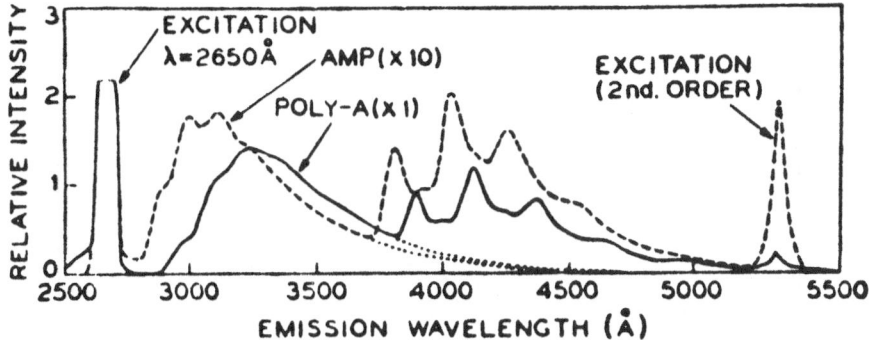

FIG. 9. Luminescence of AMP and poly A at 77°K in ethylene glycol and water glass. (From Rahn et al. 1966b. *J. Chem Phys.*, 45:2948. Courtesy of the American Institute of Physics.)

linearly with the degree of protonation. Therefore, quenching of poly-A phosphorescence is a consequence not only of protonation of the adenine subunits, but also of the ordering of the bases due to double-helix formation. Hydrogen bonding between the amino group and N_7 position of adenine, or energy transfer from a nonprotonated excited singlet to a protonated base, which then acts as a nonradiative trap, were suggested as explanations for the quenching not due to protonation.

The polymer polyadenylic-polyuridylic acid (poly-[A + 2U]) is a triple-stranded polymer, which can be prepared by mixing poly-A and polyuridylic acid (poly-U) at *pH* 7 (Felsenfeld and Rich, 1957). The available evidence suggests that the polymer is exclusively in the form poly-(A + 2U) without any poly-(A + U) in ethylene glycol and water at 77°K (Rahn, Yamane, et al., 1966). When titrating poly-A against poly-U, the phosphorescence of poly-(A + 2U) is extensively quenched at 50% poly-U, as compared to that of poly-A; however, the characteristic poly-A structure is still present in the emission spectrum of the 50:50 mixture. At 67% poly-U, which gives complete formation of triple-stranded poly-(A + 2U), the phosphorescence emission is negligible. The polymer poly-(A + 2I) also has no phosphorescence. These results confirm the conclusion that ordering, i.e., formation of double- or triple-stranded helices as a result of hydrogen bonding, quenches poly-A phosphorescence.

In order to investigate the mechanism of adenine quenching, triplet energy transfer from adenine to the pyrimidines uracil and cytosine was studied in the heteropolymers poly-A$_2$U and poly-A$_2$C, which are single-stranded polynucleotides with random sequences. Compared to the controls 2-poly-A + UMP and 2-poly-A + CMP, i.e., mixtures of poly-A with the nucleotides, there is a 50% increase in phosphorescence emission of poly-A$_2$U and poly-A$_2$C. The poly-A$_2$C phosphorescence-emission spectrum is characteristic of poly-A, yet less well resolved. Poly-A$_2$U has two decay constants, one ~0.4 sec (33%) and another 1.9 sec (66%), compared to a $\tau_d = 2.4$ sec observed for 2-poly-A + UMP (characteristic of poly-A + AMP). According to ESR measurements, τ_d for poly-A$_2$U is 1.8 ± 0.15 sec. Therefore, the shorter-lived component observed in the phosphorescence decay of poly-A$_2$U origi-

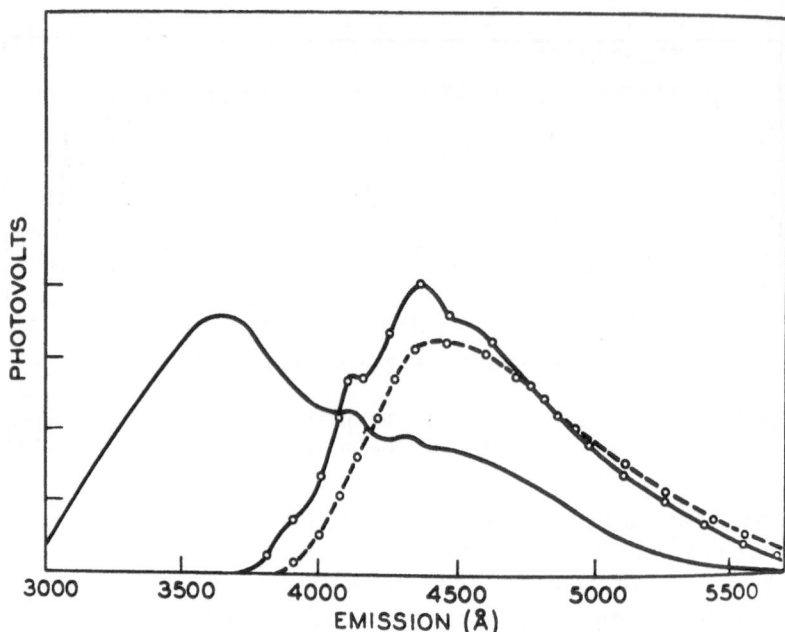

FIG. 10. Total luminescence and phosphorescence of native calf-thymus DNA; (o - - o) refers to excitation at 290 mμ, and (o—o) to excitation at 260 mμ. (From Rahn et al. 1966a. *J. Chem. Phys.*, 45: 2956. Courtesy of the American Institute of Physics.)

nates from uracil. The decrease of τ_d and the appearance of a short decay moment, both in poly-A_2U and poly-A_2C, indicate that there is some triplet energy transfer from adenine to the pyrimidines.

Studies on adenine-cytosine (AC) dinucleotides in various configurations (Hélène et al., 1965) also indicate two phosphorescence emissions, each characterized by a different lifetime: a long lifetime from adenine, and a rapid decay from cytosine. The phosphorescence intensity of solutions containing equal concentrations of solutes decreases in the order A>ApC>CpA>AppC (the designation *p* indicates nucleotide linkages). These results confirm that there is a small amount of triplet transfer between adenine and cytosine; the triplet state of cytosine is apparently reached directly by triplet-triplet transfer.

Studies on DNA luminescence date back to the work of Steele and Szent-Györgyi (1957), who observed a blue phosphorescence from a solution of DNA in glucose and water. Since then, numerous and often conflicting reports concerning the origin of DNA phosphorescence have appeared, the discrepancies resulting most likely from the presence of impurities in the DNA samples, solvent effects, conformational state, etc.

Extensively purified DNA from different sources (calf thymus, salmon sperm, *E. coli*) was studied under various conditions in 1:1 ethylene glycol and water at 77°K, and its phosphorescence behavior was compared to that of poly-d AT, which was chosen as a possible model compound for DNA phosphorescence (Rahn, Shulman, and Longworth, 1966). Using an excitation wavelength of 290 mμ, native DNA from all three sources resulted in a broad phosphorescence spectrum with an emission maximum slightly less than 450 mμ at neutral *pH*. Excitation at 260 mμ gives a more structured spectrum, with fine structure peaks at 390, 410, and 437 mμ, as shown in Figure 10. The phosphorescence quantum yield of native DNA at *pH* 7 is ~0.002. At *pH* 12, the DNA emission is characteristic of adenine, and, at *pH* 1, of guanine, as would be expected since AMP is quenched at low *pH*. The phosphorescence emission at *pH* 1 and *pH* 12 is greater than that observed at *pH* 7. Heat-denatured DNA gives an increase in phosphorescence intensity and a shift to shorter wavelengths, indicating a sensitivity of phosphorescence emission with respect to conformational state.

Decay times of native DNA (measured at 450 mμ) seem to be concentration dependent; i.e., at concentrations of 10 and 2 mg/ml, unimolecular decay times of 0.27 and 0.29 sec are observed, respectively; at 0.1 mg/ml, $\tau_d = 0.26$ sec for 85% of the intensity decay. Examination of DNA phosphorescence decay over the entire emission range reveals that the decay is composed of two components, a short-lived one, $\tau_d = 0.27$ sec, which is red-shifted from the longer-lived one, $\tau_d = 1.6$ to 1.9 sec (Rahn, Yamane, et al., 1966). Since native DNA in water at 77°K has a decay constant of ~0.3 sec (Rahn et al., 1966b), the long-lived decay component observed for DNA is considered to arise from the denaturing action of ethylene glycol. Adenine and guanine, which have decay constants of 2.5 and 1.3 sec, respec-

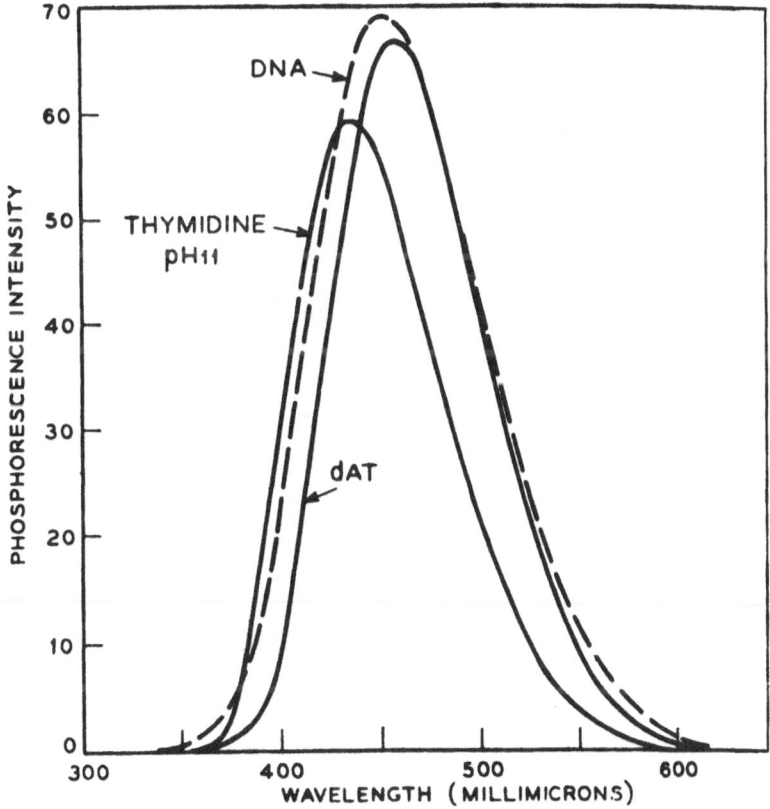

FIG. 11. Phosphorescence emission of DNA, poly dAT, and thymidine. (From Rahn et al. 1966a. *J. Chem. Phys.*, 45:2960. Courtesy of the American Institute of Physics.)

tively, give a single decay time of ∼1.6 sec when present in equimolar quantities in the same solution.

Examination of the double-stranded deoxyribonucleotide poly-d AT reveals that its phosphorescence emission is very similar to that of DNA (Rahn, Shulman, and Longworth, 1966). Both polynucleotides have an emission maximum at 448 mμ, as shown in Figure 11. Moreover, the phosphorescence decay constant for poly-d AT is 0.34 ± 0.03 sec, a value which is close to that for DNA (0.28 ± 0.03 sec). These similarities indicate a common origin for the phosphorescence of both DNA and poly-d AT, which is probably due to the triplet state of N_3-deprotonated thymine, since it is known that thymine or TMP phosphoresces only in strong basic solution. The thymidine phosphorescence emission spectrum is similar to that of DNA (see Figure 11), except that the latter is shifted to the red. The triplet decay constant for thymidine is 0.5 sec, compared to $\tau_d \simeq 0.3$ for DNA. These slight differences between the thymine and DNA phosphorescence characteristics are reasonable in view of the fact that thymine in DNA is in an altered environment, as compared to free base. ESR measurements (Rahn, Yamane, et al., 1966) agree with phosphorescence data; that is, the observed DNA triplet emission is probably due to ionized thymine, rather than adenine or guanine.

Amino Acids

Phosphorescence of the 20 naturally occurring amino acids is confined to the aromatic amino acids tryptophan, tyrosine, and phenylalanine. Tryptophan and

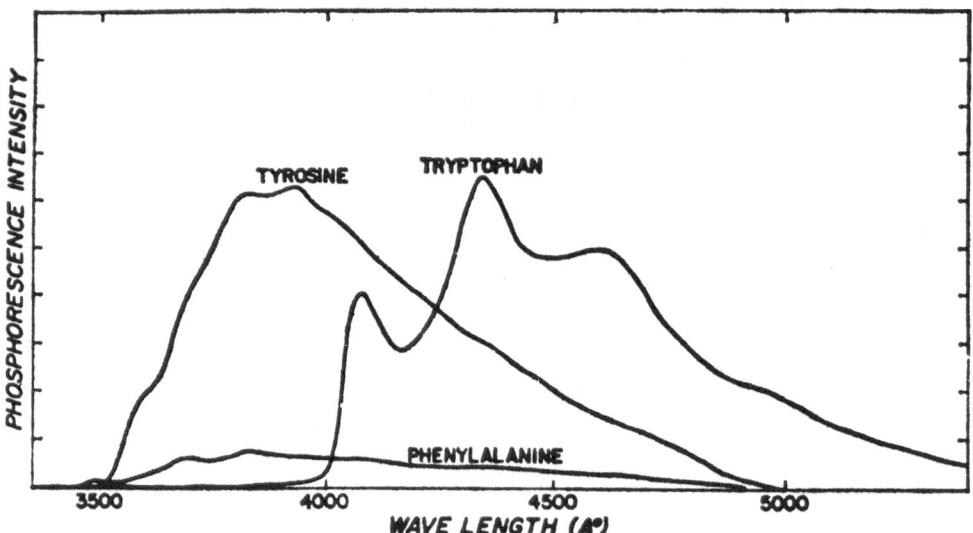

FIG. 12. Phosphorescence emission of tryptophan, tyrosine, and phenylalanine. Concentration 10^{-3} M in 0.5% aqueous glucose at 77°K; identical instrument settings for all solutions. (From Truong et al. 1967. *J. Biol. Chem.*, 242:2980. Courtesy of The American Society of Biological Chemists, Inc.)

tyrosine phosphorescence was first observed by Debye and Edwards (1952). A well-resolved phosphorescence emission spectrum of tryptophan in a 9:1 methanol–ethanol solution at 77°K exhibits maxima at 408, 438, and 460 mμ (Freed and Salmre, 1958). At −100°C, tyrosine shows a maximum at 387 mμ and a weak shoulder at 410 to 420 mμ (Vladimirov and Burshtein, 1960). Phenylalanine, which has a very weak phosphorescence compared to that of tyrosine and tryptophan, gives three maxima, 424 to 426 mμ, 448 to 450 mμ, and 490 to 495 mμ (Vladimirov and Burshtein, 1960). The phosphorescence emission characteristics for tryptophan, tyrosine, and phenylalanine at 77°K in a 0.5% aqueous glucose solution (Truong et al., 1967) are shown in Figure 12. The decay times for tryptophan, tyrosine, and phenylalanine are approximately 5.7, 2.8, and 3.2 sec, respectively (Truong et al., 1967). The tryptophan and tyrosine decay constants measured by Truong et al. (1967) are in general agreement with those found by other researchers.

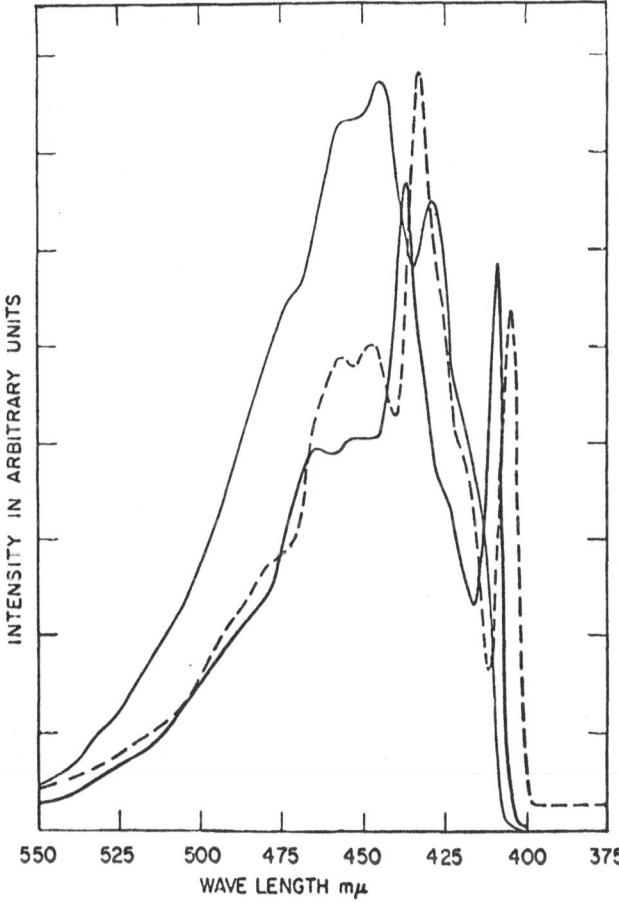

FIG. 13. Phosphorescence emission spectra of indole and indole derivatives. Tryptophan, heavy line; indole, freshly sublimed, dashed line; and serotonin creatinine sulfate, thin line. Each spectrum was taken at 77°K, in a 1:9 (v/v) ethanol-methanol solvent. (From Freed and Vise. 1963. *Anal. Biochem.*, 5:339. Courtesy of Academic Press, Inc.)

The phosphorescence of tryptophan can be traced entirely to the presence of the indole ring, since indole, tryptophan, indole acetic acid, and various other substituted indoles give almost identical emission maxima, as shown in Figure 13 (Freed and Salmre, 1958). Thus, substitution of the indole ring does not greatly affect phosphorescence; substituent effects in the fluorescence of indole derivatives are more marked (Van Duuren, 1961). Involvement of the imino hydrogen in hydrogen bonding has a pronounced effect on phosphorescence emission intensity (Konev, 1967a). In nonpolar solvents, such as hexane, the imino group is free, and intense indole-ring phosphorescence is observed. Protic solvents, e.g., methanol and ethanol, which promote hydrogen bonding, reduce the phosphorescence intensity of indole and its derivatives. Complete ionization of the imino group results in almost total quenching. Tryptophan in 0.1 M NaOH, for example, shows only very weak phosphorescence.

In contrast to the fluorescence emission of tryptophan, which occurs from two different excited singlet electronic levels (Konev, 1967b), phosphorescence polarization measurements and constancy of τ_d for the entire phosphorescence emission range indicate triplet decay from one electronic level only.

Tyrosine gives a broad, structureless phosphorescence emission in aqueous glucose solution, Figure 12, but shows sharp maxima at 354, 366, 376, 387, 397, and 412 mμ in 8 M lithium iodide (Konev and Bobrovich, 1965). The intensity of triplet emission is strongly pH-dependent and is highest in alkaline solution (Truong et al., 1967), as shown in Figure 14. The emission characteristics of tryptophan, tyrosine, and an equimolar mixture of the two were determined by Truong et al. (1967) at different pH values; the results are summarized in Table 8.

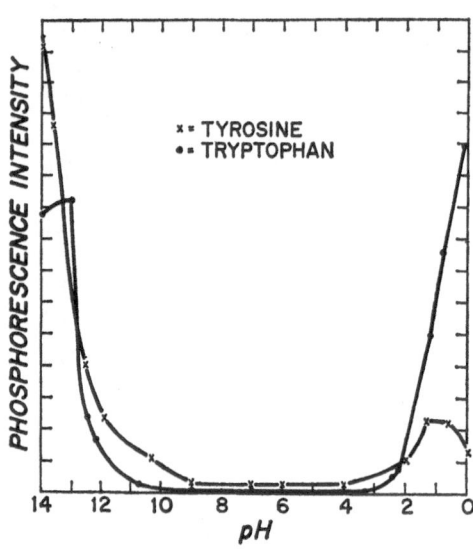

FIG. 14. Phosphorescence emission intensity of tryptophan and tyrosine as a function of pH. All measurements made at 77°K in a 0.5% aqueous glucose solution. (From Truong et al. 1967. J. Biol. Chem., 242:2980. Courtesy of the American Society of Biological Chemists, Inc.)

TABLE 8

*Phosphorescence Emission Maxima and Decay Times
of Tyrosine and Tryphophan*[a]

Compound	λ max $(m\mu)$[b]		
	pH 7	pH 1.4	pH 12.2
Tryptophan	437	434	437
Tyrosine	390	390	413
Tryptophan and Tyrosine[c]	435	423	399
	τ_d (sec)		
Tryptophan	5.4	4.7	5.1
Tyrosine	2.8	2.1	1.2
Tryptophan and Tyrosine[c]	4.7	4.4	1.6

[a]In 0.5% aqueous glucose solution at 77°K; Truong et al. (1967).
[b]Major peaks only.
[c]$10^{-4}M$ in both tyrosine and tryptophan.

Of particular interest are the results obtained for the equimolar mixture of trypto-phan and tyrosine, since both amino acids are present in many proteins, which derive their phosphorescence mainly from either one or both amino acids. In neutral solution, only tryptophan emission is observed; at pH 1.4, tyrosine and trypto-phan maxima are present but tryptophan emission is more intense than tyrosine emission, as would be expected from the titration curve, Figure 14. At both pH 12.2 and 1.4, there is an increase in the phosphorescence yield compared to that at pH 7. If the yield at pH 7 is taken as 1, then the relative phosphorescence yields at pH 7, 1.4, and 12.2 are 1.0, 2.0, and 17.0, respectively. At all three pH values, pure tryptophan has a longer decay time than pure tyrosine (Table 8). The phosphorescence characteristics of the amino acids described above are of importance in the interpretation of phosphorescence-structure relationships of proteins, discussed below.

Proteins

The phosphorescence of proteins is due mainly to the presence of tyrosine and tryptophan. Those proteins that contain tyrosine and phenylalanine, but not tryptophan, i.e., class A proteins according to Weber (1960), derive their phosphorescence from tyrosine residues. Proteins that contain tryptophan in addition to tyrosine and phenylalanine, i.e., class B proteins according to Weber (1960), show predominantly tryptophan triplet emission, with some tyrosine contribution to the total phosphorescence emission. Tryptophan incorporated into a polypeptide chain is red-shifted compared to the pure monomer in solution.

Changes in the secondary or tertiary structure of a protein are usually not

TABLE 9

Phosphorescence Emission Maxima and Relative Intensities of Fluorescence and Phosphorescence of Chymotrypsin and Casein[a]

Protein	Fluorescence Maximum (mμ)	Phosphorescence Maxima (mμ)	I_F/I_P (400 mμ)	I_F/I_P (440 mμ)	I_F/I_P (450 mμ)
Chymotrypsin					
Native	323	412, 439, 450-465	4.8	1.80	2.3
Heat denatured	322	413, 438, 450-465	3.0	2.60	3.5
Denatured, 8 *M* urea	323	412, 439, 450-465	5.3	1.80	2.5
Casein					
Native	323	390, 410, 438, 450-465	2.6	1.4	1.9
Heat denatured	323	390, 414, 440, 450-465	1.8	1.2	1.6

[a]Adapted from Konev. 1967. *Fluorescence and Phosphorescence of Proteins and Nucleic Acids*, pp. 100-101. Courtesy of Plenum Press.

reflected by any large changes in the position of the emission maxima. However, the ratio I_F/I_P, where I_F refers to the intensity of fluorescence at the emission maximum, and I_P is the phosphorescence intensity at a certain emission wavelength, is very sensitive to secondary and tertiary structure. The spectral characteristics and I_F/I_P values for chymotrypsin and casein in the native and denatured state are given in Table 9.

As discussed above for amino acids, the degree of ionization of the imino hydrogen greatly affects the phosphorescence yield of tryptophan, and complete ionization results in total quenching. Thus, the changes observed in the ratio I_F/I_P may very well reflect the degree of separation of the imino hydrogen from the nitrogen of the indole ring in tryptophan. Participation of the imino group in hydrogen-bond formation depends on the specific environment of the imino group. Thus, determination of I_F/I_P ratios for proteins could be helpful in establishing the location of tryptophan residues in the three-dimensional structure of proteins.

Studies concerning the specific environments of tyrosine and tryptophan in different solvent matrices and a comparison with similar studies on proteins containing these residues were carried out by Kuntz et al. (1969). Earlier experiments (Bishai et al., 1967; Kuntz, 1968) had indicated that phosphorescence as a function of temperature greatly depends on the nature of the solvent matrix surrounding the emitting species. Therefore, Kuntz and coworkers studied the fluorescence and phosphorescence intensity of proteins, pure tyrosine, and pure tryptophan in polyvinyl alcohol, PVA films, and aqueous glucose glasses. The PVA films were prepared by adding a glucose solution of the amino acid or protein to a 5% PVA solution and allowing the water to evaporate from a 1-mm layer adsorbed on a quartz plate or a stretched Visking membrane. The protein membranes were obtained similarly by evaporation of protein-containing glucose solutions. An iron-constantan thermocouple was either embedded directly in the glass matrices or touched the film surfaces; the temperature was measured after the liquid nitrogen had boiled off and the samples slowly warmed up. No gross melting of the matrix, glass or film, ever occurred over the entire temperature range investigated.

The changes in quantum efficiency, Q, with temperature are represented in plots of log Q versus $1/T \times 10^3$, as shown in Figure 15 for tryptophan. All plots, regardless of type of matrix and protein or amino acid, generally consist of three regions, labelled by the authors as EQ, Tr, and MQ. The MQ region, which represents measurements at the lowest temperature, consists of a flat line for both tyrosine and tryptophan, indicating a constant phosphorescence intensity. For the proteins trypsin and hyaluronidase, the MQ region is almost flat. Since there is little if any quenching in this region, the authors concluded that there was no interaction between the excited state of the emitter and the surrounding solvent matrix. This is substantiated by the fact that there are no shifts in wavelength of phosphorescence at the lowest temperatures resulting from solvent interaction.

The EQ region represents measurements at the highest temperatures possible before gross melting. It is in this region that the phosphorescence intensity decreases drastically with an increase in temperature, indicating that the environment of the emitter has "melted" sufficiently to allow interaction of the excited

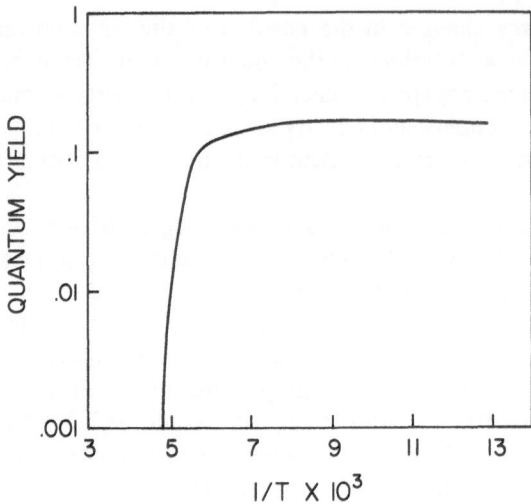

FIG. 15. Arrhenius plots for the phosphorescence quantum yields of tryptophan. 0.55% in glucose. (Adapted from Kuntz et al., 1969.)

states, leading to radiationless deactivation. Furthermore, triplet quenching is more efficient than singlet quenching in this region, as would be expected from the longer lifetimes of the triplet states.

At intermediate temperatures, there is a transition region, Tr, where the phosphorescence intensity also decreases with an increase in temperature. However, the decrease is not as drastic as that found in the EQ region. The authors interpret the Tr region as reflecting the melting of the matrix immediately surrounding the emitting species.

The results indicate that the extent of the Tr region for tyrosine and tryptophan varies from one solvent environment to another. In PVA and the aqueous glucose glass, the Tr region of tyrosine extends over a range of 30 to 40°K, and 40°K, respectively; the corresponding values for tryptophan are $\sim$100°K and 90°K. This difference in the range of the Tr region for tryptophan and tyrosine is expected, since these two amino acids have quite different molecular and three-dimensional structures and, therefore, require different solvation shells even in the same solvent. Examination of the slopes of the EQ region indicates that they are significantly different for tyrosine (or tryptophan) in PVA as compared to aqueous glucose glass. However, the slopes of tyrosine and tryptophan in the aqueous glucose glass are quite similar, and those in PVA are also almost identical. The authors therefore concluded that the quenching in the EQ region represents interaction of the amino acid with the matrix, since intramolecular conversion should not be greatly affected by the nature of the external matrix; that is, the slopes in the absence of solvent interaction should be identical in PVA and the water-glucose glass.

In addition to the three regions obtained by plotting log intensity or quantum efficiency versus $1/T$, the plots also indicate that quenching of the singlet and triplet

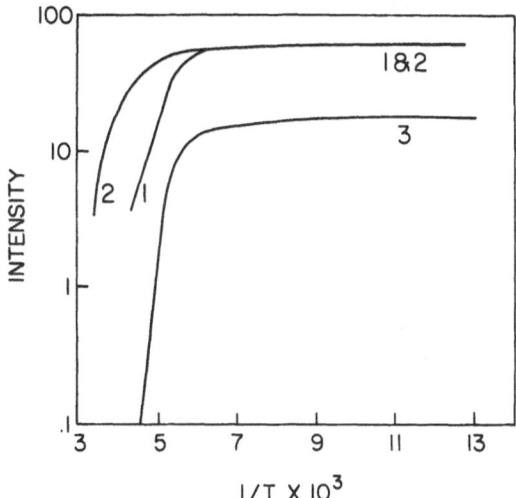

FIG. 16. Arrhenius plots for the phosphorescence intensity of tyrosine, curve 1; tryptophan, curve 2; and tryptophyl-tryptophan, curve 3. Tyrosine and tryptophan in PVA film; tryptophyl-tryptophan in 0.55% aqueous glucose glass. (Adapted from Kuntz et al., 1969.)

state of an excited species occurs at different temperatures and, therefore, at different degrees of mobility of the matrix. Moreover, the nature of the matrix (PVA or aqueous glucose glass) has a pronounced effect on the rate of intersystem crossing. In PVA films, the phosphorescence intensity of the amino acids is almost twice as great as that in an aqueous glucose glass, with no significant quenching of the total luminescence. According to the authors, different matrices impose different configurations on the solute molecules, without affecting either intramolecular or intermolecular vibronic coupling.

Examination of the dipeptides tryptophyl-tryptophan and tryptophyl-tyrosine, which give only tryptophan phosphorescence, shows a very close correspondence of the log intensity, I, versus $1/T$ plots with that of tryptophan. Furthermore, the phosphorescence and the fluorescence yields are greatly quenched as compared to that of tyrosine. The authors concluded therefore that the emitting tyrosine residues of the dipeptides are in a "micro"-environment similar to that of tryptophan in the aqueous glucose glass, and that neighbor-neighbor quenching is very efficient, as shown in Figure 16.

Hyaluronidase films, without PVA, show that the emitting tryptophan residues are in an environment similar to that in PVA. Comparison of the results for hyaluronidase in an aqueous glucose glass with those of tyrosine and tryptophan in the same solvent matrix reveals close similarities in the appearance and duration of the MQ and Tr regions, and the slope of the EQ regions. Since the interpretations of the plots obtained for hyaluronidase and trypsin in various solvent matrices is very complex, and beyond the scope of this chapter, the reader is referred to the original article (Kuntz, 1969).

Numerous phosphorescence emission spectra of proteins have recently appeared in the literature (Konev, 1967c). Truong et al. (1967), whose work

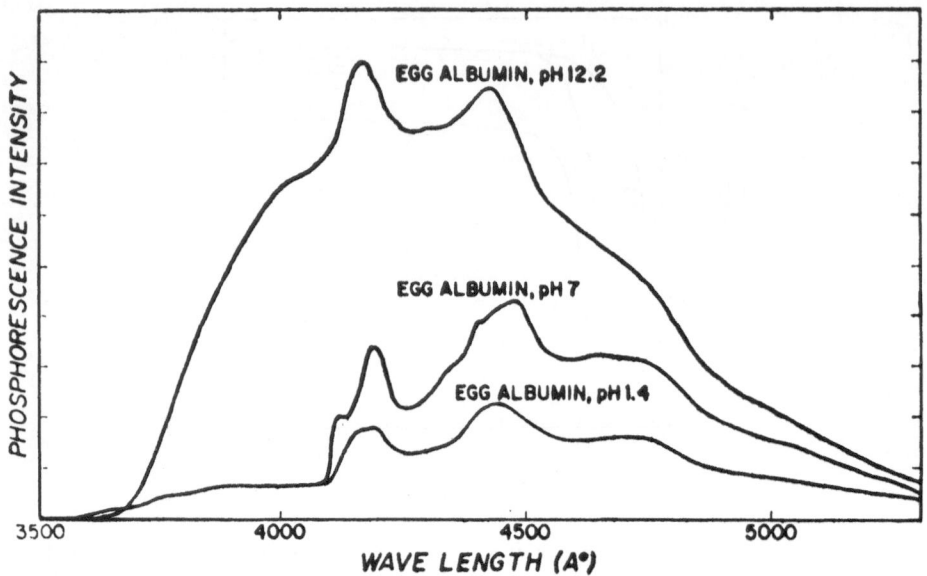

FIG. 17. Phosphorescence emission of ovalbumin at different pH values in 0.5% aqueous glucose at 77°K. (From Truong et al. 1967. J. Biol. Chem., 242:2982. Courtesy of the American Society of Biological Chemists, Inc.)

was mentioned earlier with respect to tyrosine and tryptophan triplet emission, examined the influence of pH on the phosphorescence intensity of human serum albumin, bovine serum albumin, egg albumin, globin from myoglobin and hemoglobin, and insulin. All spectra were recorded at 77°K, with the proteins dissolved in 0.5% aqueous glucose solution adjusted to the desired pH. All proteins examined emit most strongly at pH 12.2 and at that pH show mainly tyrosine triplet emission characteristics. Some tryptophan emission, however, is indicated by the presence of two small peaks at 408 and 440 mµ. These peaks, indicative of tryptophan, are present in most protein phosphorescence spectra except in that of insulin, which contains no tryptophan. As a representative example of protein emission at different

TABLE 10

Phosphorescence Emission Maxima and Decay Times of
Proteins as a Function of pH[a]

Compound	λ max (mµ)[b]		
	pH 7	pH 1.4	pH 12.2
Human serum albumin	444 (4.2)	440 (3.5)	417 (2.6)
Bovine serum albumin	446 (4.9)	440 (4.5)	414 (3.4,1.0)
Egg albumin	444 (5.5)	440 (4.6)	414 (4.0,1.2)
Globin from hemoglobin	438 (3.3)	—	410 (3.3,0.99)
Insulin	450 (1.6)	450 (1.95)	415 (0.84)

[a]Adapted from Truong et al. 1967. J. Biol. Chem., 242:2979-2985. Courtesy of the American Society for Biological Chemists.
[b]Decay times in seconds are indicated in parentheses.

*p*H values, the phosphorescence emission spectra of egg albumin are shown in Figure 17. In neutral solution, the phosphorescence of proteins is mainly due to triplet emission from tryptophan, with only a small tyrosine contribution. The emission characteristics of some proteins and the decay times as a function of *pH* are summarized in Table 10.

The role of hydrogen bonding in the phosphorescence of tyrosine and tryptophan was discussed above. The results observed with proteins were interpreted in a similar manner by Truong et al. (1967).

Analytical Applications

The analysis of drugs in biological fluids and tissues is important in several aspects of biomedical research; for example, in the study of drug metabolism and the rate of elimination from the body. Studies of this kind usually involve handling large volumes of biological fluids, extraction of the drug into a suitable solvent, and spectrophotometric determination. In some instances, a derivative of the drug has to be synthesized in order to make colorimetric determinations possible, as in the case of sulfa drugs which are converted into azo dyes. Most of these methods for drug analysis are not only time consuming, but are also of limited accuracy, since the reagents used in the extraction procedures and in conversion to suitable derivatives introduce impurities which impair the accuracy and sensitivity of the method.

Phosphorimetry as a means of drug analysis was first applied by Winefordner and Latz (1963) for the determination of acetylsalicylic acid (aspirin) in blood serum and plasma. Phosphorimetric analysis of aspirin in serum or plasma involves extraction of a small sample of serum or plasma with chloroform, removal of chloroform, and measurement of phosphorescence of the residue dissolved in EPA; the phosphorescence intensity is measured at 410 mμ and 77°K. The emission intensity is corrected for background emission, obtained by following the above procedure with samples of plasma or serum containing no aspirin. The concentration is determined by means of a concentration-intensity calibration curve. Recovery is in the range of 90 to 100% for solutions containing 5 to 50 mg of aspirin per 100 ml of serum or plasma. Standard deviations for all determinations were in the range of 5 to 10%. The presence of salicylic acid did not affect the accuracy of the results, for phosphorescence emission at 410 mμ was over 500 times weaker for salicylic acid than that of a solution of comparable concentration of acetylsalicylic acid. Using this method, rapid and accurate analyses of serum or plasma containing one to 100 mg aspirin per 100 ml of serum or plasma were obtained in less than 10 minutes.

The success of the phosphorimetric analysis of aspirin in plasma or serum led to the investigation of the determination of other drugs by means of phosphorimetry. Winefordner and Tin (1964) examined the phosphorescence characteristics of a series of organic compounds of pharmacological importance in rigid ethanol glasses at 77°K. The limits of detection of the compounds examined are listed in

TABLE 11

Limits of Detection of Drugs by Phosphorescence[a]

Compound	Limit of Detection (μg/ml)
Phenobarbital	0.1
Mebaral	0.01
Rutonal	0.02
Atropine	0.1
Benzocaine	0.007
Procaine hydrochloride	0.01
p-Aminobenzoic acid	0.004
Butacaine sulfate	0.05
Cyclaine hydrochloride	0.006
Metycaine hydrochloride	0.006
Benzoic acid	0.005
Cocaine hydrochloride	0.01
Quinidine sulfate	0.05
Quinine hydrochloride	0.04
Lidocaine	1.2
Caffeine	0.2
Ephedrine	0.2
Phenylephrine hydrochloride	0.01
Tronothane hydrochloride	0.02
Cinchophen	0.02
Physostigmine sulfate	0.03
Chlortetracyline	0.05

Table 11. The spectral characteristics of a series of drugs are included in Table 2. Calibration curves were obtained for all compounds; some of these are shown in Figure 18.

In these studies, ethanol was the solvent of choice since the solubility of most drugs in EPA, a solvent used in most phosphorimetric analyses, is very low. Most of the drugs have low limits of detectability, which indicates the feasibility of detecting trace amounts of drugs in biological fluids by means of phosphorimetry. The proper choice of excitation and emission wavelength and phosphoroscope speed allows for the simultaneous determination of two or more components present in the same solution.

The usefulness of drug analysis by way of ethanolic extraction of serum and subsequent phosphorimetric analysis was demonstrated for four sulfonamide drugs, sulfacetamide, sulfadiazine, sulfamerazine, and sulfmethazine, by Hollifield and Winefordner (1966). Sulfonamide drugs are derivatives of sulfanilic acid and are used as bacteriostatic agents. The method used for the determination of sulfonamide drugs in most clinical laboratories involves diazotization of the free amino group, subsequent coupling with N-(-1-naphthyl)-ethylenediamine hydrochloride in order to form a colored azo dye, and finally spectrophotometric analysis. This method was developed by Bratton and Marshall (1939). Since sulfonamide drugs become acetylated *in vivo*, determination of these drugs by the method of Bratton and Marshall must be preceded by a deacetylation, i.e., acid hydrolysis at 100°C. The method developed by Hollifield and Winefordner, on the other hand, is rapid,

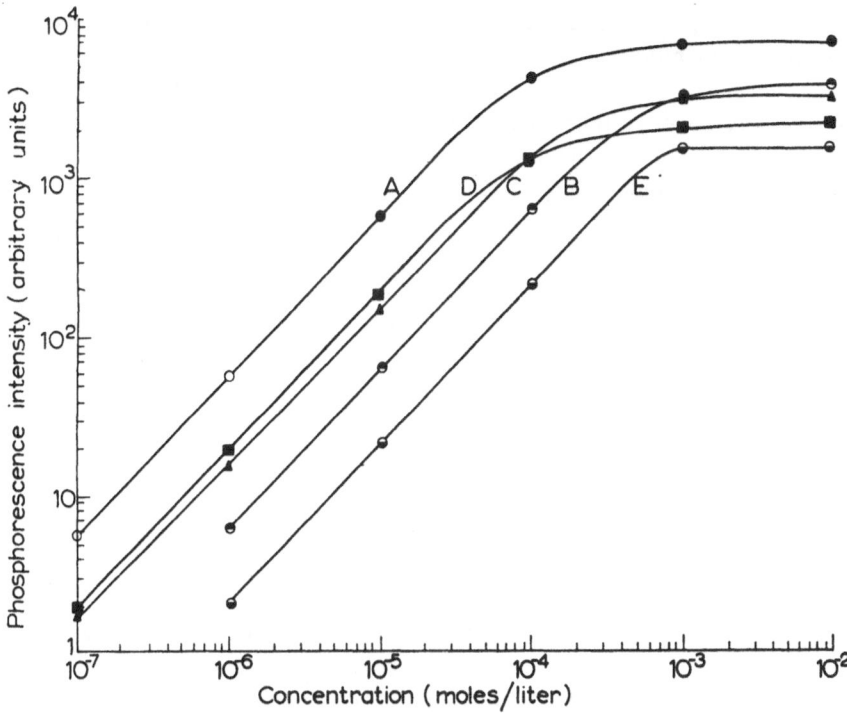

FIG. 18. Phosphorescence intensity versus concentration calibration curves for: (A) procaine; (B) quinine hydrochloride; (C) metycaine hydrochloride; (D) quinidine sulfate; (E) phenobarbital. All measurements were performed on ethanol solutions of the drugs, at 77°K. (From Winefordner and Tin. 1964. *Anal. Chim. Acta*, 31:243. Courtesy of the Elsevier Publishing Company.)

simpler, and more accurate. It consists of mixing a small sample of serum containing a known concentration of the drug with ethanol. The mixture is shaken for three minutes, and the precipitated proteins are removed by centrifugation. An aliquot of the supernatant is diluted with absolute ethanol and the phosphorescence intensity is measured. After correction for background phosphorescence, the intensity is converted to concentration by means of a calibration curve. For sulfonamide concentrations of 10 mg drug/100 ml serum and greater, the background phosphorescence due to serum is negligible. The percentage of recovery of the drugs added to plasma or serum ranged from 92 to 105.

A method very similar to that used for the analysis of sulfonamide drugs in serum was developed by Hollifield and Winefordner (1967) for the determination of anticoagulants in whole blood. One volume of citrated blood is added to nine volumes of absolute ethanol containing a known amount of the drug, and the solution is shaken for three to five minutes. The precipitated proteins are removed by centrifugation. An aliquot of the supernatant is diluted with absolute ethanol and the phosphorescence and fluorescence intensities at wavelengths of maximum emission are measured. For drug concentrations of 10 mg drug/100 ml citrated blood or at higher concentrations, the background phosphorescence is usually insignificant. The anticoagulants examined in this study were the following: dicoumarol, diphenadione, phenindione, tromexan, and warfarin; all compounds were amenable to analysis by phosphorimetry. The detection of some of these drugs by fluorimetry is more sensitive than by phosphorimetry; on the other hand, the detection of dicoumarol by phosphorimetry is 10 times more sensitive than by fluorimetry. Thus, fluorescence and phosphorescence augment each other for many drug analyses.

Winefordner and Tin (1965) also developed procedures for the phosphorimetric determination of procaine, phenobarbital, cocaine, and chlorpromazine in blood serum, and cocaine and atropine in urine. These procedures involve extraction of small samples of blood serum or urine with chloroform or ether, evaporation of the extract, and measurement of phosphorescence intensity in EPA at 77°K.

CONCLUSION

From the foregoing it is clear that phosphorescence analysis can be usefully explored for a wide variety of chemicals, polymers, drugs, and environmental agents of interest to biochemists, pharmacologists, and toxicologists. In some instances these studies reveal new information that can be obtained only by phosphorescence analysis; in other cases, the information gleaned from phosphorescence studies auguments that obtained from other spectroscopic methods. Thus, fluorescence and phosphorescence analyses reinforce each other and hence the examination of both aspects of luminescence spectroscopy provides a powerful tool not only for analytical purposes but also for basic studies on structure, electronic transitions, and studies on the configurations of complex biopolymers. Where compounds exhibit luminescence, their analysis by this spectroscopic method is frequently much more sensitive than that which can be attained by more conventional spectroscopic methods such as infrared- and ultraviolet-visible absorption spectrophotometry or nuclear magnetic resonance spectrometry. However, phosphorescence spectra are at times structureless and hence not so useful for chemical structure determination as is infrared or nuclear magnetic resonance analysis. The rapid advances made in recent years in theoretical developments, instrumentation, and application in biochemical and biomedical research suggest yet wider use in these areas in years to come.

ACKNOWLEDGMENTS

This work was supported by National Institutes of Health Grants No. CA-08946 and ES-00260 from the National Cancer Institute and National Institute of Environmental Health Sciences, respectively.

REFERENCES

General

Barenboim, G. M., A. N. Domanskii, and K. Turoverov. 1969. Luminescence of Biopolymers and Cells. New York and London, Plenum Press.

McCarthy, W. J., and J. D. Winefordner. 1967. Phosphorimetry as a means of chemical analysis. *In* Guilbault, G. G., ed., Fluorescence Theory Instrumentation and Practice, 371-442. New York, Marcel Dekker, Inc.

Konev, S. V. 1967. Fluorescence and Phosphorescence of Proteins and Nucleic Acids. New York and London, Plenum Press.

Parker, C. A. 1968. Photoluminescence of Solutions. Amsterdam, London, and New York, Elsevier Publishing Company.

Zander, M. 1968. Phosphorimetry. New York and London, Academic Press.

Text

Bäckström, H. L., and K. Sandros. 1958. The quenching of the long-lived fluorescence of biacetyl in solution. Acta Chem. Scand., 12:823-832.

———— and K. Sandros. 1960. Transfer of triplet state energy in fluid solutions. I. Sensitized phosphorescence and its application to the determination of triplet state lifetimes. Acta Chem. Scand., 14:48-62.

Becquerel, E. M. 1871. Mémoire sur l'analyse de la luminère émissé par les composés de uranium phosphorescents. Ann. Chim. Phys. (Paris), 27:539-579.

Beer, M. 1956. Electronic spectra of polyacetylenes. J. Chem. Phys., 25:745-750.

Bishai, F., E. Kuntz, and L. Augenstein. 1967. Intra- and intermolecular factors affecting the excited states of aromatic amino acids. Biochim. Biophys. Acta, 140:381-394.

Brand, J. C. D. 1954. Vibrational analysis of the low-frequency absorption system of glyoxal as a $^1Ag-^1Au$ transition. Trans. Faraday Soc., 50:431-444.

———— 1956. The electronic spectrum of formaldehyde. J. Chem. Soc., Part 1:858-872.

Bratton, A. C., E. K. Marshall, Jr., D. Babbit, and A. R. Hendrickson. 1939. A new coupling component for sulfanilamide determination. J. Biol. Chem., 128:537-550.

Corkill, J. M., and I. J. Graham-Bryce. 1961. The luminescence of some substituted naphthalenes. J. Chem. Soc., Part 3:3893-3897.

Cravitt, S., and B. L. Van Duuren. 1968. The design and performance of a new multipurpose luminescence spectrophotometer. Chem. Instrum., 1:71-93.

Dawson, W. R., and J. L. Kropp. 1969. Radiative and radiationless processes in aromatic molecules. Coronene and benzcoronene. J. Phys. Chem., 73:693-699.

Debye, P., and J. O. Edwards. 1952. A note on the phosphorescence of proteins. Science, 116:143-144.

Evans, D. F. 1957. Magnetic perturbation of singlet-triplet transitions. Part II. J. Chem. Soc., Part 3:3885-3888.

Felsenfeld, G., and A. Rich. 1957. Studies on the formation of two- and three-stranded polyribonucleotides. Biochim. Biophys. Acta, 26:457-468.

Ferguson, J., T. Iredale, and J. A. Taylor. 1954. The phosphorescence spectra of naphthalene and some simple derivatives. J. Chem. Soc., Part 3:3160-3165.

Foster, R., D. L. Hammick, G. M. Hood, and A. C. E. Sanders. 1956. Phosphorescence and fluorescence of some aromatic nitro-amines. J. Chem. Soc., Part 4:4865-4868.

Freed, S., and W. Salmre. 1958. Phosphorescence spectra and analyses of some indole derivatives. Science, 128:1341-1342.

‗‗‗‗‗‗‗ and M. H. Vise. 1963. On phosphorimetry as quantitative microanalysis with application to some substances of biological interest. Anal. Biochem., 5:338-344.

Geacintov, N., G. Oster, and T. Cassen. 1968. Polymeric matrices for organic phosphors. J. Opt. Soc. Amer., 58:1217-1229.

Hammond, G. S., and R. S. H. Liu. 1963. Stereoisomeric triplet states of conjugated dienes. J. Amer. Chem. Soc., 85:477-478.

‗‗‗‗‗‗‗ J. Saltiel, A. A. Lamola, N. J. Turro, J. Bradshaw, D. O. Cowan, R. C. Counsell, V. Vogt, and C. Dalton. 1964. Mechanisms of photochemical reactions in solution. XXII. Photochemical *cis-trans* isomerization. J. Amer. Chem. Soc., 86:3197-3217.

Heckman, R. C. 1958. Phosphorescence studies of some heterocyclic and related organic compounds J. Molec. Spectrosc., 2:27-41 (C.A. 52:10722a).

Hélène, C., P. Douzou, and A. M. Michelson. 1965. The phosphorescence of dinucleotides and the problem of energy transfer between the bases of nucleic acids. Biochim. Biophys. Acta, 109:261-267.

Herkstroeter, W. C., A. A. Lamola, and G. S. Hammond. 1964. Mechanisms of photochemical reactions in solution. XXVIII. Values of triplet excitation energies of selected sensitizers. J. Amer. Chem. Soc., 86:4537-4540.

Hoerman, K. C., and S. A. Mancewicz. 1964. Phosphorescence of calcified tissues. Arch. Oral Biol., 9:517-534.

Holcomb, D. N., and I. Tinoco, Jr. 1965. Conformation of polyriboadenylic acid: pH and temperature dependence. Biopolymers, 3:121-133.

Hollifield, H. C., and J. D. Winefordner. 1965. A phosphorimetric investigation of several representative alkaloids of the isoquinoline, morphine and indole groups. Talanta, 12:860-863.

‗‗‗‗‗‗‗ and J. D. Winefordner. 1966. A phosphorimetric investigation of several sulfonamide drugs: A rapid procedure for the determination of drug levels in pooled human serum with specific application to sulfadiazine, sulfamethazine, sulfamerazine and sulfacetamide. Anal. Chim. Acta, 36:352-359.

‗‗‗‗‗‗‗ and J. D. Winefordner. 1967. Fluorescence and phosphorescence characteristics of anticoagulants. A new approach to direct measurement of drugs in whole blood. Talanta, 14:103-107.

Hood, L. V. S., and J. D. Winefordner. 1966. Use of external heavy atom effect to increase sensitivity of measurement in phosphorimetry. Anal. Chem., 38:1922-1924.

Isenberg, I., S. L. Baird, Jr., and R. Rosenbluth. 1965. Quenching of DNA phosphorescence. Science, 150:1179-1181.

Kasha, M. 1960. Paths of molecular excitation. Radiation Res. Suppl., 2:243-275.

‗‗‗‗‗‗‗ 1950. Characterization of electronic transitions in complex molecules. Disc. Faraday Soc., 9:14-19.

Kautsky, H. 1939. Quenching of luminescence by oxygen. Trans. Faraday Soc., 35:216-219.

Kawaoka, K., A. U. Khan, and D. R. Kearns. 1967. Role of singlet excited states of molecular oxygen in the quenching of organic triplet states. J. Chem. Phys., 46:1842-1853.

Konev, S. V. 1967a. Fluorescence and Phosphorescence of Proteins and Nucleic Acids, p. 42. New York. Plenum Press.

‗‗‗‗‗‗‗ 1967b. Ibid., 29.

‗‗‗‗‗‗‗ 1967c. Ibid., 100-101.

‗‗‗‗‗‗‗ and V. P. Bobrovich. 1965. Polarization spectra of fluorescence and phosphorescence from the emission of mitochondria and the nuclei of cells. Biophysics, 10:898-901.

Krishna, V. G., and L. Goodman. 1961. Protonation effects on n→π* transitions in pyrimidine. J. Amer. Chem. Soc., 83:2042-2045.

Kuntz, E. 1968. Tryptophan emission from trypsin and polymer films. Nature (London), 217:845-846.

———— R. Canada, R. Wagner, and L. Augenstein. 1969. Phosphorescence from tyrosine and tryptophan in different microenvironments. In Lim, E. C., ed., Molecular Luminescence, 551-567. New York, W. A. Benjamin, Inc.

Lewis, G. N., and M. Kasha. 1944. Phosphorescence and the triplet state. J. Amer. Chem. Soc., 66:2100-2116.

Longworth, J. W., R. O. Rahn, and R. G. Shulman. 1966. Luminescence of pyrimidines, nucleosides and nucleotides at 77°K. The effect of ionization and tautomerization. J. Chem. Phys., 45:2930-2939.

McCarthy, W. J., and J. D. Winefordner. 1965. Use of thin-layer chromatography and phosphorimetry for rapid quantitative determination of biphenyl in oranges. J. Assoc. Offic. Agr. Chemists, 48:915-922.

———— and J. D. Winefordner. 1967. Phosphorimetry as a means of chemical analysis. In Guilbault, G. G., ed., Fluorescence Theory, Instrumentation, and Practice, 381. New York, Marcel Dekker, Inc.

McClure, D. S. 1949. Triplet-singlet transitions in organic molecules. Lifetime measurements of the triplet state. J. Chem. Phys., 17:905-913.

McGlynn, S. P., J. Daigre and F. J. Smith. 1963. External heavy-atom spin-orbital effect. IV. Intersystem crossing. J. Chem. Phys., 39:675-679.

———— B. T. Neely, and W. C. Neely. 1963. Total luminescence of organic molecules of petrochemical interest. Part 1. Naphthalene, phenanthrene and 1,2,4,5-tetramethylbenzene. Anal. Chim. Acta, 28:472-478.

———— M. R. Padhyde, and M. Kasha. 1955. Lowest triplet levels of the polyacenes. J. Chem. Phys., 23:593-594.

Moye, H. A., and J. D. Winefordner. 1965. Phosphorimetric study of some common pesticides. J. Agr. Food Chem., 13:516-518.

O'Haver, T. C., and J. D. Winefordner. 1966. The influence of phosphoroscope design on the measured phosphorescence intensity in phosphorimetry. Anal. Chem., 38:602-607.

Parker, C. A. 1968a. Photoluminescence of Solutions, 273-278. Amsterdam, London, and New York, Elsevier Publishing Company.

———— 1968b. Photoluminescence of Solutions, 404. Amsterdam, London, and New York, Elsevier Publishing Company.

———— and C. G. Hatchard. 1961. Triplet-singlet emission in fluid solutions. Phosphorescence of eosin. Trans. Faraday Soc., 57:1894-1904.

———— and C. G. Hatchard. 1962. Phosphorescence measurement in chemical analysis: Tests with a new instrument. Analyst, 87:644-676.

Porter, G., and M. R. Wright. 1959. 1. Modes of energy transfer from excited and unstable ionized states. Intramolecular and intermolecular conversion involving change of multiplicity. Disc. Faraday Soc., 27:18-27.

Rahn, R. O., R. G. Shulman, and J. W. Longworth. 1966a. Phosphorescence and electron spin resonance studies of the UV-excited triplet state of DNA. J. Chem. Phys., 45:2955-2965.

———— T. Yamane, J. Eisinger, J. W. Longworth, and R. G. Shulman. 1966b. Luminescence and electron spin resonance studies of adenine in various polynucleotides. J. Chem. Phys., 45:2947-2954.

Sawicki, E., and J. Pfaff. 1967. Analysis of compounds containing the p-nitroaniline phosphor and analogous groups by phosphorimetry and by room-temperature and low-temperature fluorimetry. Microchem. J., 12:7-25.

Scott, D. R., and J. B. Allison. 1962. Solvent glasses for low temperature spectroscopic studies. J. Phys. Chem., 66:561-562.

Shpol'skii, E. V., and L. A. Klimova. 1956. Influence of the solvent on the luminescence spectrum of aromatic hydrocarbons at low temperatures. Bull. Phys. Acad. Sci. USSR, 20:428-433.

Shull, H. 1949. Vibrational analysis of the 3400Å triplet-singlet emission of benzene. J. Chem. Phys., 17:295-303.

Shulman, R. G., and R. O. Rahn. 1966. Electron spin resonance of the excited triplet states of pyrimidines and purines. J. Chem. Phys., 48:2940-2946.

Sidman, J. W., and D. S. McClure. 1955a. Electronic and vibrational states of biacetyl and biacetyl-d_6. I. Electronic states. J. Amer. Chem. Soc., 77:6461-6470.

———— and D. S. McClure. 1955b. Electronic and vibrational states of biacetyl and and biacetyl-d_6. II. Vibrational states. J. Amer. Chem. Soc., 77:6471-6474.

Smith, F. J., J. K. Smith, and S. P. McGlynn. 1962. Low-temperature double-path absorption cell. Rev. Sci. Instrum., 33:1367-1371.

Sponer, H., Y. Kanda, and L. A. Blackwell. 1960. Triplet-singlet emission spectra of benzene in a crystalline matrix of cyclohexane at 4.2°K and 77°K. Spectrochim. Acta, 16:1135-1147.

Steele, R. H., and A. Szent-Györgyi. 1957. On excitation of biological substances. Proc. Nat. Acad. Sci. U.S.A., 43:477-491.

Streitwieser, A., Jr. 1961. Molecular Orbital Theory for Organic Chemists. New York and London, John Wiley and Sons, Inc.

Teplyakov, P. A. 1963. Quasilinear phosphorescence spectra of phenanthrene solutions. Opti. Spectr. (USSR), 15:645-650 (C.A. 60:4972d).

Terenin, A., and V. Ermolaev. 1956. Sensitized phosphorescence in organic solutions at low temperature. Energy transfer between triplet states. Trans. Faraday Soc., 52:1042-1052.

Tolmach, L. J. 1951. The influence of triphosphopyridine nucleotide and other physiological substances upon oxygen evolution from illuminated chloroplasts. Arch. Biochem. Biophys., 33:120-142.

Truong, T., R. Bersohn, P. Brumer, C. K. Luk, and T. Tao. 1967. Effect of pH on the phosphorescence of tryptophan, tyrosine, and proteins. J. Biol. Chem., 242:2979-2985.

Van Duuren, B. L. 1961. Solvent effects in the fluorescence of indole and substituted indoles. J. Org. Chem., 26:2954-2960.

———— and C. E. Bardi. 1963. Reflectance fluorescence spectra of aromatic compounds in potassium bromide pellets. Anal. Chem., 35:2198-2202.

———— T.-L. Chan, and F. M. Irani. 1968. Luminescence characteristics of aflatoxins B_1 and G_1. Anal. Chem., 40:2024-2027.

Vladimirov, Iu. A., and E. A. Burshtein. 1960. Luminescence spectra of aromatic amino acids and proteins. Biophysics, 5:445-453.

Weber, G. 1960. Fluorescence-polarization spectrum and electronic-energy transfer in proteins. Biochem. J., 75:345-352.

Wehry, E. L. 1967. Structural and environmental factors in fluorescence. In Guilbault, G. G., ed., Fluorescence Theory, Instrumentation, and Practice, 91. New York, Marcel Dekker, Inc.

Weller, A. 1961. Fast reactions of excited molecules. Progr. Reaction Kinetics, 1:187-214.

Wilkinson, F. 1962. Transfer of triplet state energy and the chemistry of excited states. J. Phys. Chem., 66:2569-2574.

Winefordner, J. D., and H. W. Latz. 1963. Phosphorimetry as a means of chemical analysis. The analysis of aspirin in blood serum and plasma. Anal. Chem., 35:1517-1522.

———— and P. A. St. John. 1963. Solvents for phosphorimetry. Anal. Chem., 35:2211-2212.

———— and M. Tin. 1964. The use of rigid ethanolic solutions for the phosphorimetric investigation of organic compounds of pharmacological interest. Anal. Chim. Acta, 31:239-245.

———— and M. Tin. 1965. Phosphorimetric determination of procaine, phenobarbital, cocaine, and chlorpromazine in blood serum, and cocaine and atropine in urine. Anal. Chim. Acta, 32:64-72.

Zander, M. 1967. Electron spectra of acene quinones. Ber. Busenges. Phys. Chem., 74:424-429 (C.A. 67:37927s).

Zudin, A. A. 1959. Phosphorescence spectra of some phenols at liquid-oxygen temperature, Izv. Akad. Nauk SSSR, Ser. Fiz., 23:142 (C.A. 53:11989i).

Chapter **4**

The Application of Circular Dichroism and Optical Rotatory Dispersion to Problems in Pharmacology

Colin F. Chignell

Laboratory of Chemical Pharmacology, National Heart and Lung Institute, National Institutes of Health, Bethesda, Maryland

And

Derek A. Chignell

Department of Biological Chemistry
University of California School of Medicine
Los Angeles, California

INTRODUCTION

The interaction which occurs between radiation and matter is greatly dependent upon both the intensity and the wavelength of radiation used. Microwaves, for example, are capable of increasing very rapidly the vibrational or translational energy of whole molecules; such energy is subsequently dissipated as heat. In contrast, radiation of short wavelength (such as x-radiation) is capable of breaking interatomic bonds within molecules very efficiently. However, at lower intensity levels, radiation will not cause irreversible changes in the material with which it is interacting over brief periods of time, but will instead provide powerful methods of exploring its architecture. The wavelength of radiation used, compared with the size of the molecules being observed, will decide quite clearly the amount of detail and the type of information that we can obtain. A simple analogy will illustrate this: electromagnetic radiation may be compared with the waves of the sea. The interaction between a molecule and microwaves would be like a number of beach balls being bounced up and down by the waves. One beach ball will move much like another without affecting the shape or direction of the waves to any measurable extent. The waves will not detect slight imperfections in the shape or the surface of the ball because they are larger than the ball itself. However, x-rays interacting with a molecular array would be more like the sea surrounding a small island. Every physical feature of the island will affect the manner in which waves break or are deflected, and the shape of the island will be clearly established because each wave is small in comparison with the whole island itself. In a similar way, x-rays have wavelengths equal to or less than the molecular dimensions within a molecule, so that much of the atomic detail of a molecule becomes available by studying the way in which the x-rays have been deflected or attenuated after passing through the material.

Most optical methods fall into the region of radiation between these two extremes and will provide valuable insights into the overall size, shape, and symmetry of the molecules, together with information about the environment of specific groups of atoms, when these have unique optical properties within the molecule which enable them to be studied separately from the rest. To complete our analogy, the use of optical methods in the infrared, visible, and ultraviolet wavelength regions would perhaps be like a small pleasure-craft at sea, undoubtedly affected by the motion of the waves, but nevertheless sufficiently large to deflect them to some extent since the dimensions of the waves and the boat are of approximately the same order of magnitude. In this chapter we will consider one way in which a beam of light may be changed by interaction with matter and the direct application of this phenomenon to the study of drug interactions with biological systems.

THEORETICAL CONSIDERATIONS

The Origin of Optical Activity

Electromagnetic radiation has associated with it electric and magnetic fields oscillating at right angles to each other in a plane perpendicular to the direction of propagation of the beam. Simple optical methods permit the dispersion and

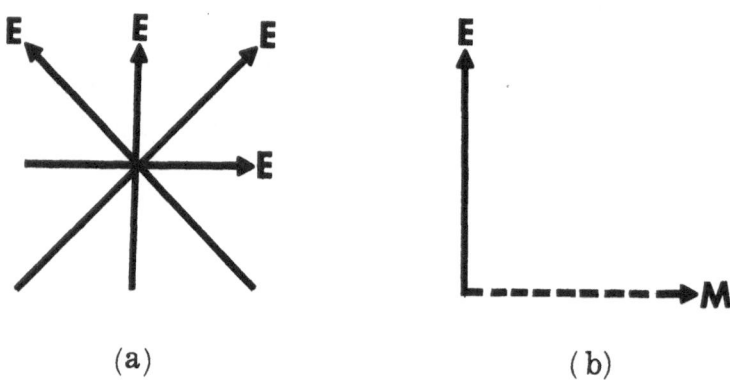

FIG. 1. Diagrammatic representation of electromagnetic radiation. *A.* Unpolarized oscillations of electric vector (**E**) in all directions within the plane (magnetic vectors **M** are not shown). *B.* Polarized radiation showing both the electric and magnetic (**M**) vectors. The direction of propagation is perpendicular to the plane of the paper.

collimation of radiation so that light of only one wavelength (monochromatic) is obtained. Monochromatic light may then be polarized to obtain an electromagnetic beam in which the electric vector E oscillates in one plane only along a determined direction in space (Figure 1). Solutions, thin films, and crystals of many substances, whether they be inorganic, organic, or biological, will interact with such a polarized beam when placed in its path. Many chemical groups have energy transitions which are of the same order of magnitude as those of the electric vector of polarized light, so that energy is freely exchanged between the two and, consequently, the resultant emerging ray may be modulated in a number of ways. A film or crystal in which the molecules are aligned in one specific direction will frequently decrease the intensity of a polarized beam of light passed through it to an extent dependent upon the plane of orientation of the molecules with respect to the plane of polarization of the incident beam (Figure 2). Such a sample is said to exhibit "linear dichroism." In the infrared region of the spectrum linear dichroism can give very valuable details about the direction of orientation of a particular chemical group such as the backbone carbonyl groups in polypeptide chains (Holzwarth et al., 1962; Fasman et al., 1970).

In a solution, the solute molecules are randomly oriented in a dynamic situation produced by thermal motion, but two extremely important physical effects can be detected when a plane polarized beam of light is passed through. First, the plane of polarization may be rotated; this is referred to as *optical rotation*. The origin of this may best be explained by considering the wave of plane polarized light to be comprised of two components of fixed magnitude rotating in an opposite sense to one another with the same center of rotation, and exactly in phase (Figure 3a). Since these components are moving along a straight line perpendicular to the plane of rotation, the resultant motion in three dimensions for each component is helical; the left-handed component is referred to as a left circularly polarized wave, E_L; and the right-handed component as a right circularly polarized wave, E_R. When radiation passes through any medium it will be retarded, the refractive index being a measure of this retardation. In a solution exhibiting no optical activity, both components of a beam of wavelength λ are retarded to the same extent (i.e., the refractive indices for the two components are the same) and the resultant emerges polarized in the same plane as it entered. However, when the polarized beam traverses an optically active solution, the two components are retarded to different

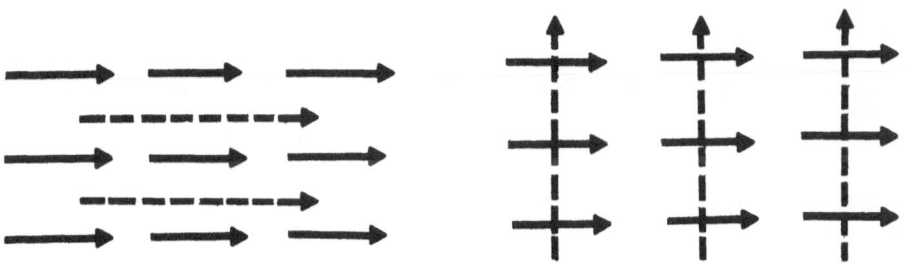

FIG. 2. The interaction of a plane polarized beam of light (- - - →) with a film or crystal containing molecules lined up in a regular ray (——→).

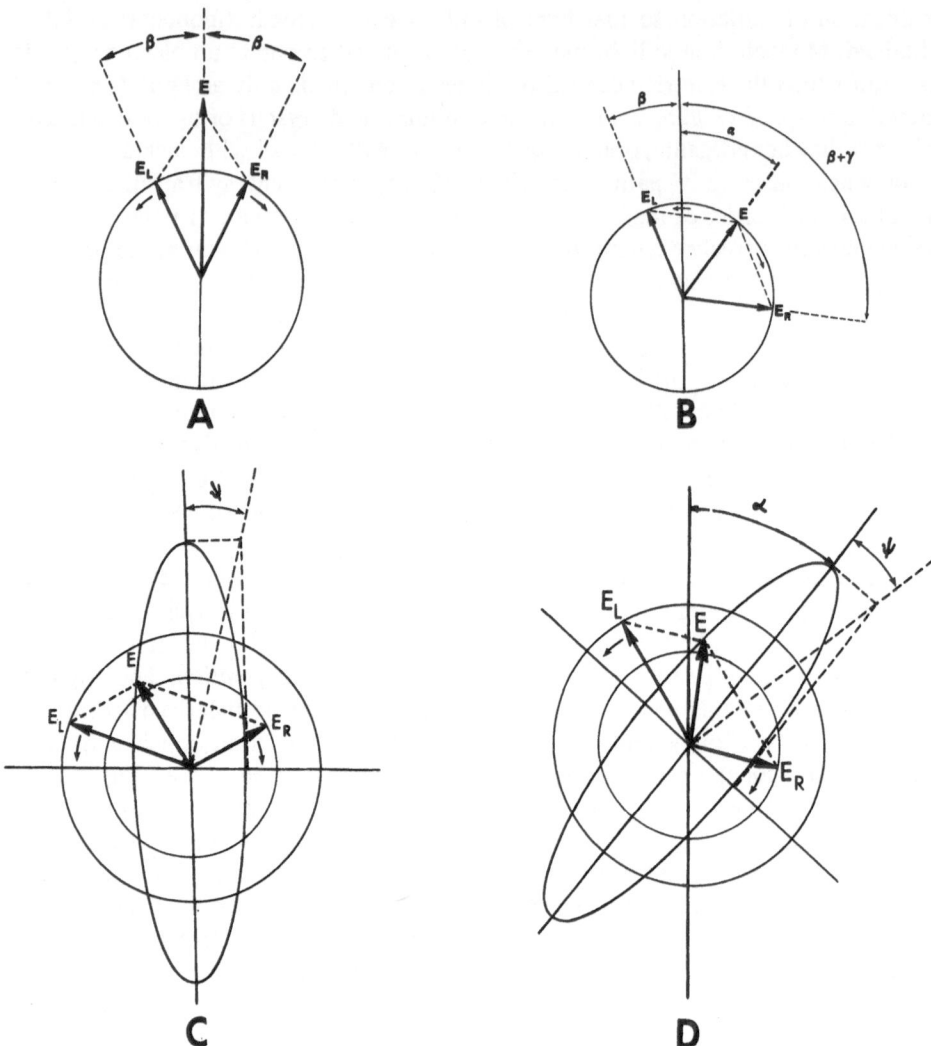

FIG. 3. *A.* Plane polarized light before it enters an optically active medium showing the elec-
tric vector, E, as the resultant of two rotating vectors $\mathbf{E_R}$ and $\mathbf{E_L}$. *B.* The rotation (α) of plane
polarized light emerging from an optically active medium. Note that the relative magnitudes of
the rotating vectors $\mathbf{E_R}$ and $\mathbf{E_L}$ are still the same but that they are out of phase by an angle
γ. *C.* The ellipticity (ψ) of plane polarized light emerging from an optically active medium at a
wavelength where light is absorbed but optical rotation is zero (see FIG. 4). Note that the vectors
$\mathbf{E_R}$ and $\mathbf{E_L}$ are in phase but have different magnitudes. *D.* The rotation (α) and ellipticity (ψ) of
plane polarized light emerging from an optically active medium in the absorption wavelength
range. The direction of propagation of the light is perpendicular to the phase of the paper.

extents; this is because the refractive indices of the solution are different for the
two components. The emergent ray will thus be composed of the two circularly
polarized components, still of the same magnitude but out of phase (Figure 3b).
The resultant of these two components, E, proves to be a plane polarized beam

emerging at an angle to the entering one. This is designated α_λ, the angle of rotation for this solution. Quantitatively, Fresnel (Crabbé, 1965) showed that the rotation (α_λ°) measured in radians per unit pathlength is related to the difference in refractive index for left (n_L) and right (n_R) circularly polarized light by the equation:

$$\alpha_\lambda^\circ = \frac{\pi}{\lambda}\,(n_L - n_R) \tag{1}$$

The second physical effect which a plane polarized beam experiences is that the two circularly polarized components may be differentially absorbed. This difference in intensity will have a profound effect on the resultant beam, which will no longer be oscillating in one direction; the end of the resultant vector will describe an ellipse, completing one revolution for every complete revolution of the two components. In the absence of optical rotation, this differential absorption would produce an ellipse with its major axis coinciding with the plane of oscillation of the entering beam (Figure 3c). This second phenomenon is called *circular dichroism* (CD). As the difference in magnitude of the two emergent components increases, so the ratio of minor axis to major axis of the ellipse will increase and this will be a measure of the circular dichroism of the solution. In Figure 3c this ratio is actually the tangent of the angle designated ψ; so to produce an analogous equation to that for optical rotation we define this angle ψ_λ as the ellipticity of the solution. To a good approximation we may write

$$\psi_\lambda^\circ = \frac{\pi}{\lambda}\,(K_L - K_R) \tag{2}$$

where ψ_λ° is the ellipticity in radians per unit pathlength at wavelength λ, and K_L and K_R are the absorption coefficients for the left and right circularly polarized components of the incoming plane polarized ray (Crabbé, 1965). At most wavelengths for a given sample, both optical rotation and circular dichroism will be observed, in which case the ellipse produced by circular dichroism will have its major axis rotated through an angle α, the optical rotation of that sample (Figure 3d).

Very little information can be obtained simply from a measurement at one wavelength. However, the profile of optical rotation over a wavelength range will enable us to recognize features belonging to various groupings within the molecule. This profile is referred to as the *optical rotatory dispersion* (ORD) of the sample. The term circular dichroism (CD) is used interchangeably for both isolated values at one wavelength, and for the whole profile over a wavelength span.

In the development of these two optical techniques, the units for measurement have changed somewhat. For the purpose of consistency, we give the modern usage and define the following units of measurement:

$$[\alpha]_\lambda = \frac{10^4 \cdot \alpha_\lambda}{l \cdot C} \tag{3}$$

where $[\alpha]_\lambda$ is "specific rotation" at wavelength λ for a given substance; α_λ is measured rotation in degrees for a solution of concentration C (gm/liter) and pathlength l (cm).

Also,

$$[\phi]_\lambda = [\alpha]_\lambda \cdot \frac{M}{100} \tag{4}$$

where $[\phi]_\lambda$ is "molecular rotation," M is molecular weight of substance,

and thus,

$$[\phi]_\lambda = \frac{100\,M\,\alpha_\lambda}{C \cdot l} \tag{5}$$

Similarly for circular dichroism, we may define the following:

$$[\psi]_\lambda = \frac{10^4 \cdot \psi_\lambda}{l \cdot C} \tag{6}$$

where ψ_λ is "specific ellipticity" at wavelength λ for a given substance.
Then also

$$[\theta]_\lambda = [\psi]_\lambda \cdot \frac{M}{100} \tag{7}$$

where $[\theta]_\lambda$ is "molecular ellipticity,"
and thus

$$[\theta] = \frac{100\,M \cdot \psi_\lambda}{C \cdot l} \tag{8}$$

One final correlation needs to be made. The relation between ellipticity and the difference between the absorption of left and right circularly polarized light has already been explained. It may be shown to a good approximation that:

$$[\theta]_\lambda \sim 3300 \cdot (\varepsilon_L - \varepsilon_R) = 3300\,\Delta\varepsilon \tag{9}$$

where ε_L, ε_R are the molar extinction coefficients for left and right circularly polarized light, respectively (Crabbé, 1965), and $\Delta\varepsilon$ is the differential dichroic absorption. This enables us to obtain $[\theta]_\lambda$ either from a measurement of ψ_λ or of $(\varepsilon_L - \varepsilon_R)$ depending on the optical system of the instrument used.

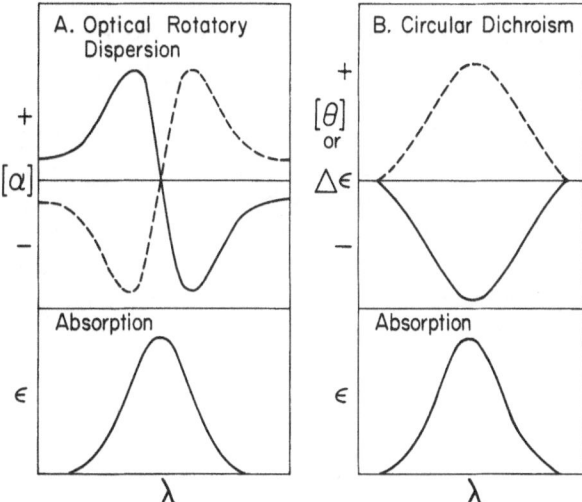

FIG. 4. Optical rotatory dispersion (*A*) and circular dichroism (*B*) curves associated with an optically active chromophore. Positive Cotton effect (- - - -); negative Cotton effect (——). The lower curves represent the absorption spectra of the optically active chromophore. Wavelength increases from left to right. (From Chignell, 1970b. *Proc. Fourth Int. Cong. Pharmacol.*, 1:218.)

The Cotton Effect

The combination of unequal absorption (circular dichroism) and unequal velocity of transmission (optical rotation) of left and right circularly polarized light in the wavelength region where an optically active absorption band occurs is called the "Cotton effect," after the discoverer of this phenomenon (Crabbé, 1965). The appearance of a simple Cotton effect, i.e., one involving a single optically active absorption band, is shown in Figure 4. Outside the wavelength region where the optically active chromophore absorbs light, the ORD curve is generally featureless (unless of course other optically active absorption bands are present in the molecule) and is therefore termed "plain." Plain dispersion curves are called positive or negative depending on whether they increase or decrease with decreasing wavelength. However, in the wavelength region where the optically active chromophore absorbs light, the ORD curve becomes anomalous, often changing sign (Figure 4). When the peak occurs at a longer wavelength than the trough, then the Cotton effect is termed positive. Conversely, when the trough occurs first, the Cotton effect is negative (Figure 4). An ORD band is characterized by (a) the breadth of the curve, i.e., the difference between the wavelengths at which the two extrema occur; (b) the wavelength at which rotation is zero and the curve inverts its sign (this is usually at or near the wavelength of maximum light absorption); and (c) the molecular amplitude, *a*, which is given by

$$a = \frac{[\phi_1] - [\phi_2]}{100} \qquad (10)$$

where $[\phi_1]$ is the molecular rotation of the extremum (peak or trough) at the longer wavelength, and $[\phi_2]$ is the molecular rotation of the extremum at the shorter wavelength.

In contrast to ORD, CD is observed only in the wavelength region where the optically active chromophore absorbs light (Figure 4). The CD band often resembles the absorption band in shape, with the extremum of CD occurring at or near the wavelength of maximum light absorption. The CD band may have a positive or negative sign (Figure 4). A CD band may be characterized by (a) the wavelength of maximum CD; (b) the half-width of the band; and (c) its "optical anisotropy" (or dissymmetry factor), g (Kuhn, 1930), which is given by

$$g = \frac{\Delta\varepsilon_\lambda}{\varepsilon_\lambda} \tag{11}$$

where $\varepsilon_\lambda =$ the molar extinction coefficient (for nonpolarized light), and $\Delta\varepsilon_\lambda$ is the differential dichroic absorption at wavelength λ.

The molecular amplitude, a, of an ORD curve for a single transition has been shown as a corollary of the Kronig-Kramer theorem (Moscowitz, 1960) to be related, to a first approximation, to the differential dichroic absorption, $\Delta\varepsilon$, of a CD curve by the equation

$$a = 40.28\ \Delta\varepsilon \tag{12}$$

and to molar ellipticity, $[\theta]$, by

$$a = 0.0122\ [\theta] \tag{13}$$

Expressions such as (12) and (13) are of obvious interest since they allow correlations to be made between ORD and CD spectra. It must be emphasized, however, that these relationships were obtained for the n-π^* transitions of a carbonyl group so that they may not be valid for other chromophores. In a situation where several transitions are involved, the more general form of the Kronig-Kramer equation should be used (Moffit and Moskowitz, 1959).

Some Theories of Optical Activity

In 1848, Pasteur (Lowry, 1964) published a classic paper in which he suggested that molecules could be divided into two classes: (a) those with superimposable mirror images, and (b) those with nonsuperimposable mirror images. He postulated that molecules belonging to the latter class had a "molecular dissymmetry" which conferred upon them an optical rotary power. Molecular dissymmetry was attributed to some form of dissymmetric grouping of atoms in a possibly helical or tetrahedral configuration. In 1874, Le Bel (Lowry, 1964) adopted the tetrahedral model for the carbon atom and associated optical activity with centers of asymmetry in the active compound. For example, the molecular dissymmetry of 3-methyl-*n*-hexane (Figure 5a,b) arises from the spatial arrangement of the hydrogen, methyl, ethyl, and *n*-propyl groups about the central or asymmetric carbon atom (often denoted by an asterisk). Van't Hoff in 1874 distinguished between two types of optically active compounds and attributed optical activity (a) to the presence of an asymmetric center in a molecule (Figure 5a,b), or (b) to the existence of an overall dissymmetry in a molecule containing no asymmetric centers (Lowry, 1964). Examples of compounds in this latter group include certain allenes, biphenyls (Figure 5c,d), alkylidenecycloalkanes, and spiranes.

In 1896, Drude formulated what was probably the first physical theory of optical activity based on the assumption that in a dissymmetric structure, charged particles are constrained to move along helical paths (Kauzmann, 1957). He suggested that the electrical and magnetic fields associated with an incident wave of electromagnetic radiation induced electronic motions, which in turn gave rise to electric and magnetic dipole moments in the molecule. Interactions between the fields produced by the helical electronic motions and the original electromagnetic wave would then result in optical activity. In 1916, Gray developed a theory which combined the ideas of geometrical molecular configuration set forth by Pasteur, Le Bel, and Van't Hoff, with the physical arguments of Drude's theory (Lowry, 1964). Gray's theory was subsequently modified by Born and Oseen (Lowry, 1964) and then presented in a somewhat simpler form by Kuhn and Braun (1930). However, although these theories were successful in explaining the phenomenon of optical activity and in deriving a useful set of empirical relations, they suffered from two serious limitations. First, the classical theory of electromagnetic radiation on which they were based did not account for the quantum nature of radiation; and second, the basic structural models employed by these theories were purely hypothetical in nature and did not correspond to the physical structure of atoms. In contrast, the quantum mechanical theory attributes optical activity to electronic transitions

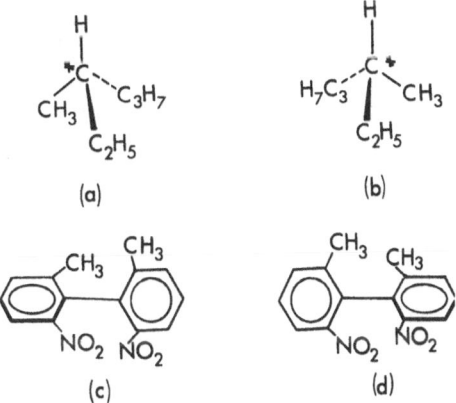

FIG. 5. The diastereoisomers of 2-methyl-*n*-pentane (a,b) and 1,1'-dimethyl-6,6'-dinitrobiphenyl (c,d).

occurring in the molecule (Moffit and Moscowitz, 1959; Rosenfeld, 1928). However, for most practical applications, a mixed theory combining the classical theory
of electromagnetic radiation and optics with the quantum mechanical concepts of
atomic and molecular structure has been found to be useful and consistent (Kauzmann, 1957).

THE OPTICALLY ACTIVE CHROMOPHORE

Moscowitz (1962) has classified optically active chromophores into two
extreme types: (a) the *inherently dissymmetric* chromophore, and (b) the inherently symmetric chromophore, which is *asymmetrically perturbed*. The optical
activity of compounds in the first class resides in the intrinsic geometry of the
chromophore. Good examples of this type of chromophore are certain biphenyls
(Figure 5c,d), allenes, as well as hexahelicine (Figure 6a). The latter compound
derives its dissymmetry from an overlap between rings 1 and 6, which confers upon
the molecule a somewhat helical form (Moscowitz, 1962).

A good example of the second type of chromophore is the carbonyl group,
which has two planes of symmetry (Crabbé, 1965). This group can, however,
become optically active if it is placed in a dissymmetric environment such as that
provided by the adjacent asymmetric carbon atom in 2-methylcyclohexanone (Figure 6b). Similarly, the optical activity of proteins and polypeptides in the random
conformation is due to perturbation of the peptide carbonyl groups (and the aromatic side chains) by the asymmetric α-carbon atoms. Alternatively, optical activity
may arise when symmetrical chromophoric groups have a dissymmetric arrangement in space. For example, the α-helical arrangement of the peptide carbonyl
groups in certain proteins and polypeptides gives rise to optical activity which is
superimposed upon that due to perturbation by the asymmetric α-carbon atoms. In
all these examples, the dissymmetric environment is provided by the molecule of
which the chromophore is a part, so that the resultant optical activity is called
intrinsic. However, if a symmetric chromophore present in one molecule interacts
with a dissymmetric environment provided by a second molecule, then *extrinsic*
optical activity is observed. For example, the carbonyl group of the symmetric drug
phenylbutazone becomes optically active when the drug binds to serum albumin

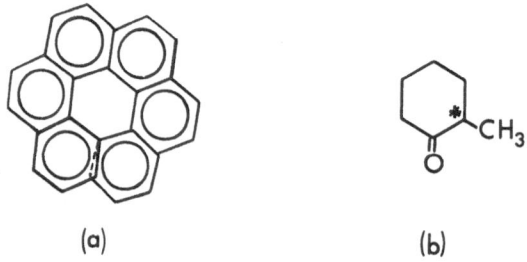

(a)   (b)

FIG. 6. Hexahelicene (a) and 2-methylcyclohexanone (b).

(Chignell, 1969a). Here, the dissymmetric environment is provided by the asymmetry of the protein binding site for the drug. Extrinsic optical activity can also be generated when the binding of a symmetrical chromophoric molecule to a macromolecule results in an asymmetric array of the chromophores in space. Blout and Stryer (1959) have reported, for example, that when acridine orange binds to α-helical poly-L-glutamic acid, the dye becomes optically active. When the α-helicity of the poly-L-glutamic acid was destroyed, then the bound dye became optically inactive.

Symmetry Rules

When a Cotton effect is generated by the interaction of a chromophore with a nearby locus of asymmetry (either in the same or another molecule), the sign of such induced optical activity is governed by the configuration of the asymmetric center and its spatial relationship to the perturbed chromophore. Schellman (1966, 1968) has shown that the space around such a chromophore may be divided into regions of positive and negative contribution to a Cotton effect, according to well-defined symmetry rules. The latter are determined by the symmetry of the perturbed transition. Examples of the simplest type of interaction are the purines and pyrimidines, which obey a planar rule, with the plane of the π-electron system as the nodal plane. Placing an asymmetric center on one side of the plane will give a Cotton effect. Moving it to the other side will reverse the effect (Schellman, 1966, 1968). The extrinsic Cotton effect induced in ATP on binding to creatine-ATP transphosphorylase is thus explainable if there is a preferred side for binding to the protein (Ulmer and Vallee, 1965). For extrinsic Cotton effects, where the asymmetric center and the perturbed chromophore are not part of the same molecule, the rigidity of the ligand-macromolecule complex is of paramount importance. A loose complex may allow this ligand sufficient freedom of movement so that the protein asymmetric may be located in regions of positive and negative contribution to a Cotton effect. Under these conditions the individual contributions may cancel out so that no optical activity is observed.

INSTRUMENTATION

Measurement of Optical Rotation and Optical Rotatory Dispersion

VISUAL POLARIMETRY.   Simple visual polarimeters usually consist of a source of monochromatic light, a polarizer (fixed), a sample cell and an analyzer (rotatable) to which is attached a circular scale graduated in degrees (Figure 7). The most usual source of monochromatic light is the sodium vapor lamp, which has its principle emission line at 589 mμ. If the mercury lamp (with main emission lines at about 436 mμ, 546 mμ, and 579 mμ) is employed, then

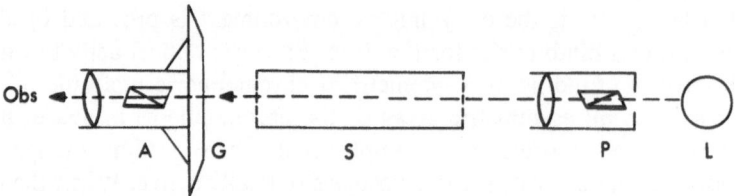

FIG. 7. Visual polarimeter. L, light source; P, polarizer; S, sample tube; G, scale graduated in degrees; A, analyzer.

filters must be used to render the light monochromatic. The Nicol prism analyzer and polarizer are made from specially cut calcite crystals which are cemented together with Canada balsam. Light entering the Nicol prism is resolved into two separate beams, the "ordinary" and the "extraordinary." The "ordinary" beam undergoes total internal reflection and is lost, while the plane-polarized "extraordinary" beam passes through the prism.

If the angle between the principal planes of the polarizer and analyzer is ϕ, the intensity of light, I, emerging from the analyzer is given by

$$I = I_0 \cos^2 \phi \tag{14}$$

where I_0 is the intensity of light from the polarizer which is incident on the analyzer. When the principal planes of the polarizer (P) and analyzer (A) are at right angles (Figure 8a) then

$$I = I_0 \cos^2 90° = 0 \tag{15}$$

so that no light emerges from the analyzer. If now a sample having a rotation of $+\alpha$ is placed between the polarizer and analyzer (Figure 8b) light will once more emerge from the analyzer with the intensity given by

$$I = I_0 \cos^2 (90° - \alpha) = I_0 \sin^2 \alpha \tag{16}$$

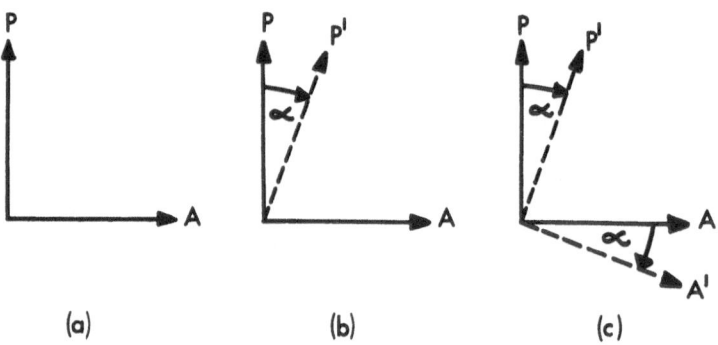

(a)   (b)   (c)

FIG. 8. The principle of optical rotation measurements. For description see text.

If the analyzer is then rotated by $+\alpha$ (Figure 8c) no light will emerge, since

$$I = I_0 \cos^2 (90° - \alpha + \alpha) = 0 \qquad (17)$$

Thus, the angle through which the analyzer must be rotated in order to reach the extinction point gives a direct measure of the optical rotation of the sample.

PHOTOELECTRIC SPECTROPOLARIMETERS. In the manual spectropolarimeter (Figure 9) the sodium lamp or mercury lamp is replaced by the xenon arc lamp, which provides continuous emission spectrum from 190 to 700 mμ. Light from the xenon lamp passes through a monochromator, which may be a single-prism (Figure 9) or a double-prism device. The monochromatic light then passes through the polarizer, the sample cell, and the analyzer, finally striking a photomultiplier tube (Figure 9). Finally the signal from the photomultiplier tube is amplified and displayed on a meter.

One of the main problems which was encountered with the first photoelectric polarimeters was the lack of precision in determining the extinction point. This is due to the small changes in light intensity per unit angle rotation of the analyzer which occur near the extinction point, as may readily be seen from the following equation

$$\frac{dI}{d\phi} = -I_0 \sin 2\phi \qquad (18)$$

so that when $\phi = 90°$, $dI/d\phi = 0$. The symmetrical angle method is now generally used to ensure a more accurate measurement of rotation angle. This is done by selecting two points having a sufficiently large value of $dI/d\phi$ positioned at angles $\pm \omega$ away from the extinction point. Since $(I = I_0 \cos^2 \phi)$ is symmetrical with respect to the extinction point $(\phi = 90°)$, the intensities of light passing through the analyzer are equal when the analyzer is rotated from the extinction point by

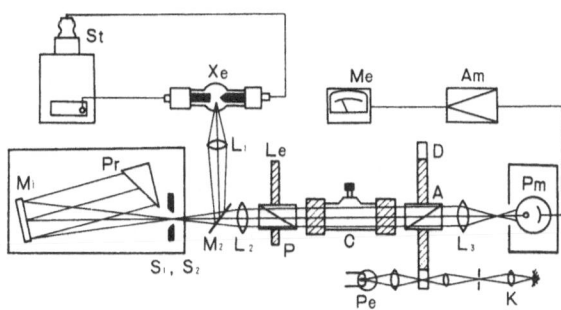

FIG. 9. Optical diagram of the Shimadzu QV 50 modified to measure optical rotatory dispersion. Xe, xenon lamp; L_1, L_2, L_3, lenses; S_1 and S_2, entrance and exit slits; M_1, collimating mirror; M_2, plane mirror; Pr, prism; P, polarizer; Le, polarizer shifting lever; C, sample cell; A, analyzer; Pm, photomultiplier; Me, zero meter; Am, amplifier; St, power supply for the xenon lamp; D, scale; K, microscope; Pe, illuminating lamp for scale. (Courtesy of Shimadzu Seisakusho Ltd.)

$+\omega$ or $-\omega$. Therefore, by measuring the angles ω_1 and ω_2 at which the intensities of light become equal, it is possible to calculate ω_0, the angle at which extinction occurs, from the relationship

$$\omega_0 = \frac{\omega_1 + \omega_2}{2} \tag{19}$$

In some instruments, e.g., Shimadzu QV-50, the polarizer is moved manually through a fixed angle (e.g., $\pm 2°$, $\pm 5°$, $\pm 10°$). The analyzer is then adjusted so that equal intensity of light passes through the analyzer when the polarizer is turned to the left or right. In this way, the angle of rotation can be read directly. In the Rudolph photoelectric polarimeter, the first device to employ the symmetrical angle principle, a motor-driven device oscillated the polarizer prism continuously at a preset symmetrical angle (Rudolph, 1955).

The first practical commercially available recording spectropolarimeter was provided by the Rudolph Company. This instrument had a single prism monochromator and operated on the symmetrical angle principle similar to that described for the manual spectropolarimeter. While the Rudolph recording spectropolarimeter is no longer available, a similar instrument, developed by the Japanese Spectroscopic Company, is currently offered by the Durrum Instrument Company. In this instrument (Figure 10) light from a xenon lamp passes through a double prism monochromator into a Rochon polarizing prism. The plane of polarization is alternately rotated left and right of the mean by a mechanical drive, which oscillates the polarizer through an angle of $\pm 1°$ at a frequency of 12 cps. The Rochon analyzing prism is fixed so that its plane of polarization is orthogonal (i.e., at right angles) to the mean angular position of the light beam from the polarizer. Since the polarizer oscillates symmetrically about its zero position, equal amounts of light are transmitted by the analyzer on oscillations to the right and left. This results in 24 equal pulses of light reaching the photomultiplier each second. When an optically active medium is placed in the sample cell, the plane of polarization of light from

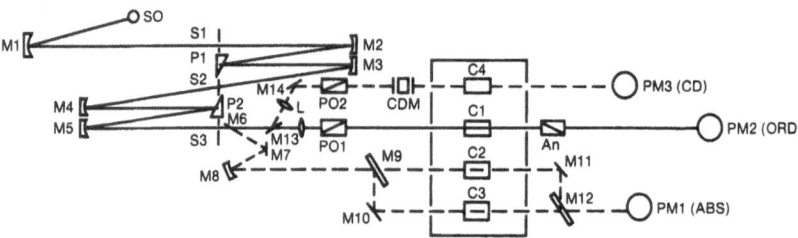

FIG. 10. Optical diagram of the Durrum-Jasco J-20 automatic recording spectropolarimeter. SO, xenon light source; M_1, source mirror; S_1, S_2, S_3, monochromator slits; $M_{2,3,4,5}$, collimating mirrors; P_1, P_2, prisms; L, lens; PO_1, ORD polarizer; C_1, ORD cell position; A_n, ORD analyzer; PM_2, ORD photomultiplier; M_6, retractable absorption mirror; M_7, plane mirror; M_8, spherical mirror; $M_{9,12}$, rotating sector mirrors; M_{10}, absorption mirror; $M_{10,11,14}$, absorption mirrors; M_{13}, retractable CD mirror; $C_{2,3}$, absorption sample and reference cell positions; PM_1, absorption photomultiplier; PO_2, CD polarizer; C_4, CD cell position; CDM, CD modulator (Pockels cell); PM_3, CD photomultiplier. (Courtesy of the Durrum Instrument Company.)

the polarizer is rotated. If the polarizer continues to oscillate about the zero position, the light pulses reaching the detector will no longer be equal. The output from the detector is then used to drive a servo system that rotates the analyzer to a new null position. The angle through which the analyzer must be rotated to reach the null point is of course the optical rotation of the sample.

In 1963, the Applied Physics Division of Varian Corporation made available the Cary recording spectropolarimeter. The main features of this instrument were a double-prism monochromator, and the use of the magneto-optical effect (Faraday effect) for modulation of the polarized ray. In the Cary 60 recording spectropolarimeter (Figure 11) a Faraday cell (consisting of a silica cylinder surrounded by an electric coil) is placed between the sample and the analyzer prism. When an alter-

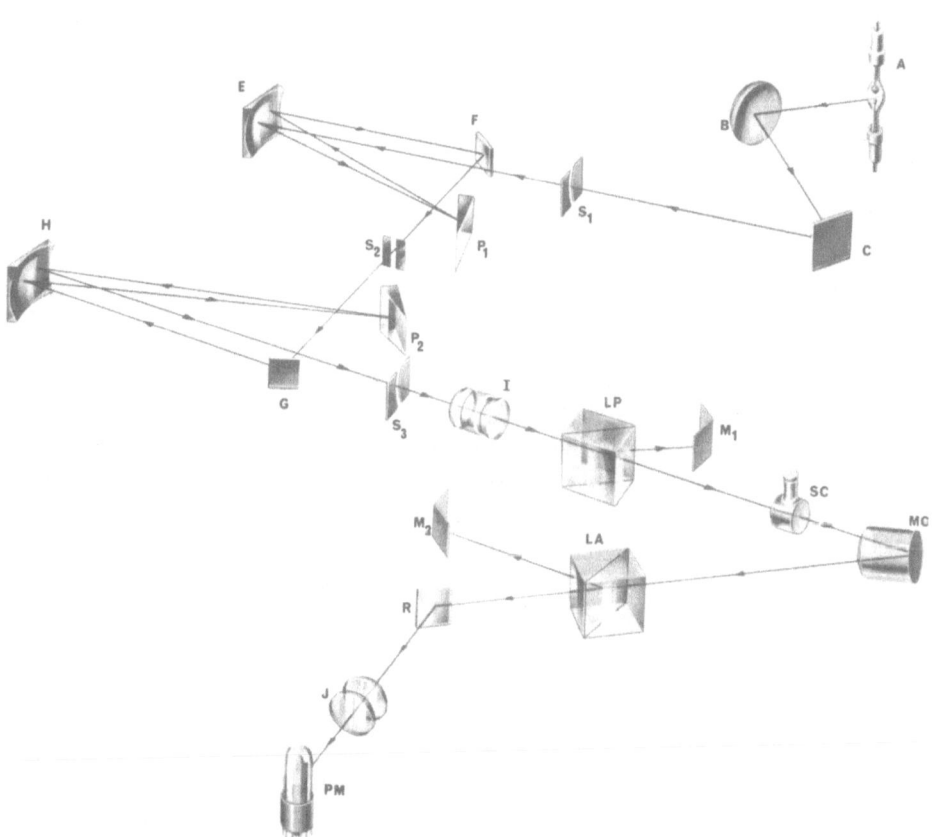

FIG. 11. Optical diagram of the Cary 60 automatic recording spectropolarimeter. A, Xenon arc lamp; B, mirror; $S_{1,2,3}$, slits; I, achromat lens; LP, linear polarizer; SC, sample cell; MC, modulator cell (Faraday cell); LA, linear analyzer; J, condensing lens; PM, photomultiplier tube. (Courtesy of Cary Instruments.)

nating current (60 cps) is passed through the coil the plane of polarization is displaced ($\pm 1.8°$ at 600 mμ) so that 120 pulses of light per second reach the detector. A motor energized by the amplified current from the photomultiplier tube moves the polarizer in a similar fashion to that described for the Durrum-Jasco instrument.

In the Spectropol 1 (F.I.C.A.) modulation of the polarized beam of light is also achieved by means of a Faraday cell (Figure 12). However, unlike the Cary 60, the polarizer and analyzer are fixed in the crossed position. Compensation is achieved by means of a second Faraday cell (Figure 12) which rotates the plane of polarization by an angle equal and opposite to that produced by the sample.

In the Bellingham-Stanley Polarmatic 62 the functions of monochromator and polarimeter are combined by using two crystalline quartz prisms which both disperse and polarize the radiation (Gilham and King, 1961). The two prisms are fixed in position and wavelength scanning is achieved by the rotation of two plane mirrors in unison about a common axis. The optical rotation of the sample is compensated for by means of a Faraday cell in a manner similar to that described for the Spectropol 1.

Some specifications of instruments for measuring ORD will be found in Table 1.

Measurement of Circular Dichroism

In a classic paper on optical activity published in 1896, Cotton described two types of apparatus which he designed and used to measure the CD of optically active copper and chromium tartrates (Abu-Shumays and Duffield, 1966). The first photographic instrument for measuring CD was described by Kuhn and Braun in 1930. Two decades later (Mitchell, 1950; Mitchell and Veitch, 1951) an accessory was designed which permitted the measurement of CD with a single-beam photoelectric spectrophotometer. An improved version of this accessory appeared in 1957 (Mitchell, 1957). The first automatic recording instrument for the measurement of CD was described by Grosjean and Legrand in 1960.

THE MANUAL CIRCULAR DICHROMETER. The only manually operated instrument currently available for the measurement of CD is supplied by Shimadzu Seisakusho Ltd. as an attachment for the QV-50 spectrophotometer. In this instrument (Figure 13) the beam of light (from a hydrogen-discharge lamp or a tungsten lamp) passes through a single prism monochromator and into the polarizer. Plane polarized light emerging from the polarizer prism enters the compensator where it is split into two orthogonally polarized components differing in phase by one quarter of a wavelength. These two components produce a circularly polarized beam of light which passes through the sample and impinges on the photomultiplier tube. The light emerging from the compensator (also known as a quarter-wave plate) may be either right or left circularly polarized depending on the angle between the principal plane of the polarizer and the principal axis of the compensator. The circular dichroism of the sample expressed as the dif-

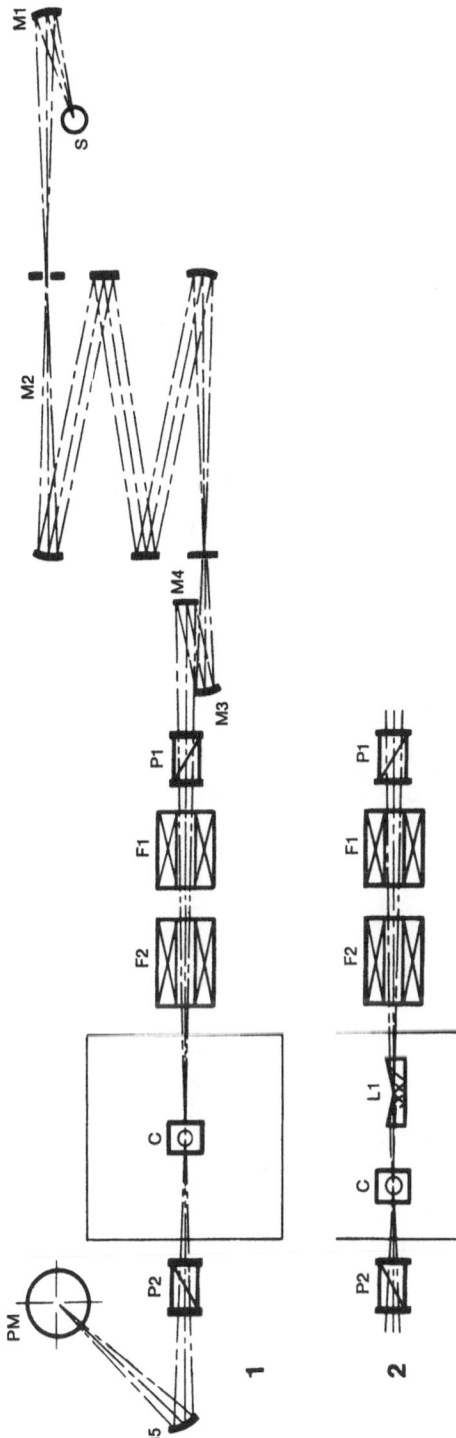

FIG. 12. Optical diagram of the Spectropol 1 automatic recording spectropolarimeter showing the optical rotatory dispersion (1) and circular dichroism (2) modes. S, light source; $M_{1,3,4,5}$, mirrors; M_2, monochromator; $P_{1,2}$, polarizers; $F_{1,2}$, Faraday cells; C, measuring cell; L_1, quarter-wave plate. (Courtesy of F.I.C.A.)

127

TABLE 1

Some Specifications of Instruments for Measuring Optical Rotatory Dispersion

Manufacturer and Name of Instrument	Type of Instrument	Wavelength Range	Sensitivity Limits	Type of Modulator	Special Features
Bellingham and Stanley Polarmatic 62	Recording Spectropolarimeter	181-666 mμ	Noise level 0.0002° at 546 mμ (5 mm pathlength methanol blank)	Faraday unit	Dispersion and polarization achieved by two quartz prisms Faraday unit used for compensation.
Cary Instruments Model 60	Recording Spectropolarimeter	185-600 mμ	RMS noise at 300 mμ, 0.0001° (30 sec pen period)	Faraday unit	Difference ORD measuring capability.
Durrum Instrument Corporation J-20	Recording Spectropolarimeter	185-800 mμ	RMS noise at 250 mμ, 0.0006° (20 sec pen period)	Oscillating polarizer (quartz Rochon)	Also records UV-visible absorption spectrum, slit width and multiplier signal
FICA Spectropol 1	Recording Spectropolarimeter	200-600 mμ		Faraday unit	Also uses a Faraday unit for compensation Magnetic ORD accessory available
Shimadzu Seisakusho QV-50	Manual Spectrophotometer with ORD attachment	210-700 mμ	± 0.002°	None (manual setting of polarization direction)	

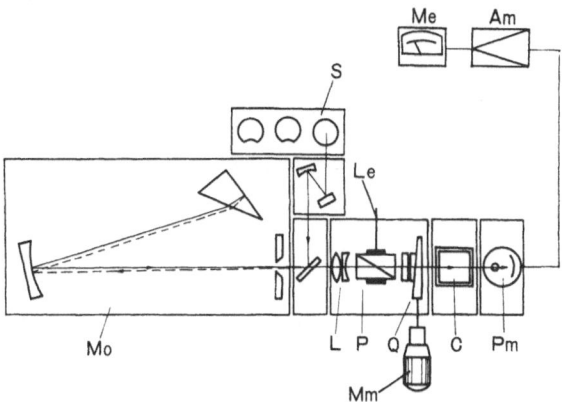

FIG. 13. Optical diagram of the Shimadzu QV-50 modified to measure circular dichroism. S, light source; Mo, monochromator; L, lens; Q, compensator; Pm, photomultiplier; Me, zero meter; Le, polarizer rotating lever; Mm, micrometer; Am, amplifier, C, sample cell. (Courtesy of Shimadzu Seisakusho Ltd.)

ferential dichroic absorption, $\Delta\varepsilon$, is calculated directly from the transmission of the left and right circularly polarized beams of light.

THE AUTOMATIC RECORDING CIRCULAR DICHROMETER. In the automatic recording circular dichrometer modulation of the direction of polarization is achieved by means of a Pockels cell, which consists of a uniaxial crystal of ammonium dihydrogen phosphate. When an electrical field is applied across the crystal it becomes biaxial and acts as a quarter-wave plate in much the same way as the compensator in the manual instrument. However, in the Pockels cell the sign of the circularly polarized light is determined by the direction of the applied field. If the applied field oscillates, then alternately left and right circularly polarized light will be transmitted through the sample (Figures 10 and 14) and, in the absence of an optically active sample, equal pulses of light reach the photomultiplier. When the light passes through a sample that exhibits a difference in absorption between left and right circularly polarized light, the output voltage of the photomultiplier tube will contain an alternating component superimposed on an average component; the alternating voltage is related to the difference in transmission of the sample for left and right circularly polarized light while the average voltage is related to the average transmission of the sample. The ratio of these two is proportional to the difference in absorption of the sample for left and right circularly polarized light. The first instrument to use the Pockels cell was described in 1960 by Grosjean and Legrand. A number of commercial instrument manufacturers, e.g., Societé Jouan, Cary Instruments (Figure 14) and the Durrum Instrument Company (Figure 10), are currently marketing spectropolarimeters capable of measuring circular dichroism employing the Pockels cell (see Table 2).

The Spectropol 1 circular dichrometer does not employ a Pockels cell but uses instead a quarter-wave plate known as a Fresnel prism (Figure 12). Plane polarized light that has traversed a Fresnel prism emerges elliptically polarized with an ellipticity of $|\psi| = |\alpha|$, where α is the angle between the plane of polar-

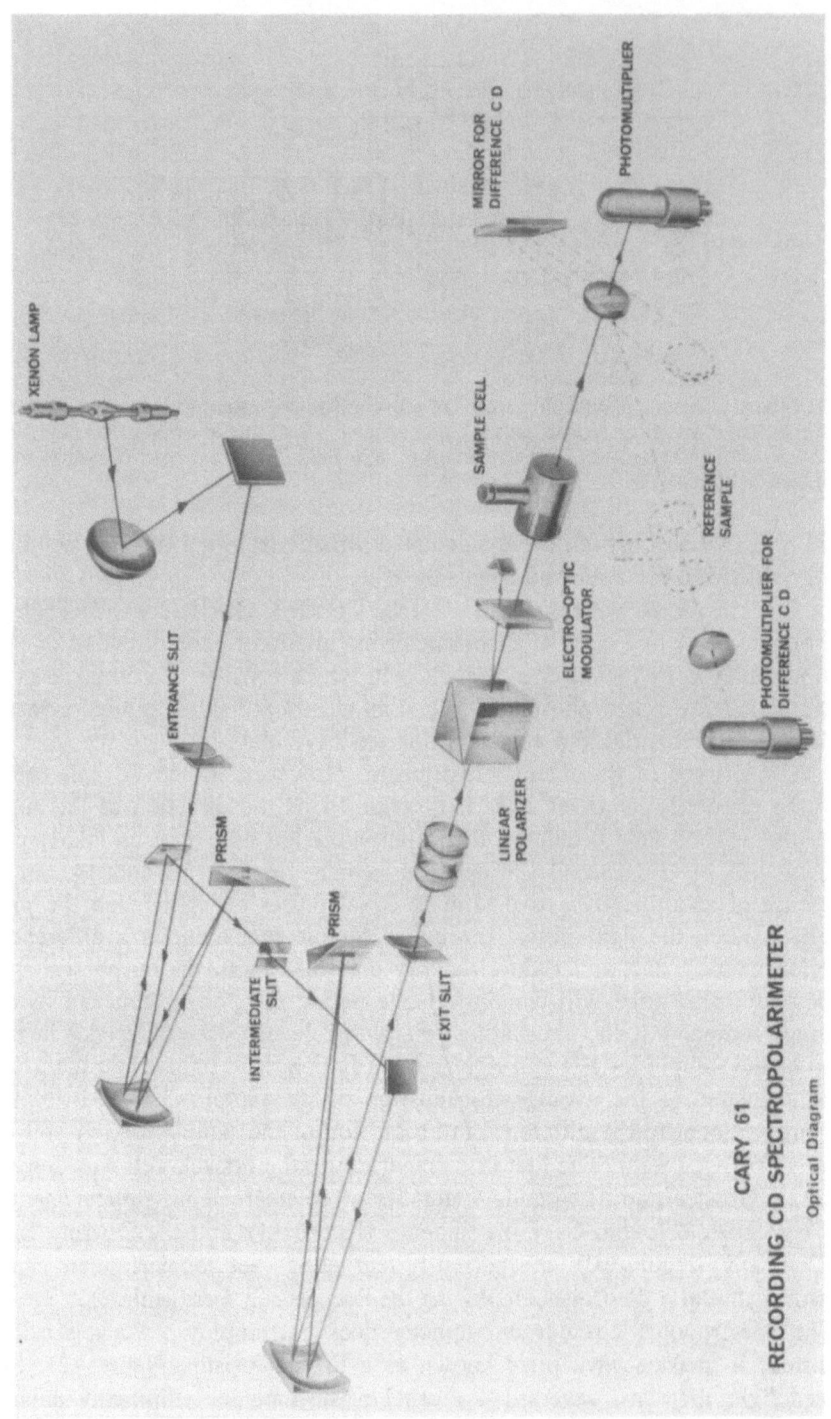

CARY 61

RECORDING CD SPECTROPOLARIMETER

Optical Diagram

FIG. 14. Optical diagram of the Cary 61 recording circular dichrometer. (Courtesy of Cary Instruments.)

TABLE 2

Some Specifications on Instruments for Measuring Circular Dichroism

Manufacturer and Name of Instrument	Type of Instrument	Wavelength Range	Sensitivity Limits	Type of Circular Polarizer	Special Features
Bellingham and Stanley Polarmatic 62	Recording circular dichrometer	181-666 mμ	Noise level 0.0002° (5 mm pathlength methanol blank)	Fresnel prism	Faraday unit used for compensation
Cary Instruments Model 60	Recording circular dichrometer	185-600 mμ	RMS noise at 250 mμ 0.0005° (10 sec time constant)	Pockels cell	Magnetic CD attachment available
Cary Instruments Model 61	Recording circular dichrometer	185-600 mμ	RMS noise at 250 mμ 0.0004° (30 sec pen period)	Pockels cell	CD difference capability All solid state
Cary Instruments Model 1402	CD accessory for Cary Model 14	200-700 mμ	2.5×10^{-4} absorbance units	Pockels cell	UV-visible absorption spectrum may be recorded with accessory mounted
Durrum Instrument Corporation J-20	Recording circular dichrometer	185-800 mμ	RMS noise at 250 mμ 0.0007° (5 sec pen period)	Pockels cell	Magnetic CD attachment available Differential CD accessory
FICA Spectropol 1	Recording circular dichrometer	200-600 mμ	± 0.001° peak to peak at 300 mμ	Fresnel prism	Faraday unit used for compensation
Roussel-Jouan Model CD-185	Recording circular dichrometer	185-600 mμ	RMS noise at 250 mμ 0.0005° (1.6×10^{-5} absorbance units)	Pockels cell	Magnetic CD (50K gauss) and controlled temperature ($-196°$ to $40° \pm 0.5°$) attachments available Flow dichroism attachment also available Vacuum type CD attachment also available for measurement in the 195mμ-1200 mμ range.
Shimadzu Seisakusho QV-50	Manual spectro-photometer with CD attachment	220-700 mμ	± 0.005 absorbance units	Babinet soleil compensator (manually adjusted)	

131

ization of the incident light and the principal plane of the prism. If this beam of elliptically polarized light now passes through an optically active sample which has an ellipticity equal and opposite to that produced by the Fresnel prism, then a plane polarized beam of light will emerge from the sample. The plane of polarization of the emerging beam will be the same as that of the beam incident on the Fresnel prism. In the Spectropol 1 the polarizer and analyzer are fixed in the crossed position. Plane polarized light passes through a Faraday cell modulator before entering the Fresnel prism. Elliptically polarized light from the Fresnel prism then enters the sample. Light emerging from the sample then passes through the analyzer and impinges on a photomultiplier tube. If the compensator rotates the plane of the polarized light entering the Fresnel prism so that light leaving the prism has an ellipticity equal but opposite to that of the sample, then light leaving the sample would once again be plane polarized and no light would reach the photomultiplier. The angle between the plane of polarization of light entering the Fresnel prism and the principal plane of the prism is then a direct measure of the ellipticity of the sample. Modulation of the beam of polarized light is achieved by means of a second Faraday cell inserted between the compensator and the Fresnel prism (Figure 12). The Fresnel prism is also employed in the Bellingham and Stanley Polarmatic 62 to permit the measurement of CD.

Some Practical Considerations

As with many instruments, the choice of conditions for maximum accuracy, sensitivity, and reproducibility is a compromise. The following factors will be of importance.
1. Choice of sample cell.
2. Absorbance of sample in comparison with its optical activity.
3. Choice of solvent.
4. Light scattering of sample.
        CHOICE OF SAMPLE CELL.   In the visual polarimeter, as well as in the early photoelectric polarimeters, 10- or 20-cm (sometimes even 40-cm) sample tubes were employed. However, the modern instruments generally have smaller sample compartments accommodating cells with 0.01- to 10-cm pathlengths. The choice of a sample cell will be determined by the following:
(1) Low strain birefringence.   As in spectrophotometry, silica is employed for the end-windows of cells to be used throughout the visible and ultraviolet wavelength ranges. Any kind of mechanical strain causes distortion of the silica crystal lattice and produces optical activity; the cell then has its own (often quite marked) optical rotation or circular dichroism, which may change considerably with wavelength. Appropriate blanks would of course allow for this, but in many cases this strain birefringence changes with time and is extremely sensitive to temperature changes and mechanical handling of the cell so that a significant decrease in reproducibility will occur.

(2) Temperature control. Thermostating of the instrument cell compartment is usually not an adequate means of keeping the sample at constant temperature, so for many purposes a jacketed cell will be important.

(3) Ease of filling. A cell with a small opening for introduction of a sample will be time consuming to fill and will also preclude titration studies where small amounts of material are added from a microburet. For drug binding studies in particular, this would be a distinct disadvantage.

Two types of sample cell are currently available. The first has a cell body made of glass or Teflon, at each end of which is a silica window held in place by plastic or rubber washers and a screw-cap device. Filling and cleaning are convenient, but the cell cannot be jacketed, and the mechanical stress necessary to hold the end-windows in place is often sufficient to cause some strain birefringence, varying with the degree of tightness of the screw-cap. The second design is a fixed window type manufactured by careful fusing and annealing processes which keep distortion to a minimum. Integral jacketed cells with a very low strain characteristic are marketed by the Opticell Corporation in a number of pathlengths and are very suitable for this purpose, though the filling entry is inconveniently small in some cases. Care must be taken not to force the ground-glass stoppers of these cells into their joints, since this may also cause strain birefringence. Some workers prefer simply to use a "Parafilm" seal and dispense with the stoppers altogether.

SAMPLE ABSORBANCE AND OPTICAL ACTIVITY. One of the basic operations in any measuring technique is to adjust the size (or pathlength) and concentration of a sample to bring the quantity measured into a range which can be adequately dealt with by the instrument. This is no less true of spectropolarimeters and circular dichrometers; if the measured rotation or ellipticity is small, base line errors due to lamp instability, cell birefringence, and so on will become a significant portion of the total signal and will therefore decrease precision. Instrument design will place an upper limit on the measured quantity also. However, solutions of biological macromolecules have a much smaller optical activity per unit absorbance at a given wavelength than most asymmetric organic compounds. Consequently, the absorbance of the sample in the wavelength region to be studied is usually the limiting factor for optical activity measurements. As absorption by the sample increases, the radiation reaching the photomultiplier tube decreases and the signal-to-noise ratio increases; at the same time stray light within the instrument may become a measurable fraction of the total flux received by the photomultiplier, causing further errors in measurement. Expressions have been derived for the optimum absorbance of a sample to give a maximum signal-to-noise ratio in both a circular dichrometer (Velluz et al., 1965) and a spectropolarimeter (Cary et al., 1964) and it is clear that it is advisable to work within optical densities of 0.5 and 1.2. In at least one early instrument, the upper limit for absorbance was even lower because of stray light problems (Resnick and Yamaoka, 1966) but subsequently increases in the output of the light source and improvements in optical deck design have reduced these errors considerably.

CHOICE OF SOLVENT. Because of the limitation on sample absorbance, it is clear that the solvent systems used for solution measurements should in general have as little absorbance as possible in the studied wavelength range. Although water is optically transparent down to 190 mμ, when buffers are employed, their selection may be critical. Acetate and carbonate buffers cannot be used in the ultraviolet region because of the absorbance of the carbonyl group, and large concentrations of chloride ion will also absorb significantly. Phosphate buffers are probably the best choice for the ultraviolet region, but even so their concentration should not be above 0.02 M. The use of very short pathlength cells and higher sample concentrations will decrease the solvent absorbance considerably (Gratzer, 1967).

LIGHT SCATTERING.   It is advisable to clarify solutions by passage through a suitable sintered glass filter or by brief centrifugation before making ORD or CD measurements. Suspended particulate matter will reduce sample transmission and cause short-term variability in measurement (if the particles are large enough) as they pass through the light beam. The extent to which suspended particles cause absolute errors in measurement of either ORD or CD is still not clear. Experiments have been carried out on samples containing suspended cell components (microsomes, cell membranes, and mitochondrial membranes) with some success (Lenard and Singer, 1966); moreover the addition of sulfur particles to DNA solutions appeared to have little or no effect on their ORD (Gratzer and McPhie, 1966). An analysis of some of the results on membranes by Urry and Ji (1968) seem to indicate possible distortion of optical activity profiles, but a recent theoretical approach (Ottaway and Wetlaufer, 1970) has shown that any contributions by light scattering are extremely small and that the observed differences are more likely to be due to structural differences in the membrane proteins themselves.

THE APPLICATION OF OPTICAL ROTATORY DISPERSION AND CIRCULAR DICHROISM TO PHARMACOLOGICAL PROBLEMS

The Interaction of Drugs and Other Small Molecules with Proteins

THE INTRINSIC OPTICAL ACTIVITY OF PROTEINS.   The ORD and CD profiles of proteins in the visible and ultraviolet wavelength region are a composite of a number of different types of contributions. We may summarize the situation as follows: The amide carbonyl group of the peptide backbone has a characteristic optical activity because of its proximity to the asymmetric α-carbon atom of the chain. Poly-α,L-glutamic acid in solution has a random-coil conformation above pH 6 (Imahori and Tanaka, 1959), and apart from some possible small contribution from γ-carboxylate groups at 243 mμ (Katchalski and Sela, 1958) may be considered to possess optical activity due only to the peptide chromophore (Figure 15). The presence of α-helix radically alters the CD and ORD spectra. The peptide chromophores are now spatially fixed in an effectively rigid structure so that the optical energy transitions are shifted and split (Figure 15). Other types of structure have been found in polypeptides, and undoubtedly these also contribute to the overall optical activity of proteins. Under certain conditions,

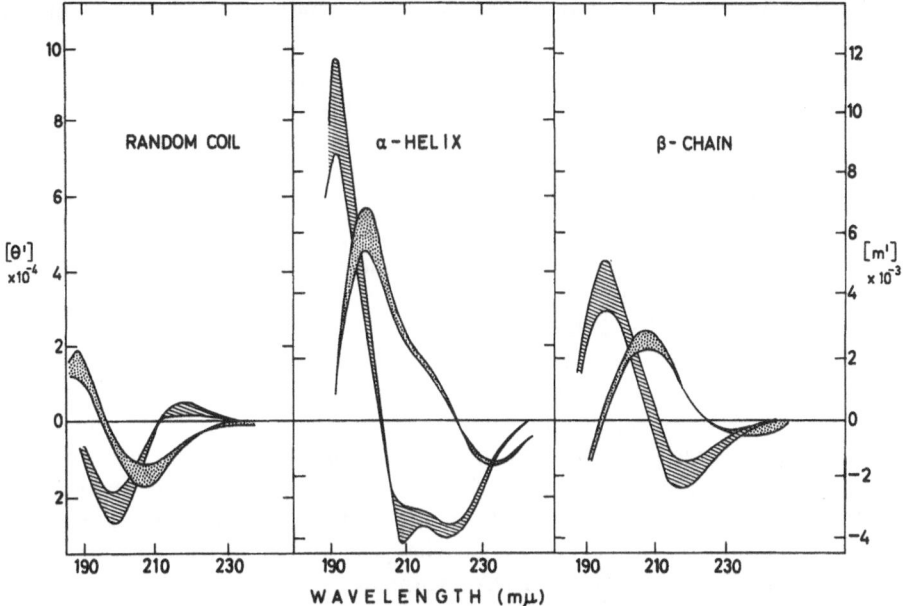

FIG. 15. Circular dichroism (cross-hatched) and optical rotatory dispersion (dotted) of homo-polypeptides in the random coil, α-helical and β-conformations. (From Gratzer and Cowburn. 1969. *Nature (London)*, 222:426. Courtesy of MacMillan [Journals] Ltd.)

polypeptides may be induced to order in a β-pleated sheet conformation (Pauling and Corey, 1951). Data from studies on poly-L-lysine (Sarker and Doty, 1966) and silk fibroin (Iizuka and Yang, 1966) is presented in a composite diagram in Figure 15.

Until recently, analysis of the ORD and CD of proteins below 240 mμ was often attempted on the assumption that only these three types of structure were present and that polypeptides were adequate models for this type of calculation. It must be pointed out, however, that although the α-helical structure is well defined and proteins consisting of all or almost all of this conformation accord well with theoretical prediction (Riddiford and Scheraga, 1962; Urnes and Doty, 1961), considerable variation occurs in the other two forms. Several types of β-conformation have already been found (Fasman and Potter, 1967), and unordered protein or polypeptide chain segments may not always be truly random-coil (Fasman et al., 1970). Specific predictions about the ORD and CD of proteins by reference to model polypeptide systems should therefore be made with much caution.

Superimposed upon these basic features may be "side-chain" Cotton effects. Tyrosine, tryptophan, and phenylalanine absorb in the ultraviolet wavelength region (270 to 290 mμ and below 240 mμ) and when these chromophores are constrained by the tertiary structure of the protein in an asymmetric environment, they may exhibit greatly enhanced optical activity based on the absorption maxima. The relative magnitude of these effects in comparison with those due to the peptide chromophore varies widely. In some cases, they are discernible only as slight discontinuities in an otherwise smooth ORD curve (Kronman et al., 1965) but they may be substantial enough to dominate the whole character of the ORD profile, such as in avidin (Green and Melamed, 1966). In addition we may note that the disulfide bond invariably exhibits optical activity (Beychok, 1965, 1968), but it is not always possible *a priori* to predict the sign or magnitude of these effects since they are modulated by the steric requirements of the groups attached; their position will be where the disulfide bond absorbs, between 240 mμ and 260 mμ. Extrinsic Cotton effects, which contribute other features to the ORD and CD spectra, are dealt with in this chapter (p. 138). A more comprehensive discussion of the optical activity of proteins and polypeptides will be found in Urnes and Doty (1961) and Gratzer and Cowburn (1969).

CHANGES IN THE INTRINSIC OPTICAL ACTIVITY OF PROTEINS DUE TO THE BINDING OF DRUGS OR OTHER SMALL MOLECULES. When a small molecule binds to a protein, changes in secondary, tertiary, or quaternary structure may result, that can often be detected as a change in the ORD or CD spectrum. The wavelength, magnitude, and character of these changes may indicate what type of transition is occurring. Pepsin, for example, has been shown to alter its optical activity in the 280 mμ region (Perlmann, 1970) presumably because an aromatic residue changes its asymmetric position, while aspartate-transcarbanylase, tyrosyl-RNA synthetase, and hemoglobin all exhibit some alteration in the peptide bond region (200 to 240 mμ). Table 3 lists these and other examples of the ligand-induced protein-conformation change.

TABLE 3

Some Enzymes and Other Proteins That Exhibit a Change
in Their Intrinsic Optical Activity on Binding
Substrate, Coenzyme, Inhibitor, or Other Ligand

Protein	Ligand	Reference
Alcohol dehydrogenase	DPNH DPNH-pyrazole DPNH-isobutyramide	Rosenberg et al. (1965)
Ribonuclease	Cytidine-3'-phosphate Cytidine-2'-phosphate Pyrophosphate	Cathou et al. (1965)
Glutamate dehydrogenase	DPNH ADP GTP	Magar (1965)
Glutamate Dehydrogenase	GTP DPNH	Bayley and Radda (1966)
Aspartate transcarbamylase	CTP Succinate Carbamylphosphate	Dratz and Calvin (1966)
Lipoyl dehydrogenase	FAD	Brady and Beychok (1968)
Tyrosyl-RNA-synthetase	RNA	Ohta et al. (1967)
Carnitine acetyltransferase	Various substrates	Tipton and Chase (1969)
Hemoglobin	Various ligands	Hanisch and Engel (1969)
Beta lipoprotein	Lipids	Gotto et al. (1968)

Both CD and ORD have been used extensively to study the interaction of detergents with proteins. Research in this particular area was pioneered by Jirgensons, who used first a manual polarimeter and then later a Rudolph spectropolarimeter. However, the interpretation of CD and ORD spectra from detergent-protein complexes is often difficult, since detergents may increase α-helical content, convert α-helical to β-structure, abolish β- but not α-helical structure, or simply act as denaturing agents. For a more detailed discussion of detergent-protein interactions, the reader is referred to a recent review by Perrin and Hart (1970).

Markus and Karush (1958) were the first to study the effect of anionic dyes on the optical rotation of HSA. Using a manual polarimeter, these workers found that the binding of several anionic azo dyes altered the specific rotation of HSA, with the strongly bound dyes causing the largest deviations. They suggested that these changes reflected alterations in the albumin molecule which involved the stabilization of configurations varying in helical content. It should be emphasized, however, that all these measurements were made at the sodium D line (589 mμ), so that these workers could also have been measuring extrinsic Cotton effects generated by the bound dyes rather than a change in the optical rotation of the protein. Indeed, one of the dyes used by Markus and Karush, 2-(4'-hydroxybenzeneazo)-benzoic acid, has been found to generate extrinsic optical activity on binding to HSA (Chignell, unpublished results). In somewhat similar experiments, Helmer et al. (1968) have measured the change in specific rotation of HSA when certain organic molecules bind to the protein, and they have related this change in optical activity to the octanol-water partition of the ligand. Once again, it is not possible to decide whether the observed change in relation is due to an alteration in protein configuration and/or to any extrinsic optical activity.

Sonenberg (1969) has reported that human growth hormone decreases the ellipticity of human red blood cell membranes at 222 mμ by 30% in phosphate buffer, but not in water. The necessity for the phosphate ion suggests that some organization of the membrane is required. Bovine growth hormone, bovine insulin, or cortisol were without effect. The possibility of studying drug interactions with membranes by measuring changes in the intrinsic optical activity of constituent proteins should be examined. Other examples of ligand induced changes in the intrinsic optical activity of proteins may be found in Table 3.

CHANGES IN THE INTRINSIC OPTICAL ACTIVITY OF A SMALL MOLECULE ON BINDING TO PROTEIN. Takagi and coworkers (1966) have reported that when flavin adenine dinucleotide binds to D-amino acid oxidase, the CD spectrum of the coenzyme changes sign from positive to negative without any appreciable shift in wavelength. This suggests that the coenzyme undergoes a specific conformational change on binding to the azoenzyme.

Since many drug molecules, particularly those of natural origin, are optically active, this particular approach may be of use in studying their interactions with biological systems. Those drugs in which there is free rotation between the chromophore and the asymmetric carbon atom would be the best candidates for such studies.

DRUGS AND OTHER SMALL MOLECULES THAT GENERATE EXTRINSIC OPTICAL ACTIVITY ON BINDING TO PROTEINS AND POLY-PEPTIDES.　A large number of small symmetrical molecules, including some dyes and drugs, that are optically inactive, become optically active when bound to certain proteins and polypeptides (Table 4). In addition, many substrates, coenzymes, and inhibitors become optically active when they interact with the appropriate enzyme (Table 4). These extrinsic Cotton effects may be divided into two distinct groups according to their origin. In the first group (Table 4, type I) optical activity results from the attachment of small molecules to a polymer in such a way that they

TABLE 4

Extrinsic Cotton Effects Generated by the Interaction of Substrates, Coenzymes, Inhibitors, and Other Ligands with Enzymes and Other Proteins

Protein	Ligand	Reference
type I		
Polyglutamic acid	Acridine orange and other dyes	Blout and Stryer (1959) Blout (1964) Blout et al. (1965) Yamaoka and Resnick (1966) Myhr and Foss (1966) Eyring et al. (1968)
type II *Noncovalent binding*		
Alcohol dehydrogenase (horse liver)	NADH	Ulmer et al. (1961)
Alcohol dehydrogenase (human liver)	NADH	Ulmer and Vallee (1965)
Alchol dehydrogenase (yeast)	NADH Zinc phenanthrolinate	Ulmer and Vallee (1961)
Creatine-ATP transphosphorylase	ATP-Mg-creatine ADP-Mg	Kägi and Li (1965)
Aspartic aminotransferase	Pyridoxal-5'-phosphate	Tochinskii and Koreneva (1964) Fasella and Hammes (1964)
Muscle phosphorylase b (rabbit)	Pyridoxal-5'-phosphate	Torchinskii et al. (1969)
Opsin	Retinaldehyde	Crescitelli et al. (1966)
Serum albumin	Bilirubin	Blauer and King (1970) Blauer et al. (1970) Woolley and Hunter (1970)
Serum albumin	Various dyes	Schechter (1969)
Serum albumin	HABA	Witiak et al. (1969)
Avidin	HABA	Chignell (unpublished results)
Covalent binding		
α-Chymotrypsin	Phenacyl group	Sigman et al. (1969)
Ribonuclease	Nitrotyrosine	Beaven and Gratzer (1968)
Glycogen phosphorylase	2,4-Dinitrophenyl group	Johnson et al. (1968)
Pancreatic trypsin inhibitor	Nitrotyrosine	Meloun et al. (1968)
Carboxypeptidase	Arsanilo group	Kagan and Vallee (1969)
Serum albumin	Various dyes	Dowben and Orkin (1967)

have an asymmetrical spatial arrangement. A good example of this type of interaction is the binding of certain cationic dyes to α-helical poly-L-glutamic acid. Here
the polyglutamate acts as a matrix to give the bound dye molecules a screw-sense. In
the second group (Table 4, type II) optical activity results from the interaction of
a single small molecule with an asymmetric locus at or near its binding site on the
protein or polypeptide. By far the large majority of extrinsic Cotton effects belong
to this second group.

Ulmer and coworkers have made an exhaustive study of the extrinsic Cotton
effects generated by the binding of coenzymes and inhibitors to alcohol dehydrogenase (see Table 4 and Ulmer and Vallee, 1965). They found that, when
reduced diphosphopyridine nucleotide (NADH) bound to horse liver alcohol
dehydrogenase (HLADH), the ORD spectrum of the complex exhibited a Cotton
effect centered at 327 mμ. Since the absorption maximum of bound NADH
appeared at the same wavelength there was little doubt that the observed Cotton
effect was extrinsic in origin (Ulmer et al., 1961). Extrinsic Cotton effects were
also generated by the binding of NADH to alcohol dehydrogenases from human
liver (Ulmer and Vallee, 1965) and yeast (Ulmer and Vallee, 1961). The interaction of the inhibitor 1,10-phenanthroline (a chelating agent) with the zinc atoms
of HLADH also generated an extrinsic Cotton effect which was centered at 297 mμ.
Further examples of extrinsic Cotton effects generated by the binding of chromophoric ligands to enzymes may be found in Table 4.

Extrinsic Cotton effects are also observed when certain acidic drugs are
bound to serum albumin (Chignell, 1968, 1969a, 1969b, 1970a). For example, the
binding of dicoumarol to human serum albumin (HSA) generates a large negative
ellipticity band at 305 mμ (Figure 16). This extrinsic Cotton effect results from

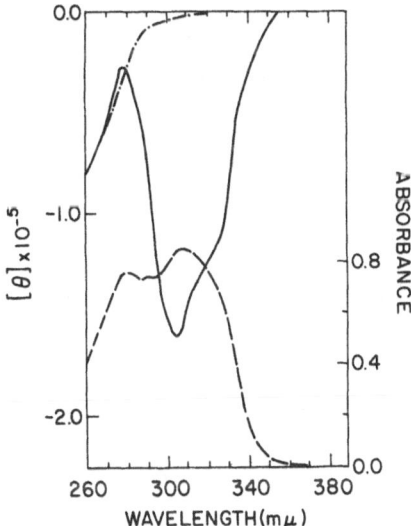

FIG. 16. Extrinsic Cotton effects generated by the binding of dicoumarol to human serum albumin. Human serum albumin (1.45×10⁻⁵M) alone (— • — • — • —); human serum albumin
(1.45×10⁻⁵M)+dicoumarol (5×10⁻⁵M) (——————); absorption spectrum of dicoumarol (5×
10⁻⁵M) (- - - - -). All solutions contained 1×10⁻¹M sodium phosphate buffer (pH 7.4).

the perturbation of π-π^* transitions in the drug molecule by an asymmetric locus at or near the HSA binding site (Chignell, 1970a). When a fixed amount of HSA was titrated with increments of dicoumarol, the ellipticity band at 305 mμ increased in amplitude up until the point where three molecules of drug had been bound per molecule of protein (Figure 17). The addition of further amounts of drug produced little increase in optical activity. Equilibrium dialysis studies showed that HSA has three high affinity sites ($K=7.7\times10^5M^{-1}$) and an indeterminate number of weaker sites ($K<1\times10^4M^{-1}$) for dicoumarol. This suggests that extrinsic optical activity is observed only when the drug-macromolecule complex is fairly rigid (Chignell, 1970a).

Although the binding of phenylbutazone to HSA generates a positive ellipticity band at 287 mμ, this extrinsic Cotton effect does not occur at the same wavelength as the absorption maximum of the drug (Figure 18). Thus, it is not the π-π^* transitions of the phenyl rings which are being perturbed but the n-π^* transition of the carbonyl group in the pyrazolidinedione ring (Chignell, 1969a). The introduction of hydrophilic groups, e.g., OH, NO_2, CH_3SO_2, into the phenyl groups of phenylbutazone drastically reduced optical activity (Table 5). In contrast, the introduction of hydrophobic substituents, e.g., Cl, F, into the phenyl rings or modification of the n-butyl side chain had a much smaller effect on the optical activity.

It has been assumed that phenylbutazone and other anionic drugs are bound to HSA by an electrostatic interaction with a cationic site on the protein. Such a one-point attachment for phenylbutazone, however, would leave the drug molecule fairly free to rotate, and it is unlikely that the extrinsic Cotton effects would be generated. On the other hand, if the electrostatic interaction was supplemented by

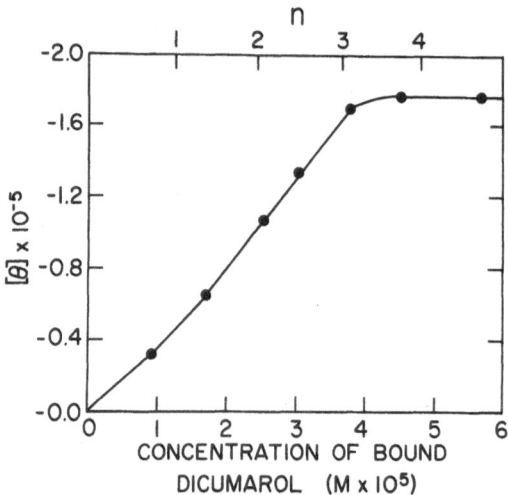

FIG. 17. Extrinsic circular dichroism at 305 mμ of dicoumarol bound to human serum albumin ($1.23\times10^{-3}M$). Solution contained $1\times10^{-1}M$ sodium phosphate buffer (pH 7.4). (From Chignell. 1970a. *Molec. Pharmacol.*, 6:1. Courtesy of Academic Press, Inc.)

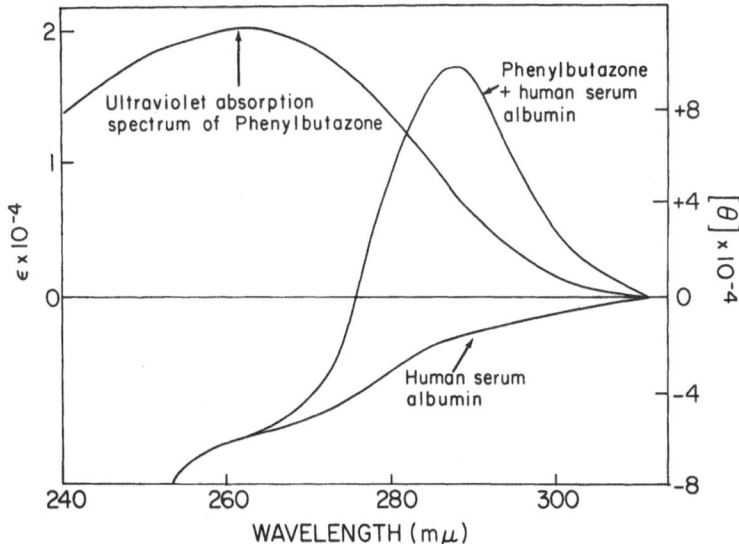

FIG. 18. Extrinsic Cotton effect generated by the binding of phenylbutazone to human serum albumin. Human serum albumin, $1.45 \times 10^{-5}M$; phenylbutazone, $5 \times 10^{-5}M$. All solutions contained $1 \times 10^{-1}M$ sodium phosphate buffer (pH 7.4). (From Chignell. 1970b. *Proc. Fourth Int. Cong. Pharmacol.*, 1:217. Courtesy of Schwabe and Co.)

van der Waals forces between the drug phenyl groups and a hydrophobic area at or near the binding site, then a rigid complex would be created. The introduction of hydrophilic groups into the phenyl rings of phenylbutazone would reduce the rigidity of the drug-protein complex by decreasing the possibility for hydrophobic interactions. The reduction in rigidity would permit the asymmetric center associated with the HSA binding site to enter regions of positive and negative contribution to a Cotton effect so that extrinsic optical activity would either be reduced or lost altogether.

When flufenamic acid, a potent anti-inflammatory drug, is bound to HSA, a large positive Cotton effect appears at 296 mμ, while a smaller negative Cotton effect is found at 345 mμ (Figure 19). These extrinsic Cotton effects result from the perturbation of two electronic transitions in the drug molecule by an asymmetric locus at the HSA binding site. Biphasic extrinsic Cotton effects were also generated by the binding of the related drugs meclofenamic acid and mefenamic acid to HSA (Table 5) (Chignell, 1969b). When comparisons have to be made between the optical activities of absorption bands with different extinction coefficients, it is customary to use the corresponding optic anisotropies or dissymmetry factors (Table 6). The results show that, as the degree of substitution in the phenyl ring increases, the dissymmetry factor decreases. This suggests that flufenamic acid is influenced by the asymmetry of the binding site to a much greater extent than meclofenamic acid. An examination of a molecular model of meclofenamic acid showed (Chignell, 1969b) that the chlorine atoms forced the N-phenyl ring

TABLE 5

Molar Ellipticities of Complexes Between Phenylbutazones and Human Serum Albumin[a]

				Wavelength maximum		
				Ultraviolet absorption	Circular dichroism	$[\theta]$ [b]
				(mμ)	(mμ)	(deg cm² dmole⁻¹) × 10⁻³
Drug	R_1	R_2	R_3			
Phenylbutazone	H	H	$CH_3(CH_2)_3$	265	287	52.2
Oxyphenbutazone	p-OH	H	$CH_3(CH_2)_3$	264	287	6.6
Sulfinpyrazone	H	H	$C_6H_5SO(CH_2)_2$	254	288	49.4
G-13838	H	H	$(CH_3)_2CH$	263	288	48.0
G-25671	H	H	$C_6H_5S(CH_2)_2$	256	286	63.0
G-30249	p-OH	H	$C_6H_5CH_2CO$	268	293	9.5
G-28234	p-NO₂	H	$CH_3(CH_2)_3$	260	—	0
G-15140	p-Cl	p-Cl	$CH_3(CH_2)_3$	265	296	28.8
G-32170	p-F	p-F	$CH_3(CH_2)_3$	262	290	29.8
G-34764	p-CH₃SO₂	H	$CH_3(CH_2)_3$	263	—	0
G-32568	m-CH₃SO₂	m-CH₃SO₂	$CH_3(CH_2)_3$	271	—	0
Ketazone	H	H	$CH_3CO(CH_2)_2$	261	287	29.0
Benzopyrazone	H	H	$C_6H_5CO(CH_2)_2$	251	287	74.0

[a]From Chignell. 1969. *Molec. Pharmacol.*, 5:244-252. Courtesy of Academic Press, Inc.
[b]Calculated with reference to the concentration of bound drug. The number of moles of drug bound per mole of HSA was kept below 2 for all measurements.

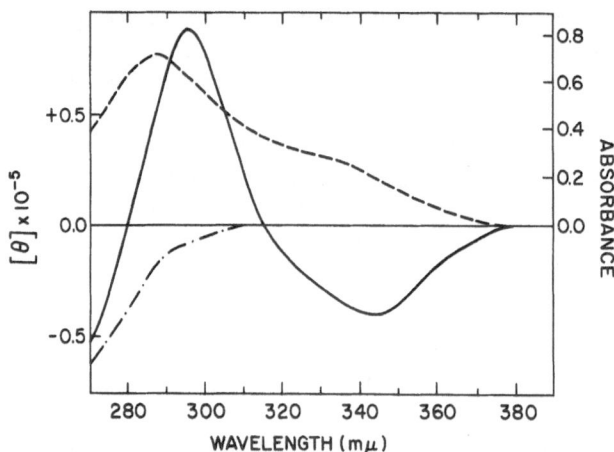

FIG. 19. Extrinsic Cotton effects generated by the binding of flufenamic acid bound to human serum albumin. Human serum albumin (1.45×10⁻⁵M) alone (— • — • — •), human serum albumin (1.45×10⁻⁵M)+flufenamic acid (1×10⁻⁴M) (————); absorption spectrum of flufenamic acid (5×10⁻⁵M) (- - -); all solutions contained 1×10⁻¹M sodium phosphate buffer (pH 7.4).

TABLE 6

Molar Ellipticities of Complexes between Fenamic Acids and Human Serum Albumin[a]

Drug	R_1	R_2	R_3	Ultraviolet Absorption Maximum Wavelength (mμ)	$\epsilon \times 10^{-4}$ ($M^{-1}cm^{-1}$)	Circular Dichroism Maximum Wavelength (mμ)	$[\theta]^{b} \times 10^{-4}$ (deg cm^2 dmole^{-1})	Dissymmetry Factor $(\Delta\epsilon/\epsilon) \times 10^4$
Flufenamic acid	H	CF_3	H	288	1.24	296	+2.01	+5.70
				322	0.54	345	−0.69	−7.04
Mefenamic acid	CH_3	CH_3	H	284	1.40	292	+2.24	+4.70
				332	0.64	340	−1.44	−6.54
Meclofenamic acid	Cl	CH_3	Cl	277	0.88	302	+0.44	+2.40
				315	0.56	332	−0.30	−2.80

[a] From Chignell. 1969. Molec. Pharmacol., 5:455-462. Courtesy of Academic Press, Inc.
[b] Calculated with reference to the concentration of bound drug.

into a plane at right angles to the anthranilic acid portion of the molecule. If the binding site in HSA consisted of a narrow hydrophobic cleft, then meclofenamic acid might have difficulty entering and hence would be less influenced by the asymmetry of the protein (Chignell, 1969b).

Flufenamic acid can also be used to probe the asymmetries of drug binding sites on different serum albumins. For example, the binding of flufenamic acid to human, porcine, equine, and bovine serum albumins generated biphasic Cotton effects (Table 7), suggesting that these proteins have similar binding sites. The flufenamic acid binding sites on canine and bovine serum binding sites were also similar, while the rabbit serum albumin binding site was unique among the albumins studied (Table 7).

Although heme has a plane of symmetry, the iron atom constitutes a center of asymmetry for prosthetic groups, since different ligands may occupy the fifth and sixth coordination sites of the metal atom and because the protein may be linked to both iron and the porphyrin side chains. Many heme-containing enzymes show extrinsic optical activity in the wavelength (Soret) region where the heme absorbs light (Ulmer and Vallee, 1965; Perrin and Hart, 1970). For example, Yong and coworkers (1970) have reported that rat-liver submicrosomal particles containing oxidized cytochrome P-450 exhibit a negative Cotton effect with a trough at 432.5 $m\mu$ and a peak at 410 $m\mu$. Reduction of the cytochrome by dithionite abolished the Cotton effect almost completely. However, the carbon monoxide complex of the reduced P-450 exhibited a negative Cotton effect with a trough at 467 $m\mu$ and a peak at 447.5 $m\mu$. No extrinsic Cotton effects were

TABLE 7

Molar Ellipticities of Flufenamic Acid Bound to Different Serum Albumins[a]

Serum Albumin	Wavelength Maximum $m\mu$	$[\theta]$ [b] (deg cm^2 dmole^{-1}) $\times 10^{-4}$	$\Delta\epsilon/\epsilon$ $\times 10^4$
Human	296	+2.01	+5.70
	345	−0.61	−7.04
Porcine	292	+1.90	+4.43
	352	−0.31	−3.92
Equine	292	+0.49	+1.14
	348	−0.36	−3.63
Bovine	305	+0.77	+2.65
	348	−0.26	−2.63
Canine	295	+1.08	+2.64
Ovine	302	+0.90	+2.84
Rabbit	297	+1.23	+3.22
	325[c]	+0.40	+1.95

[a]From Chignell. 1969. *Molec. Pharmacol.*, 5:455-462. Courtesy of Academic Press, Inc.
[b]Calculated with reference to the concentration of bound drug.
[c]Shoulder.

observed with cytochrome P-420. It was concluded that cytochrome P-450 probably undergoes a functional conformational change during mixed function oxidation. Circular dichroism measurements in our own laboratory (Chignell, Sasame, and Gillette, unpublished observations) have confirmed these results and have also shown that the binding of drugs such as hexobarbital and aniline alter the extrinsic optical activity of rat and rabbit liver microsomal P-450. However, no difference was observed between the changes induced by the binding of the type I and type II substrates described by Remmer and coworkers (1966).

The substitution of zinc by cobalt in human carbonic anhydrase is accompanied by the appearance of multiple absorption maxima in the region 500-650 mμ, reflecting the *d-d* electronic transitions of the cobalt ion (Coleman, 1965). While cobalt carbonic anhydrase is optically inactive in this wavelength region, the binding of the sulfonamide inhibitor acetazolamide generates asymmetrical anomalous rotatory dispersion with a peak at 590 mμ, a crossover point at 544 mμ, and a trough at 525 mμ (Coleman, 1965). The generation of extrinsic Cotton effects by the acetazolamide cobalt human carbonic anhydrase complex suggests that either there has been a protein conformational change at or near the active site, or that there has been a change in the ligands occupying the fifth and sixth coordination sites of the metal.

The Interaction of Drugs and Other Small Molecules with Nucleic Acids

THE INTRINSIC OPTICAL ACTIVITY OF NUCLEIC ACIDS. The optical activity of nucleosides, the monomeric components of nucleic acids, results from asymmetric perturbation of the purine or pyrimidine chromophore by the adjacent ribose or 2'-deoxyribose sugar. The sign and magnitude of this optical activity depends on the spatial relationship between the purine or pyrimidine base and the glycosidic portion of the nucleoside molecule. Although it has been generally assumed that the ORD and CD curves of nucleosides and nucleotides are due to an *anti*-conformation about the glycosidic link, it has been shown recently that some nucleosides may exist partly in the *syn*-conformation (Hart and Davis, 1969). It is not known at present whether this new information will significantly alter future thinking on the conformation of nucleic acids.

When nucleosides are joined by the 3',5'-phosphodiester linkage to form nucleic acids the optical activity of the polymer is often quite different from that of the isolated monomer. Indeed, only in the case of nucleic acids in the unordered random coil configuration does the optical activity of the polymer resemble that of its monomeric units. In the single-stranded stacked base form and in the double helical form of nucleic acids extensive interactions between adjacent bases result in an enhancement of optical activity. Such interactions are even seen in dinucleoside phosphates such as adenyl-3',5'-adenosine (ApA), which exists in aqueous solution in a stacked conformation. The CD spectrum of ApA is biphasic with a positive extremum at 270 mμ and a negative extremum at 258 mμ. At 268 mμ, the ultraviolet absorption maximum of ApA, the dinucleoside phosphate has no circular dichroism. This type of CD spectrum is typical of an "exciton" interaction between identical transition dipoles occurring in a system of ordered chromophores (Tinoco, 1968). As the chain of bases in ApA becomes longer the proportion of bases with neighbors on both sides increases so that the amplitude of the Cotton effects increases, reaching an asymptotic maximum in the high polymer, poly-A (Brahms et al., 1966).

It has long been known that in DNA optical activity is enhanced but that when the double helix is melted it reverts to something close to the constituent monomers. DNA has a Cotton effect centered at about 260 mμ, as well as other somewhat weaker Cotton effects at shorter wavelengths (Figure 20). The magnitude of the 290 mμ extremum of the ORD curve is a linear function of base composition. Two-stranded synthetic ribonucleotides, poly-(A+U), poly-(G+C), have characteristic Cotton effects in the same region which are much larger than those of DNA. The large Cotton effect observed in fully paired viral RNA (Figure 20) indicates that the geometry of RNA generates higher optical activity than that of DNA.

For a more comprehensive discussion of the optical activity of nucleic acids the reader is referred to the review of Yang and Samejima (1969) as well as to recent papers by Johnson and Tinoco (1969) and Gratzer et al. (1970).

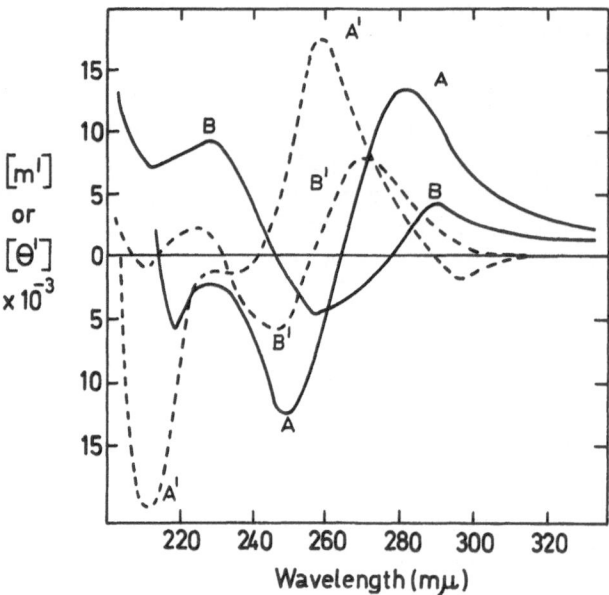

FIG. 20. Optical rotatory dispersion and circular dichroism of native salmon sperm DNA (B) and two-stranded (rice dwarf virus) RNA (A). The prime indicates the circular dichroism curves. (From Gratzer and Cowburn. 1969. *Nature (London)*, 222:426. Courtesy of MacMillan [Journals] Ltd.)

CHANGES IN THE INTRINSIC OPTICAL ACTIVITY OF NUCLEIC ACIDS BY THE BINDING OF DRUGS AND OTHER SMALL MOLECULES. Mahler and coworkers (1968) have studied the interaction of two steroidal diamines malouetine (5-α-pregnan-3-β,20-α-ylenebis [trimethyl ammonium iodide]) and irehdiamine A (pregn-5-ene-3-β,20-α-diamine) with DNA, by monitoring changes in the intrinsic optical activity of the nucleic acid. At low ionic strength, two different complexes are formed. The first, observed at low steroid/DNA ratios (<0.2), is characterized by a shift in the long wavelength (285 mμ) CD band to longer wavelengths with an increase in ellipticity. The second requires a higher steroid/DNA ratio (>0.2) when the nucleic acid displays optical activity characteristic of disoriented DNA.

Wagner (1969) has observed marked changes in the CD spectrum of calf thymus DNA on the addition of lysergic acid diethylamide (LSD). There was a decrease in the positive CD band at 276 mμ, a shift in the crossover point from 256 mμ to 260 mμ, a strengthening and broadening of the negative band at 245 mμ, and a strengthening and slight blue shift in the positive band at 220 mμ. Since similar changes were observed when ethidium bromide bound to RNA, Wagner concluded that LSD was intercalated between the bases of the nucleic acid. While it is unlikely that intercalation *per se* is responsible for the chromosal breakage ascribed to LSD, it is possible that neutralization of the DNA phosphate groups by the drug may lead to a dissociation of histones, which in turn may render the nucleic acid susceptible to enzymatic attack and breakage.

DRUGS AND OTHER SMALL MOLECULES THAT GENERATE EXTRINSIC OPTICAL ACTIVITY ON BINDING TO NUCLEIC ACIDS. Although the acridines were first used to stain nuclear materials for histological examination, it was soon found that these dyes were potent antibacterial agents and mutagens. Since the binding of many of these acridine dyes to nucleic acids generates extrinsic Cotton effects, both ORD and CD have been used extensively to study the interaction. For example, in 1965, Blake and Peacocke reported that the binding of proflavine to calf thymus DNA generated an extrinsic Cotton effect centered at 443 mμ (Figure 21). The magnitude of the Cotton effect increased until a DNA/dye ratio of 4:1 was reached. However, when the concentration of DNA was further increased, optical activity decreased and eventually disappeared (Blake and Peacocke, 1966). When the ionic strength of a solution of DNA and proflavine was lowered, the extrinsic optical activity increased above and beyond that expected from the concomitant increase in bound dye concentration. Denaturation of the DNA by either heat or acid did not change the extrinsic Cotton effect to any great extent. Blake and Peacocke (1966) attempted to explain their results on the basis of the models proposed by Blout (1964) for the acridine orange poly-L-glutamic acid system. The possibility that optical activity arose from helical aggregates of dye was rejected since optical activity was still observed at proflavine concentrations where the binding of aggregates to DNA was negligible. Since Cotton effects appeared when proflavine was bound to denatured DNA, the orientation of the dye molecules in an extended helical array was not a prerequisite

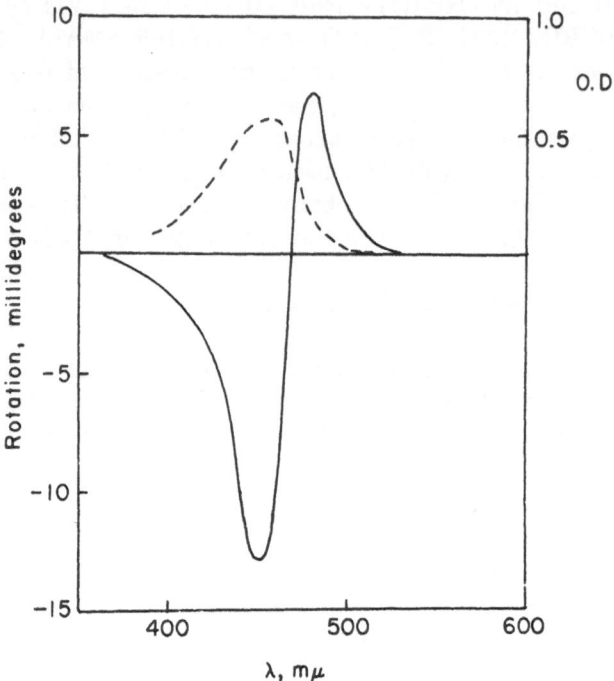

FIG. 21. Optical rotatory dispersion curve (————) of proflavine bound to native calf thymus DNA and the optical density (- - - - - - - -) of the same solution. Proflavine, $1.81 \times 10^{-5}M$; DNA phosphorus, $8.0 \times 10^{-5}M$; sodium chloride, $0.9 \times 10^{-3}M$; sodium phosphate (pH 6.6), $1 \times 10^{-1}M$. (From Blake and Peacocke. 1966. *Biopolymers*, 4:1091. Courtesy of John Wiley & Sons, Publishers).

for optical activity. On the other hand, the binding of the proflavine molecule was not in itself a sufficient criterion for binding since optical activity was dependent on the extent of binding. The decrease in optical activity at high DNA/proflavine ratios suggests that each dye molecule contributes less to the rotation when they are spread sparsely over the molecule. Some kind of nearest-neighbor effect therefore seems to be necessary for optical activity. This was confirmed by later CD measurements (Blake and Peacocke, 1967), which showed the presence of an unsymmetrical double ellipticity curve characteristic of exciton interactions. Tinoco (1968) has shown that exciton interactions in polymers occur only when two chromophores are in close proximity to one another.

Extrinsic optical activity is also generated by the binding of other dyes to nucleic acids (Table 8). The interaction of several drugs, including actinomycin D, chloroquine, quinacrine, and berberine with nucleic acids has also been studied by measuring their extrinsic Cotton effects (Table 8). In recent experiments Greenblatt and coworkers (1970) have studied the competition between the acridine and triphenylmethane dyes for binding sites on nucleic acids. They found that both crystal violet (a triphenylmethane dye) and trypaflavine (an acridine dye) generated extrinsic Cotton effects on binding to DNA. However, when both dyes

TABLE 8

Extrinsic Cotton Effects Generated by
the Binding of Ligands to Nucleic Acids

Ligand	Nucleic Acid	Reference
Acridine orange	DNA	Gardner and Mason (1967)
Methylene blue	DNA	Hahn and Krey (1968)
Methyl green	DNA	Hahn and Krey (1968)
Quinacrine	DNA	Hahn and Krey (1968)
Chloroquine	DNA	Hahn and Krey (1968)
Actinomycin D	DNA	Yamaoka and Ziffer (1968)
Aminocridines (1,2,3, and 9)	DNA	Blake and Peacocke (1967)
Berberine	DNA	Krey and Hahn (personal communication)
	RNA	Chignell (unpublished results)
Ethidium bromide	DNA	Aktipis and Martz (1970)

were present in solution, the Cotton effect due to trypaflavine disappeared, suggesting that the acridine dye had been displaced from its nucleic acid binding site. This observation may help to explain the so-called "therapeutic interference" between acridine dyes and triphenylmethane dyes, which was described in 1922 by Browning and Gulbransen. These workers found that trypanosome-infected mice injected with trypaflavine recovered, while those receiving parafuchsin (a triphenylmethane dye related to crystal violet) did not. When the mice received both drugs, they died, suggesting that the noneffective drug had prevented the effective drug from exerting its therapeutic effect.

Gabbay (1968, 1969) has synthesized reporter molecules of the type (I)

R_3

R_2

R_1

CH_3

$NH(CH_2)_n N^+ (CH_2)_3 N^+ (CH_3)_3$ $2Br^-$

CH_3

(I)

(where $n=2$ or 3, $R_1 = H$, NO_2, CH_3; $R_2 = H$, CH_3; and $R_3 = NO_2$, H), and found that extrinsic Cotton effects are generated when they bind to nucleic acids. Two of these molecules (I, $R_1 = R_3 = NO_2$; $R_2 = H$; $n = 2$ or 3) generated a positive Cotton effect on binding to RNA but a negative Cotton effect on binding to DNA. Gabbay (1969) suggested that these opposite effects resulted from a different orientation of the reporter molecule with respect to the helix axis. Studies such as these suggest that it may be possible to use reporter molecules to examine the changes in conformation which occur when drugs interact with nucleic acids.

Small Molecule–Small Molecule Interactions

Thyrum and coworkers (1968) have found that the intrinsic optical activity of adenosinetriphosphate (ATP) at 350 mμ decreases when either procaine or procaine amide is present in the solution. They attributed this decrease in optical rotation to a change in orientation between the adenine group and the sugar moiety of ATP brought about by complex formation between the drug and the nucleotide. The optical activity changes permitted calculation of association constants of 1.43×10^3 M^{-1} (procaine) and 3.6×10^2 M^{-1} (procaine amide) for complex formation between ATP and the drug molecules. Thyrum et al. (1968) suggested that procaine and procaine amide may act on nerve membranes by complexing with membrane-bound ATP and thereby interfering with the nucleotide's natural function.

In somewhat similar experiments Nakano and Higuchi (1968) have obtained evidence for complex formation between tryptophan and certain alkylxanthines. These workers found that the optical activity for tryptophan at 330 mμ increased in the presence of caffeine, theophylline, 8-methoxycaffeine, and 1,3-dimethyluracil. The association constant for the caffeine-tryptophan complex was found to be 30 M^{-1} while measurements at four different temperatures gave the heat of binding as -4.2 kcal M^{-1}.

In recent experiments Noack (1969) has reported that n-π* transition of the optically inactive ketone cyclohexanone exhibits CD in the presence of 1-menthol. Results show that a 1:1 complex is formed between the alcohol and ketone, in which hydrogen bonding appears to play an important role. The introduction of a methyl group into the 2-position of cyclohexanone reduced the extrinsic optical activity by about 30%, while a methyl group in the 3-position had little effect on the optical activity, suggesting that steric factors are also important.

The Metabolism of Optically Active Compounds and the Formation of Optically Active Metabolites

Elliott, Tao, and Williams (1965) have made an extensive study of the metabolism in rabbits of the isomeric methylcyclohexanols and methylcyclohexanones. The cyclohexanols were isolated from the urine as glucuronides, methylated, then acetylated and crystallized as triacetyl methyl esters. The esters were then hydrolyzed and the alcohol identified. Measurement of specific rotation showed that ($\pm$) cis-2-methylcyclohexanol and ($\pm$) 2-methylcyclohexanone were excreted as glucuronides of ($\pm$) trans-2-methylcyclohexanol, while the ($\pm$)-trans-alcohol was excreted unchanged. Elliott and coworkers concluded from these and other results that only one face of the NADH coenzyme took part in the reduction of the methylcyclohexanols and that the structure of the coenzyme-substrate complex was governed by stereochemical interactions. For a more detailed discussion the reader is referred to a recent review (Elliott, Jacob, and Tao, 1969).

The metabolism of (±)-*trans*-*p*-tolylcyclohexanol and (±)-*trans*-*o*-tolylcyclohexanol in the rat has been studied by Galpin and coworkers (1969). They found that about half of the urinary metabolites recovered from intraperitoneal administration of the (±) *trans*-isomer of *p*-tolylcyclohexanol had undergone aromatic methyl group oxidation, while there was no evidence for similar changes occurring in the *o*-tolyl compound. The other major metabolite from (±)-*trans*-*p*-tolylcyclohexanol was the (±)-*trans*-diastereoisomer. Optical rotatory dispersion measurements established the absolute configuration of this isomer by comparison with (±)-*trans*-2-*p*-tolylcyclohexanol obtained by resolution of racemic (±)-*trans*-2-tolylcyclohexanol.

PROGNOSIS

Circular dichroism and optical rotatory dispersion have been used to study the interaction of a wide variety of small molecules, including some drugs, with biological macromolecules such as proteins and nucleic acids. Since a vast majority of biomolecules as well as some drugs are optically active, CD and ORD should prove to be useful tools for studying the interactions of many drugs with biological systems. At the present moment, such studies are best carried out with the isolated biomolecules, since CD and ORD studies in heterogeneous cell systems containing a large amount of particulate matter are not presently feasible. However, as instruments become more sophisticated, it may yet be possible to study drug interactions with the whole cell.

REFERENCES

Abu-Shumays, A., and J. L. Duffield. 1966. Circular dichroism—theory and instrumentation. Anal. Chem., 38:29A-58A.

Aktipis, S., and W. W. Martz. 1970. Circular dichroism properties of ethidium bromide—deoxyribonucleic acid complexes. Biochem. Biophys. Res. Commun., 39:307-313.

Ballard, R. E., A. J. McCaffrey, and S. F. Mason. 1966. Electronic spectrum, optical activity, and structure of the acridine orange complex with poly-α, L-glutamic acid. Biopolymers, 4:97-106.

Bayley, P. M., and G. K. Radda. 1966. Conformational changes and the regulation of glutamate dehydrogenase activity. Biochem. J., 98:105-111.

Beaven, G. H., and W. B. Gratzer. 1968. Nitration of ribonuclease. Biochim. Biophys. Acta, 168:456-462.

Beychok, S. 1965. Side-chain optical activity in cystine-containing proteins: Circular dichroism studies. Proc. Nat. Acad. Sci. U.S.A., 53:999-1006.

———— 1968. Circular dichroism of biological macromolecules. Science, 154:1288-1299.

Blake, A., and A. R. Peacocke. 1965. Optical rotatory dispersion of complexes of proflavine with nucleic acids. Nature (London), 206:1009-1011.

———— and A. R. Peacocke. 1966. Extrinsic Cotton effects of aminoacridines bound to DNA. Biopolymers, 4:1091-1104.

———— and A. R. Peacocke. 1967. Induced optical activity of various aminoacridines bound to DNA. Biopolymers, 5:871-875.

Blauer, G., D. Harmatz, and A. N. Naparstek. 1970. Circular dichroism of bilirubin—human serum albumin complexes in aqueous solution. FEBS Letters, 9:53-56.

———— and T. E. King. 1970. Interactions of bilirubin with bovine serum albumin in aqueous solution. J. Biol. Chem., 245:372-381.

Blout, E. R. 1964. Extrinsic and intrinsic Cotton effects in polypeptides and proteins. Biopolymer Symps., No. 1:397-408.

———— J. P. Carver, and E. Schechter. 1965. Optical rotatory dispersion of polypeptides and proteins. *In* Snatzke, G., ed., Optical Rotatory Dispersion and Circular Dichroism in Organic Chemistry, 224-300. Norwich, England, Jarrold and Sons.

———— and L. Stryer. 1959. Anomalous optical rotatory dispersion of dye: Polypeptide complexes. Proc. Nat. Acad. Sci. U.S.A., 45:1591-1593.

Brady, A. H., and S. Beychok. 1968. Optical activity and conformation studies of two preparations of pig heart lipoyl dehydrogenase. Biochem. Biophys. Res. Commun., 32:186-191.

Brahms, J., A. M. Michelson, and K. E. Van Holde. 1966. Adenylate oligomers in single- and double-strand conformation. J. Molec. Biol., 15:467-488.

Browning, C. H., and R. Gulbransen. 1922. An interference phenomenon in the action of chemotherapeutic substances in experimental trypanosome infections. J. Path. Bact., 25:395-397.

Cary, H., R. C. Hawes, P. B. Hooper, J. J. Duffield, and K. P. George. 1964. A recording spectropolarimeter. Applied Optics, 3:329-337.

Cathou, R. E., G. G. Hammes, and P. R. Schimmel. 1965. Optical rotatory dispersion of ribonuclease-nucleotide complexes. Biochemistry (Washington), 4:2687-2690.

Chignell, C. F. 1968. Circular dichroism studies of drug protein complexes. Life Sci., 7:1181-1186.

———— 1969a. Optical studies of drug-protein complexes. II. The interaction of phenylbutazone and its analogs with human serum albumin. Molec. Pharmacol., 5:244-252.

———— 1969b. Optical studies of drug-protein complexes. III. The interaction of flufenamic acid and other N-arylanthranilic acids with serum albumin. Molec. Pharmacol., 5:455-462.

———— 1970a. Optical studies of drug-protein complexes. IV. The interaction of warfarin and dicoumarol with human serum albumin. Molec. Pharmacol., 6:1-12.

———— 1970b. Circular dichroism as a tool for studying the interaction of drugs with biomolecules. Proc. Fourth Int. Cong. Pharmacol., 1:217-226.

———— 1970c. Spectroscopic techniques for the study of drug interactions with biological systems. Advances Drug Res., 5:55-94.

Coleman, J. 1965. Human carbonic anhydrase. Protein conformation and metal ion binding. Biochemistry (Washington), 4:2644-2655.

Crabbé, P. 1965. Optical rotatory dispersion and circular dichroism. *In* Organic Chemistry. San Francisco, Holden Day.

Crescitelli, F., W. F. H. M. Mommaerts, and T. I. Shaw. 1966. Circular dichroism of visual pigments in the visible and ultraviolet spectral regions. Proc. Nat. Acad. Sci. U.S.A., 56:1729-1734.

Dowben, R. M., and S. H. Orkin. 1967. Extrinsic Cotton effects in dye-bovine plasma albumin adducts. Proc. Nat. Acad. Sci. U.S.A., 58:2051-2054.

Dratz, E. A., and M. Calvin. 1966. Substrate and inhibitor induced changes in the optical rotatory dispersion of aspartate transcarbamylase. Nature (London), 211:497-501.

Elliott, T. H., E. Jacob, and R. C. C. Tao. 1969. The *in vitro* and *in vivo* metabolism of optically active methylcyclohexanols and methylcyclohexanones. J. Pharm. Pharmacol., 21:561-572.

———— R. C. C. Tao, and R. T. Williams. 1965. The metabolism of methylcyclohexane. Biochem. J., 95:70-76.

Eyring, H., H.-C. Liu, and D. Caldwell. 1968. Optical rotatory dispersion and circular dichroism. Chem. Rev., 68:525-540.

Fasella, P., and G. G. Hammes. 1964. An optical rotatory dispersion study of aspartic amino transferase. Biochemistry (Washington), 3:530-535.

Fasman, G. D., H. Hoving, and S. N. Timasheff. 1970. Circular dichroism of polypeptide and protein conformations. Film studies. Biochemistry (Washington), 9:3316-3324.

———— and J. Potter. 1967. The optical rotatory dispersion of two beta structures. Biochem. Biophys. Res. Commun., 27:209-216.

Gabbay, E. J. 1968. Topography of nucleic acid helices in solutions. XI. A novel method of distinguishing between ribo- and deoxyribonucleic acids by the use of reporter molecules. J. Amer. Chem. Soc., 90:6574-6575.

———— 1969. Topography of nucleic acid helices in solutions. XII. The origin of the oppositely induced circular dichroism of reporter molecules bound to ribo- and deoxyribonucleic acid. J. Amer. Chem. Soc., 91:5136-5150.

Galpin, D. R., T. G. Cochran, and A. C. Huitric. 1969. Application of nuclear magnetic resonance and optical rotatory dispersion to studies in drug metabolism— stereoselectivity in the metabolism of trans-2-*p*-tolylcyclohexanol and trans-2-*o*-tolylcyclohexanol in the rat. Biochem. Pharmacol., 18:979-991.

Gardner, B. J., and S. F. Mason. 1967. Structure and optical activity of the DNA-aminoacridine complex. Biopolymers, 5:79-94.

Gillham, M. A., and R. J. King. 1961. New design of spectropolarimeter. J. Sci. Instrum., 38:21-25.

Gotto, A. M., R. I. Levy, and D. S. Frederickson. 1968. Observations on the conformation of human beta lipoprotein: Evidence for the occurrence of beta structure. Proc. Nat. Acad. Sci. U.S.A., 60:1436-1441.

Gratzer, W. B. 1967. Ultraviolet absorption spectra of polypeptides. *In* Fasman, G., ed., Poly-α-Amino Acids, 205-235. New York, M. Dekker.

———— and D. A. Cowburn. 1969. Optical activity of biopolymers. Nature (London), 222:426-431.

———— L. B. Hill, and R. J. Owen. 1970. Circular dichroism of DNA. Europ. J. Biochem., 15:209-214.

———— and P. McPhie. 1966. Conformational change in poly-L-lysine on reaction with polyacids. Biopolymers, 4:601-606.

Green, N. M., and M. D. Melamed. 1966. Optical rotatory dispersion, circular dichroism and far-ultraviolet spectra of avidin and streptavidin. Biochem. J., 100:614-621.

Greenblatt, C. L., N. E. Sharpless, and K. Yamaoka. 1970. Competition for polymeric binding sites between acridine and triphenylmethane dyes. Molec. Pharmacol., 6:649-658.

Grosjean, M., and M. Legrand. 1960. Appareil de measure du dichroïsme circulaire dans le visible et l'ultraviolet. C. R. Acad. Sci. (Paris), 251:2150-2152.

Hahn, F. E., and A. K. Krey. 1968. Deoxyribonucleic acid induced anomalous optical rotatory dispersion of antimalarial drugs and dyes. *In* Hobby, G. L., ed., Antimicrobial Agents and Chemotherapy, 15-20. Bethesda, Md., American Society for Microbiology.

Hanisch, G., and J. Engel. 1969. Ligand induced conformational changes in various normal and modified hemoglobins as indicated by changes in optical rotatory dispersion. Europ. J. Biochem., 9:335-342.

Hart, P. A., and J. P. Davis. 1969. The conformation of nucleosides and nucleotides. An application of the nuclear Overhauser effect. J. Amer. Chem. Soc., 91:512-513.

Helmer, F., K. Kiehs, and C. Hansch. 1968. The linear free-energy relationship between partition coefficients and the binding and conformational perturbation of macromolecules by small organic compounds. Biochemistry (Washington), 7:2858-2863.

Holzwarth, G. M., W. B. Gratzer, and P. Doty. 1962. The optical activity of polypeptides in the far ultraviolet. J. Amer. Chem. Soc., 84:3194-3196.

Imahori, K., and J. Tanaka. 1959. Ultraviolet absorption spectra of poly-L-glutamic acid. J. Molec. Biol., 1:359-364.

Iizuka, E., and J. T. Yang. 1966. Optical rotatory dispersion and circular dichroism of the β-form of silk fibroin in solution. Proc. Nat. Acad. Sci. U.S.A., 55:1175-1182.

Johnson, G. F., G. Philip, and D. J. Graves. 1968. Dinitrophenylation of glycogen phosphorylase. II. Circular dichroism of the modified enzyme. Biochemistry (Washington), 7:2101-2105.

Johnson, W. C., and I. Tinoco. 1969. Circular dichroism of polynucleotides: A simple theory. Biopolymers, 7:727-749.

Kagan, H. M., and B. L. Vallee. 1969. Environmental sensitivity of azo chromophores in arsanilocarboxypeptidase. Biochemistry (Washington), 8:4223-4231.

Kägi, J. H. R., and T. K. Li. 1965. Quoted by Ulmer and Vallee (1965).

Katchalski, E., and M. Sela. 1958. Synthesis and chemical properties of poly-α-amino acids. Advances Protein Chem., 13:243-492.

Kauzmann, W. 1957. Quantum Chemistry. New York, Academic Press.

Kronman, M. J., R. Blum, and L. G. Holmes. 1965. Estimation of helicity of proteins from optical rotation dispersion measurements. Biochem. Biophys. Res. Commun., 19:227-232.

Kuhn, W. 1930. The physical significance of optical rotatory power. Trans. Faraday Soc., 46:293-308.

_____ and E. Braun. 1930. Messung des Zirkulardichroismus im Ultravioletten. Z. Physik. Chem. B., 8:445-54.

Lenard, J., and S. J. Singer. 1966. Protein conformation in cell membrane preparations as studied by optical rotatory dispersion and circular dichroism. Proc. Nat. Acad. Sci. U.S.A., 56:1828-1835.

Lowry, T. M. 1964. Optical Rotatory Power. New York, Dover.

Magar, M. E. 1965. Conformational changes in glutamate dehydrogenase. Biochim. Biophys. Acta, 96:345-348.

Mahler, H. R., G. Green, R. Goutarel, and O. Khuong-Huu. 1968. Nucleic acid-small molecule interactions. VII. Further characterization of deoxyribonucleic acid-diamino steroid complexes. Biochemistry (Washington), 7:1568-1582.

Markus, G., and F. Karush. 1958. Structural effects of anionic azo dyes on serum albumin. J. Amer. Chem. Soc., 80:89-94.

Meloun, B., I. Fric, and F. Sorm. 1968. Nitration of tyrosine residues in the pancreatic trypsin inhibitor with tetranitromethane. Europ. J. Biochem., 4:112-117.

Mitchell, S. 1950. A photo-electric method for measuring circular dichroism. Nature (London), 166:434-435.

_____ 1957. Accessories for measuring circular dichroism and rotatory dispersion with a spectrophotometer. J. Sci. Instrum., 34:89-90.

_____ and J. Veitch. 1951. Rotatory dispersion measurements with a unicam spectrophotometer. Nature (London), 168:662-663.

Moffitt, W., and A. Moscowitz. 1959. Optical activity in absorbing media. J .Chem. Phys., 30:648-660.

Moscowitz, A. 1960. Theory and analysis of rotatory dispersion curve. *In* Djerassi,

C., ed., Optical Rotatory Dispersion; Applications to Organic Chemistry, 150-177. New York, McGraw-Hill.

———— 1962. Theoretical aspects of optical activity. Part one: Small molecules. Advances Chem. Phys., 4, 67-112.

Myhr, B. C., and J. G. Foss. 1966. Polyglutamic acid-acridine orange complexes. Cotton effects in the random coil region. Biopolymers, 4:949-952.

Nakano, M., and T. Higuchi. 1968. Determination of molecular binding in aqueous solution from optical activity measurements. Interaction of tryptophan with alkylxanthines. J. Pharm. Sci., 57:1865-1868.

Noack, K. 1969. Induktion von Circulardichroismus in einer optisch inaktiven Verbindung durch zwischenmolekulare Wechselwirkung mit einem optisch aktiven Lösungmittel. Helv. Chim. Acta, 52:2501-2507.

Ohta, T., I. Shimada and K. Imahori. 1967. Conformational change of tyrosyl-RNA synthetase induced by its specific transfer RNA. J. Molec. Biol., 26:519-524.

Ottaway, C. A., and D. B. Wetlaufer. 1970. Light-scattering contributions to the circular dichroism of particulate systems. Arch. Biochem. Biophys., 139:257-264.

Pauling, L., and R. B. Corey. 1951. Configurations of polypeptide chains with favored orientations around single bonds: Two new pleated sheets. Proc. Nat. Acad. Sci. U.S.A., 37:729-740.

Perlmann, G. E. 1970. *In* Desnuelle, P., H. Neurath, M. Ottensen, eds., Structure-Function Relationships of Proteolytic Enzymes, 261. New York, Academic Press.

Perrin, J. H., and P. A. Hart. 1970. Small molecule-macromolecule interactions as studied by optical rotatory dispersion and circular dichroism. J. Pharm. Sci., 59:431-448.

Remmer, H., J. Schenkman, R. W. Estabrook, H. Sasame, J. R. Gillette, S. Narasimhulu, D. Y. Cooper, and O. Rosenthal. 1966. Drug interaction with hepatic microsomal cytochrome. Molec. Pharmacol., 2:187-190.

Resnick, R. A., and K. Yamaoka. 1966. A precautionary note on measurements of optical rotatory dispersion. Biopolymers, 4:242-244.

Riddiford, L. M., and H. A. Scheraga. 1962. Structural studies of Paramyosin. II. Conformational changes. Biochemistry (Washington), 1:108-114.

Rosenberg, A., H. Theorell, and T. Yonetani. 1965. Optical rotatory dispersion of liver alcohol dehydrogenase and its complexes with coenzymes and inhibitors. Arch. Biochem. Biophys., 110:413-421.

Rosenfeld, L. 1928. Quantenmechanische Theorie der natürlichen optischen Aktivität von Flüssigkeiten und Gasen. Z. Physik, 52:161-174.

Rudolph, H. C. 1955. Photoelectric polarimeter attachment. J. Opt. Soc. Amer., 45: 50-59.

Sarker, P. K., and P. Doty. 1966. The optical rotatory properties of the β-configuration in polypeptides and proteins. Proc. Nat. Acad. Sci. U.S.A., 55:981-989.

Schechter, E. 1969. The circular dichroism of bovine plasma albumin-dye complexes. Europ. J. Biochem., 10:274-277.

Schellman, J. A. 1966. Symmetry rules for optical rotation. J. Chem. Phys., 44:55-63.

———— 1968. Symmetry rules for optical rotation. Accounts Chem. Res., 1:144-151.

Sigman, D. S., D. A. Torchia and E. R. Blout. 1969. Phenacyl bromides as chromophoric reagents for α-chymotrypsin. Biochemistry (Washington), 8:4560-4566.

Sonenberg, M. 1969. Interaction of human growth hormone and human erythrocyte membranes as demonstrated by circular dichroism. Biochem. Biophys. Res. Commun., 36:450-455.

Takagi, T., K. Aki, T. Isemura, and T. Yamano. 1966. Inversion and enhancement of the circular dichroic spectrum of flavin adenine dinucleotide by the combination to D-amino acid oxidase. Biochem. Biophys. Res. Commun., 24:501-505.

Thyrum, P. T., R. J. Luchi, and H. L. Conn, Jr. 1968. The complex formation of procaine and procaine amide with adenosine triphosphate. J. Pharmacol. Exp. Ther., 164:239-251.

Tinoco, I. 1968. The optical properties of polynucleotides. J. Chem. Phys., 65:91-97.

Tipton, K. F., and J. F. A. Chase. 1969. The effects of substrates on the optical rotatory dispersion of carnitine acetyltransferase. Biochem. J., 115:517-520.

Torchinskii, Y. M., and L. G. Koreneva. 1964. Anomalous rotatory dispersion of aspartate-glutamate transminase: The effects of carbonyl reagents and substrate analogs. Biochim. Biophys. Acta, 79:426-429.

———— N. B. Livanova, and V. Y. Pikhelgas. 1969. Circular dichroism and optical rotatory dispersion of muscle phosphorylase B. Molec. Biol. (English edition), 1:23-28.

Ulmer, D. D., T. K. Li, and B. L. Vallee. 1961. Anomalous rotatory dispersion of enzyme complexes. II. The asymmetric binding of coenzymes and inhibitors to liver alcohol dehydrogenase. Proc. Nat. Acad. Sci. U.S.A., 47:1155-1165.

———— and B. L. Vallee. 1961. Anomalous rotatory dispersion of enzyme-chelate complexes. I. Alcohol dehydrogenase. J. Biol. Chem., 236:730-734.

———— and B. L. Vallee. 1965. Extrinsic Cotton effects and the mechanism of enzyme action. Advances Enzym., 27:37-104.

Urnes, P., and P. Doty. 1961. Optical rotation and the conformation of polypeptides and proteins. Advances Protein Chem., 16:401-544.

Urry, D. W., and T. H. Ji. 1968. Distortions in circular dichroism patterns of particulate (or membranous) systems. Arch. Biochem. Biophys., 128:802-807.

Velluz, L., M. Legrand, and M. Grosjean. 1965. Optical Circular Dichroism. New York, Academic Press.

Wagner, T. E. 1969. In vitro interaction of LSD with purified calf thymus DNA. Nature (London), 222:1170-1172.

Witiak, D. T., T. D. Sokoloski, M. W. Whitehouse, and F. Herman. 1969. Species difference in the competitive binding of 2-(4'-hydroxybenzeneazo)-benzoic acid and α-(4-chlorophenoxy)-α-methyl-propionic acid to serum albumin. J. Med. Chem., 12:754-761.

Woolley, P. V., and M. J. Hunter. 1970. Binding and circular dichroism data on bilirubin-albumin in the presence of oleate and salicylate. Arch. Biochem. Biophys. 140:197-209.

Yamaoka, K., and R. A. Resnick. 1966. Extrinsic Cotton effect of acridine orange bound to native DNA and helical poly-α, L-glutamic acid. J. Phys. Chem., 70:4051-4066.

———— and H. Ziffer. 1968. The optical properties of actinomycin D. II. Optical activity of the deoxyribonucleic acid complex. Biochemistry (Washington), 7:1001-1008.

Yang, J. T., and T. Samejima. 1969. Optical rotatory dispersion and circular dichroism of nucleic acids. Prog. Nucl. Acid. Res. 9:224-300. New York, Academic Press.

Yong, F. C., T. E. King, S. Oldham, M. R. Waterman and H. S. Mason. 1970. Redox-dependent conformational changes of rabbit liver cytochrome P-450. Arch. Biochem. Biophys., 138:96-100.

Chapter **5**

Mössbauer Effect Spectrometry in the Study of Biological Phenomena

Jordan L. Holtzman

Clinical Pharmacology Division, Minneapolis Veterans Administration Hospital, Minneapolis, Minnesota, and Department of Pharmacology, University of Minnesota, Minneapolis, Minnesota

INTRODUCTION

Mössbauer effect spectrometry, or nuclear resonance fluorescence, represents the newest and, for biology, the least applied of all the methods presented in this volume. In 1957 Rudolph L. Mössbauer, while working on his doctoral thesis, observed an anomalous temperature sensitivity of the absorption of γ-rays from metastable iridium, [191m]Ir, by the stable isotope, [191]Ir. He correctly interpreted these results as a resonance absorption of the γ-rays from the source by the nuclei of the absorber and published them in 1958 (Mössbauer, 1962). The importance of this work to nuclear physics resulted in his receiving the Nobel award in physics in 1961. It is doubtful that this form of spectrometry will yield the wealth of very basic information to biology that it has to physics, but it is already serving as a useful adjunct to the other forms of spectrometry, particularly as an index of changes that may be occurring around central atoms during a variety of biochemical processes.

THEORETICAL BASIS

The Excited State

It is now well established that both emission and absorption spectroscopy measure the quantized interaction of electromagnetic radiation with various energy states of an atom or molecule. Such energy states may represent an excited

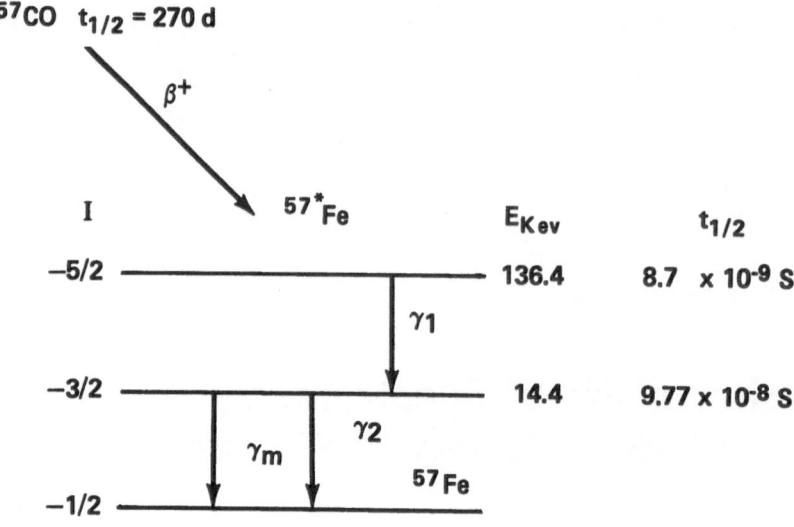

FIG. 1. Energy levels of the ^{57}Fe nucleus.

state of the nucleus, the electron shell, or the whole molecule. Mössbauer absorption spectrometry is no exception to this rule, since it is a method that measures γ-ray absorption by the nucleus. The γ-ray interaction with the atom results in changes of the spin state of the nucleus. Like elemental particles, the nucleus has an intrinsic spin, I. This spin is determined by the number and type of nucleons. A nucleus with both an even atomic number and mass has no ground state spin, while one with an odd atomic number, but an even mass, will have a spin with an integral value for I. Finally, if the nucleus has an odd mass number, I is an odd half-integer. In the case of ^{57}Fe, the most commonly studied of the Mössbauer isotopes, there are 26 protons and 31 neutrons. This means that the ground state for the nuclear spin is an odd half-integer, which in this case is $-\frac{1}{2}$. When the nucleus is excited, the spin state changes by integral units so that the first excited state is $I = -\frac{3}{2}$, the second $I = -\frac{5}{2}$, etc. (Figure 1). These excited states represent energy levels of 14.4 and 136.4 kev respectively. When the nucleus is irradiated with a 14.4 kev γ-ray, it can absorb the radiation and change its spin state to $I = \frac{3}{2}$. If this γ-ray is from another ^{57}Fe in an excited state, then the absorption is clearly a resonance phenomenon.

One of the unusual properties of the Mössbauer lines is that with the proper choice of source and absorber it is possible to demonstrate peak widths that are not appreciably greater than the width predicted by the Heisenberg uncertainty principle:

$$\Delta E \Delta t \geqslant h \tag{1}$$

where ΔE is the uncertainty in the energy of the excited states and also represents the minimal line width Γ, Δt is the mean life of the excited state, and h is Planck's constant. This can be rewritten:

$$\Delta E = (0.692\hbar)/t_{\frac{1}{2}} \qquad (2)$$

where $\hbar = h/2\pi$. In the first excited state of ^{57}Fe, where $I = -\frac{3}{2}$, the $t_{\frac{1}{2}} = 97.7$ nano-sec. The uncertainty in the energy of the transition or line width, Γ, is 4.6697×10^{-12} kev (Figure 2). If we divide this uncertainty by the energy of the transition, 14.4 kev, we find that the line width is 3.24×10^{-13} of the peak energy. For comparison, a spectral line at 8000 Å with a line width of 0.001Å has a dispersion of 1.25×10^{-7} of the peak energy. Even the international definitions of the standard units of length and time are defined only to 9 and 10 significant figures, respectively.

There are several reasons why the Mössbauer lines are so much sharper than at least the usual electronic spectra. The first is that the $t_{\frac{1}{2}}$ of the electronic transitions (10^{-13} sec) is several orders of magnitude shorter than the nuclear transitions, giving a proportionally greater value for the uncertainty in energy of the photons from electronic transitions. Secondly, the energy of these latter are much lower (only a few ev). Clearly, therefore, the ratio of the uncertainty of the energy of electronic transitions to their average energies will be much higher. Furthermore, these transitions will be much more sensitive to excited states of other molecular energy states.

Obviously, the usual techniques used for the determination of γ-ray energies, that is with proportional counters, crystal scintillators, or semiconductor detectors, can serve only as detectors, but can hardly serve to resolve any small shift in either the peak width or energy. Fortunately, these shifts in energy are sufficiently small so that it is possible to measure them by creating small shifts in the frequency of

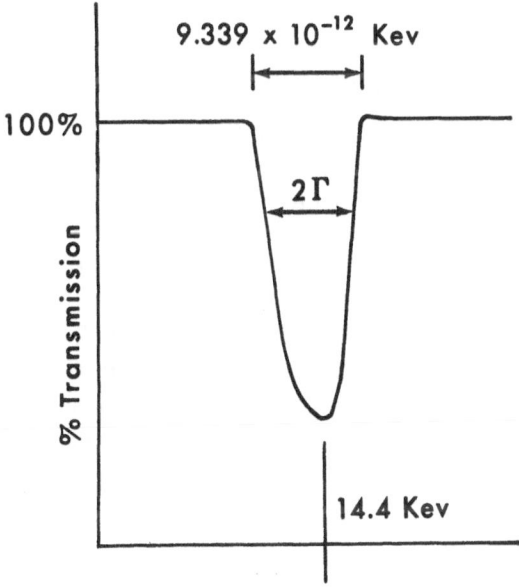

FIG. 2. Energy distribution of Mössbauer peak of ^{57}Fe nucleus ($I = -3/2 \rightarrow I = -1/2$).

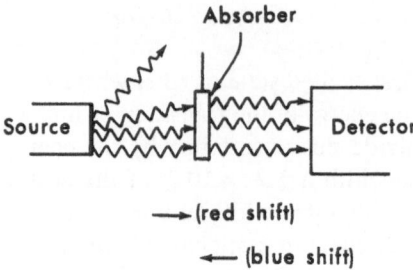

FIG. 3. Basic Mössbauer spectrometer.

the γ-ray by the use of the Doppler effect. The standard expression for Doppler shift is:

$$\nu = \nu_0 (c+v)/c \tag{3}$$

where v is the relative velocity of the emitting to the absorbing nuclei. When a correction is included to compensate for the fact that γ-rays are not truly collimated, the expression becomes:

$$\nu = \nu_0 (1+[v/c]\cos\theta) \tag{4}$$

where θ is the angle of incidence from perpendicular. In energy terms

$$E = E_0 (1+[v/c]\cos\theta) \tag{5}$$

$$\Gamma = E_0 (v/c)\cos\theta \tag{6}$$

It is clear therefore that for γ-rays perpendicular to the sample, small changes in the velocity of the absorber may well cause sufficient changes in the apparent energy of the γ-rays to be able to scan the natural peak width of the Mössbauer line. The basic arrangement of such a spectrometer is illustrated in Figure 3. In the case of ^{57}Fe the necessary change in velocity is

$$v = (\Gamma/E)c = 3.24 \times 10^{-13} \times 3.00 \times 10^{-11} = 9.72 \times 10^{-2} \text{ mm/sec} \tag{7}$$

for the half width, or 0.1944 mm/sec for the full width. This represents a velocity of 0.7 m/hr. For the usual Mössbauer isotopes studied, the maximum velocity is less than 5 mm/sec or 18 m/hr. These are clearly speeds that are readily achieved by a variety of simple techniques, as will be discussed below. A typical spectrum obtained is shown in Figure 4.

Because of the narrow line width, the lines of a Mössbauer spectrum are best described by a Lorenzian distribution:

$$I(E) = \frac{A\Gamma}{(E-E_0)^2 + (\Gamma/2)^2} \tag{8}$$

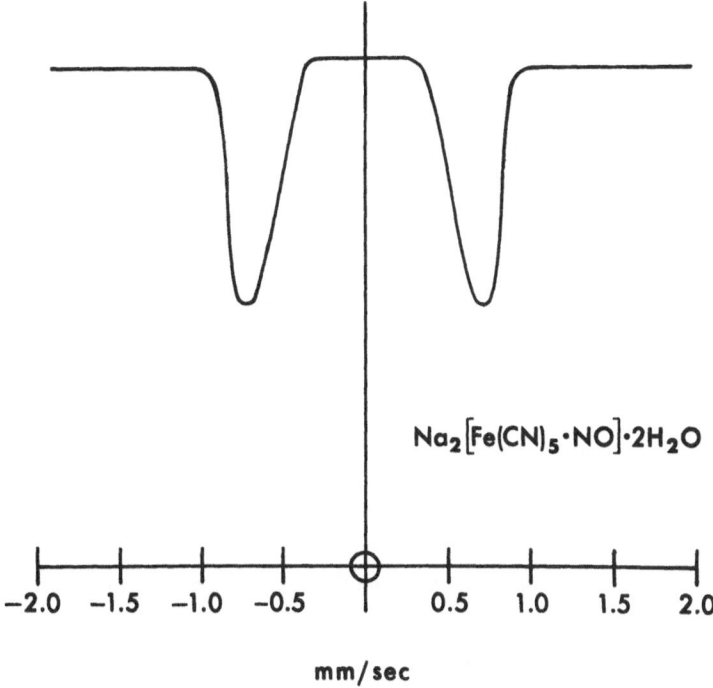

FIG. 4. Mossbauer spectrum of sodium nitroprusside.

where $I(E)$ is the intensity at energy E, A is a constant, and E_0 is the energy at the center of the peak. As these peaks are broadened by a variety of processes (discussed below), the shape becomes better approximated by the Gaussian distribution.

The Recoil-free Emission and Absorption

The above considerations might make it seem rather a simple matter to observe these spectra. One may well wonder, therefore, why they were not observed prior to 1957, especially since adequate technology had existed for at least 25 years. Furthermore, the existence of this phenomenon had been recognized almost 30 years before by Kuhn (1929). The main stumbling block was the recoil of the emitting and absorbing nuclei. When a resonant γ-ray leaves or enters the nucleus, classical mechanical considerations would predict that the overall change in momentum for the system should be zero. Therefore, the momentum of the nucleus should be equal to the momentum of the γ-ray, p. The latter is given by:

$$p = h\nu/c = E/c \tag{9}$$

This in turn should equal the momentum of the recoiling nucleus or:

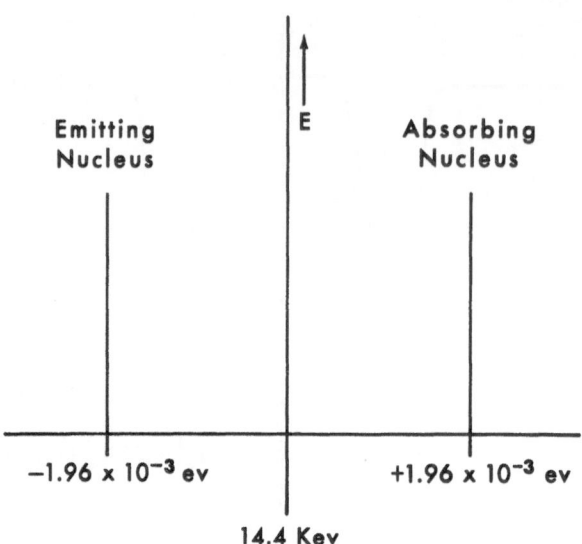

FIG. 5. Energy of emitting and absorbing ^{57}Fe nuclei when they are free to recoil.

$$p = mv_r \text{ and } E/c = mv_r \tag{10}$$

where m is the mass of the nucleus, and v_r is its recoil velocity. The energy of recoil, E_r, is then

$$E_r = \tfrac{1}{2} mv_r^2 = \tfrac{1}{2} E^2/mc^2 \tag{11}$$

For the 14.4 kev transition of ^{57}Fe, E_r is 1.96×10^{-3} ev. Now, the emitting nucleus will recoil in the opposite direction from the absorber, so that due to the recoil energy of the nucleus the emitted γ-ray will be 1.96×10^{-3} ev below the rest energy of the transition while the absorbing nucleus will be the same amount above (Figure 5). Furthermore, since their line widths are so narrow (3.24×10^{-9} ev—note change from kev to ev to correspond to the recoil energies) the two lines will not cross and there will be no absorption. Mössbauer (1962), in his studies of ^{191}Ir, had hoped that the peak widths would be sufficiently broad so that the two lines would cross, as shown in Figure 6, in spite of the recoil energy. Actually, the line width, Γ, is 3.564×10^{-6} ev, which is several orders of magnitude less than the recoil energy, 4.707×10^{-2} ev. As he cooled the samples, he began to observe absorption of the γ-rays so that at 80°K there was a 3% decrease in the total counts. He correctly concluded that the reason for the absorption was that, as the atoms were cooled, the strength of the bonding in the crystal lattice became sufficiently strong so that no recoil occurred. He postulated that the vibrations of the crystal, which must absorb the recoil energy, are quantized and that the lowest quantum level for crystal vibration was greater than the recoil energy, and hence recoil could not occur. The absorbing fraction is then the fraction of excited nuclei that do not go

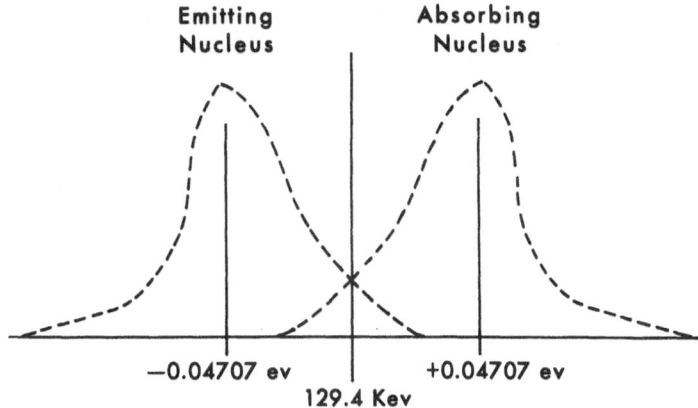

FIG. 6. Energy of emitting and absorbing ^{191}Ir nuclei when they are free to recoil.

into the first vibrational excited state of the crystal lattice. This fraction, f, is determined by the formula

$$f = \exp\left(-\frac{4\pi^2 d^2}{\lambda^2}\right) \tag{12}$$

where d is the displacement of the recoiling atom, and λ is the wavelength of the radiation. Clearly, the recoil-free fraction vanishes to zero in a liquid where the possible values of d are 0 to ∞. For crystalline materials these parameters can be estimated as a function of the Debye-Waller Factor.

Interestingly enough, absorption can be observed even in the presence of recoil if enough energy is added to the γ-ray to compensate for the recoil velocity as calculated in equation (6). In the case of ^{57}Fe, the necessary velocity is 40.8 m/sec. If the source is placed on the rim of a 10-cm ultracentrifuge rotor, absorbance should be observed at 39,000 rpm. Needless to say such a system is not likely to show the high resolution of the recoil-free system. Moon (1951) actually demonstrated such a system with ^{198}Au, an isotope for which no Mössbauer spectrum has been reported.

Mössbauer Isotopes

On the basis of the above considerations it is possible to make some prediction as to which isotopes will show the Mössbauer effect and those which will not. There are three primary factors, as follows.

(1) The nucleus must have an excited state that has a half-life of at least 10^{-11} sec. The nucleus with the shortest half-life which has been reported to have a Mössbauer γ-ray is ^{187}Re with a half-life of 1×10^{-11} sec. The Doppler shift required to observe such a large Γ resulting from the short half-life would be 12 m/min. At the other extreme is a half-life of 44 sec for ^{107}Ag. This gives

a Γ value of 10^{-20} kev for a γ-ray of 93 kev, which undoubtedly represents one of the most sharply resolved spectral lines in nature, with a dispersion of 10^{-22}.

(2) The transition must go to the ground state of the nucleus. Otherwise there will not be enough absorber nuclei in the proper state to absorb the γ-rays.

(3) The energy of the emitted γ-ray must be sufficiently low so that there remains a recoil-free fraction sufficient to observe absorption. The practical limit on the energy of the γ-ray is around 150 kev. Beyond this there is too much energy stored in the nucleus, and all the nuclei will recoil and cause vibration of the crystal lattice. The isotopes that have been shown to have Mössbauer γ-rays are listed in Table 1. Of these ^{57}Fe and ^{119}Sn have proven to be the most widely studied because of the convenient sources, the ease of equipment construction, and the general importance of these elements in chemistry and biology.

The Isomer Shift and Quadrupole Splitting

The above discussion gives no indication as to the interaction of the nucleus with the surrounding environment, for if the nucleus did not interact with extra-nuclear forces, this method would be of little interest to the chemist or biologist.

There are three ways in which the nucleus can react with the outside environment: (1), interaction with the electron cloud, or monopole interaction; (2), interaction with an electric field gradient (EFG), or quadrupole interaction; and (3), interaction with a magnetic field. The first and second of these are by far the most important in the application of this method.

The isomer shift represents the interaction of the nucleus with the electron cloud. The energy of interaction of the electrons with the nucleus is given by:

$$\Delta E = \frac{2\pi}{5} Ze^2 |\psi(o)|^2 R^2 \qquad (13)$$

where Z is the atomic number, $|\psi(o)|^2$ is the electronic density at the nucleus, R is the radius of the nucleus, and e is the electronic charge. Therefore, the difference in this interaction between the excited and the ground state will be given by:

$$\Delta E = \frac{2\pi Ze^2}{5} |\psi(o)|^2 (R_{EX}^2 - R_{GR}^2) = \frac{4\pi\,Ze^2 R_{av}^2}{5}\left(\frac{\delta R}{R_{av}}\right)|\psi(o)|^2 \qquad (14)$$

The differences in the energies of these electronic interactions for the given compound and those of a convenient standard for that isotope is the isomer shift, or δ. This is given by equation (13) as:

$$\delta = \Delta E_{Exp} - \Delta E_{Std} = \underbrace{\frac{4\pi Ze^2\,R_{av}^2}{5}\left(\frac{\delta R}{R_{av}}\right)}_{\text{Nuclear}}\underbrace{|\psi(o)\,Exp|^2 - |\psi(o)\,Std|^2}_{\text{Electronic}} \qquad (15)$$

TABLE 1

Isotopes with Reported Mössbauer Spectrum

Isotope	γ-Ray (kev)	Peak Width (mm/sec)	Source Isotope
^{107}Ag	93	6.685×10^{-11}	^{107}Cd
^{197}Au	77.3	1.966	^{197}Pt or ^{197}Hg
^{133}Cs	81.0	0.5378	^{133}Ba
^{160}Dy	86.8	1.576	^{160}Tb
^{161}Dy	25.7	0.3716	^{161}Tb or ^{161}Ho
^{166}Er	80.6	1.865	^{166}Ho
^{151}Eu	21.6	1.439	^{151}Sm
^{153}Eu	103.18, 97.43	17.55, 0.6868	^{153}Gd
^{57}Fe	14.4	0.19427	^{57}Co
^{155}Gd	60.0, 86.5	1900, 0.5142	^{155}Eu
^{158}Gd	79.5	1.434	^{158}Tb
^{73}Ge	67.0	2.520	^{73}Ge[a]
^{177}Hf	113.0	4.843	^{177m}Lu
^{127}I	57.6	2.553	^{127m}Te
^{129}I	27.8	0.6123	^{129m}Te
^{191}Ir	129.4	16.515	^{191}Os
^{193}Ir	73	0.6245	^{193}Os
^{40}K	29.4	2.386	^{39}K[b]
^{83}Kr	9.3	0.2001	^{83}Kr[a], ^{83}Br
^{61}Ni	67.4	0.7658	^{61}Ni[a]
^{237}Np	59.5	7.293	^{237}U
^{186}Os	137.2	2.374	^{186}Re
^{188}Os	155.0	2.485	^{188}Re
^{141}Pr	145.4	0.9797	^{141}Ce
^{195}Pt	8.8	17.30	^{195m}Pt, ^{195}Au
^{187}Re	134.2	203.8	^{187}W
^{99}Ru	90	0.1505	^{99}Rh
^{121}Sb	37.2	2.104	^{121m}Sn
^{149}Sm	22	1.636	^{149}Eu
^{119}Sn	23.9	0.6227	^{119m}Sn
^{181}Ta	6.25	6.436	^{181}W
^{159}Tb	58.0	36.28	^{159}Gd, ^{159}Dy
^{125}Te	35.5	5.209	^{125}I, ^{125m}Te
^{169}Tm	8.41	8.340	^{169}Er
^{182}W	100.1	1.995	^{182}Ta
^{183}W	46.5, 99.1	29.43	^{183}Ta
^{184}W	111.2	1.952	^{184}Ta, ^{184}Re
^{186}W	122.5	2.127	^{186}Re
^{129}Xe	39.6	7.016	^{129}I
^{131}Xe	80.2	7.583	^{131}I
^{170}Y	84.3	2.042	^{170}Tm
^{171}Y	66.7	8.199	^{171}Tm
^{67}Zn	93	3.129×10^{-4}	^{62}Zn[a]

[a] By coulombic excitation.
[b] After neutron irradiation.

Clearly, the first set of terms is nuclear, while the second set is dependent on the changes in the electron density at the nucleus.

Of all the orbital electrons, those which would have a significant density at the nucleus are those which are spherically symmetrical, namely the s-electrons. Yet in the case of, say, iron, these electron shells are full ($1s^2$, $2s^2$, $2p^6$, $3s^2$, $3p^6$, $4s^2$, $3d^6$), while the orbitals primarily involved in bonding are the $3d$, which have zero electron density at the nucleus. Yet changes are seen in δ because the $3d$ electron orbitals interact with the s-electron and tend to shield the latter from the nucleus. This lowers the s-electron density at the nucleus; that is, $|\psi(o)|^2$ for the s-electrons goes down. Changes in the electronic configuration which change the $3d$ shielding effect will change δ. From a series of Mössbauer spectra of iron compounds with anions of differing electronegativity, it has been possible to estimate that the value of the nuclear parameter $\dfrac{\delta R}{R_{av}}$ is -5.4×10^{-4}. It is interesting that the nucleus actually contracts in going to the excited state. To those accustomed to thinking in terms of the classic Bohr atom, with the increasing radius of the electron orbits with higher energy states, this may seem something of an anomaly. These results indicate that increased shielding of the nucleus by increased density of $3d$ electrons, as going from Fe^{3+} to Fe^{2+}, would lead to a positive δ, which it in fact does. On the other hand, ^{119}Sn has a positive $\dfrac{\delta R}{R_{av}}$ of 3.6×10^{-4}, and therefore the opposite effect would be expected for changes in $|\psi(o)|^2$.

A second interaction of the nucleus with the electrons of the atom is the interaction of the quadrupole moment of the nucleus with the electric field gradient resulting from asymmetries in the electron distribution. The quadrupole moment of the nucleus is due to the nucleus being ellipsoid rather than spherical. The existence of the quadrupole interaction would lead to the observation of two peaks in the Mössbauer spectrum. This splitting often represents, as in the case of the spectrum of sodium nitroprusside shown in Figure 7, obvious changes in the steric chemistry of the iron, since five of the six ligands are occupied by CN^-, while the sixth is occupied by NO.

From the point of view of understanding the gross symmetry of the molecules about the Mössbauer atom, the example of the nitroprusside ion is convenient, although more sophisticated molecular orbital calculations of the bonding about this atom will undoubtedly in the long run lead to a better understanding of the actual processes involved in chemical reactions. Unfortunately such considerations are beyond the scope of the training of the average investigator in the biological sciences. Furthermore, in many of the problems in biology, the necessary ancillary data, such as sequence analysis or x-ray diffraction data, are not available. But certain general comments can be made about the configuration of the electrons of the Mössbauer atom by studies of the isomer shift, δ, and the quadrupole splitting ΔE_Q. These values can also be compared to both ESR spectra and magnetic susceptibility determinations. The most fundamental information that these methods can yield is that concerning the oxidation and spin states of the Mössbauer atom; it would therefore be appropriate to discuss the significance of the electron orbital spin state.

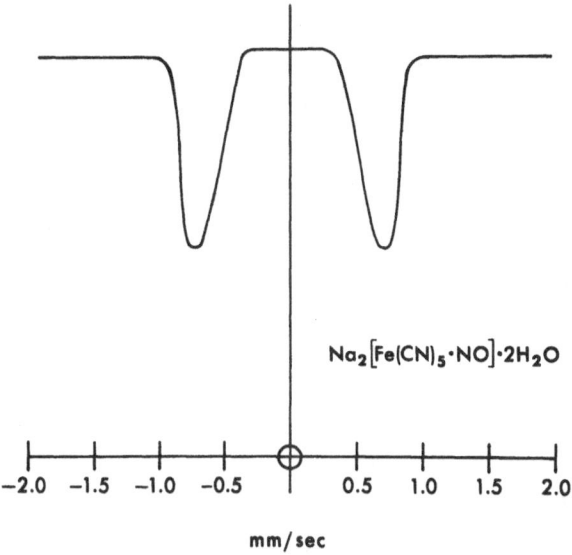

$$Na_2[Fe(CN)_5 \cdot NO] \cdot 2H_2O$$

-2.0 -1.5 -1.0 -0.5   0.5 1.0 1.5 2.0

mm/sec

FIG. 7. Mössbauer spectrum of sodium nitroprusside.

It is well known that as the atomic number increases the s- and p-orbitals are successively filled until the 4s is filled. After the filling of the 4s orbitals, the transition metal series begins with the filling of the 3d orbitals. In the case of metallic iron with $4s^2$, $3d^6$, the unpaired electrons of the 3d orbitals lead to its magnetic properties (Figure 8). When the ionic species of iron are formed, the remaining electrons can line up in a variety of arrangements. The primary effect is that the electrons are lost from the 4s shell, so that $|\psi(o)|^2$ decreases, and since $\dfrac{\delta R}{R_{av}}$ is negative, δ increases. Secondly, the remaining electrons in the d-orbitals can either pair up to give a low spin complex with a minimal number of unpaired electrons, or line up to give the maximum number of unpaired electrons in the high-spin complex. The total electron spin, S, is ½ for each unpaired electron. For example, low-spin ferric is $S=\frac{1}{2}$, while the high spin is $S=\frac{5}{2}$. The character as well as the symmetry of the ligands determines the nature of the spin state. For example, one would expect a CN⁻ complex of a ferriheme to be low spin, in spite of molecular asymmetry, since this species can participate in the π-bonding of the porphyrin ring. On the other hand, the single substitution of F⁻ or other electronegative species that cannot participate in π-bonding will give the high-spin species. Therefore the determination of the spin state gives a clue as to the nature, as well as the symmetry, of the ligands.

In dealing with pure compounds having a single iron species, such information concerning the spin state can be determined by measuring the magnetic susceptibility. This measurement indicates the number of unpaired electrons. A much more sensitive method for determining the spin state is ESR spectrometry. The low- and high-spin ferric compounds both may give spectra, since they have at least one

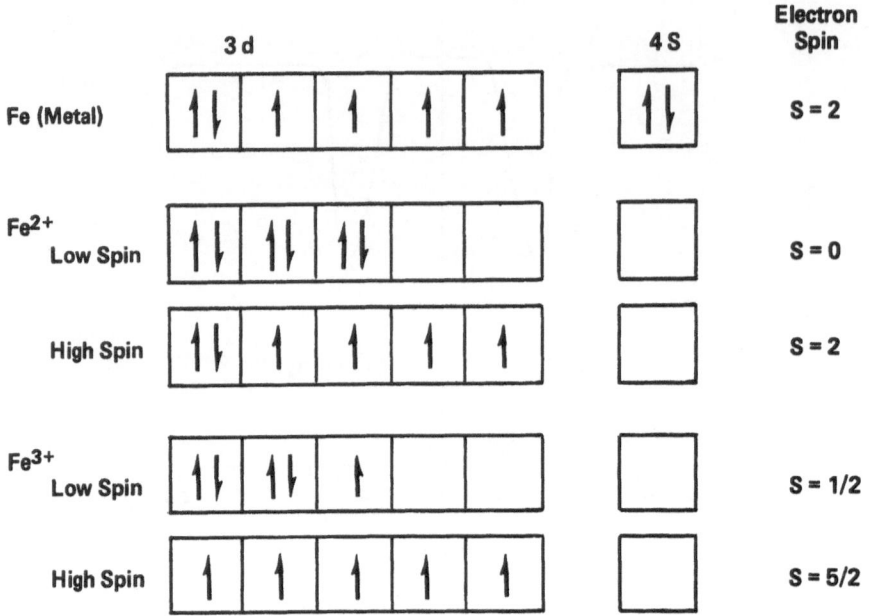

FIG. 8. Orientation of the electron spin in metallic iron and in low and high spin ferrous and ferric compounds.

unpaired electron, while only the high-spin ferrous will give a spectrum since the low-spin has no unpaired electrons. In the case of some biological reductions, though, it may be difficult to determine whether the unpaired electrons observed in the ESR spectrum are due to some free radical species, as flavine semiquinone, or are due to high-spin iron. Further problems related to the ESR spectrum of hemoproteins are discussed below.

The Mössbauer spectrum quadrupole splitting provides a means for determining the spin state of the iron. Quadrupole splitting is generally seen as two peaks in the spectrum. The isomer shift is taken as the average velocity of the two peaks, while the splitting is the distance between the peaks. At room temperature, for example, high-spin ferric may have little or no quadrupole splitting since all the orbitals are symmetrically filled and there is no electric field gradient. In fact, one would not expect to see any splitting until the sample had been brought to below 10°K, since only at this temperature are there sufficient differences in the energies of the various d-orbitals so that, in accordance with the Boltzman equation, some orbitals are more populated than others. The total spin may drop to $S = \frac{3}{2}$ or even $\frac{1}{2}$, depending on the splitting of the orbital energies.

The above considerations are important in establishing the parameters of the iron species, but from the point of view of the chemist, certain guide lines are useful in determining the oxidation and spin state of the iron atom. For this purpose a large amount of data has been collected and a general pattern established (Figure 9) for the various species as to their characteristic δ and ΔE_Q. Such graphs

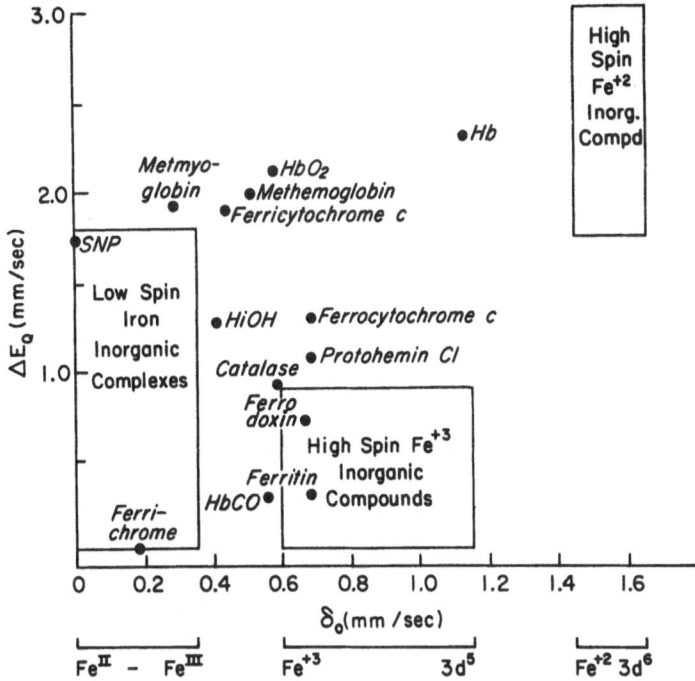

FIG. 9. Scattergram of various iron species as a function of isomer shift (abscissa) and quadrupole splitting (ordinate). The isomer shift for sodium nitroprusside (SNP) is taken to be zero. (Courtesy of L. May.)

are useful for making a tentative identification of the chemical state of the iron atom. Further studies involving changes in both the chemical and physical state of the material can lead to more definitive identification. One word of caution should be added here. All the spectra in these graphs are corrected to 25°C. There is a small effect of temperature on δ since the molecular vibrations cause a small or secondary Doppler shift in the γ-ray energies.

Magnetic Hyperfine Splitting

In the previous section the interaction of the nucleus with the electron cloud and with any electric field gradient which may be present was discussed. These effects are the ones of primary importance to the chemist, but another effect is that of the interaction with a magnetic field gradient. The nucleus, like the electron orbitals, has a magnetic moment (m). There are $(2|I|+1)$ possible states. So for $I = -\frac{1}{2}$, $m = \pm\frac{1}{2}$. For $I = -\frac{3}{2}$, $m = -\frac{3}{2}, -\frac{1}{2}, \frac{1}{2}, \frac{3}{2}$. In a transition from $I = -\frac{1}{2}$ to $I = -\frac{3}{2}$, m changes of -1, 0, or 1 are allowed. In a magnetic field, where these energy levels are no longer degenerate, the six permissible transitions will be represented by six Mössbauer lines. Such splitting may result from a magnetic field in the crystal or from an externally applied field. Although this phenomenon is of lesser importance for the biologist than those presented in the previous section, it can be used as a guide in determining the sign of the electric field gradient and can also indicate the spin state of the iron.

Line Broadening and Peak Asymmetries

There are a number of effects which may lead to an increase in the apparent or real width of the peak beyond that predicted for the natural line width, Γ. The most obvious cause of line broadening is that the spectrum may actually represent the sum of two or more peaks. For example, in the preparation of the specimen, such as hemoglobin, a certain amount of denaturation occurs and both a high- and low-spin-state species can be observed. In such a case the area represented by the various peaks is proportional to the concentration of the different species. Other examples have been observed and will be discussed below. In some of these cases, a mixed spin state has been postulated to represent a spin-spin equilibrium, in which each molecule may switch from one to another state.

A second problem is that the γ-rays are not collimated and therefore the $\cos\theta$ term of equation (6) will not be one resulting in some broadening of the peak. A second important mechanical problem is that the samples have a finite thickness so that the orbital electrons will scatter the γ-rays by Compton scatter. This results in a broadening of their energies and a reduction in the resolving power of the spectrometer. This phenomenon places a lower limit on the concentration of Mössbauer nuclei present in the sample which will give a spectrum.

Gol'danskii et al. (1963) have demonstrated that, when the recoil-free fraction is anisotropic, line-broadening or asymmetry in two separate lines may be observed. In this instance the recoil-free fraction will depend on which plane of the crystal the γ-ray is absorbed. In some planes the minimum vibrational level will be lower than in others. For example, the energy of minimum recoil should be lower if the γ-ray hits perpendicular to the plane of the porphyrin ring than if it hits parallel to it. This might be a factor in dealing with powdered crystals, but in frozen solutions, where the crystal lattice is composed of the ice crystals, isotropic behavior would be expected.

Another phenomenon which can lead to both line broadening and asymmetry is electronic spin-spin and electronic spin-nuclear relaxation. In the former, there is an exchange of spin energies between two molecules so that one may go from, say, $S = \frac{5}{2}$ to $S = \frac{3}{2}$, while the other goes in the opposite direction. If a system happens to be in an excited nuclear spin state of $I = -\frac{3}{2}$, then this change in the value of S could cause an alteration in the electron density at the nucleus with concomitant changes in the δ and ΔE_Q. As the temperature is lowered to $4.2°K$, the upper spin states become less populated. Furthermore, since these upper spin states have longer $t_{\frac{1}{2}}$'s and their net effect on the electron density at the nucleus is less likely to average to zero, when they become less populated and only the lower $S = \frac{1}{2}$ is filled, this asymmetry disappears.

DESIGN OF THE SPECTROMETER

Methods of Scanning the Energy Spectrum

As stated above, all the presently used methods for the scanning of the energy spectrum depend on the creation of a Doppler shift in the energy of the γ-rays. The original method used by Mössbauer was to attach a cone drive to a toy phonograph table on which was mounted the source (Figure 10a). By varying the angular velocity, and therefore the tangential velocity, it was possible to scan the energy spectrum, but only one velocity at a time could be employed. This method also suffers from the disadvantage that either the source is exposed to the exit port for only a small fraction of the cycle or, if the source is deposited as a ring on the rim of the table, only a small fraction of the source is exposed all the time.

A second method, which has received a great deal of attention, is to move the source at a constant velocity by a screw cam either directly or through a hydrau-

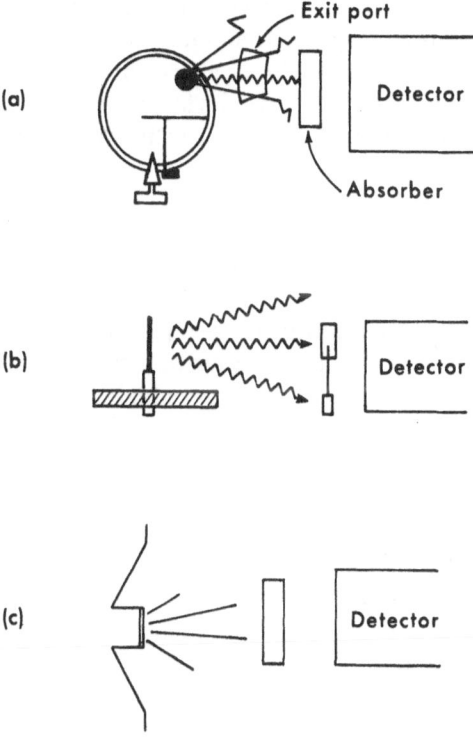

FIG. 10. Methods for creating a Doppler shift in the γ-rays. (a) The source is mounted on a rotating table (constant velocity). (b) The source is mounted on a cam drive (constant velocity). (c) The source (or absorber) is mounted on an electromagnetic drive (speaker cone) (constant velocity or constant acceleration).

lic system (Figure 10b). As with the turntable technique, only one velocity can be done at a time. Also, there will be a change in the intensity of the radiation since the source is changing its distance from the detector. The changes follow the well-known inverse square law of radiation, and it is no difficult matter to cancel out this effect either by modifying the computer program used to fit the data, or by simply running the source between the same points for each velocity and making appropriate corrections. Nevertheless, for samples with low absorption this may lead to some loss of sensitivity.

A much more ingenious method, which has now become the most widely used, is to mount either the source or the absorber on the coil of an ordinary loudspeaker (Figure 10c). The speaker can then be connected to a signal generator with a sawtooth output. This will give a linearly changing velocity (constant acceleration) so that the entire energy spectrum can be scanned and the counts at each velocity can be fed into a multichannel analyzer. It is possible to control the address in the analyzer to which the counts are sent by directly measuring the velocity of the coil. Several such feedback schemes have been used. Probably the simplest is to have a second coil wound onto the speaker. The voltage from this coil is then proportional to the velocity of the driving unit and can be used directly to control either the multichannel analyzer or the drive mechanism. It is also possible to determine the velocity by the use of optical techniques such as an interferometer lit by a He-Ne laser or Moiré grating. The fringe patterns or grating interference patterns can then be detected with a light-sensitive device, such as a semiconductor photodiode, and the output used either to control or calibrate the electronic drive or the addressing circuits of the analyzer.

Detectors and Associated Electronics

There are three major factors which are important in the choice of detectors. Clearly, the most important is that the detector be sensitive to the γ-ray photons of interest. Secondly, the detector must be usable at high count rates. And finally, the unit should be able to discriminate against unwanted radiation resulting from Compton scatter or from other nuclear transitions. At the present time the two most commonly used detectors are the proportional counter and the NaI (Tl) crystal scintillators.

The proportional counter is constructed very much like the more familiar Geiger-Müller counter and consists of a central wire anode and concentric cathode. A thin (1-mil thick) window of beryllium, aluminum, or metal-coated plastic is placed over the end. A counting gas is either sealed in or more often constantly flushed through. The sole basic difference between the proportional counter and the Geiger-Müller is the applied voltage. If the voltage across the tube is increased from zero, at first no current flows, but at about 90 to 100 volts there is an increase in current representing the total number of electrons produced by the primary interaction of the radiation with the counting gas. As the voltage is further increased, the current increases due to a cascading effect in which the free electrons formed liberate other electrons from the atoms of the counting gas. In this region, the proportional region, the number of free electrons formed is proportional to the original energy of the radiating particle. At a higher voltage, the Geiger-Müller region, the tube totally discharges irrespective of the energy of the radiation. The proportional counter, by giving pulses proportional to the energy of the radiation, permits discrimination against unwanted radiation and has an energy resolution of about 12% using a gas flow mixture of 90% A and 10% CH_4. A second advantage of the proportional counter is the high count rates which can be achieved. It is possible to achieve count rates close to 100,000 counts per second, whereas with the Geiger-Müller counter the maximum rate is about 200 counts per second. This permits the use of extremely active sources (50 mc or more). By the use of such active sources, the time to reach one or more million events in each of 200 channels can be significantly reduced. This then minimizes the error due to counting statistics. Since the interaction of γ-rays and gases is markedly reduced at energies greater than 20 kev, the proportional counters find their greatest use below this energy as with the 14.4 kev line of ^{57}Fe.

In contrast to the proportional counter, the efficiency of the thallium-activated NaI crystal scintillators is close to 100% at energies above 6 kev. These are used in the well and scanning γ-ray counters, but are limited to about 10,000 counts per second. Moreover, the resolution of these units ranges from 50% at 6 kev to about 10% of the γ-ray energy at 200 kev. These units are therefore the most commonly used at higher ranges, such as the 23.9 kev line of ^{119}Sn.

A third group of detectors, which will probably be used more in the future, are the semiconductor detectors. These units consist of germanium or silicon wafers into which lithium has been diffused. The silicon-lithium drift detector has a range of 5 to 200 kev, with a resolution of 3.5% at 100 kev. Unfortunately, such detectors are much noisier than the other two, so that they place greater demands on the associated electronic equipment and also require liquid nitrogen cooling.

An interesting detector is constructed by placing a proportional counter between the source and the absorber, or with the absorber actually in the counter. In this arrangement for ^{57}Fe, the 14.4 kev γ-ray excites the absorber ^{57}Fe. The excited state can either re-emit the 14.4 kev γ-ray or, as usually happens, emit a 6.4 kev γ-ray, which is formed by internal conversion, a process which is ten times more likely than the re-emission of the Mössbauer γ-ray. Because of the low energy of the conversion γ-ray, this method is limited to surface phenomena. It does, however, have the advantage of a low background so that absorption is observed as a small increase above background rather than the difference between two large numbers.

It may well be that in the future the resonance phenomenon itself may be used as a detector. In such a case the background due to the Compton scatter would be greatly reduced without affecting the pure Mössbauer γ-ray. Unfortunately, the problem of matching the source and detector so that the two do not require a Doppler shift to observe resonance has proven to be technically difficult to resolve.

Irrespective of the detector used, the output is fed through a preamplifier and a discriminator circuit to a 200-channel multichannel analyzer. Such a unit can be synchronized with the drive circuit, as mentioned above, so that each channel is used to record the total number of events for each small range of velocities. These individual channels usually record up to 10^6 events, so that the total number of events which can be stored is 2×10^8. As each channel reaches its full capacity, it starts over again. It is no difficult matter to calculate the total overflow number, that is how many times the channel filled up during the run.

Sources and Standard Absorbers

The preparation of the sources demands a good deal of skill and investment in equipment and personnel. Fortunately, a number of sources are commercially available including ^{57}Co for ^{57}Fe, ^{119m}Sn for ^{119}Sn, and ^{129m}Te for ^{129}I. The method by which any source is prepared depends on several considerations. The first is whether the emitter is derived by the radioactive decay of a nucleus to the excited state of the Mössbauer isotope, as in the case of ^{57}Co with a half-life of 270d, or whether the emitter is a long half-life metastable that decays to the Mössbauer excited state, as ^{119m}Sn, which has a half-life of 245d. In the first case the source isotope can be made and then diffused into and/or electroplated onto the matrix. In the latter case a tin compound, such as $BaSnO_3$, can be irradiated and used directly.

In the preparation of the source, the recoil-free fraction, f, of the source-matrix should be as close to unity as is possible at the operating temperature. This is necessary in order to achieve the highest efficiency. Another requirement is that the electron orbitals about the emitter atom must be symmetrical. This will eliminate the possibility of quadrupole splitting of the energy of the emitted γ-rays. For iron the requirement for spherical symmetry can be achieved by diffusing the ^{57}Co into a palladium foil.

Another method for the preparation of Mössbauer emitters is the direct irradiation of the source, ^{1}H, ^{2}H, neutrons or ^{16}O in a van de graaff accelerator, in order either to raise the isotope to the excited state (as with ^{61}Ni or ^{67}Zn) or to produce the excited state from a stable isotope, as in the case of producing ^{40}K by the irradiation of ^{39}K with either deuterons or neutrons. In the latter case the ^{40}K formed is highly excited and quickly decays to the Mössbauer energy level of 29.4 kev, which has a half-life of 3.7×10^{-9} sec. Although these methods permit the study of the Mössbauer spectra of isotopes for which no convenient source is available, the complexity of the system and the high background often limit their usefulness and clearly demand a great deal of skill and investment in order to obtain meaningful results.

After preparation of the source and the assembly of the equipment, it is necessary to calibrate the velocities of the drive and to determine the zero velocity position of the unit. Without such calibration, the values obtained from different sets of experiments would bear little relationship to each other. The velocity can be determined optically, as stated above, or by a variety of mechanical means, although such methods are rather complex for the routine measurement of peaks. Perhaps of greater theoretical and practical significance is that the zero isomer shift, δ, must be defined in terms of some standard. Initially, this was taken as either α-iron or stainless steel. Spijkerman et al. (1967), and Herber (1965), have found that there were significant changes dependent on the method of preparation of these standards, particularly in their carbon content. In addition, there is a wide range of alloys which are referred to as stainless steel. Therefore, for the purposes of reproducibility, a more consistent standard has been chosen, namely sodium nitroprusside ($Na_2Fe[CN]_5NO\cdot2H_2O$), and its isomer shift set equal to zero. This compound is readily obtainable and can be easily prepared with ^{57}Fe; it has the same isomer shift from one preparation to the next; and it has a well-defined pair of peaks representing a quadrupole splitting of 1.726 mm/sec$\pm$0.002 peak to peak. Therefore by running this material it is possible to determine both the channel representing zero velocity as the average of the two peaks and the channels representing $\pm$0.863 mm/sec, the velocities of each peak. If the drive velocity is linear with respect to the channel number, as it usually is to about 1%, then the velocity calibration is complete for the source-drive combination. Recently a pure preparation of iron has become available and is recommended as the standard for $\delta=0$. With regular calibration, experimental results may be obtained in which the investigator can place some confidence and can compare with those obtained by other workers.

Useful Accessory Equipment

By far the most useful piece of accessory equipment is an electronic computer. The data from the multichannel analyzer can be punched out onto a tape and fed into a computer outlet. The best fit peaks can then be determined by a least-squares program to fit the data either to a set of Lorentzian curves, if the peaks are sharp, or to a set of Gaussian curves if the peaks are broad. The programs can also be set to calculate the best fit for a predetermined number of lines. Such programs in Fortran are available and can be used with units having memories with as little as a 7000-word capacity, such as is found in some of the time-sharing systems.

A second piece of useful equipment is a low-temperature cryostat, preferably a unit that can bring the absorber to liquid-helium temperatures. In the study of solutions it is necessary to freeze the sample, since in free solution there is no recoil-free fraction. Even with solid samples, running spectra at low temperatures, particularly at liquid-helium temperatures, gives a great deal of information about the structure and spin state of the Mössbauer isotope.

A third piece of equipment that can yield a great deal of information, although it is not nearly as important as the previous two, is a high-flux magnet. With an electromagnet capable of fluxes of 5 to 100 kilogauss, it is possible to gain an enormous amount of information about the electric and magnetic field gradients about the Mössbauer atom. Furthermore, the causes of asymmetries and line broadening can be more effectively studied.

Sources of Equipment

There are at least two commercially available complete spectrometers. These consist of the drive mechanism with the associated oscillators, the counting device, and the preamplifiers and multichannel analyzer. They are available from Austin Science Associates, Inc., Austin, Texas; and Elron, Inc., Skokie, Illinois. These units cost about $10,000.

Radioactive sources are available from New England Nuclear Corp., Boston, Massachusetts; ICN Instrument Division, Oakland, California; and Amersham/ Searle Corp., Arlington Heights, Illinois. A 50-mc ^{57}Co source with a 270d half-life costs about $1,000. Such a source would give useful spectra for one or two years, depending on the counting statistics required to observe a Mössbauer effect in the samples being studied. This will depend in turn on the concentration of the element and the percentage of the Mössbauer isotope present and the recoil-free fraction, f. For example, with ^{57}Fe, which has a natural abundance of 2.19%, L. May and I have obtained a discernible spectrum with as little as 0.28 μg atoms of native iron (1.7×10^{17} atoms of iron or 3.4×10^{15} atoms of ^{57}Fe) in a half gram of lyophilized hepatic microsomes. In these studies a 10 mc source was used and each channel recorded about 3×10^6 events over 18 to 24 hours of scanning.

An alternative to the use of hotter sources or larger samples is to enrich the material with ^{57}Fe. Iron with 90 to 100% abundance of ^{57}Fe is obtainable from New England Nuclear Corp. for $7.50/mg. Lesser abundances may also be obtained at a substantial saving from Oakridge National Laboratories. In the preparation of iron-containing compounds, the substitution of high abundance ^{57}Fe iron is a simple matter. Even in the use of bacterial or yeast systems, with moderate precautions it is not difficult to achieve abundances of 50% or better for the ^{57}Fe, by culturing the organism on media containing the iron as ^{57}Fe. Unfortunately the matter is not so simple when using vertebrates. Gonser and Grant (1965) were able to obtain only about 3.5% abundance of ^{57}Fe in hemoglobin by injection of 90% ^{57}Fe citrate into anemic rats.

For those whose interests or finances do not allow such an investment in equipment, it is quite possible to assemble much of the necessary equipment and fabricate the remainder. The most important component, the multichannel analyzer, is available from a number of commercial sources for around $5,000. The remainder of the equipment, particularly the hybrid operational amplifiers, are now available from such sources as Analog Devices, Cambridge, Massachusetts, and Philbrick-Nexus, Dedham, Massachusetts, for as little as $10 to about $150 for the high-speed, low-noise preamplifiers. Because of their excellent characteristics and low cost, any investigator who is adept at electronic fabrication and has access to a machine shop can now assemble a Mössbauer spectrometer.

APPLICATIONS OF MÖSSBAUER SPECTROMETRY
TO PHYSICAL AND CHEMICAL PROBLEMS

The initial applications of Mössbauer spectrometry were related to under-standing the resonance fluorescence phenomenon itself and its implications to nuclear structure. Because of the high-line resolution, it has been used to study the gravitational effect on photons, which results in the red shift predicted by Einstein's special theory of relativity. More recently it has been suggested that it might be valuable in the detection of gravitational waves, and therefore be a further test of the general theory of relativity.

Mössbauer spectrometry has also proven to be a valuable technique in the study of the magnetic properties of alloys. Such studies, moreover, give a clue as to the crystalline structure of these materials, as well as their magnetic properties. Although these studies have provided basic information to the physicists and physical chemists, they bear little relation to the type of problem faced by the biologist.

More in line with the usual chemical problem has been the study of the oxidation state of the iron atoms in the ferri-ferrocyanides. It is possible to synthe-size these iron cyanide compound complexes, either by the addition of a ferric salt to a ferrocyanide (Prussian blue), or the addition of a ferrous salt to a ferricyanide (Turnbull's blue). The method of synthesis might suggest that these two com-pounds are different, but Mössbauer studies have unequivocally indicated that the anion is a ferric ferrocyanide in both. Furthermore, there were distinct peaks, one for a high spin Fe^{3+} and the other for a Fe^{II}, the latter being a more covalent bond than is found in ferrocyanide complexes and the metallic state. Since the peaks are distinct, there cannot be any rapid exchange of electrons between the two iron atoms, otherwise there would be equal amounts of ferro-ferricyanide and ferri-ferrocyanide, and the peaks would be broadened due to changes in the electron density occurring with transition rates greater than the life time of the Mössbauer excited state.

The number and symmetry of the Mössbauer peaks can give valuable informa-tion concerning the structure of iron compounds. An example of this has been studies on the iron dodecal carbonyl, $Fe_3(CO)_{12}$. Mössbauer spectrometry indicated that there are two different types of atoms with peak areas in a ratio of $1:2$. These results suggested two possible structures for this compound (Figure 11). Further studies showed that when a hydride ion replaced one of the CO groups, there was no effect on the spectrum. If the structure is that shown in Figure 11a, then the only place that a hydride ion could go is onto one of the end iron atoms, a replacement which would lead to radical changes in the spectrum. Therefore the only structure that fits the data is the one in Figure 11b.

Such studies have not been limited to the study of iron compounds. For example, studies on the spectra of I_2, ICl, IBr, and $I_2Cl_4Br_2$ have indicated that the last compound is not just a mixture of ICl_6 and IBr_6, but rather a true compound

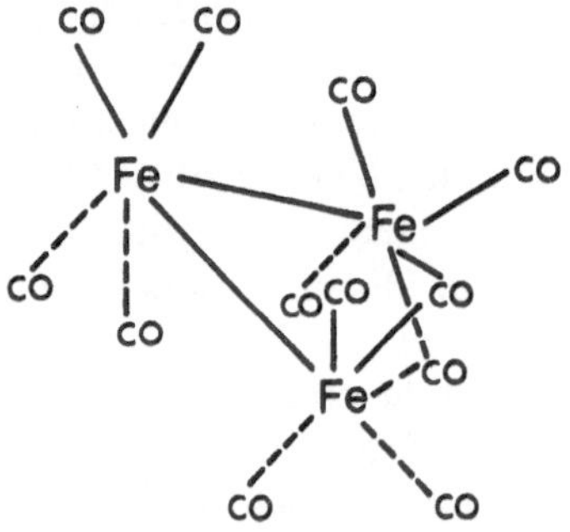

FIG. 11. Possible structures of iron dodecacarbonyl.

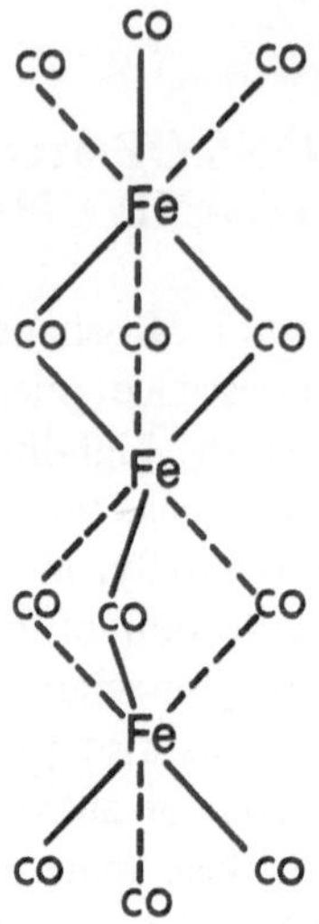

in its own right. Furthermore, these studies have indicated that this compound is linear with Cl bridges between the two iodines (Figure 12). Similar studies have been performed on Xe compounds, such as $XeCl_4$ and XeO_4 by using the ^{129}I compounds as the source. After the ^{129}I decays by electron capture to the excited state of ^{129}Xe, the resulting compound does not break up, but rather gives Mössbauer spectra characteristic of the Xe compound. As will be mentioned below, similar studies have been performed on iron derivatives of vitamin B_{12}.

These examples hardly begin to scratch the surface of the studies in physics and chemistry which have been performed with the aid of Mössbauer spectrometry, but have been presented to indicate the type of information which can be obtained by this method. One might well wonder whether such methods might be applicable to the small range of pharmaceuticals that contain iron. With this in mind we might mention the results of two sets of workers, Tsing and Wang (1963) in Taiwan, and Kisynska et al. (1968) in Russia, who have examined the Mössbauer spectrum

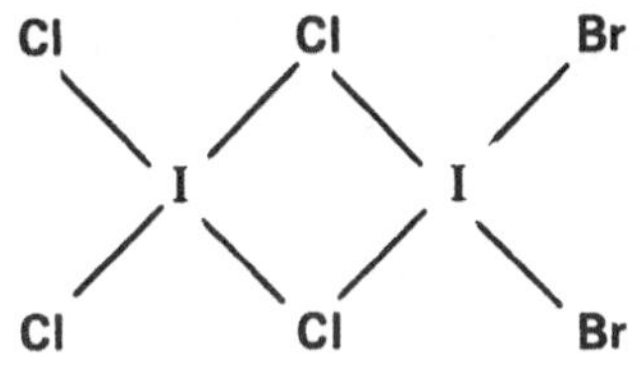

FIG. 12. Structure of $I_2Cl_4Br_2$.

of ferrous gluconate. Their results indicate the characteristic spectrum of a high-spin ferrous compound, similar to ferrous sulfate. Although such results are those which would have been expected, they are still of some interest, as was probably the authors' intent, in the creation of spectra catalogs. On the other hand, it is doubtful that such studies of these preparations will yield much basic or practical information concerning the use of such compounds as medicinal agents.

APPLICATIONS OF MÖSSBAUER SPECTROMETRY TO BIOLOGICAL PROBLEMS

Hemes and Hemoproteins

Of all the iron-containing compounds of biological interest, the most thoroughly investigated group, both chemically and spectrometrically, consists of the hemes and their protein derivatives, the hemoproteins. All of these molecules consist of the very familiar complex of iron with a porphyrin, usually protoporphyrin IX in vertebrates, to give heme (Figure 13). The iron in this compound has a coordinate number of six, of which four ligand bonds are taken up by the porphyrin and the other two (L_1 and L_2 of Figure 13) may be bound to a number of ligands. In the hemoproteins, L_1 is often coordinated to a histidyl residue on the apoprotein. The sixth ligand (L_2) may be bound to a variety of substituents as OH^- or, in the case of oxyhemoglobin, O_2. Alternatively, the sixth ligand could be tied up to some other amino acid residue in the protein. As an example of this, Dickerson et al. (1967) have suggested that the sixth ligand of ferrocytochrome-C may be a methionyl residue.

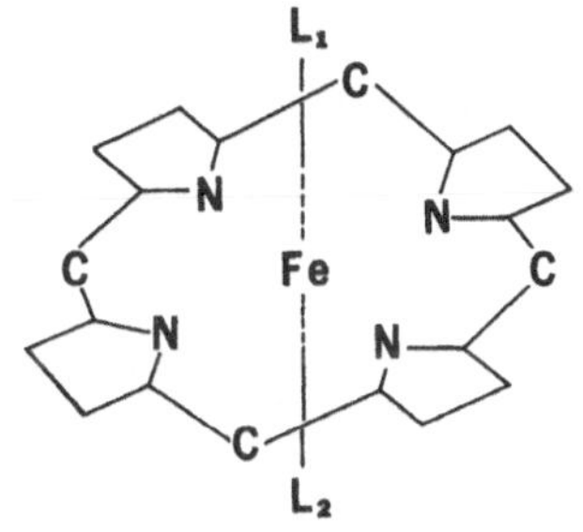

FIG. 13. Basic structure of hemes.

The physical characteristics of several hemoproteins have been well elucidated, including the resolution of the x-ray diffraction pattern of hemoproteins beginning with the classic work of both Perutz (1963) and Kendrew (1963) and their coworkers. Their work led to maps of the precise geometries of crystalline hemoglobin and myoglobin, respectively. The hemoproteins have a characteristic visible absorption spectrum with an α band around 560 nm, a β band around 530 nm, and the Soret bands around 420 nm. These spectra have been correlated with the spin state of the central iron atom; the spin state being determined from magnetic susceptibility measurements. As discussed above, magnetic susceptibility determines the number of unpaired electrons, but demands the preparation of relatively pure compounds with a fairly high concentration of the active species. Fortunately for the study of ferrihemoproteins, the high- and low-spin states of each have a characteristic ESR spectrum.

Since we and other workers have used correlations of Mössbauer spectrometry with the ESR spectra, and since the description of the methodology of ESR presented in these pages is not directed towards the study of hemoproteins, a short description of the significance of these spectra may be appropriate here. As discussed above, the high spin ferrihemoprotein has five unpaired electrons and an electron spin of $S = \frac{5}{2}$ (Figure 8). If single crystals of such a hemoprotein are placed in an ESR spectrometer, there will be different absorption peaks depending on the orientation of the crystal with respect to the magnetic field. If the crystal is oriented so that the axis is parallel to the magnetic field, then an absorption peak is observed at a $g = 2.0$. If the crystal is now rotated so that the axis is perpendicular to the field, the resulting peak will have a $g = 6.0$. Finally, if there is rhombic symmetry of the heme with the iron out of the plane of the porphyrin ring, rather than the usual octahedral symmetry, then there may be a peak at $g = 4.3$, which has less dependence on the orientation of the crystal in the magnetic field. On the other hand, the low-spin ferrihemoproteins lack such axial symmetry properties, and show peaks at $g = 2.4$ to 2.8 for the orbital contributions in the z-axis, $g = 2.2$ for those in the y-axis, and $g = 1.8$ to 1.9 for those in the x-axis. As is evident from Figure 8, the low-spin ferrohemoproteins have no unpaired electrons, that is $S = 0$, and exhibit no ESR spectrum. Therefore, since on reduction of the ferrihemoproteins the low-spin ferrohemes are usually formed, the spectrum is likely to disappear. This clearly is a serious deficiency of the method in the study of oxidation-reduction systems. A second, potentially more serious problem is that, due to the spin-lattice relaxation, many hemoproteins do not exhibit any ESR spectrum; that is, there is sufficient interaction between the unpaired electrons of the heme with the other energy states of the molecule and crystal to broaden the peaks so that they cannot be observed. In spite of these problems ESR has become one of the most important tools in the study of hemoproteins.

There are a number of studies that have attempted to correlate the Mössbauer parameters of isomer shift, δ, and quadrupole splitting, ΔE_Q, with the results of ESR and magnetic susceptibility studies, and to use the results of these studies to build simplified quantum mechanical models of the electron orbitals. Lang and Marshall (1966) as well as other workers have attempted to apply either the Hückel molecular orbital approximations or the consistent crystal field approximations to develop a complete model of the electron orbitals about the heme. Furthermore, they have determined significant parameters of these orbitals using these models. Such investigations have been particularly concerned with heme, hemoglobin, and myoglobin (Lang et al., 1970), all of which have well-known structures. These studies can predict some features of the infrared spectrum. Often in such studies, as pointed out above, ESR can offer no information, and even the magnetic susceptibility does not offer the wealth of information that can be obtained from Mössbauer studies, particularly when temperature and magnetic effects are included.

Mössbauer spectrometry can be used more directly for structural studies of hemes. One example of this is the recent studies on the structure of heme dimers in oxygenated solutions (Cohen, 1969; Sadasivan et al., 1969). Studies with molecular weight determinations established the existence of the heme dimer, while infrared spectrometry and magnetic susceptibility determinations suggested that there was an oxygen bridge between the irons of the hemes. This latter hypothesis was consistent with the Mössbauer spectra.

An interesting aspect of hemoprotein chemistry is the role of water in the structure of these molecules. In aqueous solution, for example, hemoglobin is completely in the high-spin ferrous state, as determined by both magnetic susceptibility and Mössbauer spectrometry on frozen solutions. On the other hand, when it is lyophilized, it becomes a $1:1$ mixture of high- and low-spin ferrous. There are three possible interpretations of this observation. The first is that one set of chains (either the α or the β) change their configuration to allow a group, such as another histidyl residue with strong π-bonding characteristics, to become the sixth ligand of the heme and therefore for the heme to become low spin. A second possibility is that the change in chain conformation is relatively nonspecific, and that there may be a heme-heme spin-spin equilibrium where no single heme is necessarily in one spin state or another all the time. A third possibility is that there is water bound to the sixth ligand of the heme. Its removal, rather than changes in the conformation of the protein, may be the major effect. This latter possibility seems unlikely, at first, because of the x-ray evidence, which indicates that there is no water in this position in the crystalline state. This is not very strong evidence, since the x-ray data are taken in the essentially dry state.

To examine this problem further, the spin states of dried myoglobin and metmyoglobin were studied. This makes an excellent model since the protein sequence of this monomer is considered to be the phylogenetic precurser of the α-chain of hemoglobin. The high-spin ferrous of myoglobin is not altered by drying. Since there is no change in the spin of the myoglobin on drying, the change in spin would appear to occur only in the β-chains of the hemoglobin.

Leopold May and I (May and Holtzman, 1970) have performed similar studies on the cytochrome P-450 of the hepatic microsomes. This cytochrome, unlike hemoglobin and myoglobin, cannot be obtained in the pure state and, in fact, is not soluble. As soon as this cytochrome is detached from the lipoprotein matrix of the microsomal membrane, it becomes completely denatured and is essentially undetectable. We have made microsomal preparations from animals that

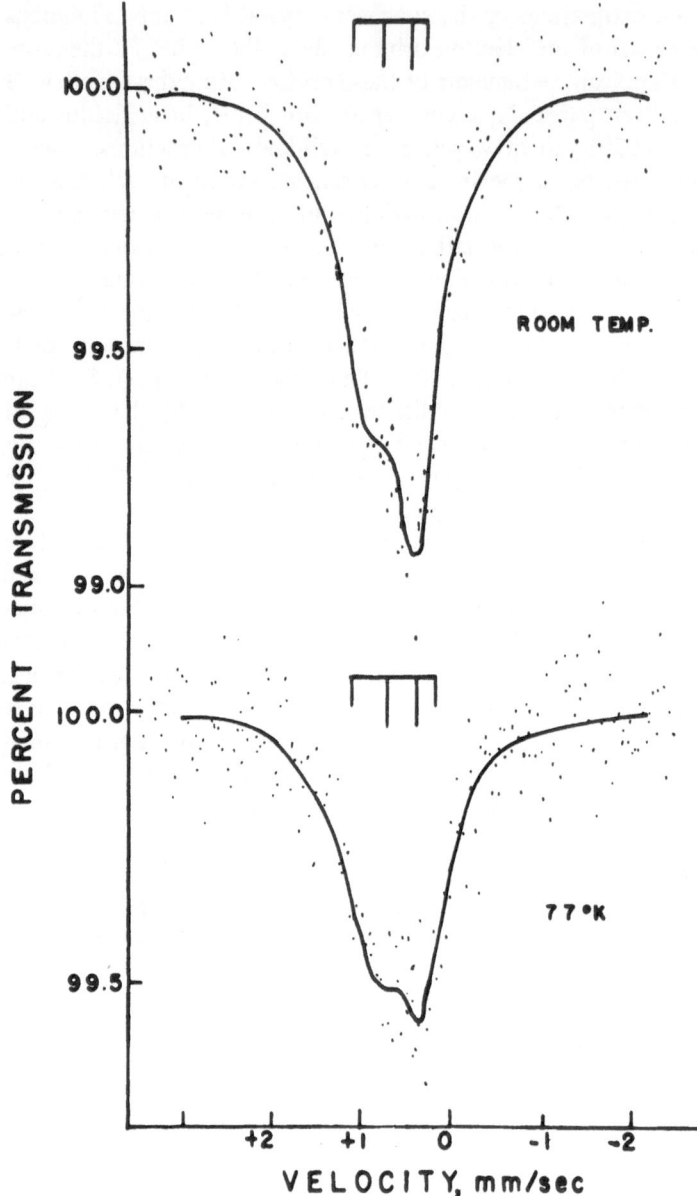

FIG. 14. Mössbauer spectrum of lyophilized rat hepatic microsomes. (From May and Holtzman. 1970. *Biochem. Biophys. Research Commun.*, 39:296.)

have received phenobarbital for several days to induce the accumulation of this cytochrome. The microsomes were lyophilized either in distilled water initially to avoid possible contamination by iron in the buffers, or in KCl-tris buffer. In both cases, the spectra indicated a high-spin ferric or a mixed-spin state (Figure 14). Yet, the ESR spectrum of this cytochrome in frozen solution has been found by Mason

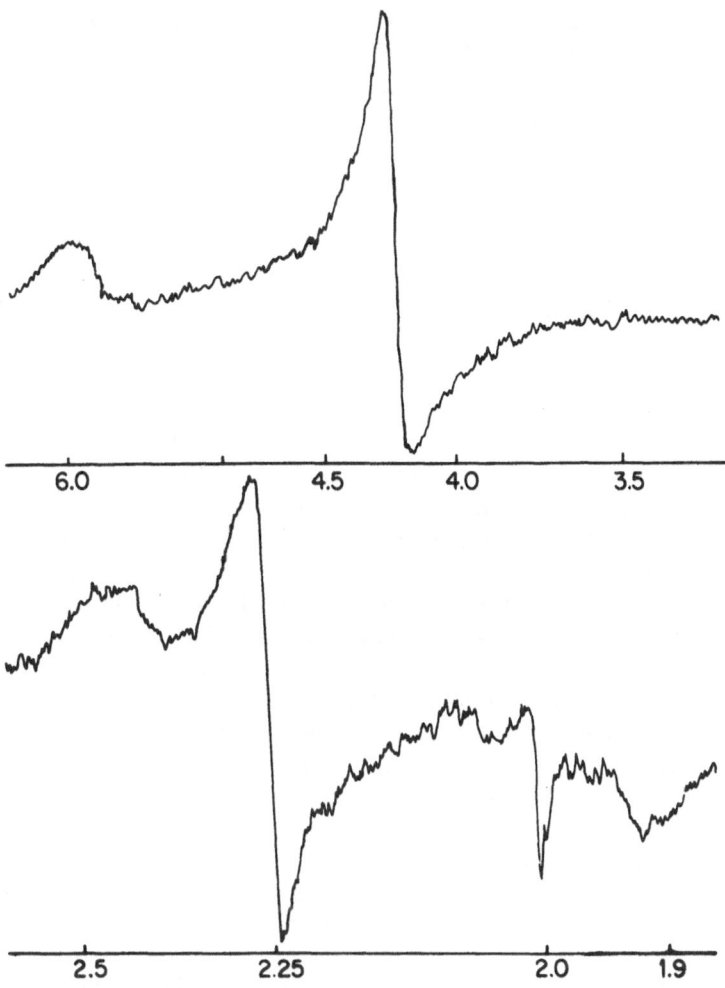

FIG. 15. ESR spectrum of lyophilized rat hepatic microsomes. (From May and Holtzman. 1970. *Biochem. Biophys. Research Commun.*, 39:296.)

and coworkers (1965) to have $g_z = 2.4$, $g_y = 2.25$, and $g_x = 1.92$, values characteristic of low-spin ferrihemes. Further ESR studies on a lyophilized preparation from distilled water showed a $g = 6.0$, 4.3, and 2.0, as well as the low-spin lines; while from buffer they showed only the low spin (Figure 15). It is not clear at this time whether this failure to observe the mixed spin state in the ESR spectrum of the buffer-suspended microsomes is due to differences in the lattice relaxation of the differently prepared hemes, or whether there is a real difference in the spin states of the microsomes. The Mössbauer data would indicate the former, since there was no difference in this spectrum of the two types of preparations. Furthermore, Peisach and Blumberg (1970) have demonstrated the existence of the high-spin form in whole microsomes from a 3-methylcholanthrene-treated rabbit by the use of ESR at 16°K, where lattice degeneration is less important.

There are two interesting implications of these data. The first is that this may represent further evidence that the cytochrome in question is not a single species, but like the α- and β-chains of hemoglobin, is really several closely related species. There is a vast body of evidence to indicate this, but since this cytochrome cannot be solubilized and separated into its various component species, we may have here the first physical evidence for the existence of these multiple species in animals not receiving aromatic hydrocarbons.

A second interesting implication is that the water does bind to this cytochrome in spite of the fact that it is buried in a lipid membrane. In fact, it has long been considered that, on the basis of the high enzymatic activity of this cytochrome for lipophilic substrates, the active sites are not exposed to water. Yet, the changes observed would indicate that some regions must be well hydrated. Furthermore, if the lyophilization is performed in buffer, this hydration is quite reversible. Recent studies in our laboratory with D_2O have tended to substantiate the probable importance of hydration of the cytochrome near or on the active sites. The question of whether the heme itself is hydrated still remains unanswered.

Maeda and Morita (1968) have also used Mössbauer spectrometry to study the oxidation state of horseradish peroxidase. This compound does not give an ESR spectrum. In the native state it appears, from the Mössbauer spectrum, to be in the low-spin ferric state. On the addition of peroxide, a series of three compounds, I, II, and III, are formed. It has been assumed that I has a Fe^{4+}-O which goes to the Fe^{5+} on the formation of II. Mössbauer spectra indicated that no such shift occurred, but that both I and II had typical values of δ and ΔE_Q, indicating a high-spin ferric. These data are consistent with the presence of the Fe^{4+} in both I and II, so that the transformation must occur by the removal of an electron from some region of the molecule other than the iron. Compound III has a Mössbauer spectrum with values of δ and ΔE_Q that are found in a high-spin ferric or a low-spin ferrous such as oxyhemoglobin. In view of the similarities of the parameters to those of oxyhemoglobin, it has been suggested that compound III is an oxy-ferrous heme.

Recently Pasternak et al. (1970) have examined the bonding of ^{129}I and ^{125}Te to heme. They observed that these bonds are essentially covalent unlike the fluoride bond. Furthermore, they found that the bonding of histidine had no effect on the spectrum of the iodine-heme complex. These data suggest that the histidine does not significantly participate in the π-bonds of the heme.

A more unusual study of the oxidation state of hemes has been reported by Champion and Drickamer (1967), who have examined the effect of pressure on the Mössbauer spectrum of ferric heme. They found that the spectral parameters of the iron reversibly went from those of a typical ferric state at atmospheric pressure to those of a ferrous state at 165 kilobars. It is not quite clear whether this change represents a genuine change in the oxidation state of the iron, or whether the high pressure merely distorted the electronic configuration of the iron to give these strange results.

Recently several workers have used ^{57}Co cyanocobalamin as the source for the Mössbauer spectrometer (Nath et al., 1968; Mullen, 1970). As the ^{57}Co decays, the highly excited atom of ^{57}Fe is not ejected from the molecule, but merely loses several electrons. There is a rapid (10^{-13} sec) readjustment of the iron to the ferrous state, so that by the time the Mössbauer γ-ray is emitted, the iron atom is in an electronically unexcited state. They found that the recoil-free fraction was as high (greater than 0.9) as would be expected if the iron had been chemically incorporated.

Even from this rather sketchy review of the Mössbauer studies of hemes and hemoproteins, it should be evident that a vast body of information concerning the effects of various factors on the spectra of these compounds has been obtained. At the present time Mössbauer spectroscopy is being used along with other spectrometric and chemical methods to establish the homogeneity of the iron species in these compounds.

Nonheme Iron-Sulfur Proteins

The nonheme iron-sulfur proteins represent a second and very important component of many electron chains found in all phyla of living organisms investigated so far. These compounds are, among others, important constituents of the mitochondrial electron chain, the chloroplasts, and the hydroxylating systems of steroid hormone producing organs. They have a characteristic absorption at 450 and 550 nm and, in the reduced state, have an ESR absorption peak at $g = 1.94$, although only a few have the nonspecific $g = 4.3$ in the oxidized state, representing rhombic symmetry. A final interesting property is that these compounds, which contain 2 to 8 iron atoms per molecule, will not transfer more than one electron per two iron atoms. For example, ferridoxin, with two iron atoms, will accept only one electron.

Among questions which may be examined by Mössbauer spectrometry is whether the transfer of electrons through these molecules is through the iron atoms or whether the actual reduced species is a sulfur atom. If the iron atoms are involved, it would be of interest to know whether the electron is shared by both atoms or whether one atom is reduced and the other remains unaffected. Finally, it is hoped that eventually these data, along with the available sequence analysis, may give a clue as to the coordination chemistry of the iron.

The present evidence seems to indicate that nonheme iron-sulfur proteins, although very similar, are not entirely the same. For example, the nonheme iron component of oxidized xanthine oxidase would appear to be high-spin ferric, while the oxidized ferridoxins and putidaredoxin appear to be low spin. Unfortunately, there appears to be some confusion in the literature, even for a single type as spinach ferridoxin, as to whether the iron atoms in the reduced state are equivalent or whether there is the reduction of one atom of the molecule and the other remains oxidized. But clearly the reduction does involve a change in the oxidation-reduction of the iron atoms, and does not require the involvement of the sulfur.

Two groups of Russian workers have examined the spectra of a nonheme iron system that seems to be involved in the fixation of atmospheric nitrogen by *Azobacter vinelandi* (Moshkovskii et al., 1967; Novikov et al., 1968). They have demonstrated an interaction of this enzyme with N_2, which does not occur in an inert atmosphere of pure argon. Recently Kelly and Lang (1970) have studied the Mössbauer spectra of the two purified components of the nitrogenase system from *Klebsiella pneumoniae*. Their studies on the spectra of these iron-containing proteins in the presence of substrates and inhibitors confirms and extends the above observations concerning the importance of the iron in this process.

Other Studies of Biological Interest

Mössbauer studies have also been reported for the iron core of ferritin, an iron-binding protein found both in the intestinal mucosa and liver. The iron appears to be a ferric hydroxide, of which there are four mineral forms, α, β, γ, and δ. When the core iron was compared to the mineral forms, it was found that the Mössbauer spectrum was closest to that of the δ form, which is a mineral called lipidocrocite (Gilchrist et al., 1966).

The interaction of ferric iron with nucleotides and nucleic acids showed that, at low pHs, the iron binds to the phosphate while at higher pHs it binds to the amino groups of the adenine (Rabinowitz et al., 1966).

The absorption properties of cellulose and bone have been studied by the interaction with ferric salts in the first case, and with ^{133}Ba in the latter case, in which the ^{133}Ba was adsorbed onto the bone. It decays to ^{133}Cs, and this isotope was used as the Mössbauer source (Ianakieva et al., 1968; Marshall, 1968).

Lest the reader think that only chemical or crystallographic studies lend themselves to the use of Mössbauer spectrometry, it should be mentioned that the method can be used for more macroscopic studies. In one case, SnO_2 absorbers were glued onto ants and the effect of temperature on the line width examined (Bonchev et al., 1968). It was found that as the temperature was raised there was a broadening, which the authors attributed to increased breathing of their subjects. This method therefore offered a measure of the average movement of the ants. Similar studies have been performed on the middle ear of the anesthetized guinea pig (Gilad et al., 1967).

POTENTIAL APPLICATIONS TO BIOCHEMICAL AND PHARMACOLOGICAL PROBLEMS

Since this has been a rather abbreviated account of the various theoretical, mechanical, and chemical aspects of Mössbauer spectrometry, the reader may well wonder of what value this method may be to the average investigator, whose most likely *modus operandi* will initially be to search out a physicist or physical chemist and try to convince him that these studies could be both fruitful and of mutual interest. Clearly, in the study of iron-containing proteins, a vast amount of work has been done and more undoubtedly will be done in order to elucidate the mechanisms involved in electron transport. Related to this, it might be of interest to examine the Mössbauer spectra of ^{119}Sn in relation to the ability of alkyl tins to uncouple mitochondrial phosphorylation. Such a study would be greatly enhanced if the iron spectra could be obtained concurrently.

Another metal which may be of some interest is ^{67}Zn. There are a number of enzymes and protein hormones that require this element for activity. Similarly, the binding of ^{133}Cs and ^{40}K to membranes or other active proteins might well lend themselves to studies of this nature.

One of the most tantalizing subjects for study is the interaction of Xe with membrane and respiratory proteins. Either ^{129}I or ^{131}I could be used as a source material, since the resulting ^{129}Xe and ^{131}Xe both are reasonably abundant in the native gas (26% and 21%, respectively). The ^{129}I has a very long half-life (1.6×10^7 yr), so that only low activities can be obtained, but the ^{129}Xe has a large cross-section. Such studies may well give some information as to how Xe can act as an anesthetic agent.

Another isotope which might seem of potential value is ^{127}I, the only stable isotope of iodine. A convenient commercial Mössbauer source, ^{127m}Te ($t_{1/2} = 105$d), is available. The iodination of proteins would provide a convenient probe of the importance of tyrosine residues in the interaction of antibodies and antigens, and of enzymes with their substrates. The only difficulty with the use of iodine or xenon is that both have less resolution than iron. Since the half-life of the Mössbauer-excited state is of the order of 10^{-9} to 10^{-8} sec, the line widths are about 2 mm/sec. Because of the large peak width for ^{127}I, ^{129}I would be preferred since its natural width is one-fourth that of ^{127}I. The source for this, ^{129}Te ($t_{1/2} = 33$d), is also commercially available.

One final note. As has been emphasized above, the ability of an isotope to absorb the resonant γ-rays is dependent on its recoil-free fraction as well as the energy of the γ-rays. In all the studies discussed above, the recoil-free fraction, f, was brought close to unity by either freezing a solution or by using a dry material. Craig and Sutin (1963) have investigated the effect of viscosity on the recoil-free fraction. They have found that by the addition of glycerol to a solution of ^{57}CoCl$_2$, it was possible to increase the viscosity of the solution to a point at which the recoil-free fraction was very high. In view of these results, it may well be possible to study the viscosity of membrane-bound constituents by the estimation of the recoil-free fraction. Other methods for examining movement in membranes, such as differential thermal analysis, allow for the determination of phase changes in the bulk material, but do not offer the fine probe that Mössbauer spectrometry may offer, either by the examination of native iron-containing enzymes, or by the binding of iodine, or one of the rare earths, to the membrane protein. If iron is to be used in such a dilute state, it will be necessary to study methods for increasing the abundance of ^{57}Fe in the whole animal.

ACKNOWLEDGMENT

I wish to thank Dr. Leopold May for his helpful criticism and comments in the preparation of this manuscript.

REFERENCES

General

A. BOOKS
Wertheim, G. K. 1964. Mössbauer Effect, Principles, and Applications. New York, Academic Press.

Gol'danskii, V. I., and R. H. Herber. 1968. Chemical Applications of Mössbauer Spectroscopy. New York, Academic Press.

May, L., ed. 1970. An Introduction to Mössbauer Spectroscopy. New York, Plenum Press.

B. REVIEWS
DeVoe, J. R., and J. J. Spijkerman. 1966-1970. Mössbauer spectrometry. Anal. Chem., 38:382R-393R (1966); 40:472R-489R (1968); 42:366R-388R (1970).

Greenwood, N. N. 1967. The Mössbauer spectra of chemical compounds. Chemistry in Britain, 3:56-72. (This excellent review is available gratis from the New England Nuclear Corporation, Boston, Massachusetts 02118.)

Mössbauer, R. L. 1962. Recoilless nuclear resonance absorption of gamma radiation. Science, 137:731-738. (This is Professor Mössbauer's Nobel Prize acceptance speech.)

Lang, G. 1970. Mössbauer spectroscopy of heme proteins. Quart. Rev. Biophys., 3:1-60.

C. SYMPOSIA AND SOURCE BOOKS
Gruverman, I. J., ed. 1970. Mössbauer Effect Methodology. Vols. 1-5. New York, Plenum Press.

Gould, R. F., ed. 1967. The Mössbauer Effect and Its Application in Chemistry. Advances in Chemistry Series, No. 68. Washington, American Chemical Society.

Muir, A. H. Jr., K. J. Ando, and H. M. Coogan. 1966. Mössbauer Effect Data Index 1958-1965. New York, Wiley/Interscience.

Index of Publications in Mössbauer Spectroscopy of Biological Materials. (Available from Dr. Leopold May, Department of Chemistry, The Catholic University of America, Washington, D.C.)

Text

Bonchev, T., I. Vassilev, T. Sapindzhiev, and M. Evtimov. 1968. Possibility of investigating movement in a group of ants by Mössbauer effect. Nature (London), 217:96-98.

Champion, A. R., and H. G. Drickamer. 1967. The effect of pressure on the Mössbauer resonance in hemin and iron phthalocyamine. Proc. Nat. Acad. Sci. U.S.A., 58:876-883.

Cohen, I. A. 1969. The dimeric nature of hemin hydroxides. J. Amer. Chem. Soc., 91:1980-1983.

Craig, P. P., and N. Sutin. 1963. Mössbauer effect in liquids: Influence of diffusion broadening. Phys. Rev. Letters, 11:460-462.

Dickerson, R. E., M. L. Kopka, J. E. Weinzierl, J. C. Varnum, D. Eisenberg, and

E. Margoliash. 1967. An interpretation of a two-derivative, 4 Å resolution electron density map of horse heart ferricytochrome c. *In* Okunuki, K., M. Kamen, and I. Sekuzu, eds., Structure and Function of Cytochromes. Tokyo, University of Tokyo Press.

Gilad, P., S. Shtrikman, P. Hillman, M. Rubinstein, and A. Eviatar. 1967. Application of Mössbauer methods to ear vibration. J. Acoust. Soc. Amer., 41:1232-1236.

Gilchrist, J. L., W. H. Orme-Johnson, and R. L. Collins. 1966. Mössbauer studies of ferritin. Bull. Amer. Phys. Soc. (ser. II), 11:50 (abstract cc 13).

Gol'danskii, V. I., E. F. Makarov and V. V. Khrapov. 1963. On the difference in two peaks of quadrupole splitting in Mössbauer spectra. Physics Letters, 3:344-346.

Gonser, U., and R. W. Grant. 1965. Mössbauer effect in hemoglobin and some iron containing biological compounds. Biophys. J., 5:823-844.

Herber, R. H. 1965. Mössbauer spectroscopy: Some recent applications to chemical problems. *In* Gruverman, I. J., ed., Mössbauer Methodology, vol. 1:3-12. New York, Plenum Press.

Ianakieva, M., J.-P. Quiles, M. Chêne, T. Christov, R. Chevalier, and M. Belakhovsky. 1968. Applications de l'effet Mössbauer à l'étude de la cellulose. C. R. Acad. Sci. (Paris), 267c:1013-1016.

Kelly, M., and G. Lang. 1970. Evidence from Mössbauer spectroscopy for the role of iron in nitrogen fixation. Biochim. Biophys. Acta, 223:86-104.

Kendrew, J. C. 1963. Myoglobin and the structure of proteins. Science, 139:1259-1266.

Kisynska, K., M. Kopecewicz, S. J. Hiigenza, and Prekaszewski. 1968. Mössbauer effect in ferrous gluconate. Nukleonika, 13:969-974.

Kuhn, W. 1929. Scattering of Thorium C″ γ-radiation by radium G and ordinary lead. Philos. Mag. (series 7), 8:265-636.

Lang, G., T. Asakura, and T. Yonetani. 1970. Mössbauer spectroscopy of mesohaem and protohaem myoglobin and their fluoride complexes. Biochim. Biophys. Acta, 214:381-388.

———— and W. Marshall. 1966. Mössbauer effect in some hemoglobin compounds. Proc. Amer. Phys. Soc., 87:3-34.

Maeda, Y., and Y. Morita. 1968. Mössbauer effect in peroxidase. *In* Okunuki, K., M. D. Kamen, and I. Sekuzu, eds., Structure and Function of Cytochromes. Baltimore, University Park Press.

Marshall, J. H. 1968. The Mössbauer effect from crystal surfaces. Phys. Med. Biol., 13:15-22.

Mason, H. S., J. C. North, and M. Vanneste. 1965. Microsomal mixed-function oxidations: The metabolism of xenobiotics. Fed. Proc., 24:1172-1180.

May, L. 1970. An Introduction to Mössbauer Spectroscopy. New York, Plenum Press.

———— and J. L. Holtzman. 1970. Mössbauer spectroscopy of lyophilized rat liver microsomes. Biochem. Biophys. Res. Commun., 39:296-300.

Moon, P. B. 1951. Resonant nuclear scattering of gamma-rays: Theory and preliminary experiments. Proc. Phys. Soc., 64:76-82.

Moshkovskii, Y. S., I. D. Ivanov, R. A. Stukan, G. I. Matkhannov, S. S. Mardanyan, Y. M. Belov, and V. I. Gol'danskii. 1967. Application of the Mössbauer effect to the study of the role of iron in biological nitrogen fixation. Dokl. Biol. Sci. Akad. Nauk S.S.S.R., 174:215-217 (Russian); 343-345 (English).

Mössbauer, R. L. 1962. Recoilless nuclear resonance absorption of gamma radiation. Science, 137:731-738.

Mullen, R. T. 1970. Mössbauer studies of vitamin B_{12} and some related cobalamine. *In* Gruverman, I. J., ed., Mössbauer Methodology, 5:95-105. New York, Plenum Press.

Nath, A., M. Harpold, and M. P. Klein. 1968. Emission Mössbauer spectroscopy for biologically important molecules. Vitamin B_{12}, its analogs, and cobolt phthalocyanine. Chem. Phys. Letters, 2:471-476.

Novikov, G. V., L. A. Syrtsova, G. I. Likhtenshtein, V. A. Trukhtanov, V. F. Rachek, and V. I. Gol'danskii. 1968. Investigation of the iron containing paramagnetic protein of non-heme nature contained in the nitrogen fixing system of *Azotobacter vinelandii* by the method of nuclear γ resonance. Dokl. Akad. Nauk S.S.S.R. (Phys. Chem.), 181:1170-1173 (Russian); 590-592 (English).

Pasternak, M., P. G. Debrunner, G. DePasquali, L. P. Hage, and L. Yeoman. 1970. Application of ^{129}I Mössbauer effect to biological systems: Studies with heme models. Proc. Nat. Acad. Sci. U.S.A., 66:1142-1147.

Peisach, J., and W. E. Blumberg. 1970. Electron paramagnetic resonance study of the high- and low-spin forms of cytochrome P-450 in liver and in liver microsomes from a 3-methylcholanthrene treated rabbit. Proc. Nat. Acad. Sci. U.S.A., 67:172-179.

Perutz, M. F. 1963. X-ray analysis of hemoglobin. Science, 140:863-869.

Rabinowitz, I. N., F. F. Davis, and R. H. Herber. 1966. Mössbauer effect on metal binding in purine compounds. J. Amer. Chem. Soc., 88:4346-4354.

Sadasivan, N., H. I. Eberspaecher, W. H. Fuchsman, and W. S. Caughey. 1969. Substituted deuteroporphyrins. VI. Ligand-exchange and dimerization reactions of deuterohemins. Biochemistry (Washington), 8:534-541.

Spijkerman, J. J., D. K. Snediker, C. F. Ruegg, and J. R. DeVoe. 1967. Mössbauer spectroscopy standard for the chemical shift of iron compounds. National Bureau of Standards Miscellaneous Publications, 260-13. Washington, United States Government Printing Office.

Tsing, P.-K., and S.Y. Wang. 1963. Mössbauer absorption lines of ferrous gluconate. Chinese J. Phys., 1:81-2.

Chapter **6**

Nuclear Magnetic Resonance with Applications to Pharmacology

Donald P. Hollis

Department of Physiological Chemistry, The Johns Hopkins University, School of Medicine, Baltimore, Maryland

INTRODUCTION

Nuclear magnetic resonance (NMR) was discovered in 1946 by two groups of physicists, one with Bloch (1953) at Stanford, the other with Purcell (1948, 1953) at Harvard. The magnetic properties of nuclei were already known at that time and had been measured using difficult atomic and molecular beam techniques. The work of Bloch and Purcell had the great advantage that it made possible precise observations of nuclear magnetism in ordinary bulk samples such as water and paraffin. The initial experiments were intended to benefit the study of nuclear physics, and this aim has been realized. However, due to the influence of many features of the nuclear environment on the characteristics of nuclear magnetic resonance spectra, it has proved possible to use certain magnetic nuclei as probes for the investigation of molecular structure. Such chemical applications of nuclear magnetic resonance soon overshadowed the original intent of the physicists, and by now thousands of publications concerning the use of NMR in organic chemical structural studies have appeared and such applications have become almost routine. On the other hand, the application of NMR to biochemical problems has proceeded more slowly, partly because of certain inherent difficulties in obtaining useful NMR spectra for the high molecular weight polymers which characterize biochemical systems. During the past few years several new techniques have been developed to enhance the feasibility of studying biochemical systems by NMR, and an increasing number of publications dealing with such systems have appeared. Although the use of NMR in biochemical systems is potentially of interest in pharmacology, the application of NMR to problems of direct pharmacological interest is still in its infancy. In this area as well, however, increased activity is evident and some interesting and provocative studies have appeared. Results to date certainly seem to make desirable further exploration and more frequent use of NMR in pharmacology.

TABLE 1

Biochemical Aspects of Nuclear Magnetic Resonance

I.   Chemical shifts and electron coupling of nuclear spins
  A. Structure and conformation of proteins and nucleic acids
  B. Qualitative and quantitative analysis
  C. Dynamic processes: kinetics of enzyme-substrate interactions, changes in molecular configuration and conformation
  D. Inter- and intramolecular associations, hydrogen bonding, ion binding
  E. Structure of enzyme active sites

II. Relaxation Times
  A. Structure of enzyme-substrate complexes
  B. Interaction of molecules and ions with biological membranes
  C. Mechanism of association of protein subunits
  D. Interaction of small molecules with macromolecules
  E. Conformation of proteins and nucleic acids
  F. State of water and ions in physiological systems such as muscle and nerve

Table 1 lists some of the biochemically oriented aspects of NMR, and although not all of these are of immediate interest in pharmacology, it does seem likely that many of them will find at least limited and perhaps widespread use. Many publications of a general or review type have discussed in great detail the principles of NMR (Abragam, 1961; Carrington and McLachlan, 1967; Pople et al., 1959) and several publications dealing specifically with biochemical and pharmacological applications have appeared (Fischer, 1971; Jardetzky, 1964; Jardetzky and Jardetzky, 1962; Kowalsky and Cohn, 1964). New applications and methods are developing quite rapidly, however, and therefore this chapter will emphasize those aspects which are presently, or which seem most likely to prove, useful to pharmacology.

NMR is closely related to electron spin resonance, which is discussed by Griffith and Jost in Chapter 7 of this volume. Both are examples of several types of radio-frequency and microwave spectroscopy developed since World War II. NMR is basically similar to the more familiar spectroscopic techniques which use infrared, visible, and ultraviolet radiation. Each sample has a set of energy levels that are characteristic of its structure. Under appropriate experimental arrangements, the sample absorbs electromagnetic energy at characteristic frequencies, giving a spectrum which corresponds to the allowed transitions among the energy levels. Since various types of interaction can perturb the energy levels and thus change the appearance of the spectrum, information can be obtained about the structure of an unknown sample from the details of its spectrum. NMR differs from the other spectroscopic methods in that the interactions studied are magnetic while the frequencies involved usually fall in radio-frequency range from less than 1 MHz[1] up to a few hundred MHz.

The purpose of this chapter is to survey several types of NMR phenomena observable in biochemical systems, to describe some experimental methods and techniques applicable to biochemical systems, and finally to discuss several representative applications of NMR which are of direct or potential interest in pharmacology.

NUCLEAR MAGNETIC RESONANCE

Nuclear magnetic resonance owes its existence to the fact that, in addition to their familiar properties of mass and charge, atomic nuclei may also possess spin angular momenta and magnetic moments. For present purposes, a sufficient insight into these properties can be obtained in terms of the nuclear mass and charge by means of a simple model. Assume that both the mass, M, and the charge, e, of a nucleus, the proton for example, are uniformly distributed over a thin spherical shell and that the shell is spinning about an axis through its center with a constant angular velocity. The spinning of mass produces an angular momentum, $\mathbf{P}$, a vector pointing along the axis of rotation.[2] The spinning of the charge produces an electric current circulating about the rotational axis and it in turn generates a magnetic field which is symmetrical about the rotational axis. A magnetic field can be described conveniently by its magnetic dipole moment, μ, which is the product of the magnetic pole strength and the distance between the two poles necessary to produce the field. Since the spinning motion is common to both charge and mass, the magnetic moment and angular momentum are collinear and in direct proportion. Calculation using this simple model shows that μ and $\mathbf{P}$ are related by the equation

$$\mu = (e/2Mc)\,\mathbf{P} \tag{1}$$

where c is the speed of light. This equation does not describe accurately the behavior of actual nuclei. In addition to certain other anomalies the proportionality constant between μ and $\mathbf{P}$ is not $e/2Mc$. However, the magnetic moment of a nucleus is always proportional to its angular momentum, so equation (1) can be written as

$$\mu = g\,(e/2Mc)\,\mathbf{P} = g\,(e/2Mc)\,h\mathbf{I} \tag{2}$$

where g, the magnetogyric ratio, is a dimensionless constant of the order of unity, and M is the mass of the proton. The nuclear angular momentum is usually designated as $\mathbf{I}$, with units of $\hbar/2\pi$ so that $h\mathbf{I}$ can be substituted for $\mathbf{P}$ in equation (2), where $\hbar = h/2\pi$, and h is Planck's constant.

---

[1] One Hertz (Hz) is one cycle per second; one megahertz (MHz) is 10^6 Hz.
[2] Vector quantities are given in boldface type; components for vectors and properties for which only the magnitudes are significant are given in italics.

In the absence of magnetic fields the energy of the nuclear magnet is independent of its orientation. In an external magnetic field, however, the magnetic dipole experiences a torque which tends to align the magnetic moment parallel to the field. According to elementary magnetic theory the torque, $\mathbf{L}$, produced on a magnetic moment μ in a field $\mathbf{H}$ is

$$\mathbf{L} = \mu \times \mathbf{H} \tag{3}$$

The potential energy of the magnetic moment μ in a magnetic field $\mathbf{H}_0$, whose value is fixed, is

$$E = -\mu_H H_0 \tag{4}$$

where μ_H is the component of μ along the direction of $\mathbf{H}_0$.

Although equation (4) allows a continuous range of energies between $-\mu H_0$ and $+\mu H_0$ for a classical system, nuclei have a discrete set of magnetic energy levels. General laws of quantum mechanics require that the angular momentum be quantized along any defined direction in space. Since the interaction of μ with $\mathbf{H}$ defines a direction in space for the nuclei, the nuclear angular momentum $\mathbf{I}$ is quantized along the direction of the magnetic field. The allowed components of $\mathbf{I}$ along H are determined by the magnetic quantum number, m, whose values are I, $I-1, \ldots, -I$ for a total of $2I+1$ states. Each nucleus has a particular integral or half-integral value of I. Observed values range from 0 to 7. The most important nuclei including ^{1}H, ^{19}F, ^{31}P, and ^{13}C have $I = \frac{1}{2}$.

Because of the collinearity and proportionality of μ and $\mathbf{I}$, quantization of I leads to quantization of μ through equation (2),

$$\mu = g(e/2Mc)\hbar m = mg\mu_0 \tag{5}$$

where $e\hbar/2Mc$ is denoted by μ_0. Using this result for μ in equation (4) gives

$$E = -mg\mu_0 H_0 \equiv -m\gamma\hbar H_0 \tag{6}$$

which corresponds to a set of $2I+1$ nuclear orientations and energy levels. These are shown in Figure 1 for $I=1$. γ is used to express the magnetogyric ratio in units of $g/\hbar$. The selection rule for transitions among the energy levels given by equation (6) is that m changes by ± 1. Therefore

$$\Delta E = \pm g\mu_0 H_0 \tag{7}$$

By the Bohr frequency condition $\Delta E = h\nu$ we find the frequency, ν_0, in Hz corresponding to an allowed transition to be

$$\nu_0 = g\mu_0 H_0/h \tag{8}$$

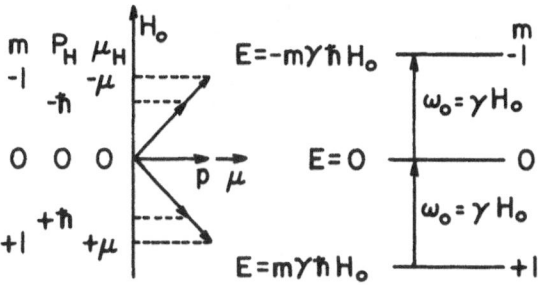

FIG. 1. The orientations and energy levels of a magnetic nucleus of I=1 in a magnetic field. Both the angular momentum and the magnetic moment are quantized along the magnetic field.

which in angular frequency units becomes

$$\omega \equiv 2\pi\nu_0 = g\mu_0 H_0/\hslash = \gamma H_0 \tag{9}$$

This equation can also be obtained by considering the dynamic aspects of nuclear magnetization. It is found that the transitions require radio-frequency magnetic fields that are circularly polarized in a plane perpendicular to H_0. Equation (3) states that the magnetic field exerts a torque on the nuclear magnetic moment tending to align it with the field. This, however, would also reorient the angular momentum, **P**. For such a reorientation, Newton's law requires that the time rate of change of the angular momentum equal the torque,

$$dP/dt = L \tag{10}$$

Replacing **L** by $\mu \times H$ as given in equation (3) and converting μ to **P** by equation (2) we obtain

$$dP/dt = g\,(e/2Mc)\,P \times H_0 \tag{11}$$

This equation describes the precession of **P** about H_0 with an angular velocity

$$\omega = g\,(e/2Mc)\,H_0 \equiv \gamma H_0 \tag{12}$$

the same as equation (8), which resulted from the nuclear magnetic energy levels. Figure 2 illustrates the precession of the spinning nucleus about H_0. A familiar example of precession is the wobbling of a spinning top in the earth's gravitational field.

The precession of the nuclear spin axis about a magnetic field suggests a way to change the orientation and, therefore, the magnetic energy of μ. A small magnetic field H_1 is placed in the xy plane which is perpendicular to H_0, whose direction is along the z-axis. The torque which H_1 exerts on μ will cause the spin axis to precess around H_1, changing the orientation of the nucleus with respect to H_0. Whether the angle between μ and H_0 increases or decreases depends on the relative orienta-

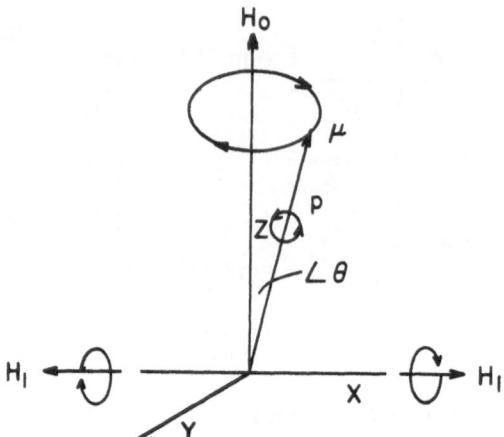

FIG. 2. The magnetic interaction between μ and H_0 produces a torque on the spinning nucleus causing it to precess about H_0 at a constant frequency and a constant angle θ. When a small magnetic field H_1 is applied in the xy plane, μ also tends to precess about H_1, thereby changing θ and the magnetic energy. Since the direction of precession depends on the relative orientation of μ and H_1, H_1 produces no net effect unless this orientation is kept constant by rotating H_1 in the xy plane in the same direction and at the same frequency as μ precesses around H_0.

tions of μ and H_1, as implied by equation (11), and shown in Figure 2. There will therefore be little or no effect unless H_1 maintains its orientation with respect to μ a condition which can be accomplished by rotating H_1 about H_0 at the same rate that μ precesses about H_0. Thus, H_1 must rotate in resonance with the precession of μ about H_0. The rotating magnetic field corresponds to circularly polarized radiation at the frequency ω_0. In practice, the circularly polarized radiation is obtained by passing a radio-frequency (r.f.) current through a small coil mounted perpendicular to H_0, producing a magnetic field oscillating along the coil axis. Such a field is mathematically equivalent to two equal circularly polarized fields rotating in opposite directions. The component rotating in the correct sense will automatically be in resonance, while the other component will have negligible effect. More exact treatments of this vector model from both the classical and quantum mechanical viewpoints have been given elsewhere (Andrew, 1955).

We have seen that consideration of the behavior of a spinning magnetic nucleus in a magnetic field from either the standpoint of nuclear energy levels or from a classical dynamical viewpoint leads to the same result, namely, that

$$\omega_0 = \gamma H_0 \tag{12}$$

This result clearly implies the following:
(1) For each nucleus, the resonance frequency is directly proportional to the applied field, H_0. Proton resonance, for example, is observed at 60 MHz, 100 MHz, and 220 MHz in fields of 14,100, 23,400, and 51,500 gauss, respectively.
(2) In any given field, nuclei with larger magnetogyric ratios, γ, will have larger

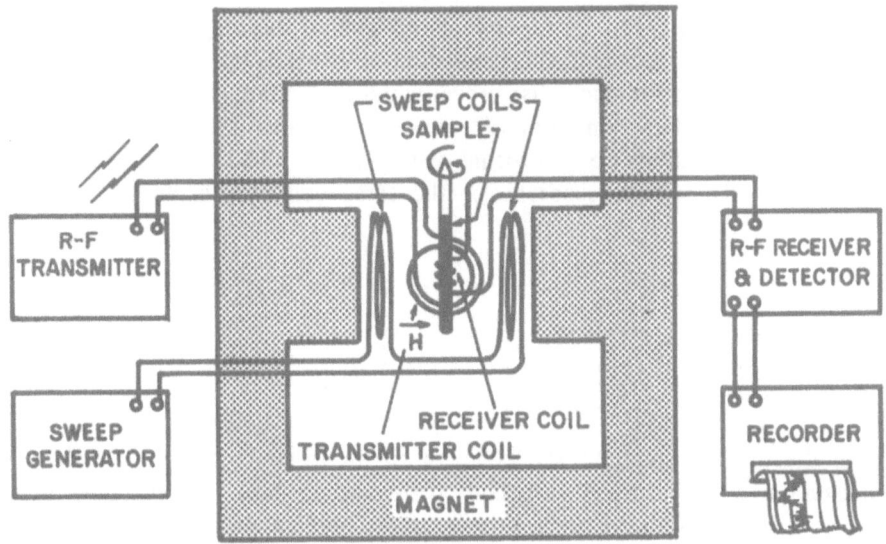

FIG. 3. Simplified block diagram of a basic NMR spectrometer. See text for details.

resonance frequencies. Thus, in a field of 23,400 gauss, the resonance frequency for protons is 100 MHz as compared to 40 MHz for ^{31}P in the same field.

(3) On the other hand, at a fixed frequency, nuclei with larger magnetogyric ratios will come into resonance at smaller applied fields. For example, a field of about 9,460 gauss is required to observe proton resonances at 40 MHz, while 23,400 gauss is necessary for observation of ^{31}P resonance at the same frequency.

DETECTION OF MAGNETIC RESONANCE—THE BASIC NMR SPECTROMETER

The previously mentioned precession of a nuclear dipole about the rotating field H_1 makes possible the detection of resonance by placing a pick-up coil anywhere in the plane in which H_1 is rotating. The changing magnetic field associated with the reorienting dipole induces a current in such a coil, and this current can be amplified and recorded. A block diagram of a basic NMR spectrometer is shown in Figure 3. Three component systems are required:

(1) The magnet, usually consisting of an iron core electromagnet (although superconducting magnets and permanent magnets are also used), including a power supply and controls allowing the field to be swept by varying the current through the magnet coils. The field is generated in a gap between two cylindrical pole pieces, the axis of which defines the z direction (i.e., the direction of the field intensity vector H_z) of a Cartesian coordinate system to which all the dynamic variables describing the NMR phenomenon can be referred.

(2) The transmitter, which consists of an oscillator to serve as a source of radiation (i.e., the field $\mathbf{H}_1$) and a coil placed so that the magnetic component of its field oscillates in a plane perpendicular to H_z, thus defining the x direction. The remaining coordinate, y, is perpendicular to x and z.

(3) The detector system, consisting of a detector coil, one or more amplifiers, and a recorder or oscilloscope for visual display of the signal. The transmitter and receiver coils may be separate, or the same coil may serve as transmitter and receiver.

RELAXATION TIMES AND
RELAXATION MECHANISMS

In the previous sections the behavior of an isolated, spinning nucleus has been examined. When NMR is actually observed in bulk matter, the observed signal represents not the reorientation of an isolated nucleus but that of a large number of identical nuclei. These nuclei may interact among themselves and with their surroundings. The behavior of the isolated magnetic nucleus must be related to the behavior of a set of nuclei taking these interactions into account.

Consider an assembly of identical nuclei of spin $I = \frac{1}{2}$, in identical environments so that all of the nuclei in the assembly experience the same total magnetic field. Such an assembly constitutes a *magnetically equivalent set*. All of the remaining particles in the sample constitute the lattice. Only two magnetic energy levels are accessible to each nucleus in such a system and these correspond approximately to alignment of the nuclear magnetic moment either with or against the magnetic field. At equilibrium the nuclei are distributed between the two energy levels and the ratio of the number of spins in each level is given by the Boltzmann factor

$$n+/n- = e^{-\Delta E/kT} \tag{13}$$

where $n+$ and $n-$ are the populations of the upper and lower states respectively, $\Delta F = 2\mu H$ is the energy difference between the two states, k is the Boltzmann constant, and T is the absolute temperature. For a given ΔE, increasing the $n+/n-$ ratio corresponds to raising the temperature of the spin system, equal populations corresponding to an infinitely high temperature. At equilibrium at any finite temperature the number of nuclei in the lower state always exceeds that in the upper state. At moderate temperatures in the magnetic fields normally used for NMR studies the excess number of nuclei in the lower state is relatively very small. In the case of protons, for example, an excess of about five nuclei per million would be typical. That is, in a sample of about 2×10^6 protons, 10^6 might be in the upper state and 10^6 plus 10 in the lower state. If the system is irradiated at a frequency $\nu = \Delta E/h$, the system absorbs energy from the radiation field with a consequent increase in the ratio $n+/n-$. Since the probability per unit time per nucleus of absorption is identical to that for induced emission, absorption will exceed emission only so long as excess nuclei remain in the lower state. This excess will obviously dwindle away in the absence of mechanisms allowing radiationless transitions from the upper to the lower energy states. When the system absorbs sufficient energy to equalize the population of the two states it is said to be *saturated* and the temperature of the spin system is infinite. Only a small amount of energy is required to do this heating, since the heat capacity of the spin system is very small.

A saturated or partially saturated spin system will tend to return to thermal equilibrium if left to itself. Two simultaneous processes are involved in the return of a saturated system to equilibrium: (1) flow of energy from the spin system to the lattice, resulting in the cooling of the spin system by transitions of nuclei from the higher to the lower state and a heating of the lattice (this process is called *spin-lattice relaxation*); and (2) redistribution of the absorbed energy among the nuclei by mutual exchange of nuclei between the higher and lower states, the total energy of the spin system being constant (the latter process is called *spin-spin relaxation*). These two processes, having different mechanisms, need not occur at the same rate. Their rates can be determined separately for a given spin system.

The difference between these relaxation processes can also be discussed in terms of the dynamic vector model by discussing the motion of a macroscopic magnetization vector, **M**, which is the vector sum of all the individual magnetic moments making up the system. At equilibrium **M** is aligned with the external magnetic field H_0, and thus there is no magnetization in the xy plane. Momentary application of the irradiating field, H_1, will tip **M** away from the z axis, and **M** will then have a component, M_{xy}, in the xy plane as well as a component M_z in the z direction. Left to itself the system will now return to equilibrium and there will again be a magnetic moment, **M**, aligned in the z direction and there will be no magnetization in the xy plane.

The magnetization component in the xy plane (M_{xy}) evidently cannot last for a time longer than that required for the magnetization to return to its equilibrium value. However, it is possible for the component M_{xy} to disappear faster than the magnetization in the z direction reaches its equilibrium value, as illustrated in Figure 4. M_{xy} can decay because the individual magnetic moments get out of phase in their precession. Obviously this can occur with no resultant change in M_z and without any energy change between the spin system and the lattice. For example, when two nuclei undergo a mutual reorientation of their moments with respect to the external field, they lose their phase coherence. Spin-spin relaxation is also called, for obvious reasons, *transverse relaxation*, while spin-lattice relaxation is also called *longitudinal relaxation*.

For the two-state spin system such as we are discussing, both longitudinal and transverse components change with time according to a single exponential function involving characteristic time constants called T_1, the *longitudinal* or spin-lattice relaxation time, and T_2, the *transverse* or spin-spin relaxation time, respectively. The relaxation time T_2 is sometimes called the line-width parameter because it is related to the line width of the Lorentzian shaped absorption line by $1/T_2 =$

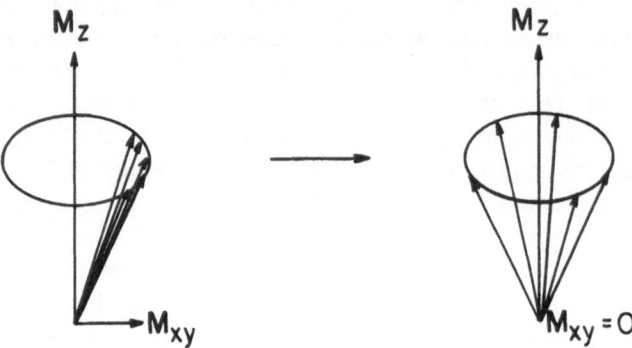

FIG. 4. The resultant magnetization in the *xy* plane shown at left can decay due to independent precession of individual nuclei as shown at right. The process can occur without affecting the net magnetization in the *z* direction.

$\pi \Delta \nu_{\frac{1}{2}}$, when $\Delta \nu_{\frac{1}{2}}$ is the width in Hz of the resonance at one-half maximum intensity. When defined in this way, T_2 is composed of three parts:

$$1/T_2 = 1/T_2' + (1/T_2'')_{loc} + (1/T_2'')_{mag}$$

where $1/T_2$ is the observed relaxation rate as determined from the line width, $1/T_2'$ is the contribution from spin exchange, $(1/T_2'')_{loc}$ is the contribution from the local field inhomogeneities due to the sample, and $(1T_2'')_{mag}$ is the contribution from the inhomogeneity of the applied external magnetic field. In order to obtain meaningful results in terms of molecular events in the sample, $(1/T_2'')_{mag}$ must be reduced to as low a value as possible placing stringent requirements on the homogeneity of the magnet and accounting in large part for the expense of modern NMR spectrometers. Alternatively, a correction for $(1/T_2'')_{mag}$ can be made if its value is constant and known during a particular experiment. Clearly, $1/T_2'$ and $1/T_2''$ also measure the rate at which the nuclei lose their precessional phase coherently, since field inhomogeneity, regardless of its source (that is, from the sample itself or from an inhomogeneous applied field), will result in the nuclei in different parts of the sample precessing at different rates, thus getting rapidly out of phase and giving a broad resonance.

GENERAL FEATURES OF NMR SPECTRA

Four parameters characterize the absorption of radio frequency radiation by atomic nuclei placed in a magnetic field: (1) the *chemical shift*, which expresses the frequencies of absorption relative to some arbitrary standard absorption line; (2) the *coupling constants*, which describe the interactions between neighboring nuclei and which lead to multiplicity of the lines originating from a given group of nuclei; (3) the *intensities of absorption lines*, described by their integrated areas, which are proportional to the number of nuclei contributing to each line; and (4) the *relaxation times* T_1 and T_2, defined earlier, which describe the return of excited nuclei to a lower energy state. The correlations of chemical structure to NMR spectra are based almost entirely on the observed chemical shifts, coupling constants, and intensities. Pharmacological and biochemical studies on the other hand are likely to involve interactions between molecules and these are most sensitively reflected in the relaxation process.

The Chemical Shift

In the fundamental equation for the resonance condition, $\omega_0 = \gamma H_0$, derived above, H_0 refers to the magnetic field actually present at the site of the magnetic nucleus. This field is not simply the externally applied magnetic field, because local fields generated by induced electronic currents may add to or subtract from the applied field. The local field, H_{loc}, at a particular site can be expressed in terms of the externally applied field as $H_{loc} = H_0(1-\sigma)$, where σ is called the *shielding constant*. The resonance condition then becomes

$$\omega = \gamma H_{loc} = \gamma H_0 (1-\sigma) \tag{14}$$

where σ is a characteristic of each nuclear environment and may be positive or negactive. As a result, an NMR experiment carried out on a molecule or mixture of molecules causes the signals from the various nuclei to be spread out in a spectrum according to their chemical environments. The chemical shift between two sets of nuclei is defined as the difference in their resonance frequencies measured at constant field. This difference is directly proportional to the magnitude of the applied field and is most conveniently expressed in field-independent units as parts per million (ppm) of the constant field or frequency:

$$\delta = \frac{(\nu_2 - \nu_1)}{\nu_1} \times 10^6 \tag{15}$$

where δ is the chemical shift, and ν_1 and ν_2 are the resonance frequencies for the two groups of nuclei. Note that frequency and field strength have equal status and are readily interconvertible through equation (12). Either field or frequency may be kept constant and the other varied to obtain the spectrum. For protons, the normal range of chemical shifts covers about 12 ppm. Since it is impossible to measure a large magnetic field to sufficient accuracy for absolute chemical-shift determinations, chemical shifts are measured relative to an arbitrary reference, which for protons is almost always tetramethylsilane (TMS). For the aqueous solution of most interest to biochemists, an ionic derivative of TMS must be used since TMS is insoluble in water. Most commonly used is the sodium salt of dimethylsilapentane-sulfonic acid (DSS). Figure 5 shows the spectrum of a mixture of compounds each having only a single-proton environment.

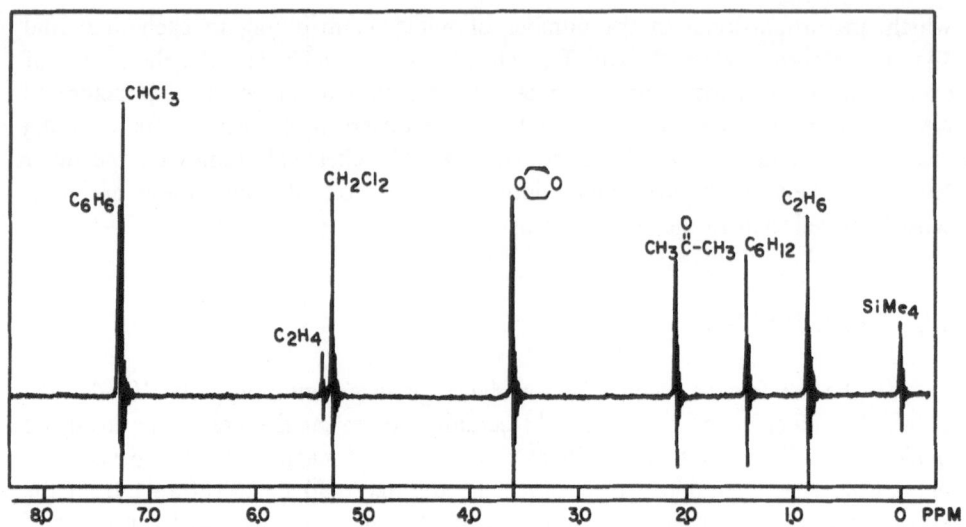

FIG. 5. The NMR spectrum of a mixture of compounds each having only a single proton environment.

The Coupling Constant

In addition to the lines accounted for by chemical shift differences, the high resolution spectra of many compounds contain patterns of lines that arise from interactions with neighboring magnetic dipoles. These patterns are accounted for by an indirect coupling between the nuclei, transmitted by the electrons of intervening chemical bonds. The mechanism of transmission can be understood by considering that the magnetic field of a nuclear dipole will tend to orient the valence electrons antiparallel to the nuclear spin. Simultaneously the spins and magnetic moments of the electrons in a covalent bond must be paired so that the valence electron on the neighboring atom will tend to be oriented parallel to the nucleus of the first atom. This results in the creation of a magnetic field at the second atom, whose direction reflects the orientation of the first atom, and whose magnitude reflects the extent of polarization of the electrons; this in turn depends on the characteristics of the chemical bond. At the same time the second nucleus exerts a similar effect on the first one through the same bonding electrons. The magnitude of the interaction is expressed in terms of a coupling constant J, which is expressed in frequency units and which measures the interaction energy between two spins. Figure 6 shows the NMR spectrum of ethyl ether and is a simple example of the effect of spin-spin coupling. The arrows above each component line in the spectrum show the orientation of the protons of the neighboring group that produces that component. The relative intensities of the components of each multiplet are determined by the statistical weights of each arrangement of neighboring spins. The separation between the components of each multiplet is the coupling constant J. Since the coupling energy arises from an intramolecular effect, it is not surprising

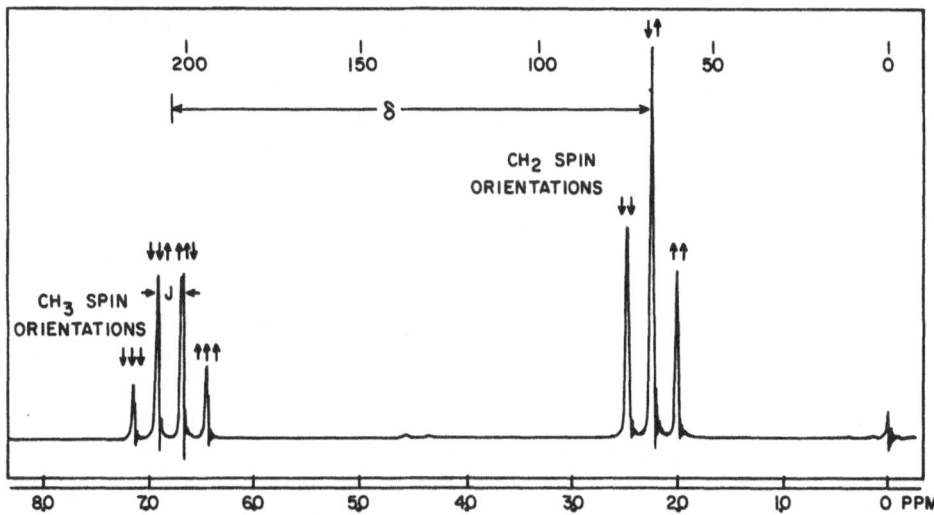

FIG. 6. The NMR spectrum of ethyl ether illustrating the effects of spin-spin interactions.

that the J-value and hence the observed splittings, in contrast to chemical shifts, are independent of the applied field.

Figure 6 also illustrates the fact that the areas under the absorption lines are proportional to the number of protons contributing to the absorption. Thus the ratio of the area of the methyl triplet to the methylene quartet in Figure 6 is 3:2. In terms familiar to conventional spectroscopists, one might say that the NMR extinction coefficients for all protons are the same at a given resonance field. If the field is swept while the frequency remains constant, the extinction coefficients will still be practically the same because the field is changed only a few parts per million.

As the ratio of the chemical shift to the coupling constant, δ/J, becomes smaller, the spectrum becomes more complicated and cannot be interpreted in the simple way shown in Figure 6. In these cases the spectrum can be analyzed by the methods of quantum mechanics to yield the chemical shifts and coupling constants (Pople et al., 1959).

THE DEPENDENCE OF SPIN-LATTICE AND SPIN-SPIN INTERACTIONS UPON LATTICE MOTIONS

With respect to biochemistry and pharmacology the principle importance of NMR relaxation measurements is their applicability to the study of intermolecular interactions such as the binding of drugs or other small molecules to proteins and other macromolecules. These interactions cause changes in the relaxation times of the protons in the small molecule, which in some cases can be interpreted so as to shed light on the details of the mechanism of interaction. The primary reason that the relaxation times of the small molecule change on binding is that the relaxation times depend on the rates of motion of various magnetic entities present in the sample, and these rates are affected when the rapidly moving small molecule is bound to a sluggishly moving macromolecule. The purpose of this section is to discuss in more detail the relaxation mechanism and its relationship to the molecular motion. An extensive quantitative treatment of relaxation theory is outside the scope of this chapter, but it is hoped that the simple physical picture to be presented here will make the reader aware of the rather intricate theory underlying relaxation, allow him to recognize possible advantages and pitfalls of magnetic relaxation studies in biochemical systems, and prepare him for a more sophisticated treatment of the subject. More extensive general treatments of NMR relaxation are to be found in the references (Abragam, 1961; Jardetzky, 1964). The latter reference deals specifically with biochemical and pharmacological applications.

In our discussion of the basic NMR phenomenon we found it necessary to include the effects of energy transfer between the nuclear spin system and its surroundings as well as energy transfers within the spin system. The time constants T_1 and T_2 were introduced in order to measure the time scale for attainment of thermal equilibrium in these two processes. This matter is usually unimportant in other types of spectroscopy because electronic, vibrational, rotational, and translational energies are rapidly interchanged in various kinds of collisions and the resulting relaxation times are very short compared to the time required to obtain the spectra. Nuclei, on the other hand, are insulated from their surroundings by the atomic electrons and by other atoms in the molecule, with the result that the transfer of magnetic energy from the nucleus to other degrees of freedom in the sample is a relatively slow process. Spontaneous emission is negligible, and induced transitions require a magnetic field oscillating at the resonance frequency as discussed above. For energy transfer between the nuclei and the lattice the required oscillating magnetic fields must be produced by the thermal motion of the lattice. Unless these fields are reasonably effective, making T_1 short, detection of the NMR phenomenon is hampered or even made impossible due to the saturation effect discussed earlier. If either T_1 or T_2 is extremely short on the other hand, the spectra become undetectably broad as will be explained below.

In the systems of interest here the magnetic fields producing relaxation usually come from the magnetic nuclei themselves although in some cases other magnetic entities such as paramagnetic ions and free radicals are important. The local field H_{loc} of a magnetic dipole μ is illustrated in Figure 7. If the position of the dipole μ is held fixed, the local field H_{loc} can be divided into a static and rotating component. The static component arises from the component of μ along the external magnetic field, and the rotating component arises from the precession of μ around the static field. The magnitude of the local field produced at a point P by a dipole μ depends on the distance r between P and the dipole, and on the direction of P from the dipole. A typical value for H_{loc} is a few gauss. The proton, for example, produces a field of about 50 gauss at a distance of 1 Å. Molecular motions such as rotation and translation will change r and θ and will therefore cause the local magnetic field at any given point to fluctuate. The fluctuating magnetic fields can produce transitions among the nuclear magnetic energy levels leading to transfer of energy

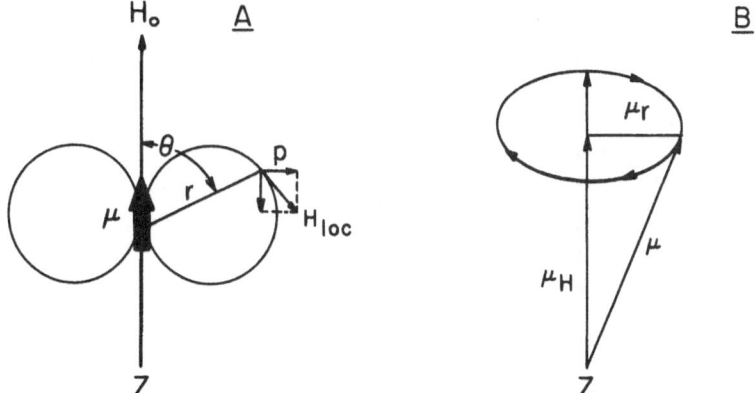

FIG. 7. The local magnetic field due to a precessing nuclear magnet may be divided into a static component μ as shown in A and a rotating component, μ_r, in a plane perpendicular to H_0 as shown in B. The value of the static part of the local field depends on the distance r and the angle θ.

between the thermal degrees of freedom of the lattice and the magnetic energy levels of the nuclei, thus allowing relaxation and reducing T_1 and T_2. Two main factors determine the effectiveness of a particular lattice motion in causing relaxation: (1) the amplitude of the local field fluctuations produced by the motion, and (2) the probability that the motion occurs at the resonance frequency and thus is able to induce transitions. In order to calculate the relaxation times in terms of the time-dependent local magnetic fields, it is necessary to know how the total power involved in each type of molecular motion is distributed among all the possible frequencies so that the strength of the fluctuations at the resonance frequency can be determined. In the cases of interest here it is molecular rotation which is the dominant mechanism of relaxation. Assuming random motion and considering only rotation it can be shown that

$$J_{(\omega)} \propto 2\tau_c / (1 + \omega^2 \tau_c^2) \qquad (16)$$

where $J_{(\omega)}$ is the power present as rotational motion at a frequency ω and τ_c is the correlation time for rotation. The correlation time arises naturally from a mathematical treatment of the power spectrum of a randomly varying force. The physical meaning of τ_c is not precisely defined but it is a rough measure of the time required for an average fluctuation in the local field to die away. τ_c also characterizes the frequency at which the power goes to zero, i.e., it characterizes the upper frequency limit of the motion. Knowing the power spectrum as a function of the correlation time, one can obtain the relaxation times in terms of τ_c. The results are

$$1/T_1 = \gamma^2 (H_x^2 + H_y^2) [\tau_c / (1 + \omega_0^2 \tau_c^2)] \qquad (17)$$

$$1/T_2 = \gamma^2 [H_z^2 \tau_c + (H_x^2 + H_y^2)]/2[\tau_c / (1 + \omega_0^2 \tau_c^2)] \qquad (18)$$

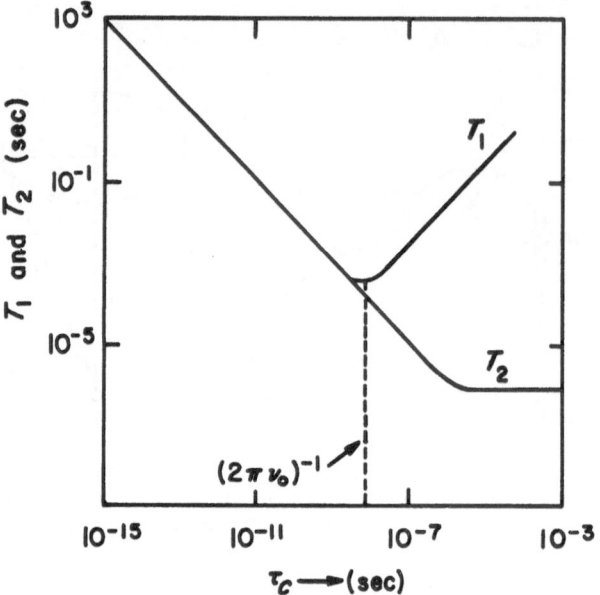

FIG. 8. A schematic representation of the dependence of the relaxation times T_1 and T_2 on the correlation time τ_c assuming that all interactions have the same τ_c. See text for discussion.

where $\mathbf{H}_x^2\ \mathbf{H}_y^2$ and $\mathbf{H}_z^2$ are the mean square values of the perturbing fields along the three coordinates. Since the molecular motion is isotropic, these mean square averages are equal. Evidently, when molecular motion is very rapid $\omega_0\tau_c$ will be small and $T_1 = T_2$; that is

$$1/T_1 = 1/T_2 = \gamma^2 2\mathbf{H}_x^2 \tau_c \tag{19}$$

On the other hand if the molecular motion is slow, the $1 + \omega_0^2\tau_c^2$ terms become large and $T_2 < T_1$. T_2 cannot of course be greater than T_1. The dependence of T_1 and T_2 on the correlation time is shown in Figure 8. Note the appearance of a minimum in the T_1 curve, while T_2 continues to decrease, eventually reaching a constant value characteristic of a solid. This occurs because the intensity of the motion at ω_0 must become less when the motion becomes either very fast or very slow, passing through a maximum when $\omega_0\tau_c = 1$, thus producing a minimum T_1. T_2, however, continues to decrease linearly with τ_c until the motion is completely frozen. One might say the T_1 relaxation is favored by frequencies around $\omega = \omega_0$, while T_2 relaxation is favored by frequencies around $\omega = 0$.

It can also be seen from equations (17) and (18) that although T_1 and T_2 might at first seem to be independent quantities this is not so. In fact,

$$1/T_2 = \gamma^2 \mathbf{H}_x^2 \tau_c + \tfrac{1}{2}T_1 \tag{20}$$

Apparently any mechanism contributing to T_1 relaxation also contributes to T_2, but there are additional mechanisms that contribute to T_2 but not to T_1. These latter are the static part of the dipole-dipole interaction and the mutual spin exchange mechanisms. The former results because the static part of the local field is not averaged out when molecular motion is slow. This is best appreciated by considering the situation in a solid where the random orientation of neighboring spins will produce a different net local field at the site of each spin. This will give a spread of resonance frequencies for different nuclei according to $\omega_0 = \gamma H_{loc}$. This results in a short T_2 and a broad resonance. The mutual spin exchange mechanism is the result of two identical nuclei precessing at the same frequency mutually irradiating each other's energy levels with a resultant exchange of orientations. Although energy is conserved in this process, phase coherence is lost between the involved nuclei and others in the same orientation, resulting in a shorter T_2. Another way to view this is that the lifetime of the two energy states involved are shortened, leading to line broadening by the Heisenberg Principle.

SOME APPLICATIONS OF NUCLEAR MAGNETIC RESONANCE TO PHARMACOLOGICAL PROBLEMS

Interaction of Small Molecules with Proteins

The application of relaxation measurements to the study of the interactions between small molecules and macromolecules as in drug-protein interactions depends on the fact that the large molecules rotate more slowly in solution than small molecules, i.e., they have longer rotational correlation times. When a small molecule is rigidly bound to a large one, it takes on the correlation time of the large molecule with the result that the relaxation times of its protons are shortened and their NMR linewidths increased.

Zimmerman and Brittin (1957) have developed a theory dealing with the case in which a small molecule exists in equilibrium between two or more phases (i.e., bound and free) having different characteristic relaxation times and hence different line widths. It is predicted that the observed line widths depend on the rate of exchange of molecules between the bound and free phases as well as on the equilibrium binding constant. Particularly simple behavior is predicted for two limiting cases in which the average lifetimes of a molecule in the two states are either very long or very short as compared to the corresponding relaxation times. For the slow-exchange case

$$(1/T)_{exchange} < (1/T_2)_{free} < (1/T_2)_{bound} \qquad \text{Case I}$$

where T is the average lifetime of a molecule in either the free or bound states, and $(1/T_2)_{free}$ and $(1/T_2)_{bound}$ are the relaxation rates of protons in the free and bound phases, respectively; molecules in the two phases relax independently and two separate relaxation times should be experimentally observable. Thus, the NMR spectrum should show a broad line and a narrow line corresponding to the bound and free phases, respectively. These lines need not be superimposed since a chemical shift difference may also exist between the bound and free molecules. The integrated intensity of each line will be proportional to the number of molecules in the corresponding phase.

For the fast-exchange case

$$(1/T_2)_{free} < (1/T_2)_{bound} < (1/T)_{exchange} \qquad \text{Case III}$$

only a single, average relaxation time can be observed, which is given by

$$1/T_{av} = P_F/T_{2F} + P_B/T_{2B}$$

where P_F and P_B are the fractions of the molecules in the free and bound phases and T_{2F} and T_{2B} are the corresponding relaxation times. The NMR spectrum will then show only one line whose width will be intermediate between those corresponding to the free and bound species and whose integrated intensity will represent the total concentration of free and bound molecules.

For the case in which the exchange rate is intermediate between the relaxation rates of the two phases

$$(1/T_2)_{free} < (1/T)_{exchange} < (1/T)_{bound} \qquad \text{Case II}$$

the nuclei in the bound phase will relax normally but the relaxation rate of the free molecules will be influenced by the exchange process. If most of the molecules are free, the relaxation rate of the free phase will be determined by the exchange rate.

It is possible that the nuclei located in different portions of a complex molecule may experience differential changes in relaxation rate upon binding, depending on the extent of involvement of the various portions of the molecule in the binding mechanism. Such selective broadening effects have been used in several cases to elucidate the mechanism of binding of small molecules to proteins. In such applications it must be kept in mind that, if the results are to be interpreted simply in terms of selective changes in the rotational correlation times due to binding of the small molecule, then all other sources of line broadening both nonspecific and specific should be eliminated insofar as possible. Possible nonspecific mechanisms include (1) changes in the macroscopic viscosity of the solution of the small molecule upon addition of protein; (2) an increase in inter- and/or intramolecular interactions among the small molecules caused by addition of protein which could affect the activity of the small molecule; (3) the possibility of direct relaxation effects on the small molecule caused by the protein but not requiring the formation of a complex; (4) the existence of paramagnetic ions in the solution which could also lead to line broadening; (5) if the bound form of the small molecule has its protons chemically shifted from those free in solution, then rapid chemical exchange can lead to line broadening; (6) if a proton in the bound state of the small molecule resides at a site whose microscopic magnetic susceptibility is anisotropic, i.e., dependent upon the orientation of the site with respect to the applied field, H_0, then molecular rotation will cause fluctuation of the local field experienced by the bound proton and thereby provide a relaxation mechanism. In the case of magnetic anisotropy the relaxation rate depends upon H_0^2 and the effect of magnetic anisotropy can be detected or eliminated by carrying out the measurements at two field strengths, for example 24,000 gauss and 50,000 gauss for protons. Elimination of this factor has not been mentioned in several published experimental studies of the binding of small molecules to macromolecules, probably because sensitivity requirements dictate use of the highest possible fields. This mechanism is quite likely to be important for small molecules bound to proteins as evidenced by the extreme high and low field chemical shifts which have been observed in globular proteins and which are attributed to the effect of aromatic rings on nearby proton containing groups. These effects are anisotropic. Since modulation of the scalar spin-spin coupling can produce line broadening and therefore change T_2 but not T_1, it is preferable where possible to measure T_1 rather than just the linewidth, or to show that $T_1 = T_2$.

Just how these possible complicating factors are to be eliminated depends on the particular system under study but some examples are given in the following sections describing specific applications. In general, the effect of viscosity can be determined by substituting for the protein of interest a similar noninteracting protein to produce a solution of the required viscosity. If this protein produces considerably less broadening, then specific interaction is indicated for the system under study. The effect of interaction among the small molecules themselves can be determined by a concentration study in the absence of protein or by addition of further quantities of the small molecule to a solution containing both small molecule and protein. In the usual case where the small molecule is in large excess and the exchange rate conforms to Case III as described above, addition of further quantities of the small molecules will cause a *narrowing* of the resonance lines of the small molecule, whereas intermolecular interaction among the small molecules induced by the protein would cause line *broadening*. The possible effects of protein-small molecule interactions other than complex formation can also be estimated by a control experiment using a nonbinding protein. The presence of paramagnetic ionic impurities in the solution can generally be detected by its effect on the linewidth of the residual proton peak in the deuterated solvent. The possibility of specific binding of paramagnetic impurities by the protein in such a way that some portions of the bound small molecule lie closer to the paramagnetic center is very difficult to eliminate. Such effects could arise even though the paramagnetic impurity is not present in directly detectable amounts. The effect of chemical exchange between environments in which the protons of the small molecule have different chemical shifts can usually be avoided by using concentrations such that the free form of the small molecule is in great excess over the complexed form. Chemical exchange affects only T_2, which is another reason that T_1 measurements are preferred. The possibility of varying the fraction of the small molecule that is bound has the additional advantage of placing the linewidth under experimental control making it unnecessary to deal with inconveniently broad lines.

The application of NMR relaxation measurements to a problem of pharmaco-

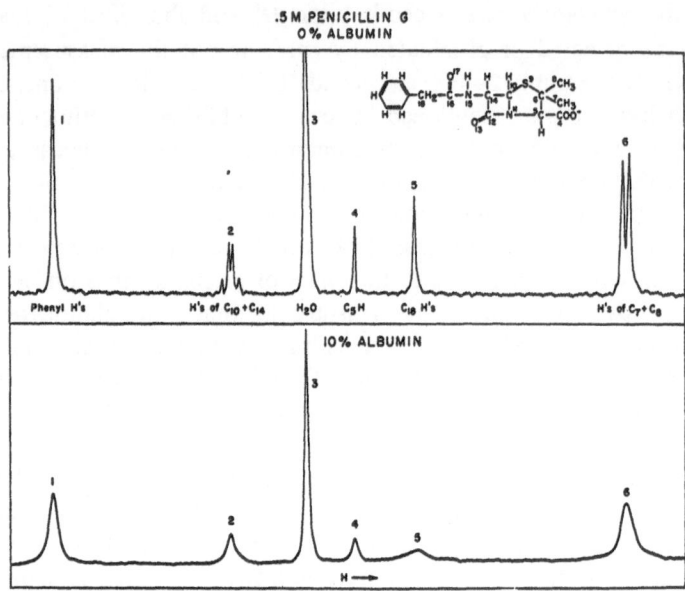

FIG. 9. A. (Top) NMR spectrum of 0.5M penicillin G in D₂O. B. (Bottom) Same as A but 10% albumin added. (From Fischer and Jardetzky. 1965. *J. Amer. Chem. Soc.*, 87:32. Copyright © 1965 by the American Chemical Society. Reprinted by permission of the copyright owner.)

logical interest is exemplified by the pioneering study of Fischer and Jardetzky (1965) on the binding of penicillin to bovine serum albumin (BSA). It was desired to determine which portion of the penicillin molecule was involved in the binding to serum albumin. Several possibilities exist, *a priori,* since there is an ionic group which could be involved in electrostatic binding; there are several possible hydrogen-bonding sites on both ring structures and on the sidechains; and there is a large aromatic sidechain which could be involved in hydrophobic interactions. Although several techniques including equilibrium dialysis, ultracentrifugation, and drug activity assay can measure the extent of binding, they do not give information about the binding mechanism.

The proton NMR spectrum of 0.5 M penicillin G in D₂O is shown in Figure 9a along with the structural formula and numbering system. The peaks in the spectrum are assigned and numbered. The effect of added albumin on the penicillin spectrum is shown in Figure 9b. Although all lines are noticeably broadened, the extent of broadening varies from proton to proton. In order to interpret the selective broadening of the proton peaks in terms of changes in the rotational correlation times of different parts of the penicillin molecule, it is first necessary to eliminate all possible sources of broadening that are nonspecific, that is, unrelated to the formation of the drug-protein complex. Possible nonspecific mechanisms include penicillin-penicillin interactions which could conceivably be increased by addition of protein, an increase in the macroscopic viscosity and the possibility of inter-

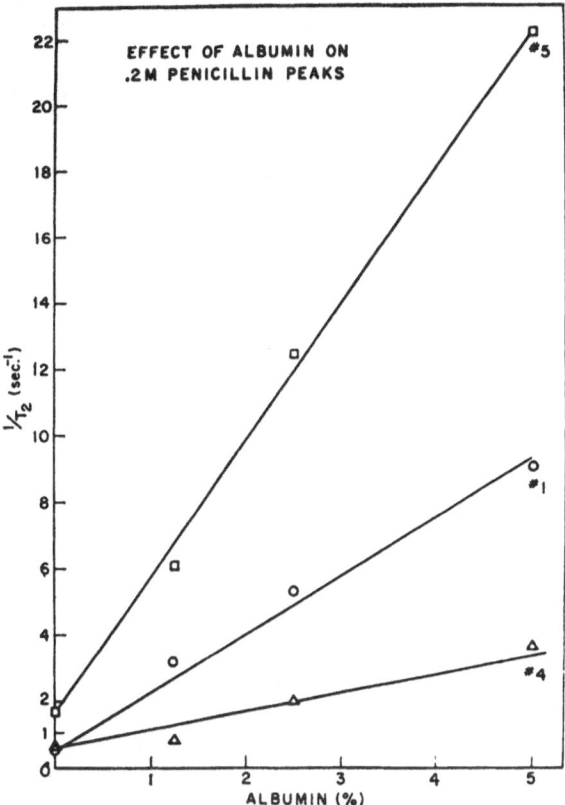

FIG. 10. Effect of albumin on the relaxation rates of different peaks in the NMR spectrum of penicillin G. (From Fischer and Jardetzky. 1965. *J. Amer. Chem. Soc.*, 87:3237. Copyright © 1965 by the American Chemical Society. Reprinted by permission of the copyright owner.)

molecular relaxation effects caused by the protein could occur in the absence of complex formation. It proved possible to eliminate each of these possibilities by suitable control experiments. Drug-drug interactions were eliminated by a concentration study of the penicillin spectrum, which showed that large relaxation rate changes were observed in the absence of protein only at much higher drug concentrations than those used in the binding studies and that furthermore these changes were accompanied by chemical shift changes not observed when protein produced the broadening. Furthermore, addition of more penicillin to a given penicillin-albumin solution *decreased* the widths of all lines although it increased the viscosity and any drug-drug interactions, while probably having little influence on any intermolecular effect of the protein on the drug. Viscosity effects were further eliminated by experiments using γ-globulin, which does not bind penicillin, but does increase the viscosity of the solution to a similar degree. γ-Globulin had little effect on the linewidth when corrections were made for viscosity changes, further supporting the idea of specific interaction.

The effect of varying the albumin concentration at constant penicillin concentration on the linewidths of the spectrum of Figure 9 is shown in Figure 10. Although peak 5 is broadest, the relaxation rate of peak 1 has evidently been changed by a larger fraction than that of either peak 4 or 5. It is this relative increment, not the absolute linewidth, which is related to the relative degree of rotational stabilization of the different moieties comprising the penicillin molecule. The absolute linewidths reflect the number, types, and distances of the magnetic neighbors of a given proton in the free and bound environments in addition to depending on the correlation times. For rotational relaxation, the relaxation rate due to each individual magnetic neighbor is proportional to r^{-6}, where r is the distance from the protein of interest to the neighbor causing the relaxation. Since peak 1 corresponds to the resonance of the phenyl group, it was concluded that this group was the primary binding site of the penicillin to bovine serum albumin.

Studies similar to the one just discussed have also been carried out on the binding of sulfonamides to bovine serum albumin, which has only one binding site for sulfonamides (Jardetzky and Wade-Jardetzky, 1965). It was found that with sulfacetamide, sulfathiazole, and sulfamethylisoxazole the aromatic ring was the primary binding site, while sulfaphenazole, which has two phenyl rings, was bound at both rings. It is interesting that competitive binding experiments showed that one phenyl ring could be displaced while the other remained bound, suggesting that the two binding sites on the BSA were distinct.

This technique has also been used to study a number of enzyme substrate interactions including the enzymes cholinesterase (Kato, 1968a,b), alcohol dehydrogenase (Hollis, 1967), and chymotrypsin (Gerig, 1968), as well as in the study of the interactions of haptens with antibodies (Burgen et al., 1967).

Another important NMR method for detecting and studying binding is to monitor any chemical shifts occurring in the spectrum of the bound molecule. When the chemical shift for a given proton is different in the bound and free forms, the three cases of slow, intermediate, and rapid exchanges are possible. Space limitations prohibit a detailed discussion of the various possibilities and the reader is referred to Pople et al. (1959) for further details. Only the fast exchange case seems to have been observed in the small molecule-protein interactions studied to date. As a prototype of this method, the elegant studies by Dahlquist and Raftery (1968b) on lysozyme, which hydrolyzes certain hexosamine-containing glycosides and is inhibited by many hexosamines including N-acetylglucosamine (NAG), will serve. In the presence of lysozyme the single acetyl methyl peak of the NAG spectrum is replaced by two peaks which are shifted upfield, as shown in Figure 11. The two upfield peaks have been assigned to the α and β anomers of NAG. That their chemical shifts are different in the bound state indicates a difference in the geometrical relationships of the two inhibitors to the enzyme active site. Further information on this system has been obtained by a study of the effects of chemical exchange on the relaxation times of the inhibitor protons (Sykes, 1969). Such studies allow the measurement of the lifetimes and formation rates of the complexes and these in turn suggest some features of the reaction mechanism.

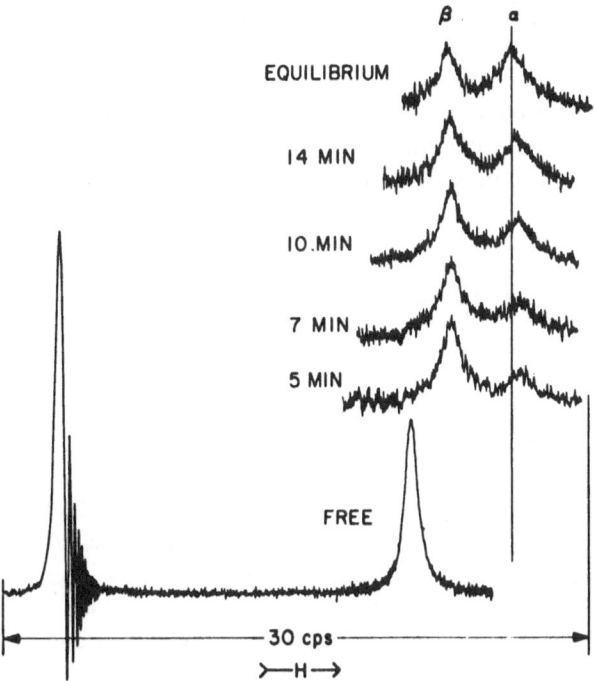

FIG. 11. NMR spectra of the acetamido methyl protons of NAG free in solution and of β-NHG during mutarotation in the presence of lysozyme. Strong resonance at left is from acetone. (From Dahlquist and Raftery. 1968a. *Biochemistry*, 7:3269. Copyright © 1968 by the American Chemical Society. Reprinted by permission of the copyright owner.)

Interaction of Drugs with Biological Membranes

Some success has been attained in the application of NMR relaxation measurements to the study of biological membranes. The principles involved are identical to those discussed in the section on small molecule-macromolecule interactions.

Metcalfe et al. (1968) have studied the interaction of anesthetics such as benzyl alcohol with erythrocyte membranes. Either binding or insertion of the anesthetic molecule into the membrane would be expected to restrict the molecular motion and result in line broadening. With increasing anesthetic concentration (benzyl alcohol, for example) the relaxation rate of the benzyl protons first decreases and then increases after passing a minimum. Such results reflect changes in membrane structure brought about by the small molecule and can be correlated with physiological effects such as hemolysis and nerve fiber blockage.

Fischer and Jost (1968) have observed line broadening and chemical shifting of the phenyl groups of epinephrine in the presence of isolated mouse liver cells. Although some type of specific and saturable interaction is indicated, this study illustrates some of the difficulties in studying these more complex systems. For example, the elimination of possible paramagnetic ions associated with the cell and the elimination of possible effects of chemical shifts and exchange on the line-widths, the latter in the absence of any knowledge of the number of binding sites present, do not seem possible. Even with these limitations, however, some interesting information can be obtained, and the use of NMR to study more complex biological systems is expected to increase.

NMR Spectra of Proteins

Although amino acids and small peptides give sharp and simple NMR spectra, native proteins generally show only a broad series of envelopes with most spectral detail smeared. This broadening is caused by two factors: (1) the motional freedom of the amino acid residues is hindered in the native protein conformation, (2) the protons of different residues of the same amino acid can, in the folded, native state, be exposed to a range of environments having different chemical shifts. Which of these factors predominates for a given kind of resonance depends on the detailed properties of the particular protein, including its molecular weight. Heating or otherwise unfolding the protein causes line narrowing by counteracting the two line-broadening effects just mentioned. This general broadening is the prime difficulty in obtaining useful information from NMR studies about the structure of proteins and the involvement of specific amino acid residues in the formation of complexes. Although one immediately thinks of going to higher magnetic fields in order to resolve the spectra, a simple calculation shows that frequencies of at least 1000 MHz are required in order to make significant improvement of protein spectra. The highest frequency currently in use is about 250 MHz.

For these reasons, most progress to date in obtaining really new information from protein NMR spectra has centered on the study of a few resonances that for various reasons have extreme chemical shifts lying outside the overall spectral envelope. The spectrum of ribonuclease, for instance, at about pH 5.4 shows four small peaks downfield from the usual aromatic proton region. It has proved possible to assign these to the imidazole C-2 protons of the four histidine residues of the protein. In fact, careful chemical manipulations have actually shown each peak to be connected to a specific histidine, and this in turn has made it possible to determine the pK values of the four histidines individually! The interaction of an inhibitor 3'cytidylic acid affects the resonances of histidine residues 12, 48, 105, and 119 differently. The C-2 peak of histidine 119 shifts downfield by 60 Hz, while histidine 12 undergoes a smaller shift. Histidine 105 is not affected at all, while histidine 48 is hardly affected. Residues 105 and 48 therefore are not involved in complex formation, while 12 and 119 are. On the other hand, binding to 5'-cytidylic acid does not affect residue 119, indicating a different binding mechanism. This brief discussion only suggests the extent to which NMR has contributed to the structure activity correlation for ribonuclease. For full details the reader is referred to the original papers, Meadows et al. (1969) and references therein. The point, however, is that significant information can be gleaned from protein NMR spectra when the spectra of the specific residues involved in the binding are in a clear region of the spectrum. Biosynthetic deuteration has been used to simplify the spectrum of staphylococcal nuclease (Markley et al., 1968) and this approach seems most promising even for higher molecular weight enzymes. By deuterating all but selected residues of interest, only their proton spectra are allowed to remain, since the deuteron absorbs at a far different frequency than the proton.

Some success has been attained in the study of the overall protein NMR spectral envelope. In a study of chymotrypsin and some of its slightly modified chemical derivatives, it was possible to demonstrate by NMR linewidth measurements a different degree of unfolding for the several species and to show that one derivative, which was partially inactivated by partial unfolding, reassumed a nearly completely folded conformation in the presence of a pseudosubstrate capable of binding to the enzyme (Hollis et al., 1967). This seems to be an example of an extreme case of Koshland's induced-fit hypothesis.

Interactions Between Small Molecules

NMR has been used to study interactions between small molecules of pharmacological interest. One case which has been studied in some detail by relaxation time measurements is the structure of the weak complex formed between catecholamines and nucleotides (Jardetzky, 1964). It was found that, when epinephrine forms a 1:1 complex with adenosine triphosphate (ATP), there was a more pronounced broadening of the proton peaks of the sidechains than from the aromatic rings, suggesting preferential stabilization of this portion of the molecule.

Chemical shift measurements have also proved useful in the study of small molecule interactions, especially those involving nucleotides. We have recently reviewed the contribution of NMR in the study of nucleic acids (Ts'o, Kondo, et al., 1969) and we have shown how chemical shift data can be used to construct a general conformational model for dinucleoside mono- and diphosphates (Ts'o, Schweizer, and Hollis, 1969). The reader is referred to these references and those cited therein for details. For present purposes, suffice it to say that the aromatic purine ring is strongly magnetically anisotropic so that any molecule interacting with it to form a complex will experience strong perturbations in its NMR spectrum due to the large chemical shifts resulting upon complexation.

Sternglanz et al. (1969) have utilized this method to investigate the interaction of the antimalarial drug chloroquine diphosphate with adenosine-5'-phosphate (AMP) and other nucleotides. Chemical shifts in both the drug and AMP NMR spectra definitely established the existence of ring-ring interactions in this system and they also gave some indication that, in accord with previous conclusions, ring-ring interactions between chloroquine and pyrimidine nucleotides are considerably less than those between the drug and purine nucleotides.

INSTRUMENTATION AND TECHNIQUES

General Remarks

Owing to the small energy difference between the nuclear magnetic energy levels giving rise to NMR spectra, NMR suffers from an inherent lack of sensitivity simply because the Boltzmann distribution favors the lower state only slightly so that only a small magnetic polarization results at usual temperatures of biochemical reactions, i.e., $-10°C$ and above. This lack of sensitivity has been one of the major impediments to the use of NMR methods in biochemical systems. Increased sensitivity has therefore been a major goal in the design of NMR instrumentation. A second important property of the NMR spectrometer, however, is its resolution, which, in practice, is determined by the degree of homogeneity of the magnetic field over the volume of the sample. Unfortunately, but not unexpectedly, the magnet improvements, which increase sensitivity, also tend to decrease resolution so that a compromise must be reached. In this section, some of the factors influencing the sensitivity and resolution of the instrument will be discussed as well as techniques for sensitivity improvement based on time-averaging rather than improved instrument design.

Considering resonance at a fixed value of the polarizing field, an obvious method for increasing sensitivity is to use a bigger sample. Commercial high resolution spectrometers accommodate sample tubes of only 5 mm diameter, and an active sample volume of about 0.4 ml. The tube size which can be accepted by a given instrument it determined by the width of the gap between the magnet poles. As this gap is made larger, it is necessary to increase the pole diameter and the overall size of the magnet in order to maintain the resolution. This approach has proved feasible and commercial instruments are available in the 90 to 100 MHz range, which by virtue of using pole diameters of 15 or 18 inches are able to combine excellent resolution with the use of sample tube diameters of up to 15 mm. Such spectrometers can detect proton resonances in the millimolar concentration range under favorable conditions.

The use of stronger magnetic fields is a second method by which one can in principle increase the polarization and therefore the NMR sensitivity. In addition, the stronger field also increases the chemical shifts in proportion to the field strength [equation (14)]. Theoretically, the sensitivity increases in proportion to $H_0^{3/2}$, where H_0 is the strength of the polarizing field. For protons a commercial instrument is available which operates at 220 MHz, employing a superconducting solenoid magnet (Figure 12). Unfortunately, the full theoretical increase in sensitivity has not been attained owing to special problems in the detection of high radio frequencies.

Figures 12 and 13 show examples of modern NMR spectrometers.

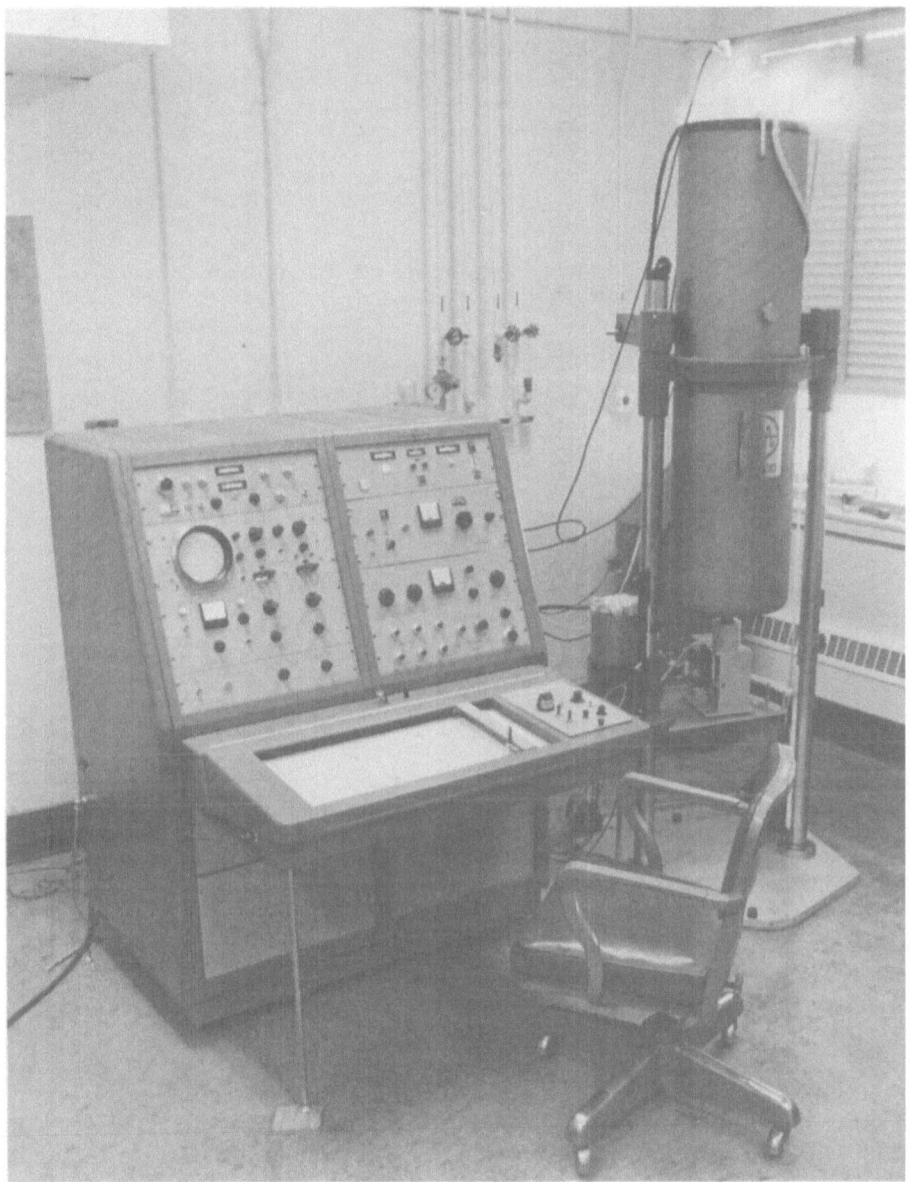

FIG. 12. The Varian HA 220, a 220 MHz spectrometer using a superconducting magnet, which is shown on the right. (Photograph courtesy of Varian.)

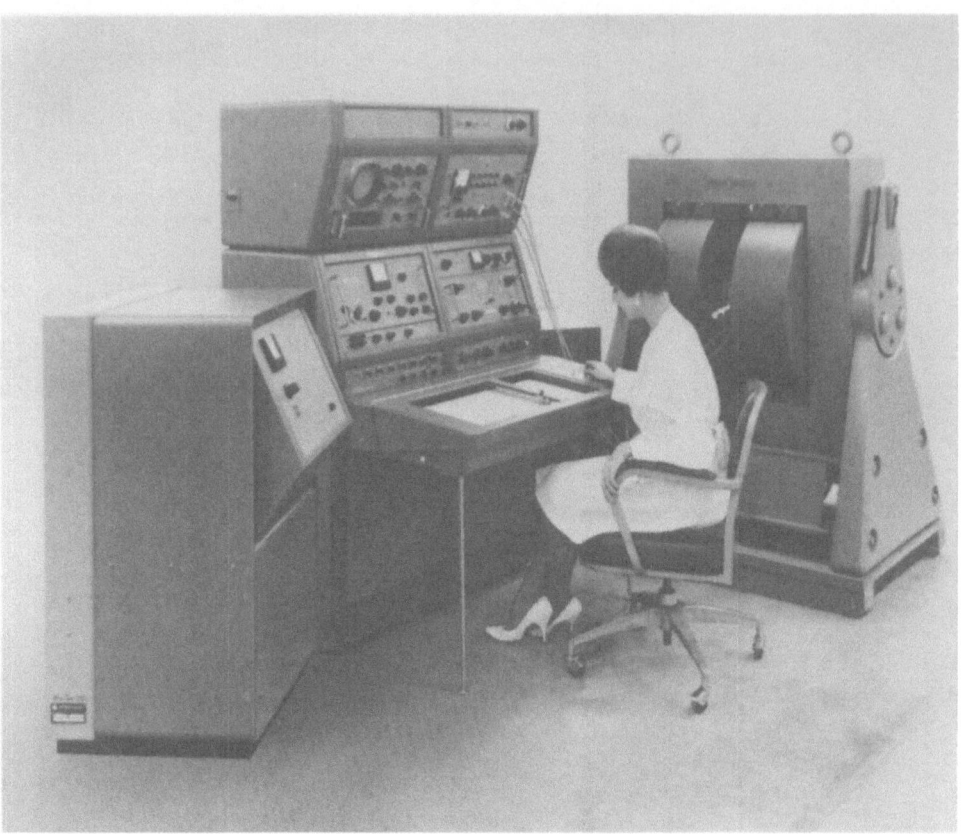

FIG. 13. The Varian HA 100, a conventional high-resolution NMR spectrometer using an iron-core electromagnet. The magnet power supply is at the left, the magnet is at the right. The console contains the recorder and radiofrequency oscillator as well as an oscilloscope, field sweep devices, field stabilization unit, and magnet homogeneity controls. (Photograph courtesy of Varian.)

Sensitivity Enhancement

A number of possibilities exist for improving the signal-to-noise ratio in NMR spectra and this rather complex subject has been discussed in detail by Ernst (1966). Two methods which are extraordinarily well suited for NMR are the *method of time averaging,* and the *Fourier transform method.* These methods are being used with increasing frequency in NMR experiments on biological systems, and commercial equipment is available allowing their use. In this section the basic principles underlying these methods will be discussed briefly.

THE TIME-AVERAGING METHOD. In principle, the signal-to-noise ratio can be increased at will by taking a sufficiently long time to do the experiment and using suitable filters to suppress the noise. In practice, it may not be possible to realize the higher sensitivity of an experiment over a longer time because of low frequency instability of the spectrometer and because the long relaxation times encountered in NMR result in saturation at low scanning rates. For these reasons time-averaging can be advantageous. Instead of a single long-term measurement, a number of relatively rapid scans of the spectrum are made and the results added together so that the signals add coherently while the noise adds randomly. In practice, the summation of the different traces can be made in one of several commercially available digital storage devices having a sufficient number of channels adequately to represent the spectrum, each channel corresponding to a single point in the spectrum. Since the signal adds up proportionally to the number of scans while the noise adds up as the square root of the number of scans, a net gain in signal-to-noise ratio proportional to the square root of the number of scans is achieved. This technique has been used frequently in biochemical applications of NMR.

FOURIER TRANSFORM SPECTROSCOPY. In the sweep method just discussed one resonance in the spectrum is excited at a time as the radio frequency is slowly varied over the spectrum. It is possible by the use of short bursts or pulses of radio-frequency power to produce a much broader frequency spectrum of the irradiation. It is, in fact, possible in effect to irradiate the entire spectrum simultaneously by using sufficiently short pulses offering the possibility of gathering information simultaneously from all or several parts of the spectrum. In practice, the sample is irradiated with a series of short, equally spaced pulses, and the response of the system to each pulse, i.e., the time decay of the system toward equilibrium, is stored in a time-averaging computer and added to previous pulses. This is continued until a sufficiently good signal-to-noise ratio is obtained. The response to the radio-frequency pulse and the usual NMR absorption spectrum form a Fourier transform pair (Lowe and Norberg, 1957). By calculating the Fourier transform of the stored sum of the responses using a computer, the absorption spectrum with enhanced sensitivity is obtained. This technique has been developed only very recently but its increasing use in biochemical applications of NMR is definitely to be anticipated. A full discussion of the Fourier transform method as applied to NMR has been given by Ernst and Anderson (1966).

REFERENCES

Abragam, A. 1961. The Principles of Nuclear Magnetism. New York, Oxford University Press.

Andrew, E. R. 1955. Nuclear Magnetic Resonance. New York, Cambridge University Press.

Bloch, R. 1953. The principle of nuclear induction. Science, 118:425-430.

Burgen, A., O. Jardetzky, J. C. Metcalfe, and N. Wade-Jardetzky. 1967. Investigation of a haptene-antibody complex by NMR. Proc. Nat. Acad. Sci. U.S.A., 101:67-68.

Carrington, A., and A. D. McLachlan. 1967. Introduction to Magnetic Resonance. New York, Harper and Row.

Dahlquist, F. W., and M. A. Raftery. 1968a. A nuclear magnetic resonance study of association equilibria and enzyme bound environments of N-acetyl-D-glucosamine anomers and lysozyme. Biochemistry (Washington), 7:3269-3276.

———— and M. A. Raftery. 1968b. A nuclear magnetic resonance study of enzyme-inhibitor association. The use of pH and temperature effects to probe the binding environments. Biochemistry (Washington), 7:3277-3280.

Ernst, R. R. 1966. Sensitivity enhancement in magnetic resonance. In Waugh, J. S., ed., Advances in Magnetic Resonance, 2:1-135, New York, Academic Press.

———— and W. A. Anderson. 1966. Application of Fourier transform spectroscopy to magnetic resonance. Rev. Sci. Instrum., 37:93-102.

Fischer, J. J. 1971. Nuclear magnetic resonance as applied to pharmacology. In Schwartz, A., Methods in Pharmacology, 1:431-453. New York, Appleton-Century-Crofts.

———— and O. Jardetzky. 1965. Nuclear magnetic relaxation study of intermolecular complexes. The mechanism of penicillin binding to serum albumin. J. Amer. Chem. Soc., 87:3237-3244.

———— and M. C. Jost. 1968. NMR studies of drug-receptor interactions. The binding of epinephrine to isolated mouse liver cells. Molec. Pharmacol., 5:420-431.

Gerig, J. T. 1968. NMR studies of the interaction of tryptophan with α-chymotrypsin. J. Amer. Chem. Soc., 90:2681-2686.

Hollis, D. P. 1967. A NMR study of substrate binding to alcohol dehydrogenases. Biochemistry (Washington), 6:2080-2087.

———— G. G. McDonald, and R. L. Biltonen. 1967. Nuclear magnetic resonance studies of proteins. I. Conformational variance among members of the chymotrypsinogen family. Proc. Nat. Acad. Sci. U.S.A., 58:758-765.

Jardetzky, O. 1964. The study of specific molecular interactions by nuclear magnetic relaxation measurements. In Duchesne, J., ed., Advances in Chemical Physics, vol. 7:499-531. New York, Wiley/Interscience.

———— and C. D. Jardetzky. 1962. Introduction to magnetic resonance spectroscopy methods and biochemical applications. In Glick, D., ed., Methods of Biochemical Analyses, vol. 9:235-410, New York, Wiley/Interscience.

———— and N. G. Wade-Jardetzky. 1965. On the mechanism of the binding of sulfonamides to bovine serum albumin. Molec. Pharmacol., 1:214-230.

Kato, G. 1968a. Studies on serum cholinesterase kinetics by nuclear magnetic resonance spectroscopy. Molec. Pharmacol., 4:640-644.

———— 1968b. NMR study of the interaction between acetylcholine and horse serum cholinesterase. Molec. Pharmacol., 5:148-155.

Kowalsky, A., and M. Cohn. 1964. Application of NMR in biochemistry. Ann. Rev. Biochem., 33:481-518.

Lowe, I. J., and R. E. Norberg. 1957. Free induction decays in solids. Physical Review, 107:46-61.

Markley, J. L., I. Putter, and O. Jardetzky. 1968. High resolution nuclear magnetic resonance spectra of selectively deuterated staphylococcal nuclease. Science, 161:1249-1251.

Meadows, D. H., G. C. K. Roberts, and O. Jardetzky. 1969. NMR studies of the structure and binding sites of enzymes. VIII. Inhibitor binding to ribonuclease. J. Molec. Biol., 45:491-511.

Metcalfe, J. C., P. Seeman, and A. S. V. Burgen. 1968. The proton relaxation of benzyl alcohol in erythrocyte membranes. Molec. Pharmacol., 4:87-95.

Pople, J. A., W. G. Schneider, and H. J. Berstein. 1959. High Resolution Nuclear Magnetic Resonance. New York, McGraw-Hill Book Company.

Purcell, E. M. 1948. Nuclear magnetism in relation to problems of the liquid and solid states. Science, 107:433-440.

———— 1953. Research in nuclear magnetism. Science, 118:431-436.

Sternglanz, H., K. L. Yielding, and K. M. Pruitt. 1969. NMR studies of the interaction of chloroquine diphosphate with adenosine 5'-phosphate and other nucleotides. Molec. Pharmacol., 5:376-381.

Sykes, B. D. 1969. A transient NMR study of the kinetics of methyl N-acetyl-D-glucosamide inhibition of lysozyme. Biochemistry (Washington), 8:1110-1116.

Ts'o, P. O. P., N. S. Kondo, M. P. Schweizer, and D. P. Hollis. 1969. Studies of the conformation and interaction in dinucleoside mono- and diphosphates by proton magnetic resonance. Biochemistry (Washington), 8:997-1029.

_____ M. P. Schweizer, and D. P. Hollis. 1969. Contribution of NMR to the study of the structure and electronic aspects of nucleic acids. Ann. N.Y. Acad. Sci., 158:256-297.

Zimmerman, J. R., and W. E. Brittin. 1957. Nuclear magnetic resonance studies in multiple phase systems: Lifetime of a water molecule in an adsorbing phase on silica gel. J. Phys. Chem., 61:1328-1338.

Chapter **7**

Electron Spin Resonance
and the Spin Labeling Method

Patricia Jost and O. Hayes Griffith

Institute of Molecular Biology and Department of Chemistry,
University of Oregon, Eugene, Oregon

INTRODUCTION

Electron spin resonance (ESR) is a spectroscopic technique that detects unpaired electrons present in paramagnetic atoms or molecules. The experimental technique employs a microwave source, but is similar in many ways to other spectroscopic methods such as nuclear magnetic resonance, optical absorption, fluorescence and infrared spectroscopy. ESR has a range of biological applications including studies of free radicals, triplet states, and paramagnetic metal ions.

The earliest and one of the most extensive applications of ESR to biochemical problems utilized the inherent paramagnetism of free radicals already present in biological systems. Free radical intermediates in biochemical reactions were detected in the first application of ESR to biology by Commoner and coworkers in 1954. They observed ESR signals in lyophilized tissues and suggested that free radicals were associated with metabolic activity. Since then ESR has been a widely applied spectroscopic technique used in the detection and identification of free radical intermediates in various enzyme reactions, including photosynthesis. Free radicals are also produced by high energy electrons or by x-, γ-, or UV-irradiation. In these studies ESR is used to identify the free radicals present, determine the free radical concentrations, and measure rates of radical formation and decay.

The second area of application, triplet states, is more troublesome for a variety of technical reasons. However, a few applications involving proteins have been reported, and the phosphorescent state of a number of organic molecules of biological interest have been examined in detail. (In addition, certain dinitroxide free radicals exhibit electron correlation and can be thought of as triplet states. These diradicals are discussed below.) The third area of application of ESR capitalizes on the inherent paramagnetism of biomolecules that contain paramagnetic metal atoms such as iron, copper, molybdenum, cobalt, or manganese. Examples are the heme proteins myoglobin, hemoglobin, and the cytochromes. Studies of iron (usually as Fe^{3+}) have led to information regarding the heme orientation with respect to the crystalline axes, energy levels associated with the d orbitals of iron, the symmetry of the electric field near the iron site, and changes in electronic structure accompanying protein denaturation.

In spite of the occurrence of occasional free radicals and paramagnetic metal ions, paramagnetism is an uncommon state in biology. To turn this apparent difficulty into an advantage, one may *introduce a paramagnetic center* by labeling with a reporter group that contains an unpaired electron (early examples include Mn^{++} or nitric oxide). The general concept of binding reporter groups to biological macromolecules has been extensively used to obtain information about biomolecular structure and function. In the widest sense, this technique encompasses such diverse approaches as isomorphous replacement in x-ray crystallography, conjugation with fluorescein in antibody studies, and even the use of radioisotopes. In spectroscopic studies the label is usually an organic molecule, with properties appropriate for detection by such techniques as fluorescence, optical absorption, or electron spin resonance. Such a label may be covalently attached at highly specific sites on the macromolecule or may be constructed so that it binds noncovalently in a region of interest.

Spin labeling refers to the use of stable free radicals as reporter groups or labels, and was first used by Ohnishi and McConnell (1965) and Stone et al. (1965), who coined the term "spin label." Spin labels (stable free radicals) are now usually molecules containing the nitroxide moiety

$\cdot$ (a)   (b)

which contain an unpaired electron localized on the nitrogen and oxygen atoms (the adjacent methyl groups indicated by straight lines are necessary to stabilize the free radical). The first free radical of class (a) was reported in 1960 (Lebedev and Kazarnovskii), and many of the basic nitroxides were developed and their spectroscopic properties characterized by the pioneering efforts of Hoffman, Rozantsev, Nieman, Rassat, and others. (See, for example, Hoffman and Henderson, 1961; Rozantsev and Nieman, 1964; Brière et al., 1965b; Rozantsev and Krinitzkaya, 1965; Rozantsev and Kokhanov, 1966). Nitroxides of class (b) were introduced by Keana and coworkers in 1967 as a general method for converting ketones into nitroxides.

The resulting nitroxides can be named as 4',4'-dimethyloxazolidine-*N*-oxyl derivatives of the ketone precursors, but for simplicity this nitroxide group will be referred to as the "doxyl" moiety.

A representative selection from the large number of nitroxides synthesized in the past decade is given in Figure 1, and some useful references to them are included in the Appendix. In each structure the relatively unreactive N-O group contains the unpaired electron necessary to produce the ESR signal. However, it is the reactive functional group on other parts of many of the smaller molecules that permits the synthesis of the final spin labels with the desired shapes and chemical properties. For example, the ketone nitroxide IV can be converted to the dinitrophenyl spin label XXXIX by textbook procedures for preparing dinitrophenylhydrazones. Similarly, the alcohol nitroxide V will undergo standard esterification reactions to yield esters such as XXVI, XLIII, XLVI, LII, or LXXV. Thus, conventional chemical reactions can frequently be utilized to attach a small nitroxide to produce the final spin label. The chemistry of nitroxides has recently been treated in considerable detail by Rozantsev (1970) and by Forrester et al. (1968). Rozantsev's book also includes useful details of preparation of many of the smaller nitroxides that can then be attached chemically to the remainder of the spin label.

The nitroxide moiety is reasonably unreactive, remaining stable in aqueous solutions on moderate heating (up to 70° or 80°C) and with changes in *p*H over the range of *p*H 3 to 10. It can be reversibly reduced to the *N*-hydroxylamine by many mild reducing agents, but reduction to the corresponding secondary amine requires treatment with stronger reducing agents than are usually encountered in biological systems.

Biological applications of ESR, including spin labeling, have been well reviewed in recent years. As a general (but quantitative) introduction to ESR, Bersohn and Baird (1966) and Carrington and McLachlan (1967) are useful. Books and monographs focusing on biological applications of ESR include Ehrenberg et al. (1967), Ingram (1969), Feher (1970), and Bolton et al. (1971). For those interested in the application of ESR in biochemistry utilizing the inherent paramagnetism of metal atoms or transient free radicals, two earlier chapters on methods have appeared (Jardetsky and Jardetsky, 1962; Palmer, 1967).

Review articles dealing specifically with spin labeling have been written by Hamilton and McConnell (1968), Griffith and Waggoner (1969), McConnell and McFarland (1970), Smith (1971), and Jost et al. (1971c). However, there appears to be a need for a methods article describing the collection and treatment of data,

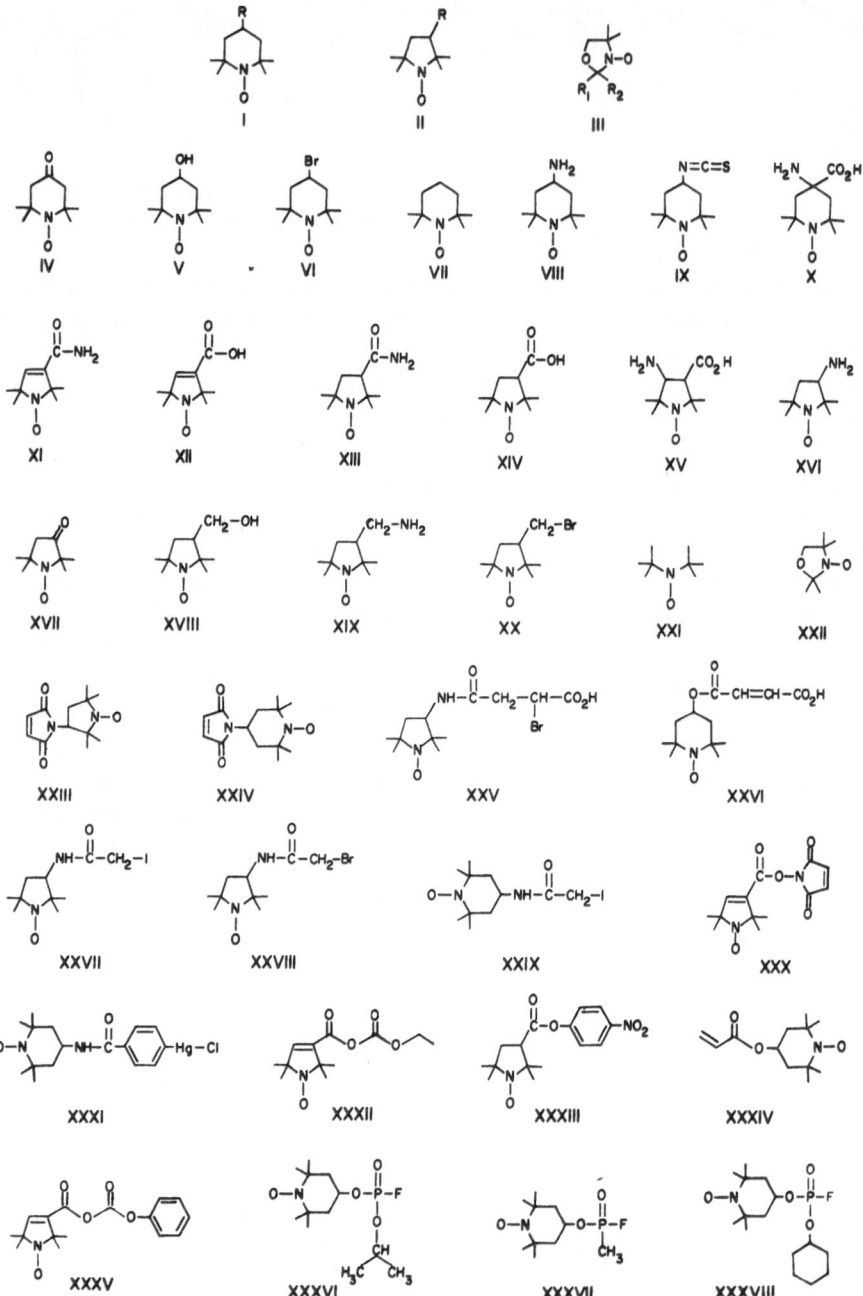

FIG. 1. Some examples of nitroxide molecules that have been used as spin labels or synthetic intermediates for spin labels. Methyl groups adjacent to the N–O moiety are shown as short lines. Useful references giving syntheses or applications are listed in the Appendix.

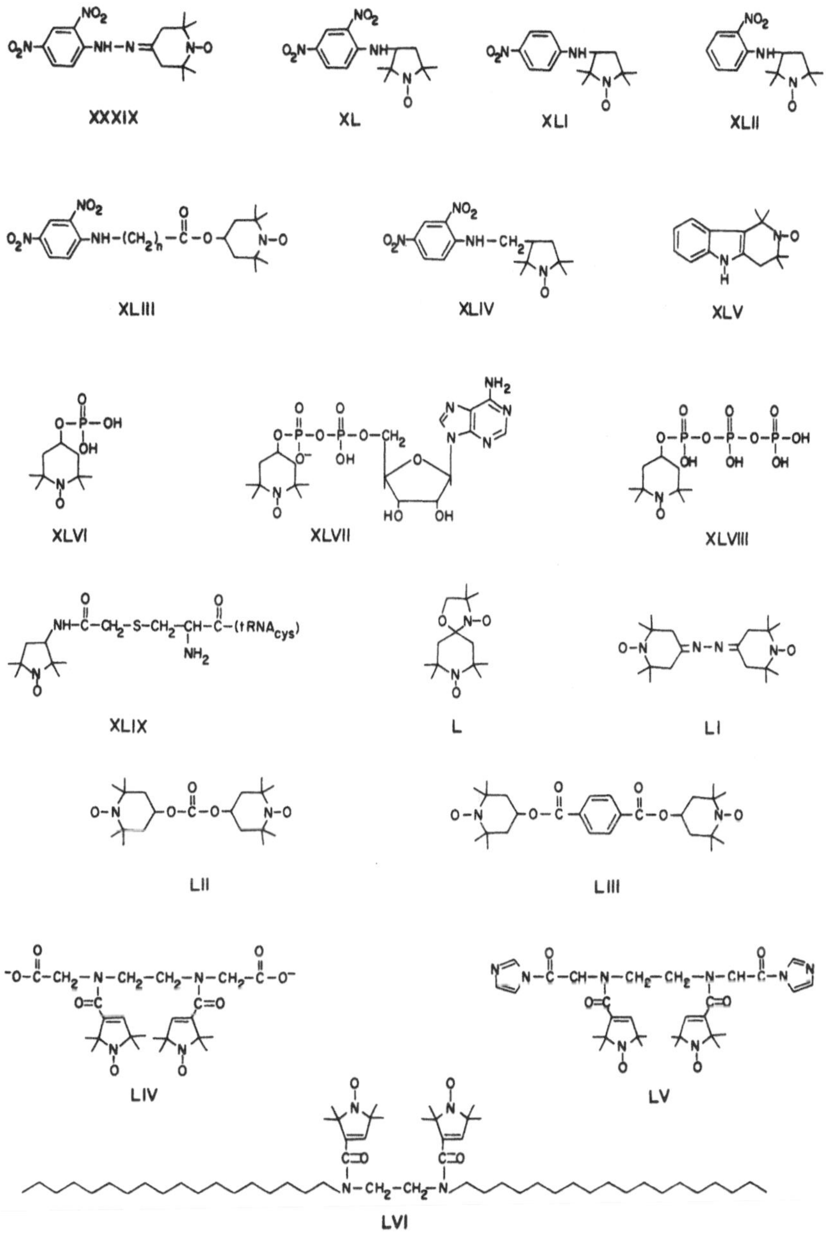

FIG. 1. (Cont.)

instrumental variables, and common errors along with a few applications to illustrate the technique. The present chapter was written with this goal in mind. No attempt has been made to cover the literature on spin labeling, and the above review articles should be consulted for a more complete list of applications. Commercial

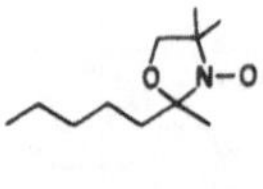
LVII

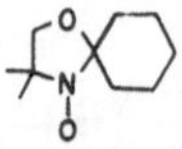
LVIII

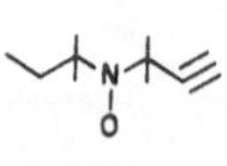
LIX

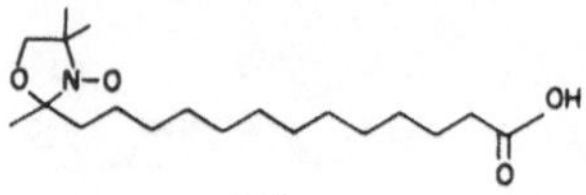
LX

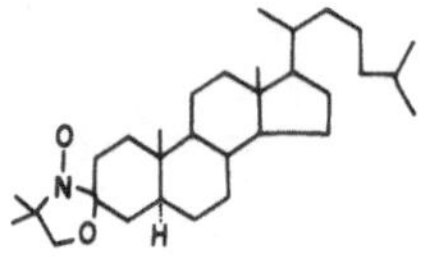
LXI

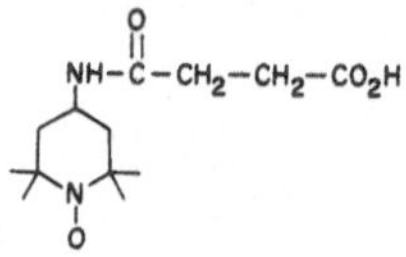
LXII

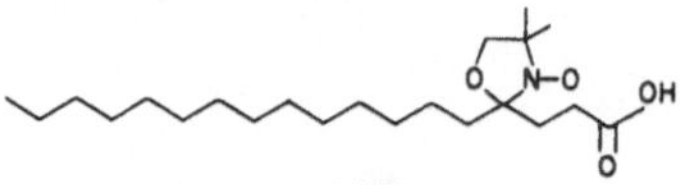
LXIII

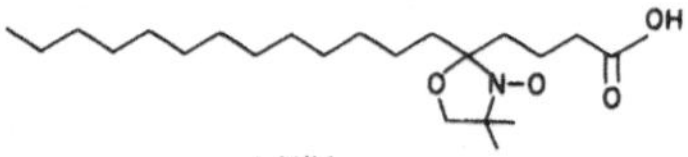
LXIV

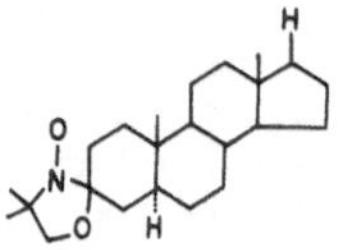
LXV

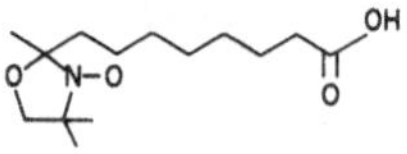
LXVI

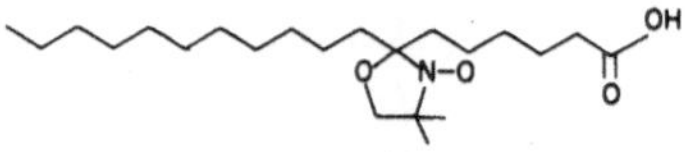
LXVII

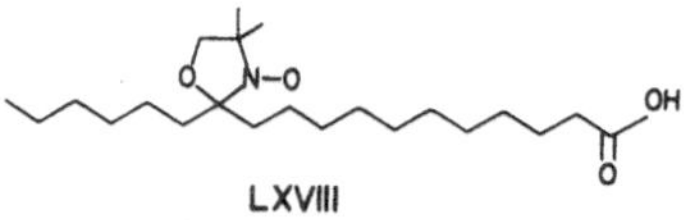
LXVIII

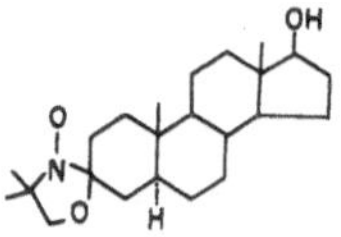
LXIX

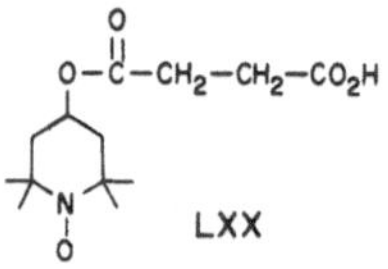
LXX

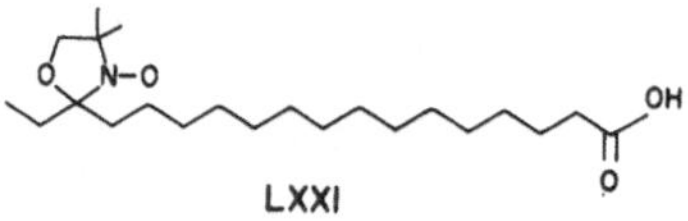
LXXI

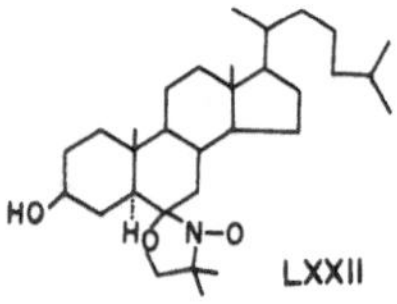
LXXII

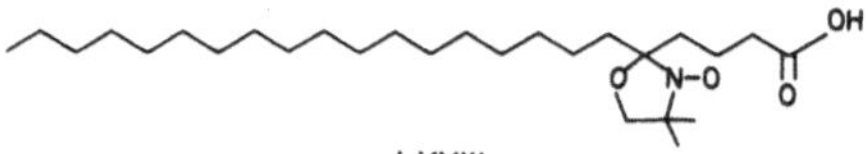
LXXIII

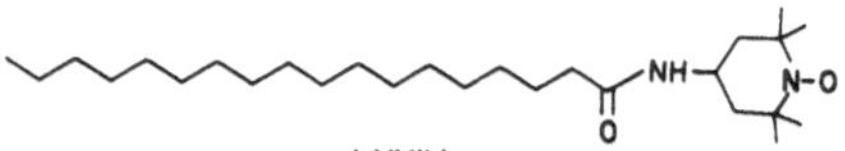
LXXIV

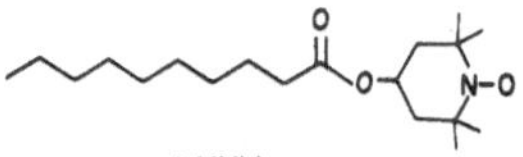
LXXV

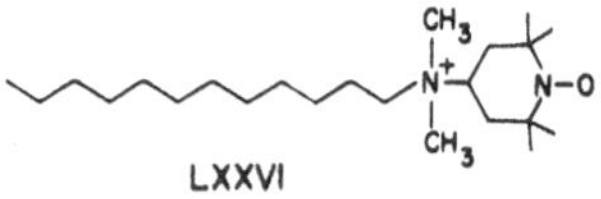
LXXVI

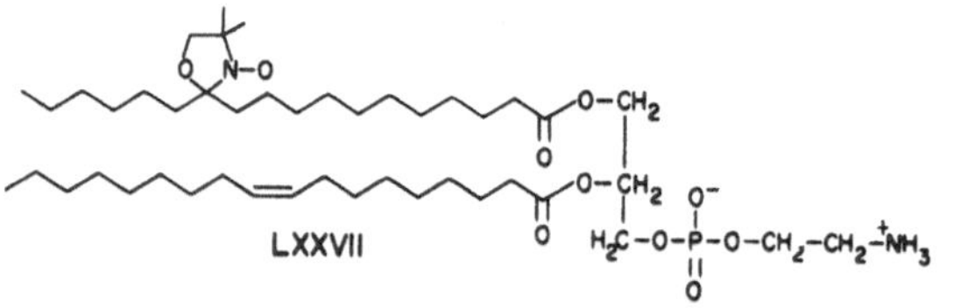
LXXVII

FIG. 1. (*Cont.*)

ESR spectrometers are now available at most institutions. It is hoped that the information presented here will help the nonexpert to use ESR and the spin-labeling method without investing the time required to master a comprehensive book on ESR until it is clear the technique will provide useful information about the system under investigation.

ELECTRON SPIN RESONANCE OF NITROXIDE FREE RADICALS

Spin Hamiltonian and Definition of Parameters

The appropriate spin Hamiltonian, $\hat{\mathcal{H}}$, required to describe a collection of nitroxide free radicals, is

$$\hat{\mathcal{H}} = |\beta| \mathbf{H} \cdot \mathbf{g} \cdot \hat{\mathbf{S}} + \hat{\mathbf{S}} \cdot \mathbf{A} \cdot \hat{\mathbf{I}} + \begin{bmatrix} \text{electron-electron} \\ \text{dipole and exchange terms} \end{bmatrix} \tag{1}$$

where β is the electron Bohr magneton, $\mathbf{H}$ the laboratory magnetic field, $\mathbf{g}$ the g-value tensor, $\hat{\mathbf{S}}$ the electron spin operator, $\mathbf{A}$ the electron-nuclear hyperfine tensor (frequently denoted by $\mathbf{T}$), and $\hat{\mathbf{I}}$ the nuclear spin operator. The nuclear Zeeman term is not important in most work (Libertini and Griffith, 1970) and has been omitted. The electron-electron dipole and exchange terms are significant only when dinitroxides or very high local concentrations of nitroxides are encountered.

For the typical nitroxide free radical rapidly tumbling in solution, the Hamiltonian takes the familiar form

$$\hat{\mathcal{H}} = g_0 |\beta| H \hat{S}_z + A_0 \hat{\mathbf{S}} \cdot \hat{\mathbf{I}} \tag{2}$$

where g_0 and A_0 are the isotropic components of g and A. The first term in equations (1) and (2), the electron Zeeman term, represents the large interaction of the electron spin with the laboratory magnetic field. This term yields the useful relation

$$h\nu = g_0 \beta H \tag{3}$$

where h is Planck's constant and ν is the microwave frequency of the ESR spectrometer. Nitroxide g values are very nearly equal to 2.00, and equation (3) may be reduced to ν (in GHz) $= 2.8H$ (in kG). Most commercial ESR spectrometers operate at $\nu = 9.5$ GHz (X-band), and thus $H = 3.4$ kG. A few spectrometers operate at higher frequencies, for example at $\nu = 35$ GHz, where $H = 12.5$ kG. The higher frequencies have some advantages (see next section) but the experiments are slightly more troublesome, and most studies are performed at 9.5 GHz.

The unpaired spin responsible for the ESR spectrum is confined largely to the N-O group. The significant magnetic interaction is between the unpaired electron and the ^{14}N nucleus (the nuclear spin of ^{16}O is zero). This electron-nuclear interaction is represented by the second term in equation (1) or equation (2). Since $I = 1$ for ^{14}N, the result is $2I + 1$ or three lines of equal intensity, separated by the coupling constant. The relationships of the important A_0 (also designated by a_0) and g_0 parameters are shown in Figure 2 along with the line widths and line heights. Figure 2 also points out the problem of phase reversal in ESR spectra. The ESR spectrum can be recorded with positive or negative phase. Spectra can, of course,

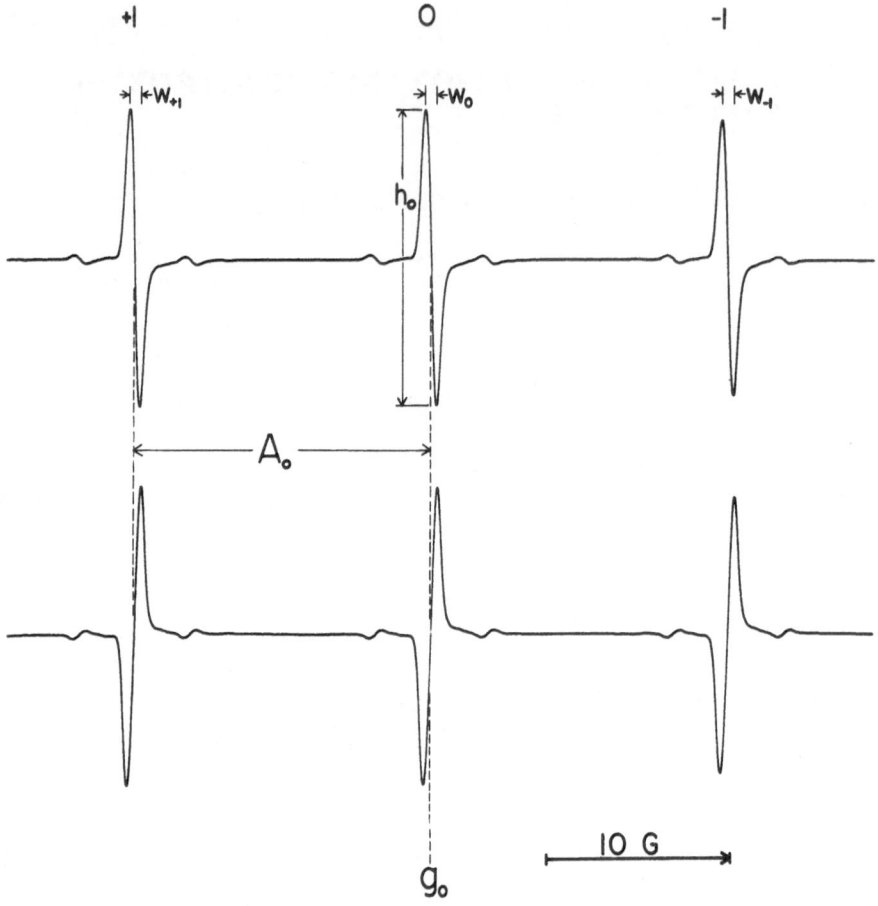

FIG. 2. Typical 9.5 GHz ESR spectra of a nitroxide spin label in solution illustrating the measurement of parameters. The most useful parameters are the coupling constant (A_0) and the g value (g_0). The peak-to-peak line widths W_{+1}, W_0 and W_{-1} are defined as shown. The subscripts $+1$, 0, -1 refer to the z components of the ^{14}N nuclear spin. Only one of the corresponding heights, h_0, is shown for clarity. The two very small peaks on either side of each of the three main ESR lines are ^{13}C peaks resulting from a natural abundance of this isotope in carbons adjacent to the N–O moiety. The top and bottom spectra are identical except for the choice of phase.

also be displayed with the magnetic field increasing from left to right or from right to left. The current literature abounds with all four permutations of these two variables. The advent of small computers and integration of spectra renders the positive phase illustrated in the top spectrum of Figure 2 more attractive and consistent with the presentation of NMR data (see pp. 253–256). As a matter of convention, all spectra from this laboratory are now scanned with the magnetic field increasing from left to right and are of positive phase. For instrumental reasons spectra are sometimes inadvertently recorded with negative phase. These data are easily phase reversed by retracing or by computer if the data are stored on tape (see pp. 253–256).

Spectral Anisotropy

Figure 3 illustrates the spectral anisotropy that is observed when nitroxides are ordered in a crystalline matrix. Both the g value (g) and the coupling constant (A) are angular dependent. The extremes in g and A lie along the principal molecular x, y, and z axes. The x axis is parallel to the N-O bond, z is parallel to the nitrogen $2p$ orbital, and y is perpendicular to the xz plane as shown below.

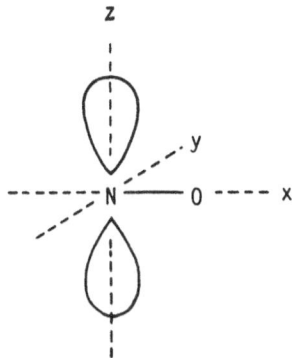

A number of nitroxides have been studied by incorporating a small amount of the spin label in a suitable host crystal and orienting the crystal in a magnetic field. Several nitroxides have been studied in the host crystal tetramethyl-1,3-cyclobutane-dione (TMCB). The principal values for di-t-butyl nitroxide XXI in TMCB are A_{xx} =7.6 G, A_{yy}=6.0 G, A_{zz}=31.8 G, g_{xx}=2.0088, g_{yy}=2.0062, and g_{zz}=2.0027 (Libertini and Griffith, 1970). The variation in tensor elements among nitroxides examined thus far is not great. For example, the small doxyl nitroxide XXII in TMCB yields the values A_{xx}=5.9 G, A_{yy}=5.4 G, A_{zz}=32.9 G, g_{xx}=2.0088, g_{yy}= 2.0058, and g_{zz}=2.0022 (Jost et al., 1971b). Small variations arise from differences in electronic structure, polarity of the environment, and some residual molecular motion in the host crystals. However, the essential features are (1) the largest splitting is observed when the magnetic field is along the z molecular axis (see Figure 3), and (2) $A_{xx} \sim A_{yy}$.

In studying anisotropic effects, it is necessary to be able to determine A and g at a given orientation of the magnetic field. Libertini and Griffith (1970) have examined the exact solution of the Hamiltonian and a number of approximate analytical expressions for A and g. The most useful equations are:

$$A = A_{xx}\sin^2\theta + A_{zz}\cos^2\theta \tag{4}$$

or

$$A = [(A_{xx})^2\sin^2\theta + (A_{zz})^2\cos^2\theta]^{1/2} \tag{5}$$

and

$$g = g_{xx}\sin^2\theta\cos^2\phi + g_{yy}\sin^2\theta\sin^2\phi + g_{zz}\cos^2\theta \tag{6}$$

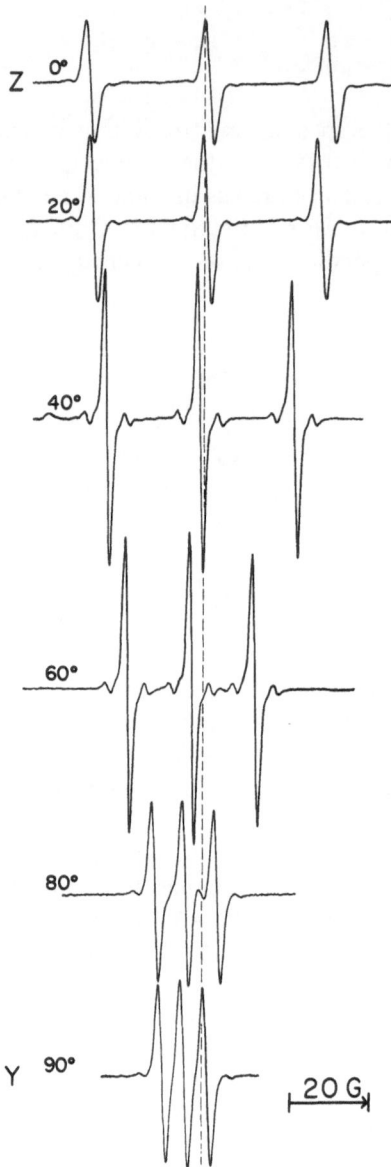

FIG. 3. Example of the very large A and g anisotropy which can be observed with an oriented nitroxide spin label. These 9.5 GHz spectra were recorded for di-t-butyl nitroxide XXI oriented in the host crystal, tetramethyl-1,3-cyclobutanedione. The crystal was rotated in the molecular yz plane. The orientations $\theta=0°$ and $\theta=90°$ correspond to the magnetic field along the z and y axes, respectively. The dashed line marks the position ($g=2.0036$) of a 2,2-diphenyl-1-picryl-hydrazyl reference sample. All spectra were recorded at room temperature.

where θ and ϕ are the usual polar coordinates of the laboratory, magnetic field direction relative to the molecular coordinate system. Equations (4) and (5) have utilized the simplifying assumption of axial symmetry of the hyperfine tensor (i.e.,

$A_{xx} = A_{yy}$). The corresponding equations in the absence of axial symmetry are given elsewhere (Libertini and Griffith, 1970). Equation (6) does not assume axial symmetry because, in general, $g_{xx} \neq g_{yy} \neq g_{zz}$. Before leaving this topic it is instructive to consider a specific example. In Figure 3, the third spectrum from the top was recorded with the magnetic field 40° from the z axis in the zy plane ($\theta = 40°$, $\phi = 90°$). The A and g values measured from this spectrum are 24.5 G and 2.0042. Equation (4), using $A_{xx} = (7.6 + 6.0)(1/2) = 6.8$ G and $A_{zz} = 31.8$ G yields 21.5 G. Equation (5), and the same A_{xx} and A_{zz}, gives 24.7 G. Equation (6) with $g_{xx} = 2.0088$, $g_{yy} = 2.0062$, and $g_{zz} = 2.0027$, yields 2.0042, in agreement with the experimental result. Of the two expressions for A, equation (5) is the more accurate approximation. However, the simple form of equation (4) is attractive when considering approximate models for anisotropic motion or a distribution of orientations. The accuracy of equation (4) improves near the principal directions of the molecule. In fact, equations (4) and (5) give the same results along the molecular axes (i.e., $A = A_{xx}$ or A_{zz}). This follows from the nature of the spin Hamiltonian. The quantities A_{xx}, A_{yy}, A_{zz} and g_{xx}, g_{yy} and g_{zz} are measured from spectra recorded with the magnetic field along the molecular axes. For example, the top spectrum of Figure 3 yields A_{zz} and g_{zz} directly.

Effects of Isotropic and Anisotropic Motion

Different nitroxide free radicals have very similar ESR spectra in water at room temperature, as shown in the top row of Figure 4. This is in marked contrast to optical reporter groups, where each chromophore has its own characteristic spectrum. The A_0 and g_0 parameters of the sharp three-line solution ESR spectrum are related to the single crystal data of the previous section by the simple equations $A_0 = (1/3)(A_{xx} + A_{yy} + A_{zz})$, and $g_0 = (1/3)(g_{xx} + g_{yy} + g_{zz})$. As these relations suggest, the fast isotropic molecular motion almost completely averages out the anisotropic dipolar terms, leaving only the isotropic interaction between the ^{14}N nuclear spin and the unpaired electron (i.e., the Fermi contact term).

When the viscosity of the solution is increased, the ESR lines gradually broaden and the spectra become asymmetric, as shown in Figure 4. In Figure 4, the increase in viscosity was brought about by dissolving each of the four spin labels in glycerol and then lowering the temperature of the solutions. Care was taken in collecting the data to insure that spectra in each row of Figure 4 could be directly compared. It is interesting to note that the ESR spectra broaden at different rates. Thus, as the temperature is lowered, the molecular motion of the alcohol nitroxide V, 2,2,6,6-tetramethylpiperidinol-1-oxyl, is reduced more readily than the motion of di-t-butyl nitroxide, XXI. It is not yet possible to assign accurate rotational correlation times to most spectra of Figure 4. However, progress in this direction is being made, and at present it is possible to simulate ESR spectra covering a wide range of rotational correlation times (Itzkowitz, 1967; Alexandrov et al., 1970; R. Melhorn and A. Keith, University of California, Berkeley, personal communication).

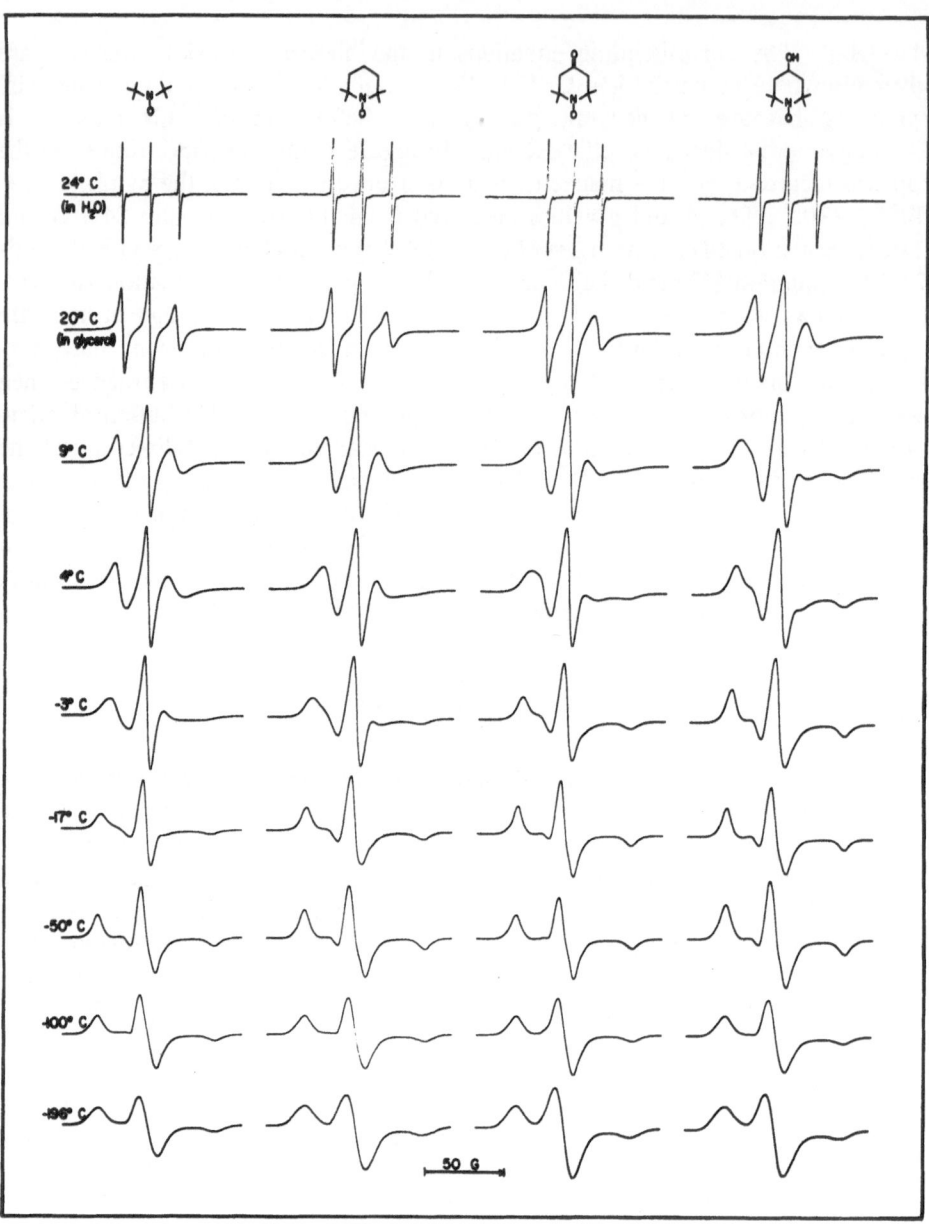

FIG. 4. The effect of viscosity on 9.5 GHz ESR spectra. The structure of each of the four spin labels used is given at the head of the corresponding column of spectra. The top row of spectra represent $10^{-4}M$ spin label in water at 24°C. All other spectra were recorded using $5\times10^{-4}M$ spin label in reagent grade glycerol (Mallinckrodt, $>95\%$ glycerol by volume, exact concentration not determined). The samples were sealed in quartz tubes in order to exclude water vapor. To obtain spectra of each row, the gas flow temperature regulator was stabilized at the desired temperature. The four samples were then run in succession before resetting the temperature regulator. The viscosity of glycerol is extremely temperature dependent and this procedure was chosen to minimize errors in resetting the regulator. Samples at liquid N_2 temperature were run in a special dewar and at reduced microwave power.

As the temperature approaches $-200°C$ the spectra of all four nitroxide free radicals in Figure 4 again become almost indistinguishable. This limiting line shape is the well-known rigid glass, powder, or polycrystalline spectrum. This spectrum can be thought of as a simple sum of all spectra of Figure 3 and spectra at all other orientations. As a result, the splitting between the outermost peaks of the rigid glass spectrum is $2A_{zz}$, corresponding to the top spectrum of Figure 3. The rigid-glass spectrum will be encountered whenever the spin label is randomly oriented and molecular motion is either absent or very slow on the ESR time scale; that is, when $\tau^{-1} \ll |A_{zz} - A_{xx}| \sim 7 \times 10^{7} \mathrm{sec}^{-1}$, and $\tau^{-1} \ll |g_{xx} - g_{zz}| \beta H h^{-1} \sim 3 \times 10^{7} \mathrm{sec}^{-1}$ (at 9.5 GHz), where τ is the rotational correlation time.[1] Spectra approaching the rigid glass limit are frequently observed in dried biological samples or when spin labels are rigidly bound to large proteins or membrane vesicles.

Molecular motion is not necessarily isotropic. Preferential motion about one axis is likely to occur for any elongated free radical, but the effects are particularly evident when the surrounding medium is anisotropic. Anisotropic motion has been observed in numerous ESR studies. Some early examples are x-ray produced ester free radicals in urea inclusion crystals (Griffith and McConnell, 1962; Griffith, 1964), and 2,2-diphenyl-1-picrylhydrazyl and other stable free radicals in the nematic phase of p-azoxyanisole (Carrington and Luckhurst, 1964; Luckhurst, 1966; Glarum and Marshall, 1966). A number of other long chain free radicals trapped in inclusion crystals have been reported, the emphasis being more on radical identification than on anisotropic motion (see, for example, Lai et al., 1970, and references contained therein). The first report of anisotropic motion of a nitroxide was made by Falle and coworkers in 1966. These authors examined two dinitroxide free radicals aligned in the liquid-crystalline phase of p-azoxyanisole. The field has developed rapidly and there is additional work on nitroxides in liquid crystals (Ferruti et al., 1969; Corvaja et al., 1970), studies of phospholipid vesicles (Hubbell and McConnell, 1969a, b) and of oriented lipids (Libertini et al., 1969; Seelig, 1970; Hsia et al., 1970a; Butler et al., 1970; and Jost et al., 1971b).

Anisotropic rotation about one molecular axis (R) combined with motion in other directions can lead to complex line shape analyses beyond the scope of this methods article. However, there are limiting cases of interest. For example, if the only motion is rapid rotational movement about R, an axis of symmetry is introduced. The problem is particularly simple when R is parallel to one of the three principal molecular axes, x, y, or z. In this case the observed coupling constant is simply an average of the principal values involved. For example, if R is parallel to the y molecular axis, then $A_{\parallel} = A_{yy}$ and $A_{\perp} = (1/2)(A_{xx} + A_{zz})$, where $A_{\parallel}$ and $A_{\perp}$ are the coupling constants observed with $H \parallel R$ and $H \perp R$, respectively (the g value is treated in a similar fashion). The coupling constant A at an arbitrary orientation of H can be estimated from the axially symmetric expression $A = A_{\parallel}$

---

[1] $|A_{zz} - A_{xx}| = (32.9 \mathrm{\ G} - 5.9 \mathrm{\ G}) 2.8 \mathrm{\ MHz/G} = 75 \mathrm{\ MHz} = 7.5 \times 10^{7} \mathrm{\ sec}^{-1}$, and $|g_{xx} - g_{zz}| \beta H h^{-1} = (2.0088 - 2.0027) (0.927 \times 10^{-20} \mathrm{\ erg/G}) (3400 \mathrm{\ G}/6.62 \times 10^{-27} \mathrm{\ erg\ sec}) = 2.9 \times 10^{7} \mathrm{\ sec}^{-1}$. The inequalities are only approximations. To be more accurate, it is the maximum shift in the line positions that is important. For the high and low field lines, the shifts represent sums or differences in the A and g anisotropies (see Figure 3).

$\cos^2\theta_1 + A_\perp \sin^2\theta_1$, where θ_1 is the angle between H and R. As a specific example, the familiar carboxylic acid radical (R-ĊHCO$_2$H) is known to have an α-proton tensor with principal values $A_{xx} = 21$ G, $A_{yy} = 32$ G, and $A_{zz} = 10$ G, where x is parallel to the carbon $2p$ orbital associated with the unpaired electron, z is along the C-H bond, and y is very nearly parallel to the long axis of the extended aliphatic chain (McConnell et al., 1960; Pooley and Whiffen, 1961). When radicals of this type are trapped in urea inclusion crystals, the long axes are aligned in the tubular cavities formed by the host. Defining $A_{||}$ and $A_\perp$ to be the coupling constants observed with H parallel and perpendicular, respectively, to the direction of the tubular cavities (the crystalline needle axis), the measured values are $A_{||} = 29.2$ G and $A_\perp = 15.1$ G (Griffith, 1964). Since $R||y$, the predicted values are $A_{||} = A_{yy} = 32$ G, and $A_\perp = (1/2)(21 + 10) = 15.5$G, in surprisingly good agreement with the experimental results. The small differences may be caused by a slight angle of tilt of the molecular y axis or small amplitude out-of-plane motion. It is clear that the hydrocarbon radicals execute large amplitude motion about an axis R and this motion averages out all anisotropy in the plane perpendicular to R. The result is an apparent (rotational) axis of symmetry that disappears at very low temperatures when the motion about R is slow or nonexistent. At room temperature, however, R is a well-defined axis, and spectra at all orientations can be interpreted using axially symmetric relations similar to equations (4) and (5).

Anisotropic motion of nitroxide free radicals has not yet been studied in a system as well ordered as an inclusion crystal. The preferred axis of rotation R will be, in general, parallel to the long axis of the spin label. The effect on the ESR spectra depends on the relationship between the nitroxide x, y, and z axes and the axis R. This can frequently be determined from molecular models. For example, if the fatty-acid spin label LXVIII were rotating about its long axis (i.e., as in an inclusion compound), $z||R$, so that $A_{||} = A_{zz} = 32.9$ G, $A_\perp = (1/2)(A_{xx} + A_{yy}) = (1/2)(5.9 + 5.4) = 5.6$ G, $g_{||} = 2.0022$, and $g_\perp = (1/2)(g_{xx} + g_{yy}) = (1/2)(2.0088 + 2.0058) = 2.0073$. In contrast, the z axis of the steroid spin label LXI is nearly perpendicular to R, so that $A_{||} \sim 5$ to 6 G, and $A_\perp = (1/2)(5.6 + 32.9) = 19.2$ G. (The exact relationship between x, y, and R depends on the disastereoisomer of LXI present and is not important to the present discussion.) Each of these labels has advantages. The only effect of motion about the long axis of the fatty acid spin label is to average the g tensor (since $A_{xx} \sim A_{yy}$). In general, spectra of the steroid label LXI reflect motion about R, whereas spectra of the fatty acid labels, such as LXVII, are more sensitive to motion of the axis R itself.

The preferential axis of rotation (R) may or may not be parallel to one of the principal axes, x, y, or z. Two more general relations are $A_{||} = A_{xx}\sin^2\beta + A_{zz}\cos^2\beta$, and $A_\perp = (1/2)A_{xx}(1 + \cos^2\beta) + (1/2)A_{zz}\sin^2\beta$, where β is the angle between R and A_{zz} (Hubbell and McConnell, 1969a; Seelig, 1970). The first equation follows from equation (4) by inspection. The second relation is obtained from the first, using the identity $A_{xx} + A_{yy} + A_{zz} = 2A_\perp + A_{||}$ (i.e., the trace of the tensor is invariant). For a discussion of this approach and anisotropic motion see McConnell and McFarland (1970). Other simple models are being used. For example,

Libertini et al. (1969) considered a distribution of orientations (and an angle of tilt), and Jost et al. (1971b) interpreted ESR data in terms of a model in which $R \parallel z$, but the axis of rotation is allowed to execute a rapid random walk within a cone defined by an angle γ. In the latter example, the resulting equations give $A_{\parallel}$ and $A_{\perp}$ as functions of γ, A_{zz}, and A_{xx}. There are two reasons why these various simple equations are useful. First, $A_{\parallel}$ and $A_{\perp}$ are generally measured from ESR spectra, and the equations allow a parameter with some physical significance to be extracted from the experimental data. Secondly, computer programs that calculate ESR spectra based on random orientations of rigid nitroxides or on a Gaussian distribution of orientations are available. These programs yield remarkably good computer simulations of anisotropic motion providing the proper $A_{\parallel}$, $A_{\perp}$ and g parameters are chosen (for example, see Figure 17). The simple expressions above provide a rational method of varying the parameters. A word of caution is in order here. All of the simple expressions derived thus far are limited by the simplicity of the assumption used. The membrane model systems such as phospholipid multilayers and vesicles are complex. Distributions of motion and environments undoubtedly occur, and it is unwise to place too heavy an emphasis on the precise value of the angular parameters obtained until more exact mathematical treatments have been made. A review of some approaches to understanding anisotropic rotational diffusion as well as isotropic motion is given by Hudson and Luckhurst (1969).

Solvent Effects

The solvent effects on the ESR spectrum are characterized by changes in the A_0 and g_0 parameters. Di-t-butyl nitroxide (DTBN) in water, for example, yields $A_0 = 16.7$ G and $g_0 = 2.0056$, whereas DTBN in hexane is characterized by $A_0 = 14.8$ G and $g_0 = 2.0061$ (Kawamura et al., 1967). In general, A_0 decreases and g_0 increases as the solvent polarity is decreased. These changes can be a nuisance or a valuable asset depending on the spin labeling experiment. In line shape studies of moderately immobilized spin labels, the solvent dependence is troublesome because it is difficult to estimate the effects on principal values of the A and g tensors. However, when small, rapidly tumbling spin labels are used, the solvent effects can be exploited in much the same way as with optical reporter groups. It is important to keep in mind that A_0 is the distance between lines and the g_0 value determines the center of the spectrum. Increasing or decreasing A_0 will expand or contract the pattern without changing the position of the center line and, similarly, increasing or decreasing the g_0 value will shift the entire three-line spectrum to lower or higher fields respectively without altering the distance between lines (ignoring small second order effects). An unknown g value can be obtained directly from equation (3) if ν and H are accurately determined. However, it is common practice to measure g relative to a known reference ESR line. From equation (3), $h\nu = g_1\beta H_1$, and $h\nu = g_2\beta H_2$, where subscripts 1 and 2 refer to the reference and unknown, respectively. Since the microwave frequency is constant it follows that

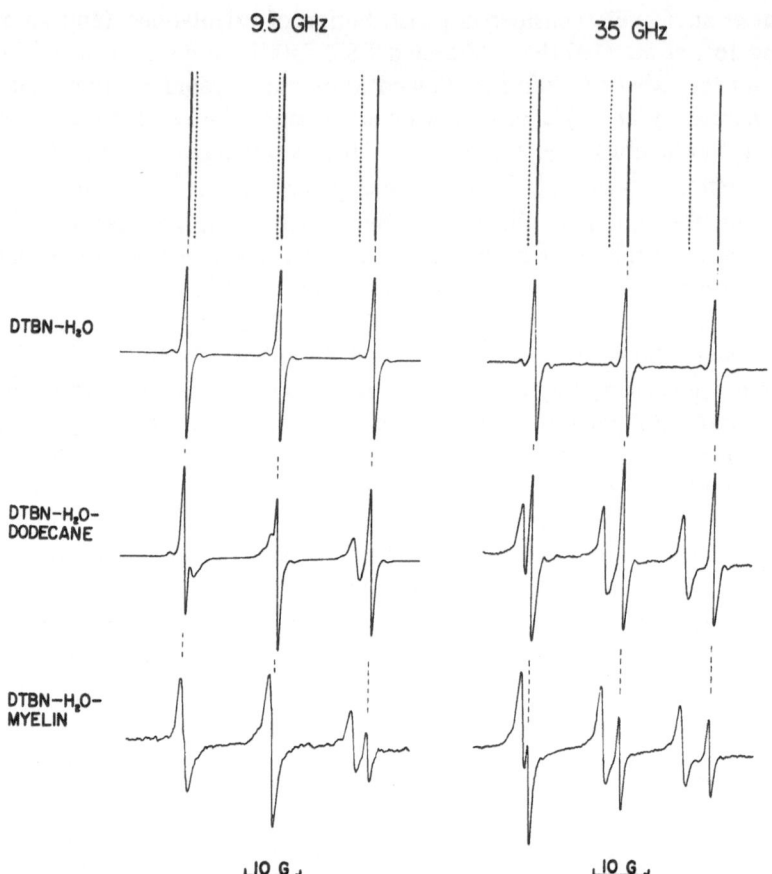

FIG. 5. Solvent effects on 9.5 and 35 GHz ESR spectra of di-*t*-butyl nitroxide (DTBN, XXI) at room temperature. Top row: the relative ESR line positions of DTBN in water (solid lines) and dodecane (dotted lines). Second row: the ESR spectra of DTBN in water. Third row: ESR spectra of DTBN in water and in degassed dodecane, using separate capillary samples (since the capillaries were undoubtedly not inserted equal distances into the cavity, the relative peak heights are not significant). Bottom row: spectra of DTBN partitioning between phases in an aqueous suspension of a crude myelin preparation from beef brain. All spectra are aligned using the aqueous DTBN signals as a reference.

$g_2 H_2 = g_1 H_1$. Defining $\Delta H_{21} = H_2 - H_1$ and substituting into the previous expression for H_1 yields the well-known expression

$$g_2 = g_1 \left(1 - \frac{\Delta H_{21}}{H_2}\right) \tag{7}$$

A typical application involves the top spectrum of Figure 3. Here $\Delta H_{21} = 1.5$ G, $g_1 = 2.0036$, $H_2 \sim 3,400$ G. Using these values in equation (7), $g_2 = 2.0027$.

An interesting situation occurs when a rapidly tumbling spin label exists in two environments of different polarity. Hubbell and McConnell (1968) found when nitroxide VII is diffused into aqueous phospholipid dispersions or a rabbit vagus nerve fiber in Ringer's solution, the high-field line of the normal three line 9.5 GHz ESR spectrum is replaced by two lines. The relative intensities of the two lines provide a measure of the amount of spin label in the hydrocarbon and aqueous environments. It would be very useful if the nitroxide A_0 and g_0 values were available to characterize the hydrocarbon regions. However, the A_0 and g_0 parameters cannot be measured if only one of the three lines is resolved. Griffith et al. (1971) recently found that complete resolution can be obtained at 35 GHz. Some results for DTBN (XXI) are illustrated in Figure 5. In these spectra the three lines of DTBN in water serve as a useful reference. To interpret these data quantitatively it is convenient to define $\Delta g_{21} = g_2 - g_1$ and substitute for g_2 in equation (7). The result is $\Delta H_{21} = - (H_2/g_1) \Delta g_{21}$ or simply (with $g_1 \sim 2$ and $H_2 = H$)

$$\Delta H_{21} = - \left(\frac{H}{2}\right) \Delta g_{21} \tag{8}$$

The shift in the center line position yields ΔH_{21} and hence the unknown g_2. The distance from the center line to either outside line gives A_0 directly and the position of the third line serves as a check. DTBN A_0 and g_0 values in dodecane measured from the appropriate spectrum in the right hand column of Figure 5 are $A_0 = 14.8$ G and $g_0 = 2.0061$. In the crude beef brain myelin preparation, $A_0 = 14.6$ G and $g_0 = 2.0061$. As judged by these criteria, the spin label diffused into myelin is in a remarkably hydrocarbon-like environment. It will be interesting to examine proposed models of drug binding in terms of possible shifts in A_0 and g_0 parameters.

Nitroxide-Nitroxide Interactions in Dinitroxides

Linking together two nitroxide free radicals adds a new dimension to spin labeling experiments. Dinitroxides such as L-LVI, in which a single molecule contains two nitroxide moieties, provide a means of sensing the relative positions of the two labels even when the specimen is not oriented. The interactions between the two nitroxides result from two terms, the electron-electron exchange Hamiltonian ($\hat{\mathcal{H}}_E$) and the electron-electron dipole interaction ($\hat{\mathcal{H}}_D$).

$$\hat{\mathcal{H}}_E = J\, \hat{\mathbf{S}}_1 \cdot \hat{\mathbf{S}}_2 \tag{9}$$

and

$$\hat{\mathcal{H}}_D = \frac{g^2 \beta^2}{r_{12}^3} \left\{ \hat{\mathbf{S}}_1 \hat{\mathbf{S}}_2 - \frac{3\,(\hat{\mathbf{S}}_1 \cdot \mathbf{r}_{12})\,(\hat{\mathbf{S}}_2 \cdot \mathbf{r}_{12})}{r_{12}^2} \right\} \tag{10}$$

where J is the exchange integral $\hat{\mathbf{S}}_1$ and $\hat{\mathbf{S}}_2$ are spin operators of electrons 1 and 2, and r_{12} is the vector joining the two electrons. $\hat{\mathcal{H}}_E$ arises from electrostatic inter-

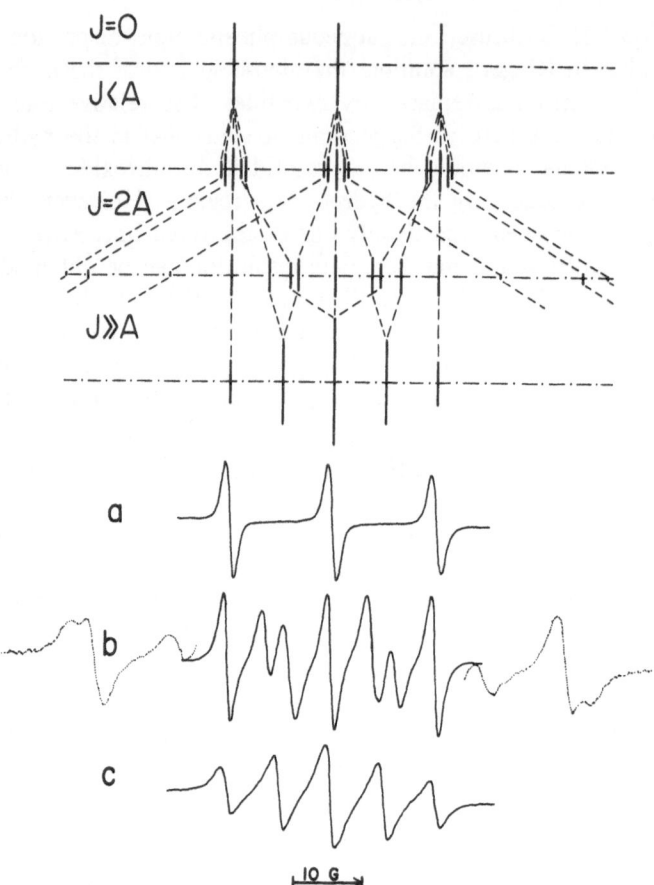

FIG. 6. *Top.* Calculated line positions of nitroxide biradicals as a function of the relative magnitudes of J and A. *Bottom.* Experimental ESR spectra of various nitroxide biradicals. Spectra *a*,
b, and *c* were recorded for dilute solutions of LIII, LII, and LI, respectively, in diethyl formamide
at room temperature. The dotted outermost lines of *b* have been amplified by increasing the
spectrometer gain. (From Brière, et al. 1965a. *Bull. Soc. Chim. France*, p. 3290. Courtesy of
the authors and the Societe Chimique de France.)

actions and does not depend on the orientation of the dinitroxide with respect to
the external magnetic field. Like all magnetic dipole terms, $\hat{\mathcal{H}}_D$ is anisotropic, and
the effects of $\hat{\mathcal{H}}_D$ will be average to zero when the dinitroxide tumbling frequency
is large compared to the maximum anisotropy. This is normally the case in solutions of low viscosity at room temperature[1]. Typical spectra are shown in Figure
6. The total Hamiltonian includes the electron Zeeman term, the electron-nuclear
term of equation (2) (now $\hat{\mathbf{S}} = \hat{\mathbf{S}}_1 + \hat{\mathbf{S}}_2$ and $\hat{\mathbf{I}} = \hat{\mathbf{I}}_1 + \hat{\mathbf{I}}_2$), and $\hat{\mathcal{H}}_E$. The appearance
of the spectrum depends on the relative magnitudes of A_0 and J. Clearly, if the two

[1] Occasionally, a dinitroxide may be encountered where the dipolar interactions are too large
to be averaged out by molecular motion in solution. Severe line broadening could result, making the spin label difficult to observe at room temperature.

nitroxides are far apart and $J \ll A_0$, the dinitroxide behaves as two independent spin labels. In this case the familiar three-line spectrum is observed (Figure 6a). As the two nitroxide moieties are brought closer together, J will eventually become much larger than A_0 and the spectrum will consist of $2nI + 1 = 2(2)1 + 1 = 5$ lines with relative intensities of $1:2:3:2:1$, separated by $A_0/2$ gauss, as shown in Figure 6c. (Notice that for a large cluster of nitroxides, say 1,000 monomers, the result is $2(10^31 + 1 = 2,001$ lines of varying intensities, each separated by only $A_0/1,000$ gauss. The individual lines would not be resolved and the result is one "exchange-narrowed" line. This effect occurs at high concentrations of spin labels and is illustrated in Figure 15.

Between the two limits of $J \ll A_0$ and $J \gg A_0$ the spectrum of a dinitroxide can consist of from three to fifteen lines, three of which remain at fixed positions as shown in the upper part of Figure 6. The ratio J/A_0, and hence J, can be calculated from the relative line positions. For example in spectrum b of Figure 6, the positions of the dotted lines relative to the three invariant lines can be used to calculate $J/A_0 = 1.85$ (Brière et al., 1965a; see also Glarum and Marshall, 1967: Ohnishi et al., 1970; Luckhurst and Pedulli, 1970). The coupling constant $A_0 = 15.6$ G is easily measured from the three invariant lines, yielding $J = 15.6$ G$\times 1.85 = 28.9$ G for spectrum b. However, it is not possible at present to relate J quantitatively to molecular geometry. The exchange interaction may be transmitted through intervening chemical bonds or by direct overlap of the orbitals containing the unpaired spins; thus the calculation of J as a function of distance is not a simple task. Nevertheless, the fact that a spectrum can exhibit three lines or five to fifteen lines, depending on the structure or conformation of the molecule, renders J an important parameter in spin labeling experiments.

The electron-electron dipole interaction is of particular value when the sample is either partially oriented or when molecular motion is essentially absent. $\hat{\mathcal{H}}_D$ is usually rewritten in the form

$$\hat{\mathcal{H}}_D = D\,(\hat{\mathbf{S}}_z^2 - \tfrac{1}{3}\hat{\mathbf{S}}^2) + E\,(\hat{\mathbf{S}}_x^2 - \hat{\mathbf{S}}_y^2) \tag{11}$$

where $\hat{\mathbf{S}}_x$, $\hat{\mathbf{S}}_y$, and $\hat{\mathbf{S}}_z$ are the components of the total spin operator $\hat{\mathbf{S}}$, and D and E are experimental parameters (Carrington and McLachlan, 1967). Ignoring temporarily the electron-nuclear interaction, the effect of equation (11) is to split the electron Zeeman line into a doublet ($\Delta m = \pm 1$ transitions) and to introduce a weak third line ($\Delta m = 2$ transition) at approximately one half the normal magnetic field setting. The form of the equations needed to measure D and E from these lines depends on whether the dipole interaction is much stronger or weaker than the electron Zeeman interaction. Useful expressions have been derived in classical papers on triplet states (see Hutchinson and Mangum, 1961, and Chestnut and Phillips, 1961, for the two extremes of large and small D and E values, respectively). If, as is usually the case, the dipolar splitting is a few hundred gauss or less, then an oriented sample will exhibit measurable doublet separations of $2D$, $D + 3E$, and $D - 3E$ along the principal z, x, and y axes, respectively. In practice $2D$ is frequently set equal to the largest splitting and this defines the z axis of the dinitroxide. The quantity $2D$ is directly related to the distance between the unpaired spins. If the two spins are assumed to be at two points separated by the distance r_{12}, then $2D/g\beta = 3g\beta/r_{12}^3 = 5.56 \times 10^4/r_{12}^3$ where r_{12} is in Å, $g = 2.00$, and $2D/g\beta$ is simply the maximum splitting in gauss. For example, unpaired spins separated by 4, 6, 8, 10, or 12 Å would yield 869, 258, 109, 56, or 32 G maximum splittings, respectively (for applications see Hirota and Weissman, 1964; Falle et al., 1966).

Reintroducing the electron-nuclear interaction at this point is straightforward. If $J \gg A_0$ and $2D/g\beta = 100$ G, then two five-line patterns with relative intensities of $1:2:3:2:1$ and exactly 100 G apart would be observed when the magnetic field is directed along the molecular z axis. Spectra of this general type have been observed from two molecules of di-t-butyl nitroxide XXI trapped in adjacent lattice sites of host crystals (L. J. Libertini and O. H. Griffith, work in progress). The unpaired spins are not, of course, point dipoles, and accurate calculations must take into account the distribution of unpaired spin density over the two N-O groups. Additional complications arise when dealing with randomly oriented samples. Triplet state ESR is a well-developed field, however, and these problems have largely been solved (see Carrington and McLachlan, 1967, Chap. 8, and Bersohn and Baird, 1966, Chap. 8, and references cited by these authors).

Thus, spin labeling with dinitroxides introduces more variables but provides new information regarding local geometry. The use of dinitroxides will increase, particularly in experiments where the spin labels tumble rapidly, when the labels are partially oriented, or where it is possible to freeze the sample to remove complications arising from intermediate or slow molecular motion.

TECHNICAL ASPECTS OF ESR

ESR Instrumentation and Instrumental Artifacts

ESR SPECTROMETERS. A number of books are available which describe the design, construction, and sensitivity of ESR spectrometers (Ayscough, 1967; Poole, 1967; Alger, 1968; Wilmhurst, 1968). These are useful to the expert in the field but most potential users have a commercial ESR spectrometer available and must use it as it is. Our aim here is to provide the nonexpert with background to help him use the ESR spectrometer as a black box. Particular emphasis is placed on instrument settings since most operator errors are made here. Any comparison between the many commercial spectrometers is purposely avoided because the various spectrometers are constantly being upgraded and because the authors have not made a careful comparison of the various instruments available. All spectra displayed in this chapter were recorded on Varian ESR spectrometers, most of them on a Varian E-3.

A schematic diagram of a simple ESR spectrometer is shown in Figure 7. The basic parts are the klystron, magic tee, cavity, detector-amplifier combination, and a recording device. The klystron, in conjunction with the fixed isolator and adjustable attenuator, provides the operator with a variable source of microwave energy.

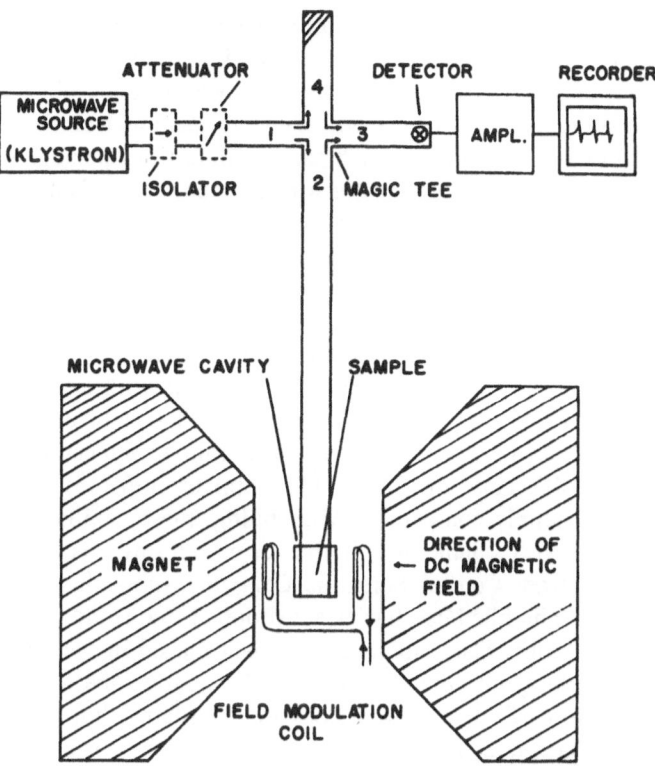

FIG. 7. A block diagram of a simple ESR spectrometer showing the essential components.

The magic tee is the microwave equivalent of the familiar Wheatstone bridge. The spectrometer is constructed so that the impedances of arms 2 and 4 are nearly matched and very little power reaches the detector on arm 3. The sample is situated in the microwave cavity, a region of high microwave field, H_1. The klystron frequency is fixed during the experiment and the magnetic field is scanned. As the resonance condition is approached, the sample absorbs microwave energy, creating an imbalance in the bridge. This imbalance is detected as increased power in arm 3 and is amplified and displayed on a recorder. The modulation coils also play an important role. They are needed in the conversion of the DC signal to an AC voltage, which can then be easily amplified using the powerful methods of phase sensitive detection. The modulation coils are frequently imbedded in plastic and fastened to the sides of the microwave cavity, out of sight of the operator. The use of modulation causes the spectra to appear as a first derivative of the microwave absorption, and provides the operator with one more control which must be adjusted properly, the modulation amplitude control.

THE MICROWAVE CAVITY AND THE SAMPLE. The cavity and sample are of special importance. Many cavity designs are available including rectangular cavities, cylindrical cavities, and special slow-wave structures. Rectangular cavities are the most common type at present and all spectra presented here were recorded using a standard Varian rectangular cavity. However, any high quality (high Q) cavity can be used in spin labeling studies. The user should be aware of which type of cavity is available to him since this determines the geometry of the sample holder. A typical cavity will have an opening 1 cm in diameter, but the actual liquid or solid sample is much smaller than this opening. As one might expect, the optimum sample geometry for a rectangular cavity is a flat rectangular cell and the best geometry for a cylindrical cavity is a cylindrical sample tube. More care must be exercised when dealing with aqueous samples than organic materials because the dielectric loss of water tends to lower the spectrometer sensitivity by lowering the cavity Q. Commercial quartz flat aqueous sample cells have approximate dimensions 6 cm×1 cm×0.3 mm ID. These useful cells are equipped with stoppered ports at the top and the bottom. When dealing with moderate concentrations of spin label, 10^{-3} M to 10^{-6} M, less expensive cells may be used. For example, the aqueous samples may be drawn into 0.4 mm ID thin-walled capillary tubes made of ordinary flint (soft) glass or Pyrex. The capillary tubes are available from standard laboratory supply companies. After filling, these capillary tubes may be sealed at the dry end with a flame or at both ends with a soft wax such as Universal Red Wax available from Central Scientific Company (note that some nitroxides are soluble in wax). The filled capillaries are dropped into standard 2 to 4 mm ID quartz ESR sample tubes. The combination is then placed in the cavity. After the experiment the capillary tube is discarded and the quartz tube is ready for reuse. The quartz tubes are easily made from stock quartz tubing, but special care must be taken since standard quartz tubing frequently has an intrinsic ESR signal. It is more convenient to avoid this problem by purchasing the quartz ESR sample tubes.

Dry tissues, powders, hydrocarbon solvents, and other samples that do not contain water are less troublesome. Large diameter flint glass or Pyrex capillaries make useful sample tubes. Disposable pipettes sealed at the small end make inexpensive tubes that are easy to degas. Of course, the quartz flat cells and ESR sample tubes may be used with organic samples as well as aqueous samples.

Many special sample holders have been constructed. These range from a simple glass cover slip used to support phospholipid multilayers, to the complex arrangement shown in Figure 8. The sample holder of Figure 8 was designed to permit simultaneous nerve excitation and ESR signal recording. Note that the sample itself (the lobster nerve) is quite small and most of the supporting structure is made of thin plastic and other dielectric materials. With reasonable care, electrodes and other small objects may be placed in the cavity. The presence of moderate quantities of metal can drastically alter the characteristics of the microwave cavity.

RECEIVER GAIN, FIELD MODULATION AMPLITUDE, AND MICROWAVE POWER. The gain, modulation amplitude, and microwave power controls are grouped together because they strongly influence the signal amplitude. If any or all three of these controls are set at zero, no signal will be observed. As each variable is increased, the signal amplitude increases, passes through an optimal range, and then either decreases or becomes distorted. The optimal range will depend on the sample and, to a lesser extent, on the ESR spectrometer. The receiver gain needs no elaboration since this control is encountered in all chemical

NERVE CHAMBER FOR STIMULATING AND RECORDING
THE ACTION POTENTIAL IN THE ESR CAVITY

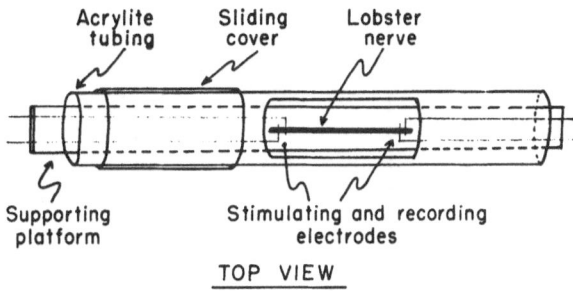

TOP VIEW

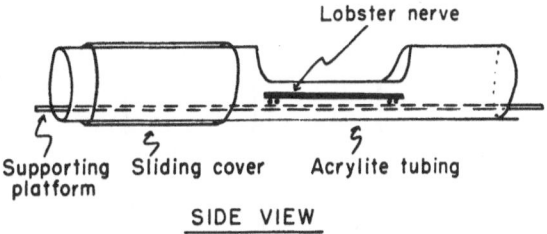

SIDE VIEW

FIG. 8. One example of a specialized ESR sample cell. This sample configuration permits the observation of spin labeled nerves during nerve stimulation. (From Calvin et al. 1969. *Proc. Nat. Acad. Sci. U.S.A.*, *63:1*. Courtesy of the authors and the National Academy of Sciences.)

instruments. The receiver gain (also called amplifier gain or signal level control) may be increased until the amplifier becomes unstable and the signal-to-noise ratio decreases. The effect of modulation amplitude is more dramatic, as illustrated in Figure 9. As the modulation amplitude increases, the ESR lines first increase in height, then broaden and finally become greatly distorted. A useful rule-of-thumb is to set the modulation amplitude equal to or less than the ESR line width in gauss. In Figure 9 the peak-to-peak line width is ∼0.5-1.0 G. As seen in Figure 9, the best choice for the modulation amplitude is also 0.5 G. (For convenience, spectra for this chapter were usually recorded at 1.0 G modulation amplitude. For very accurate line shape studies slightly lower settings may be optimal.) A word of caution is needed here. This rule-of-thumb and other generalizations mentioned in this chapter can be misused. If careful line shape measurements are being made, the investigator should always decrease the modulation amplitude (or other instrument setting) and determine if this has an effect on the line shape. Only if the change in line shape or relative peak heights is insignificant can the setting be considered correct.

The effects of microwave power on nitroxide ESR spectra have not been carefully investigated. In any system, relaxation processes are present that allow the spins to return to the ground state after absorption of microwave energy. If the power becomes too large, however, the relaxation processes are unable to return the spin system to equilibrium, and saturation takes place. The power required to saturate depends on the spin lattice relaxation time. Saturation and relaxation

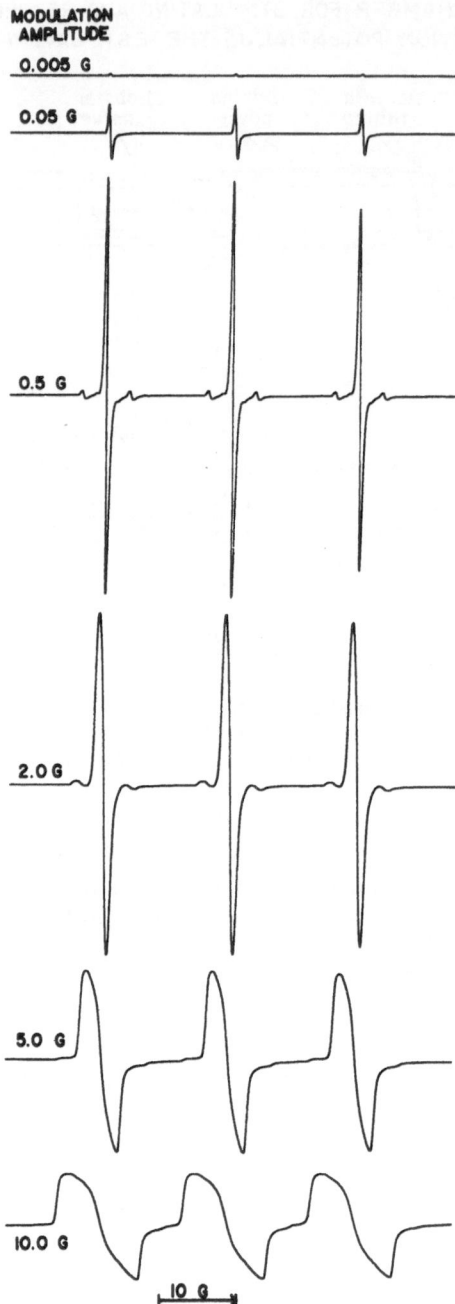

MODULATION
AMPLITUDE

0.005 G

0.05 G

0.5 G

2.0 G

5.0 G

10.0 G

10 G

FIG. 9. The ESR spectrum of a typical nitroxide as a function of field modulation amplitude. The sample is an aqueous solution containing 5×10^{-4} M ketone nitroxide IV at room temperature. The microwave power, scan time, scan range, and filter time constant are 5 mW, 4 min, 100 G, and 0.3 sec, respectively.

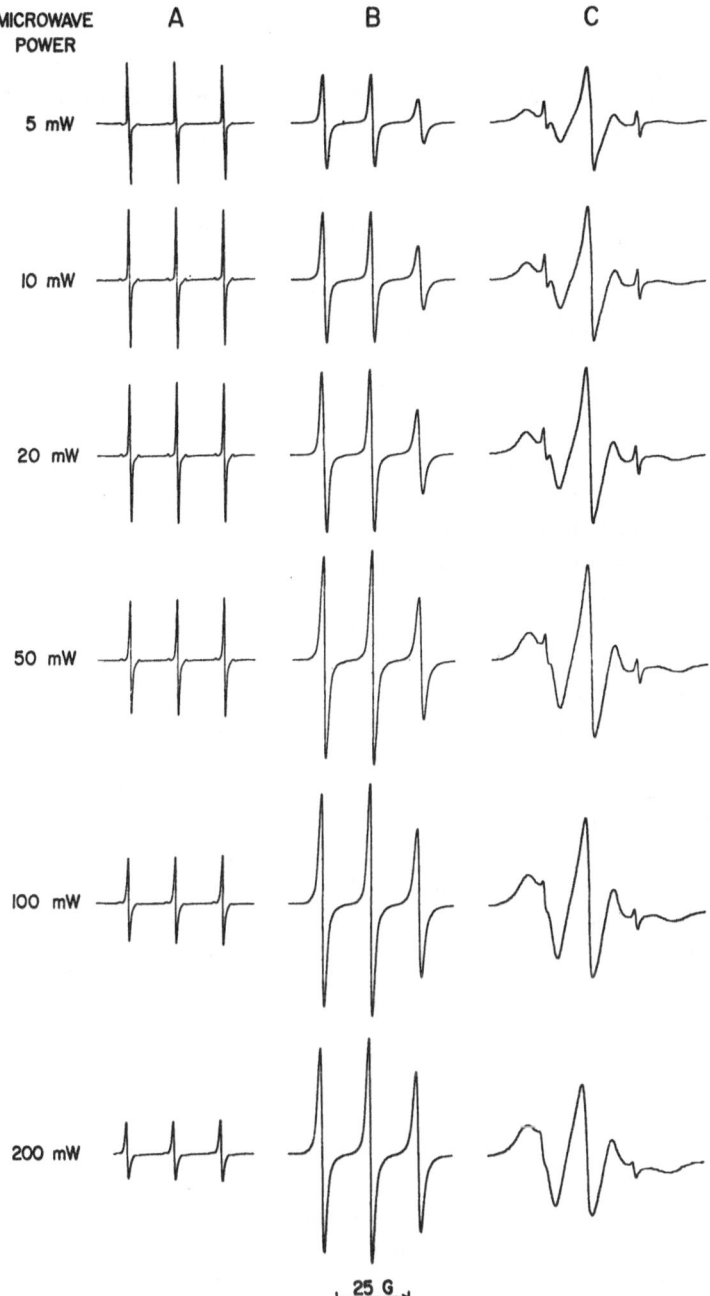

MICROWAVE POWER   A   B   C

5 mW

10 mW

20 mW

50 mW

100 mW

200 mW

25 G

FIG. 10. The effects of increasing the microwave power on the ESR spectra of nitroxides in different environments at 18°C. The spectra in the left column were recorded for 10^{-4} M ketone nitroxide IV in water. The center column is for 10^{-4} M lauryl nitroxide LXXV in 5% aqueous sodium dodecyl sulphate. The spectra on the right are of an aqueous dispersion containing 1.5×10^{-3} M 12-doxylstearic acid LXVIII and 20 wt % egg lecithin in water (pH=7). The temperature was stabilized using a commercial gas flow temperature regulator to avoid possible effects of microwave heating at high power levels. The modulation amplitude, scan time, scan range, and filter time constant for all spectra are 1 G, 4 min, 100 G, and 0.3 sec, respectively.

effects will play an important role in future spin labeling experiments involving electron-nuclear and electron-electron double resonance. In most conventional ESR studies, however, saturation should be avoided. It is difficult to determine precisely the point at which saturation becomes significant. One test involves measuring the signal height as a function of the microwave power. Below saturation, the amplitude of the signal varies linearly with the power. As saturation sets in, the amplitude increases at a lower rate and eventually either flattens out or decreases as the power is increased. Some effects of saturation are illustrated in Figure 10. The left and the center columns represent nitroxides at room temperature in water and in an aqueous sodium dodecyl sulfate solution, respectively. The relative peak heights change with increasing microwave power. Rotational correlation times are calculated from peak heights (or line shapes) and will be in error if saturation occurs. The right column of Figure 10 illustrates another possible pitfall. These spectra were recorded for a nitroxide stearic acid in an aqueous phospholipid dispersion. The pH of the solution was adjusted so that the nitroxide is present in both the aqueous phase (sharp lines) and in the phospholipid vesicles (broad lines). As the microwave power is increased, the sharp lines saturate more rapidly than the broad lines. Equilibrium constants based on data at higher powers would underestimate the nitroxide concentration in the aqueous phase. Microwave power of from 1 mW to 5 mW appears to be acceptable for room temperature spin labeling studies. Some saturation may be occurring at these power levels, but the effects evidently are not serious. Once again, the investigator should check his results by decreasing the power and looking for changes in the ESR spectrum.

SCAN TIME, FILTER TIME CONSTANT, AND FIELD INHOMO-GENEITY.   Improper adjustments in these three experimental parameters produce similar line shape distortions. The scan time or sweep time is the time required to vary the DC magnetic field slowly over a specified interval (the scan range). The effect of varying the scan time on a typical nitroxide ESR spectrum with a 100 G scan range is illustrated in the left column of Figure 11. The 4.0 min and 8.0 min scans are almost superimposable, whereas the 0.5 min scan is badly distorted. There is a trade off here between the quality of the spectrum and the amount of time required to record it. In this example a 4.0 min scan appears to be a good choice, but if the spin labeled sample is stable, the investigator may choose the 8.0 min scan time. It is interesting to note that the same effect is evident in the much broader spectrum of a membrane model system (Figure 11, right-hand column). Of course, in both samples the distortion caused by shortening the scan time can also be obtained by increasing the scan range while holding the scan time constant.

Nearly all chemical instruments have filter networks to increase the signal-to-noise ratio, and an ESR spectrometer is no exception. The effect of varying the filter time constant, given a fixed scan time and scan range, is shown in Figure 12. In this example distortion occurs in all but the top spectrum. The rule to follow is that the time constant must be much shorter than the time required to sweep through the ESR line. In this example the scan time was 4 min and the scan range was 100 G. One ESR line covers about 2 G. Therefore it takes about (4/100)

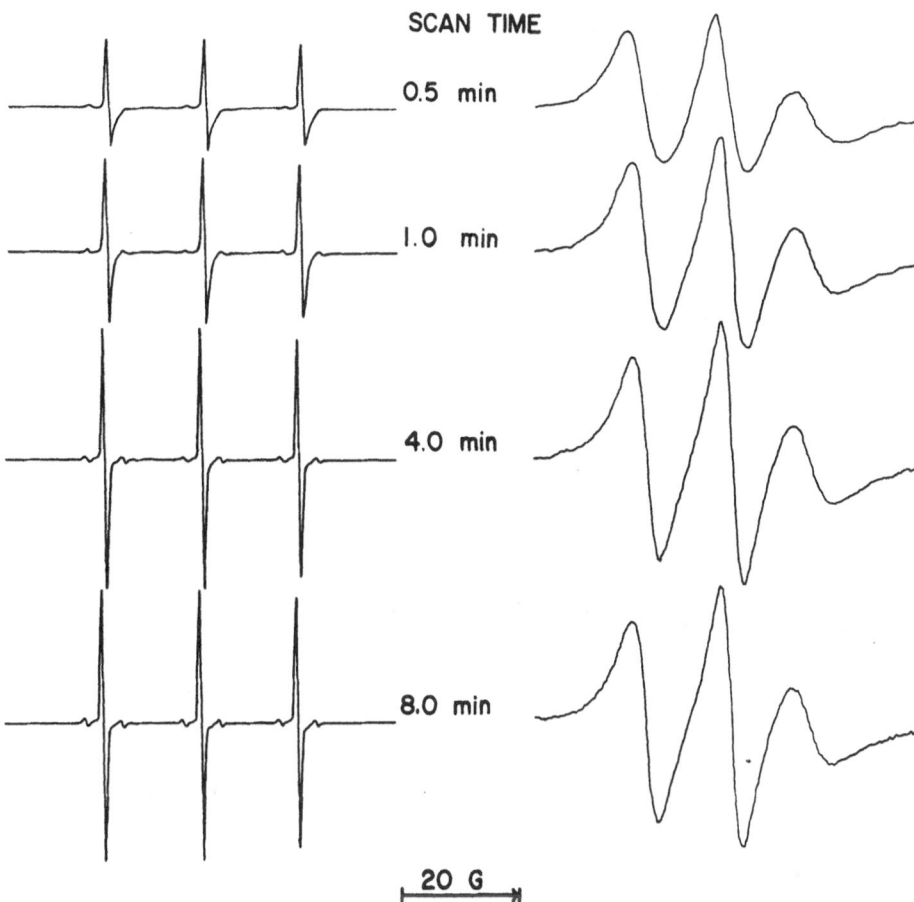

FIG. 11. The dependence of nitroxide ESR on scan time. The spectra in the left column are for 5×10^{-4} M ketone nitroxide IV in water at room temperature. The sample giving rise to the spectra on the right is a room-temperature aqueous dispersion containing 10^{-4} M 12-doxylstearate, methyl ester, and 10 wt % egg lecithin (pH = 7). For all spectra the microwave power, modulation amplitude, scan time, scan range, and filter time constant are 5 mW, 1 G, 4 min, 100 G, and 0.3 sec, respectively. The gain setting is the same for all spectra.

$\times 60 = 2.4$ sec to scan through each ESR line. It is easy to see why the 0.1 sec time constant was the only reasonable choice. To avoid distorted spectra it is good practice to check the time constant, scan time and scan range experimentally. The bottom spectrum of Figure 12 represents a special case of signal distortion. In this example the time constant of the filter network is so large that the line shape approximates the integral of the first derivative curve. This behavior is expected of a simple filter circuit (consider, for example, a resistor in series with a capacitor). However, as discussed below, the digital computer provides a better method of integration.

The distortion caused by field inhomogeneity is illustrated in Figure 13. The inhomogeneity of the DC magnetic field increases from the top spectrum to the

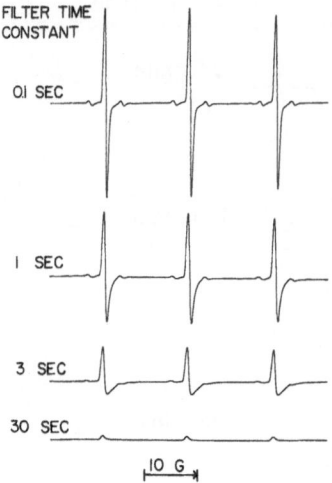

FIG. 12. An example of distortions introduced through improper choice of the time constant. The sample is the same as in the spectra in the left column of Figure 11. The microwave power, modulation amplitude, scan time, and scan range for all spectra are 5 mW, 1 G, 4 min, and 100 G, respectively.

bottom spectrum. The inhomogeneity was created by moving the cavity various distances from the center of the magnet. Field inhomogeneity of this magnitude is not ordinarily observed in commercial 9.5 GHz instruments. In 35 GHz spectrometers, special dual cavity applications, or when using older magnet systems, the

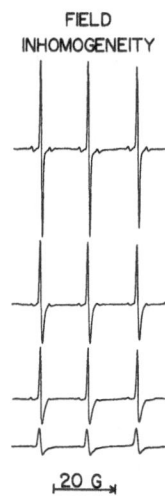

FIG. 13. Nitroxide spectra distorted by an inhomogeneous magnetic field. The sample is 5×10^{-4} M nitroxide IV in water at room temperature. The microwave power, modulation amplitude, scan time, scan range, and filter time constant are 5 mW, 1 G, 4 min, 100 G, and 0.3 sec, respectively. The gain setting is the same for all spectra, and the field inhomogeneity increases from top to bottom.

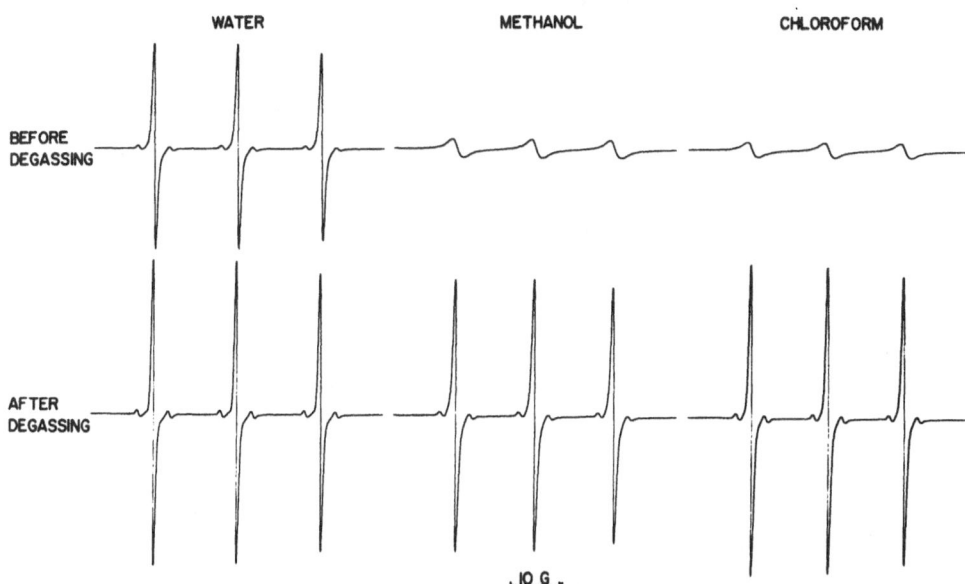

FIG. 14. Effects of oxygen broadening on the ESR spectrum. The spectra in the left, center, and right-hand columns were taken on 10^{-4} M solutions of ketone nitroxide IV in water, methanol, and chloroform, respectively. The top three spectra were recorded on samples equilibrated with the atmosphere. The bottom row of spectra were recorded after nitrogen was bubbled through the solutions at room temperature for 30 sec. The microwave power, modulation amplitude, scan time, scan range, and filter time constant are 5 mW, 1 G, 4 min, 100 G, and 0.3 sec, respectively. All spectra were recorded at room temperature and at the same gain setting. Reversibility was tested by bubbling air through the sample, to verify that concentrations were not altered by the degassing procedure.

problem is common. It can usually be corrected by adjusting the position of the microwave cavity. The reason for including this effect is to point out that the bottom spectrum of Figure 13 is almost identical to the top left spectrum of Figure 11 and the third spectrum of Figure 12. Fortunately, this is one of the few examples of a line distortion that has several possible causes.

DEGASSING AND CONCENTRATION EFFECTS.   Anyone performing spin labeling experiments soon encounters oxygen-nitroxide interactions and nitroxide-nitroxide interactions. The ground state of molecular oxygen is a triplet and oxygen is therefore paramagnetic. It is rarely observed directly by ESR, but oxygen does interact with the spin label through the exchange and dipolar mechanisms mentioned earlier. The result is the well-known oxygen broadening, illustrated in Figure 14. The top three spectra are of the ketone nitroxide IV dissolved in water, methanol, or chloroform at room temperature. Although it is not obvious from the spectra, the three solutions contain approximately equal concentrations of the nitroxide. Considerably more oxygen broadening is observed in methanol and chloroform (and other hydrocarbon solutions) than in aqueous solutions. The oxygen may be removed by either the freeze-thaw method or by bubbling a good grade of nitrogen or argon gas through the samples. The bottom three spectra of Figure 14

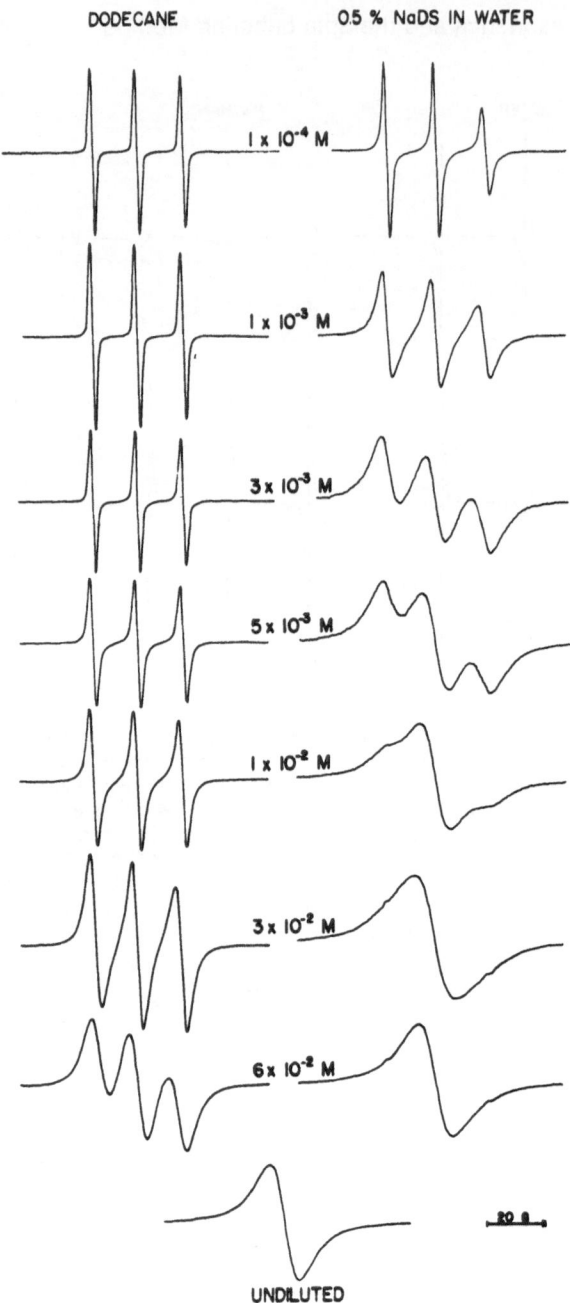

DODECANE   0.5 % NaDS IN WATER

1×10^{-4} M

1×10^{-3} M

3×10^{-3} M

5×10^{-3} M

1×10^{-2} M

3×10^{-2} M

6×10^{-2} M

UNDILUTED

FIG. 15. Concentration effects on nitroxide ESR spectra. The spectra in the left-hand column were recorded on varying concentrations of the long chain nitroxide LXXV in dodecane (degassed) at room temperature. The spectra of the right-hand column were taken using varying concentrations of the same nitroxide in an aqueous solution containing 0.5 wt % sodium dodecyl sulphate at room temperature. The nitroxide concentration is the same for the two spectra in each row and the actual value is written between the two spectra. The microwave power, modulation amplitude, scan time, scan range, and filter time constant for all spectra are 5 mW, 1 G, 4 min, 100 G, and 0.3 sec, respectively, with variable gain settings.

were recorded after nitrogen gas was passed through the solutions for approximately 30 sec. The effects are completely reversible. After passing air through these same samples, the spectra are indistinguishable from the top row of Figure 14.

Nitroxide-nitroxide interactions also occur via the familiar dipolar and exchange mechanisms. Examples of intramolecular nitroxide interactions (e.g., in dinitroxides) were discussed above. Intermolecular nitroxide interactions are also important. The effect of increasing the nitroxide concentration of the long chain nitroxide LXXV in degassed dodecane at room temperature is shown in the left column of Figure 15. The sharp three-line spectrum remains essentially unchanged until the concentration exceeds 10^{-3} M. As the concentration is increased beyond this point, the three lines gradually broaden and move together. At 6×10^{-2} M, the three lines are still evident. The exchange-narrowed, single-line spectrum of the pure nitroxide is shown at the bottom of the figure for comparison.

The values given down the center of Figure 15 represent average concentrations. Local concentrations can exceed these average values, producing unusual results. For example, if the nitroxide were not soluble to the extent of 1×10^{-3} M, solid flakes of nitroxide would be present and a superposition of three sharp lines and a single broad line would result. A more subtle example is given in the right column of Figure 15. In this case the same water-insoluble nitroxide (LXXV) is introduced into an aqueous solution containing small clusters (micelles) of sodium dodecyl sulfate. The equilibrium concentration of nitroxide molecules is very much higher in the micelles than in the aqueous phase. The net result is that the local concentration of nitroxide is much greater than the average bulk concentration, and nitroxide-nitroxide broadening is observed at lower concentrations. At 1×10^{-4} M the spectrum consists of three sharp lines. The heights are unequal due to slower rates of tumbling, but this effect is not of primary concern here. At 1×10^{-3} M all three lines are already greatly broadened. At 5×10^{-3} M, the three lines are disappearing, and the 3×10^{-2} M solution gives a spectrum very similar to that of the pure nitroxide. The point is that it is important to watch for nitroxide-nitroxide interactions even when the average concentration of nitroxide is low. With reasonable care, errors in interpretation can be avoided and nitroxide-nitroxide interactions will provide valuable information about the system under investigation.

The Use of Small Digital Computers in ESR

Small computers appropriate for interfacing with spectrometers are commercially available, and the use of these computers in spin labeling can be very profitable. Many choices are available, but our experience has been only with the Varian 620/i computer, equipped with 8K memory, teletype, and general interface, connected directly to the ESR spectrometer. The computer controls the ESR spectrometer through commands from the teletype, and digitalizes the data as the spectrum is collected. Various data treatments described below can be performed, either as the points are collected or immediately after collection. The data can also be transferred to paper or magnetic tape and re-entered into the computer for later processing.

The best known use of small computers is in time averaging, and was first used in ESR by Klein and Barton (1963). In this application, several approaches are possible, and all improve the signal-to-noise ratio in a very noisy spectrum by repeated scanning. The change in signal-to-noise ratio is proportional to $n^{1/2}$, where n is the number of scans. We have found most useful the procedure of adding successive scans, dividing each point by the number of scans, and instructing the computer to list the number of scans on the teletype. The resulting spectrum can be plotted out at any time during the repeated scans, either on an external recorder or on the spectrometer recorder itself. It is preferable to increase the signal-to-noise ratio by introducing more label or concentrating the sample, but, if this is not feasible, time averaging can be very useful in improving the quality of the spectrum and revealing otherwise inaccessible details.

With ESR spectra reduced to digital form by the small dedicated computer, it is possible to perform a number of operations that are tedious or impossible to perform by hand. Spectral subtraction is one application of the small computer that is useful when heterogeneous samples are encountered in such preparations as aqueous dispersions of macromolecules. The nitroxide probe is frequently partitioned into two environments, tumbling freely in the aqueous phase, but with its motion hindered when it binds to the macromolecules. This gives a complex spectrum arising from equilibrium concentrations of free and bound spin label. A simple example of this can be seen in the upper right-hand spectrum of Figure 10, although in this example the rapidly tumbling free nitroxide is not as prominent a feature of the spectrum as is frequently encountered. Spectral subtraction requires that a spectrum of one component be obtained separately. This is usually very simple to do by making up a sample of the spin label in the appropriate solvent (in this example, water) at any convenient concentration. Both digitalized spectra, the complex spectrum and the spectrum of the freely tumbling spin label, are placed in different memory locations in the computer. If necessary, the spectra can easily be shifted relative to each other, so that the sharp peaks of the free spin label are in register. Then successive increments of the reference spectra are subtracted from the complex spectrum until only the bound signal remains. It is important to realize that the nitroxide concentration present varies as the product of the width squared times the height of the first derivative ESR lines. Thus, if the ESR line width increases by a factor of 10 upon binding, the height of the bound spectrum will be reduced 100-fold, and small concentrations of freely moving spin label can almost obscure a much greater concentration of the bound spin label present.

One of the most useful applications of the small computer in ESR is integration. The ESR spectrum, as recorded, is usually the first derivative of the absorption spectrum. The bottom row of Figure 16 consists of the familiar first derivative ESR spectra, representing examples of three different mobilities of nitroxide spin labels. Integrating once yields the absorption spectra, analogous to the familiar absorption spectra of optical absorption or nuclear magnetic resonance spectroscopy (middle row of Figure 16). A second integration (i.e., integrating the absorption

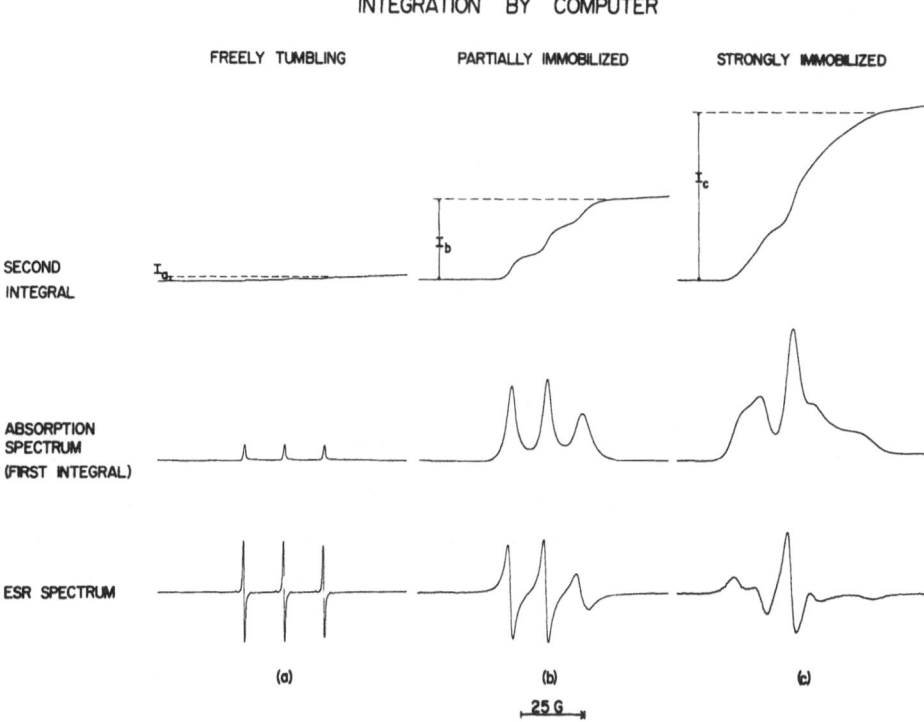

INTEGRATION   BY   COMPUTER

FREELY TUMBLING   PARTIALLY IMMOBILIZED   STRONGLY IMMOBILIZED

SECOND
INTEGRAL

ABSORPTION
SPECTRUM
(FIRST INTEGRAL)

ESR SPECTRUM

(a)   (b)   (c)

25 G

FIG. 16. Integration by small computer. (a) Freely tumbling nitroxide is aqueous sample of ketone nitroxide IV; (b) moderately immobilized nitroxide is 16-doxylstearic acid LXXI in an aqueous dispersion of lecithin; (c) strongly immobilized nitroxide is 5-doxylstearic acid LXIV in an aqueous dispersion of lecithin:cholesterol, molar ratio 2:1. All spectra were recorded at room temperature. $I_a:I_b:I_c=1:19:40$, which represents the relative concentrations of the three nitroxides. The middle lines of all three first derivative ESR spectra are of the same height.

spectrum) has been performed to determine relative concentrations, and the results are shown in the top three spectra of Figure 16. The heights, I_a, I_b, and I_c, are proportional to the concentrations of the probe, and $I_a:I_b:I_c$ is approximately $1:19:40$. For purposes of illustration, the middle line of each of the three first derivative spectra (Figure 16a, b, c) has been arbitrarily adjusted to the same height before integration. When this height is held constant, the relationship between ESR line width and concentration is dramatically evident. A small concentration of freely tumbling nitroxide has a relatively large first derivative peak height. It can be readily seen from Figure 16 that quite a low concentration of unbound spin label in the presence of bound label may dominate the composite spectrum obtained. Combinations of spectral subtraction and subsequent double integration can be used to determine equilibrium constants.

If a computer is not available, concentrations of "bound" nitroxide can sometimes be determined by assuming that the bound signal contributes very little to the
height of the free signal in the composite spectrum. The best choice is usually the
height of the high field line. Thus, as a protein is added, the height of the free
signal will diminish in proportion to the amount that is bound. An interesting use
of this approach was made by Weiner (1969) and is briefly discussed in the next
section.

We have found other useful applications of the small computer. For example,
small successive changes in the position of an oriented sample with respect to the
magnetic field causes changes in the positions and relative magnitudes of the peaks.
The computer can be asked to find the minima and maxima in the spectrum and to
print out on the teletype the positions and relative intensities of each line. Then, in
one of the programs we use, the computer integrates once and prints out the position and relative intensities of the peaks of the ESR absorption spectrum. The positions of these latter peaks correspond to the points at which the first derivative line
crosses the baseline; therefore, the distance in gauss between these peaks is the
experimental coupling constant, A. Although all of these values (the line heights,
widths, and positions) can be measured directly by hand, the computer removes
the tedious aspects when some parameter such as orientation or temperature is
being varied systematically and when many spectra must be analyzed.

The ease with which digitalized spectra can be plotted back, adjusting both the
vertical and horizontal dimensions, makes comparison between spectra much easier.
For example, experimental spectra a and b in Figure 17 (see page 260) have been
replotted to match the horizontal scale as well as the height of the spectral simulations (c and d) generated on a large central computer. The data were originally at
100G/40 cm and were replotted at 100G/8 inches. It is often useful to adjust two
closely related experimental spectra either to the same intensity or to adjust the
first derivative spectra to reflect the same concentrations, as determined by double
integration. Subtraction of the first integrals, after such an adjustment for concentration, would yield an absorption difference spectrum, analogous to difference
spectra widely used in optical spectroscopy.

While the small computer at present lacks the capability of simulating complex
line shapes, it can be used to simulate spectra where several unknown free radicals
contribute to the spectrum. We have recently used this small computer capability
to identify unknown free radicals (Birrell et al., 1971; Birrell and Griffith, 1971).
The small computers can also be on-line to a large central computer, so that the
large computer capabilities can be used when needed. We have included a more
detailed discussion of these applications in Jost et al. (1971c).

The programs we use for acquiring and processing data are written in CLASS
(Conversational Language for Spectroscopic Systems), a macro language designed
by Mr. Russell Wolfe of Cary Instruments Division of Varian especially for use
with chemical instrumentation. It has been implemented for the Varian 620/i
computer by the Cary group, and was kindly supplied to us by them. Professor
Charles Klopfenstein of the University of Oregon replaced the routines for operation of CLASS designed for optical spectrophotometers with routines to drive the

ESR spectrometer. Professor Klopfenstein also developed for us the programs we are now using.

APPLICATIONS OF SPIN LABELING TO MEMBRANE AND PHARMACOLOGICAL PROBLEMS

General Considerations and Biological Reactivity

The sensitivity of the spin labeling method using ESR lies between the highly sensitive fluorescence techniques and the considerably less sensitive NMR techniques. The practical limits of useful detection without special accessories or time-averaging techniques lie in bulk concentrations of the spin label between 10^{-7} M and 10^{-5} M, depending on the mobility of the label. This means that as little as 10^{-10} to 10^{-12} moles in a 10 μl sample volume can readily be studied. The fact that the sample can be optically opaque increases the usefulness of the technique. The few examples of applications below were selected primarily to illustrate the variety of approaches which have been used, and the kinds of information which either have been obtained or, in principle, could be obtained. They are not intended to represent a summary of spin label studies, which have become very diverse and numerous over the past few years.

Before discussing specific applications, however, it is desirable to consider briefly the compatibility of nitroxides and biological systems. The addition of some biological systems to solutions containing nitroxides can result in ESR signal loss. As an example, the small ketone nitroxide IV, when exposed to washed cells of the mycoplasma *M. laidlawii* suspended in buffer, loses most of the detectable signal in less than an hour at room temperature. Nitroxides exposed to isolated membranes from the same cells have a similar fate. A decrease in signal amplitude has been reported in spinach leaf preparations (Corker et al., 1966), suspensions of *Chlamydamonas* (Weaver and Chon, 1966), and *Escherichia coli* in buffer (Griffith and Waggoner, 1969). The phenomenon appears to be fairly general so far as aerobic tissues and cells are concerned, although the rates of destruction differ, depending both on the physiological state of the cells and the specific nitroxide present. Membrane systems, such as sarcoplasmic reticulum (Landgraf and Inesi, 1969), which lack dehydrogenase activity, apparently do not cause appreciable signal loss. Various sulfhydryl blocking agents also prevent or decrease signal loss in *Mycoplasma* and *E. coli* (Jost, unpublished). Although dehydrogenases would appear to be implicated in this signal loss, it is not clear that a simple protonation of the N-O group is involved, since this would be expected to be reversible, and reversibility has not yet been demonstrated in most of these systems.

The chemical reaction involving signal loss can be used to advantage, however, in determining the local environment of a probe by measuring the accessibility of the spin label to the reducing agent. For example, Hubbell and McConnell (1969a) diffused the lipid spin labels LXIX and LXXVI into nerves, and used the relative rates of signal loss when sodium ascorbate was added as a measure of the location (e.g., hydrophobic or polar) of the nitroxides.

Nitroxides appear to be relatively nontoxic to biological systems, and injection of quite high concentrations of one of several nitroxides into fertilized chick eggs does not seem to affect development or viability (Jost, unpublished). Growth rates of E. coli and Mycoplasma laidlawii are unaffected by nitroxide concentrations as high as 10^{-3} M. This is an area in which there are few data, and in our limited experience the only injurious effect was found when E. coli cells in buffer (i.e., without a carbon source) were exposed to a dilute concentration (5×10^{-6} M) of the small ketone nitroxide IV. In this case, the colony-forming ability decreased with time of exposure, as compared to the control. Over 90% of the colony-forming ability of log phase cells was lost in two hours, although the same concentrations of stationary phase cells lost only 50% of the colony formers. Again there may be advantageous uses for such a phenomenon.

In studies involving equilibrium determinations it will be important to evaluate the possible contribution of signal loss, since compartmentalization of the probe into two chemical environments may result in signal loss in one environment and not in the other. The diamagnetic species so produced could affect the equilibrium and lead to erroneous conclusions. If such a situation is recognized, useful information about such environments might be obtained. In general nitroxides are readily reduced or oxidized. Among reducing agents that result in loss of signal are ascorbic acid, sodium dithionite, hydroxylamine, glutathione, mercaptoethanol, cysteine, and phenylhydrazine (Hoffman and Henderson, 1961; Rozantsev et al., 1965). Some of these are reversible by oxidation with air, and water-soluble reducing agents can be useful in determining the accessibility of a spin label to the aqueous environment, for example. The studies briefly described below for the most part avoid this complicating phenomenon of signal loss. With further extensions of the spin label method, however, the possibility of fairly rapid signal loss will play a role either as a disadvantage to be circumvented or as a tool with which to approach an appropriate problem.

Anisotropy in Membrane Models and Membranes

The ESR spectrum of a spin label is sensitive to the orientation of the label, the rotational mobility of the label, and the polarity of the solvent surrounding the label. Any of these effects can be used to advantage in spin labeling studies. To take full advantage of the orientation effect, the labeled system should be aligned with respect to the laboratory magnetic field. The primary impetus for this type of experiment in membrane studies has been the need for new methods of examining membrane models. In the unit membrane model, for example, the phospholipids are aligned in a bimolecular leaflet (Robertson, 1966). ESR has the capability of determining the degree of orientation of the labels and is useful in testing membrane models and examining the effects of drugs and other additives. Some well-known model systems may not be useful in conjunction with spin labeling because of sensitivity limitations. For example, it would be difficult to study monolayers or isolated phospholipid bilayers. Recently, however, simple techniques have been developed (or rediscovered?) for preparing relatively thick oriented phospholipid multilayers (Libertini et al., 1969; Levine and Wilkins, 1971; Hsia et al., 1970a). The resulting multilayers are physically large, and ESR spectra can be observed when the probe concentration is still relatively small.

Libertini et al. (1969) prepared egg lecithin multilayers containing the fatty acid label LXVIII or the steroid label LXI. The z axis of the fatty acid label is parallel to the long hydrocarbon chain. Thus the observation of a large splitting with the magnetic field perpendicular to the phospholipid film provides evidence that an ordered multilamellar structure exists with the hydrocarbon chains perpendicular to the supporting surface. In the steroid label the z axis is nearly perpendicular to the long axis of the steroid and a small splitting is observed in the perpendicular orientation. In both cases the spectra are highly anisotropic (Libertini et al., 1969). Hsia et al. (1970a) have also studied the steroid label LXI in egg lecithin multilayers and they report effects of adding cholesterol to the preparations. From x-ray diffraction data, Levine and Wilkins (1971) also conclude there is considerable orientation of the fatty acid chains in egg lecithin multilayers.

This orientation makes it possible to examine further the behavior of the lipids in a bilayer region. When lecithin multilayers were spin labeled by incorporation of one of several positional isomers of the doxylstearic acids (LXIV, LXVII, LXVIII, LXXI, with the nitroxide moiety at carbons 5, 7, 12 or 16), the relative anisotropy of segments along the length of the lipids within the bilayer regions could be determined (Jost et al., 1971b). All four doxylstearic acids oriented in the multilayers, but there was a pronounced systematic variation in anisotropy as the nitroxide moiety was moved away from the carboxyl end of the spin label. This was interpreted as due to rapidly increasing molecular motion near the center of the bilayer region. Such a model system can also be used to examine environmental effects such as temperature and hydration (Jost et al., 1971b).

Examining biological membranes for ordered lipid structure is experimentally difficult because of the need for relatively large, physically oriented samples. Progress in this direction has been made by Hubbell and McConnell (1969b), who diffused the androstan spin label (LXIX) and 12-doxylstearic acid (LXVIII) into erythrocytes. The labeled erythrocytes were oriented by flowing through a small gap between two quartz plates. The spectra obtained were somewhat altered by changing the orientation of the sample with respect to the laboratory magnetic field. This indicated some degree of orientation of the lipid spin labels, as judged by the criteria discussed above in connection with the model systems. The spin labels are evidently reflecting ordered lipid regions. Similar observations have recently been made in bovine retinal rod outer segments (A. S. Waggoner and L. Stryer, Yale University, personal communication).

Figure 17 illustrates how spin labeling can be used to examine the effects of chemical treatments of membrane models (Jost et al., 1971a). Spectra *A* and *B* of Figure 17 are of the fatty acid label LXIV in an egg lecithin multilayer before and after exposure to osmium tetroxide vapors. Spectra *B* are the familiar rigid glass

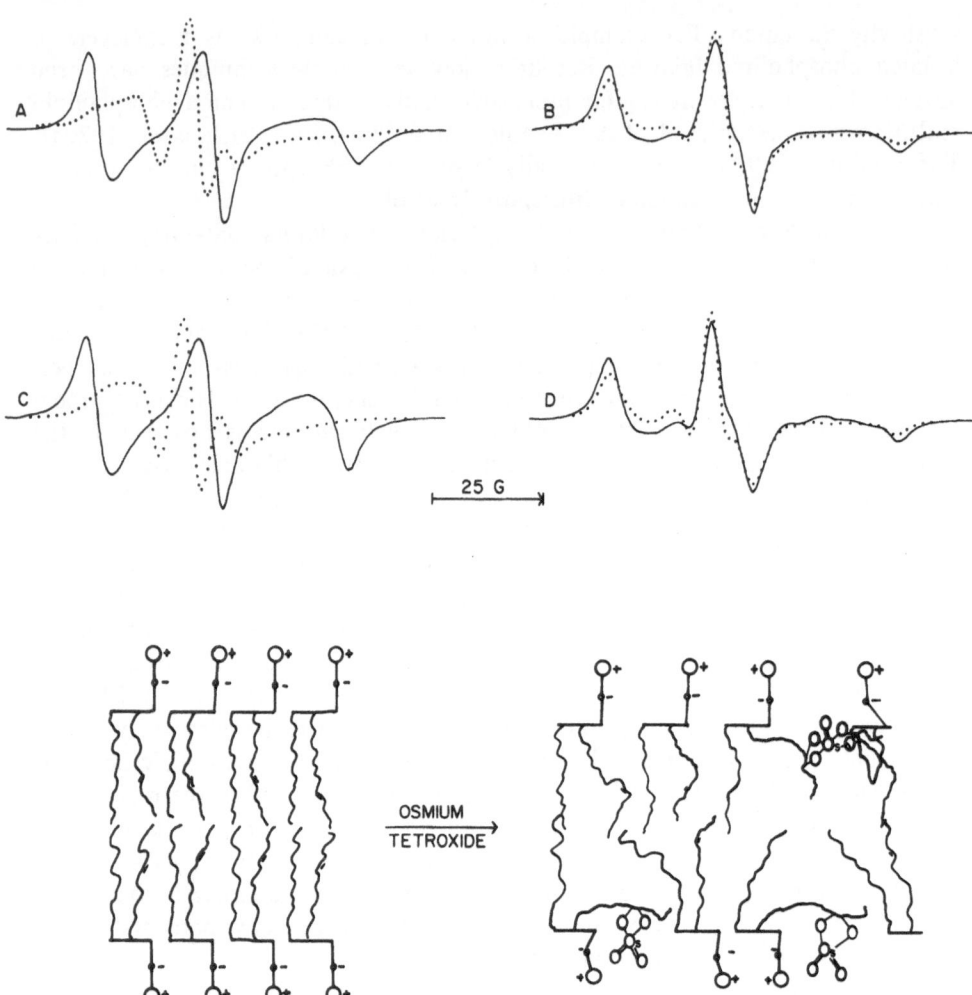

FIG. 17. Effect of osmium tetroxide on the lipid structure of an oriented model membrane system. A. ESR spectra of 5-doxylstearic acid LXIV in an oriented lecithin multilayer with the supporting slide perpendicular (solid line) and parallel (dotted line) to the magnetic field; B. The same sample after 4 min exposure to osmium tetroxide vapors; C. and D. Computer simulations of A and B, respectively. The spectra are consistent with the lipid structures illustrated schematically in the bottom sketches.

spectra observed for randomly oriented samples. Osmium tetroxide evidently destroys the ordered nature of the multilayer and at the same time increases the rigidity of the structure. The effect is depicted schematically at the bottom of Figure 17. Similar effects have been observed in biological membranes. One other development is illustrated by spectra C and D of Figure 17. These are computer simulations of anisotropic spectra based on a Gaussian distribution of orientations (Libertini et al., 1969; Jost et al., 1971b). The agreement between the experimental spectra A and B and the corresponding simulated spectra C and D of Figure 17 is surprisingly good. It is not necessary to be this quantitative in many studies, but the use of spectral simulations is becoming more widespread as more detailed information is sought.

Geometry of Binding Sites

Any molecular site exhibiting specificity of binding can, in principle, be explored with reporter groups. Antibody combining sites, and enzyme active sites all fall in the category of molecular regions suitable for spin labeling studies.

ANTIBODY COMBINING SITES. The use of spin labels to look at the binding site of antibodies was introduced by Stryer and Griffith (1965), who applied it to the study of interaction of the dinitrophenyl nitroxide XXXIX with antibodies specific for the dinitrophenyl group. ESR and fluorescence quenching experiments independently confirmed that there are two binding sites per antibody molecule. The ESR spectrum of bound hapten is very broad, indicating that the tumbling motion of the spin label is greatly reduced upon binding to the antibody. It was pointed out that the sharpness of the ESR spectrum of rapidly tumbling nitroxides makes it feasible to detect small amounts of unbound hapten in the presence of the hapten-antibody complex.

More detailed exploration of the dinitrophenyl antibody binding site was carried out by Hsia and Piette (1969a) in a fashion which has wide applicability in approaching the geometry of binding or receptor sites in general. Electron microscope studies of antibody-hapten complexes indicate that the antibody active site is located in a cleft (Valentine and Green, 1967), and Hsia and Piette used spin labels to measure the depth of the cleft. They synthesized a series of dinitrophenyl spin labels (see XLIII, where $n = 1, 2, 3, 5$; XLIV; XL). In this series the length of the hydrocarbon chains formed a series of molecules calculated to have 8, 10, 12, 13.4, 14.7 and 17.4 Å between the *para*-nitro group of the hapten and the nitroxide. When each of these spin labeled haptens was reacted with dinitrophenyl specific antibodies, the mobility of the spin label varied from highly immobilized to relatively unrestricted motion (see, for example, effects of motion in Figure 4).

By comparing the experimental spectra with those of a small nitroxide in glycerol of differing viscosities, they assigned relative correlation time values. A plot of these values shows an abrupt increase in the mobility of the spin label as the effective length of the molecule was increased. When the length was 10 Å or less, the spin label was apparently rigidly held. However, at effective lengths greater than 10 Å the label was more mobile, and further increases in the motion were observed as the distance was increased to 13.4 Å. The highly mobile character of the spectra changed only slightly as the distance was further increased from 13.4 Å to 17.4 Å. From the break in the curve the authors concluded that the depth of the cleft in the antibody molecule is 9 to 11 Å. They further suggested on the basis of composite spectra obtained only with haptens in the length range of 10 to 12 Å that there is structural heterogeneity within this range, which might be associated with high and low binding constants. They attempted to explore this structural heterogeneity (Hsia and Piette, 1969b) with a series of molecules that varied in the hapten (XL,

XLI, XLII), and tentatively suggested that the region of the cleft nearer the surface of the antibody might vary in its dimensions or hydrophobic characteristics in different antibody molecules.

The binding of spin labeled haptens is the basis of a new immunological assay technique for drugs in body fluids (Leute et al., 1971). Morphine specific antibodies were prepared in rabbits by injection of carboxymethylmorphine-BSA in complete Freund's adjuvant. The antibodies bind a spin labeled morphine (see structure below).

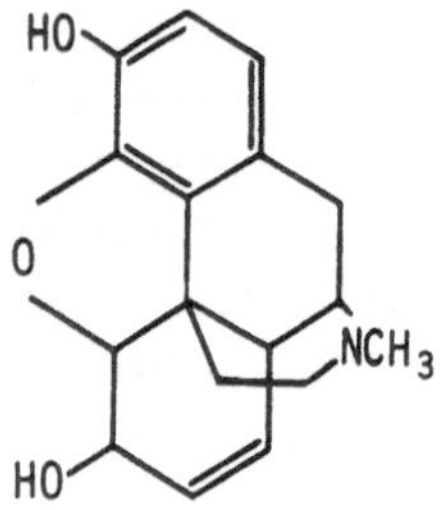

morphine

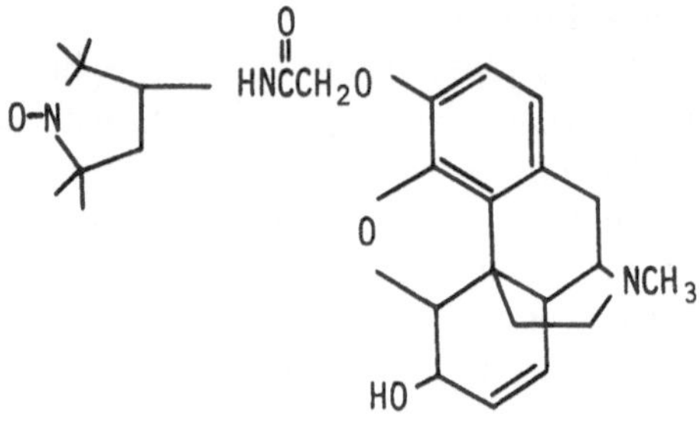

spin labeled morphine

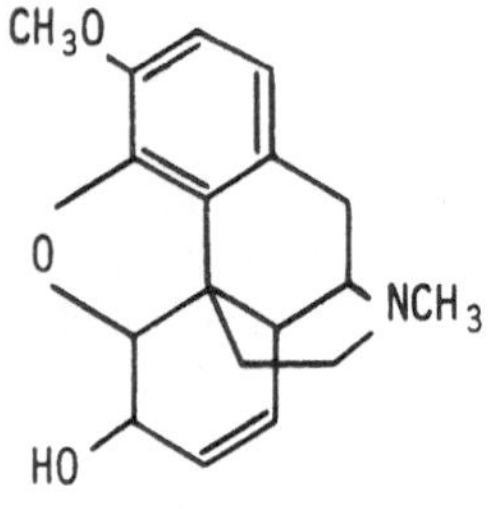

codeine

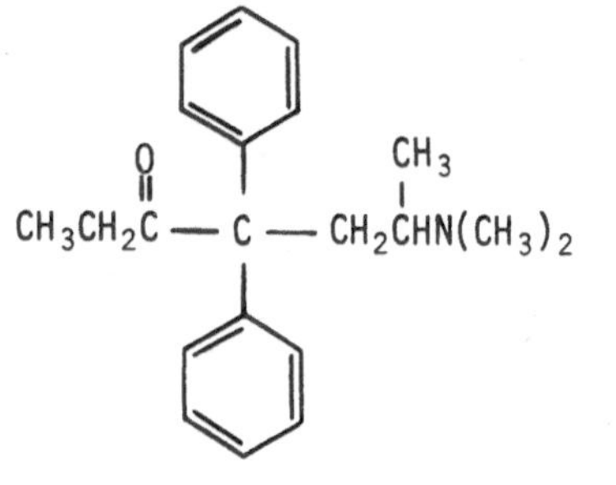

methadone

A broad ESR spectrum results due to the immobilization of the spin label. A small amount of sharp three-line spectrum arising from equilibrium concentrations of unbound spin labeled morphine is usually superimposed on the broad ESR spectrum. In the new technique, a solution of this loaded antibody is the assay reagent. When mixed with aqueous solutions containing morphine, codeine, or certain related morphine analogs, the spin label is displaced and the height of the sharp three lines increases greatly. The increase in sharp three-line signal intensity is directly related to the morphine concentration in the added solution. The assay is reported to determine morphine concentrations as low as $10^{-7}M$ (0.03 μg/ml) in 10 μl of a test sample. Methadone, amphetamines, barbiturates, cocaine, and propoxyphene (Darvon) do not competitively displace the spin labeled morphine. Thus, the assay can be used in a methadone program. The new technique has been named Free Radical Assay Technique (FRAT) (Leute et al., 1971). Because of the specificity and sensitivity, attempts will undoubtedly be made to extend this rapid immunological technique to the assay of other drugs in body fluids.

MEMBRANE-BOUND ACTIVE SITES AND INHIBITORS. Another class of highly specific interactions is represented by the binding of inhibitor molecules. Thus, spin labeled analogs of inhibitors can be used to explore and titrate accessible membrane-bound receptors or active sites as well as those of active centers in solution. Morrisett et al. (1969) have synthesized a spin label inhibitor of acetylcholinesterase, the nitroxide organophosphonofluoridate XXXVII. They have reported that this spin label inhibitor selectively spin labels the reactive serine residue of acetylcholinesterase. Organophosphonofluoridates cause rapid inactivation of this enzyme, and less than 1% of acetylcholinesterase activity remained after reacting with the spin label. They concluded that the spin label did not appear to attach to other residues or other esterases to any degree. The mobility of the spin label after labeling membrane preparations (human and bovine red cells, rat nerve ending particles) is relatively high, suggesting that the active site of the membrane-bound enzyme is exposed on the surface of the enzyme molecule, on its periphery, and not buried in a crevice. This is in contrast to esterases not normally attached to membranes, such as α-chymotrypsin, lysozyme, and ribonuclease, which are known to possess active sites in deep clefts extending into the interior of the molecule. In these enzymes this spin label would be expected to have its mobility restricted. For example, when α-chymotrypsin was spin labeled with the same label, the spectra showed a relatively high degree of immobilization (Morrisett et al., 1969).

Somewhat similar preliminary results have been reported by Hsia et al. (1969) for the organophosphate spin labels XXXVI and XXXVIII. In addition they have reported a dinitroxide spin label of this type, which inhibits α-chymotrypsin and also shows immobilization of the spin label on binding, but they have not reported on its specificity or effect on membrane-bound esterases.

If a spin label is indeed highly specific for the active site, this kind of approach makes it possible to look at changes in conformation at the active sites that may occur with various treatments. For example, does solubilizing a normally membrane-bound enzyme result in a conformational change in the active site? Another application would be to try to detect changes in the active site when lipid-requiring enzymes are activated with various lipids.

CONFORMATIONAL CHANGES IN MACROMOLECULES

If a protein undergoes conformational changes as it interacts either with small molecules or with other protein molecules, the most sensitive and generally useful label would be one attached specifically near the region of association with substrate, coenzyme, or with another protein subunit. Conformational changes with binding of substrates and coenzymes, or with protein-protein interactions, could be studied. This requires that a spin label have a reactive chemical group with high specificity for the residue to be labeled and that nonspecific labeling be absent or minimal. Several interesting problems have already been tackled using this general approach.

PROTEINS.   The best studied example of this approach is the series of studies on hemoglobin by McConnell and his coworkers (Ogawa and McConnell, 1967; Ogawa et al., 1968; McConnell et al., 1969). They took advantage of the fact that the sulfhydryl of cysteine 93 in the β-chain of hemoglobin is very reactive to alkylating agents. Hemoglobin reacted with the iodoacetamide spin label XXVII gives an ESR spectrum indicating that the spin label is highly immobilized. On oxygenation the spectral changes observed led to the conclusion that only two local protein conformations were sensed by this probe. The spectral changes observed were linear with degree of heme group oxygenation, which was interpreted to indicate that each spin label reflects the structure of the β subunit to which it is attached.

When the closely related spin label iodoacetamide XXIX was reacted with the β chains of hemoglobin, the results obtained were interpreted as evidence for the existence of a local region in the molecule that has a structure dependent on the oxygenation of more than one heme group. As these studies point out, even given the required specificity, more than one label may have to be tried in order to find one whose spectrum is sensitive to the presumptive change being studied.

Ho et al. (1970), by using human hemoglobin variants that differ in oxygen affinity and Hill coefficients, have investigated further the ESR changes in spin labeled (XXIX) hemoglobins when oxygenation occurs, and also concluded that the spin label is accurately sensing conformational changes. They further suggest that the spin label is not only detecting structural changes around the heme group but also sensing the subunit-subunit interactions in the cooperative oxygenation process.

Another example of this interesting approach is the detection of conformational changes in the structure of myosin produced by adenosine triphosphate, reported by Seidel et al. (1970). The spin label iodoacetamide XXIX binds to two rapidly reacting thiol groups in the myosin molecule under appropriate conditions, giving a strongly immobilized spectrum and yielding myosin with altered adenosine triphosphatase activity, characteristic of the reaction of myosin with sulfhydryl modifiers. The spin labeled myosin molecule contains two heavy meromyosin chains, each having an adenosine triphosphatase binding site and a nitroxide attached to the nearby reactive sulfhydryl. If ATP is added to the spin labeled myosin, the mobility of the bound nitroxide increases, becoming maximal with 2 moles of ATP per mole of protein. This effect can be reversed on removal of the ATP by dialysis. On the basis of this and supplementary experiments, the changes in the ESR spectra produced by ATP are interpreted to be the result of a conformational change in the myosin molecule when ATP binds, and these changes are near the nitroxide radicals. The authors concluded that the spin label is detecting a change in a relatively small region, since optical rotatory dispersion is reported to detect no gross change when ATP is bound to myosin.

NUCLEIC ACIDS. The approach of attempting to spin label by covalently attaching a spin label to a unique reactive group has recently been applied to the important problem of the conformation of transfer RNA in solution. Schofield et al. (1970) have capitalized on the fact that aminoacyl tRNA's have a strongly basic α-amino group, while the other amino groups and heterocyclic nitrogen atoms present in free amino acids and uncharged tRNA are much less basic. Thus, unfractionated mixtures of tRNA's can be charged enzymatically with a single amino acid and then spin labeled. They synthesized the N-hydroxysuccinimide spin label XXX, reacted it chemically with a mixture of tRNA's that had been charged with phenylalanine or valine, and then removed the unreacted spin label. The specificity of aminoacylation allows investigation by ESR of those species of tRNA specific for the amino acid used (if only the aminoacyl tRNA reacts with the spin label under the conditions used). In this example, however, the background of nonspecific labeling was high enough to require a further fractionation procedure. They then performed ESR "melting curves," using relative peak heights and an assumption of isotropic motion. Calculations based on these parameters, plotted on an Arrhenius plot, showed a discontinuity at 51° for labeled valine-tRNA, whereas similar calculations from spectra of poly-L-lysine labeled on the ε-amino groups varied linearly over the same temperature range. The ESR denaturation temperature of the labeled val-tRNA does not correspond to the optical absorption denaturation temperature, but does show a dependence on ionic strength paralleling that of the optical absorption denaturation temperature. The tentative interpretation of these results is that physical changes limited to regions near the nitroxide are being observed, whereas the optical changes involve the entire molecule. Kabat et al. (1970) reacted cysteine-charged tRNA with the spin label iodoacetamide XXVII. This gave a spin labeled cys-tRNA (see XLIX) with the label attached to the -SH group rather than the α-NH_2 group. The ESR melting temperature of this cys-tRNA was 39°, however the conditions of melting differed from those used by Schofield et al. (1970).

As chemical methods are developed to specifically label other portions of the tRNA molecule, spin labeling can provide a tool to approach secondary and tertiary structure in solution to complement the x-ray crystallographic data being collected with tRNA crystals.

This general approach also illustrates another possible advantage of the spin labeling technique. Since normally the only paramagnetic signal present is the characteristic signal from the added spin labels, it is possible to look at a single class of compounds present in a mixture if they undergo a unique reaction with the label. The limitation here is, of course, the specificity of the labeling, which must be demonstrated in each case, and the removal of the unreacted spin label especially if it dominates the spectrum.

Enzyme Mechanisms

Enzyme mechanisms that are dependent on the binding of a coenzyme can be approached using an appropriate spin labeled coenzyme analog. Weiner (1969) has

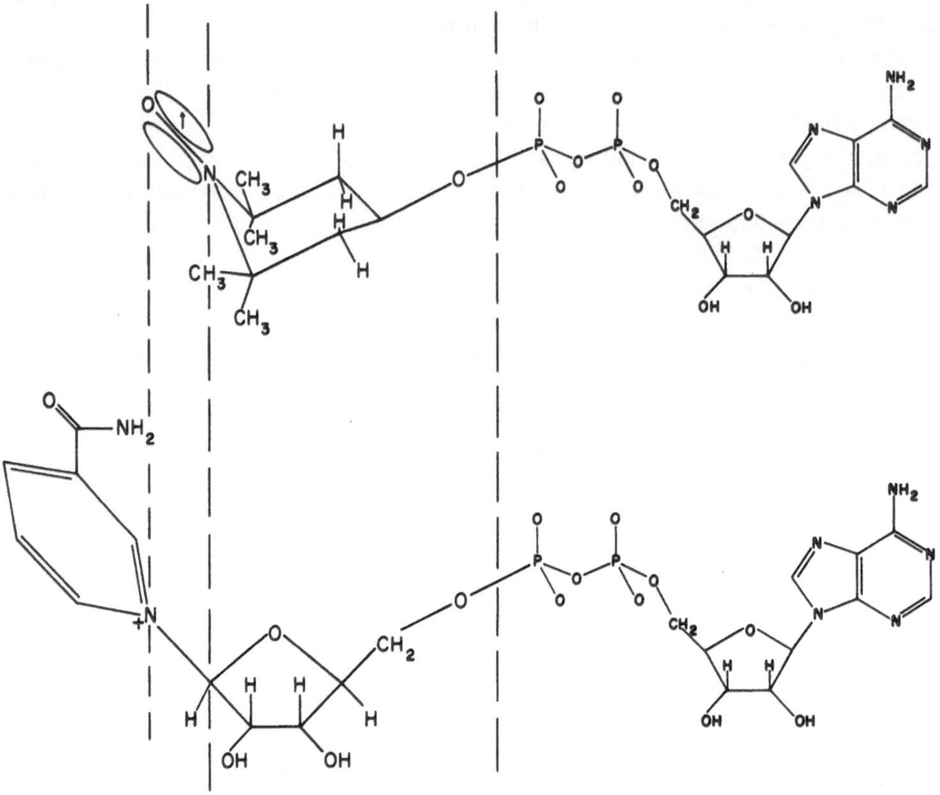

FIG. 18. Comparison of the structures of the spin label NAD analog and of NAD, showing the location of the unpaired electron. (From Mildvan and Weiner. 1969a. Courtesy of the authors and the American Chemical Society.)

synthesized a spin label that is the analog of nicotinamide-adenine dinucleotide (see Figure 18 and XLVII). This spin labeled NAD is a competitive inhibitor of liver alcohol dehydrogenase with respect to NAD, competing for the same sites on the enzyme molecule. It binds as tightly as the known competitive inhibitor ADPribose.

When the spin labeled NAD was added to the enzyme (liver alcohol dehydrogenase) in solution, a marked decrease in signal amplitude resulted, and the spectrum became more bound. Using the assumption that the ratio of signal amplitudes in the presence and absence of enzyme would be proportional to the concentration of the free probe (i.e., that the bound signal made little contribution to the total peak height), Weiner titrated the enzyme with increasing probe concentrations. A Scatchard plot from concentrations determined in this fashion could be made to measure the dissociation constant and the moles of spin label per mole of enzyme. The biphasic plot indicates that two tight binding sites exist for the spin labeled NAD and five to six weak binding sites. Reduced coenzyme displaces the spin label from the strong binding sites but not from the weak ones. These ancillary binding sites are no longer seen when the metal atom (zinc) is removed to make the catalytically inactive apoenzyme. Only the tight binding sites remain in the apoenzyme.

The presence of a paramagnetic species, either an organic free radical or a metal such as the manganous ion, is known to affect the nuclear magnetic relaxation rate of the solvent protons. Mildvan and Weiner (1969a,b) capitalized on the presence of the nitroxide free radical in the spin labeled NAD-enzyme complex to explore the structural and thermodynamic properties of both the binary complex and of the ternary complex that forms in the presence of substrate. While the NMR methods used are outside the scope of this chapter, it is interesting to summarize their conclusions here, since it is the effect of the presence of the spin label that gives the experimental handle for the NMR studies.

The results of the pulsed NMR studies indicate that there is an enhancement of the relaxation rate of water protons by a factor of at least 15 when the spin labeled NAD is bound to the enzyme. As the occupancy of the binding sites is increased, from 0 to 2, this enhancement decreases from a factor of 60 to a factor of 15, and this continuous variation is interpreted to indicate site-site interactions that have not been detected thermodynamically. In the presence of one of several substrates, the ternary spin label NAD-enzyme-substrate complex forms, and a decrease in the water proton relaxation rate is observed. This decrease suggests that the substrates bind on the "water-side" of NAD, and provide a basis for an estimate of the distance between the NAD and the substrates on the enzyme molecule. By conventional NMR technique it was determined that the resonance of the alcohol methyl protons is broadened by interaction in the active site with the nitroxide. Apparently the substrate binds close to the nitroxide moiety of the spin label and such binding limits the access of water to this region of the active site. Mildvan's group has recently (Mildvan et al., 1970) extended the same approach to mitochondrial malate dehydrogenase. Here the spin label appears to occupy the NADH binding sites and the substrates appear to alter the enzyme affinity for the coenzymes. It is evident that the general approach of combining ESR and NMR techniques with spin labels can be useful in studying enzyme mechanisms.

The examples in this chapter were chosen to illustrate *kinds* of approaches, rather than to review information obtained about a given system. This selection necessitates omission of many interesting areas of spin labeling, and the reader should consult the recent reviews available, Hamilton and McConnell (1968), Griffith and Waggoner (1969), McConnell and McFarland (1970), Smith (1971), and Jost et al. (1971c).

PROGNOSIS

The advantages of spin labeling are illustrated in the applications discussed above. It is, of course, equally important to assess the limitations of the method. Any reporter group technique carries with it the inherent disadvantage of perturbing the system by the addition of the reporter molecule (the "price of peeking"— L. Stryer). There is no question that, at the molecular level, the nitroxide group represents a bulky addition. However, it is comforting to find that spin labels are sensitive to known phase changes in lipid dispersions and that in phospholipid multilayers the spin labels are not sufficiently large perturbations to cause gross local disorder. Nevertheless, this limitation of the reporter group technique should always be kept in mind. Other shortcomings of spin labeling include the concentration of probe required and the stability of the probes. The concentration of spin label needed is somewhat greater than in fluorescence labeling and far greater than required for radioisotope experiments. The stability of nitroxides is adequate for most experiments but free radicals are inherently less stable than are most optically absorbing or fluorescent probes. The relative ease of reduction can be an advantage in determining the position or accessibility of the spin labels (see previous section).

One of the most direct approaches to pharmacological problems is the synthesis of spin labeled drug molecules. The addition of a nitroxide group might be expected generally to alter the pharmacological activity of the molecule. As an analogy, for example, the substitution of the nitroxide moiety in place of the pyrimidine in nicotinamide-adenine dinucleotide (see Figure 18) produces a molecule that behaves as a competitive inhibitor of liver alcohol dehydrogenase. Nevertheless, the binding of the spin label NAD to the enzyme appears to be highly specific, and the molecule has been very useful (see pp. 265–267).

The chemical route used in making many spin labels is to synthesize a nitroxide with a reactive functional group that can participate in preparing the desired spin label. For example, the spin labeled NAD was prepared by phosphorylating the alcohol nitroxide V and reacting the product with AMP (Weiner, 1969). It is possible to react nitroxides or their precursors with a number of reactive groups (see Figure 1 and Appendix for some of the references). Nitroxides useful for such reactions are generally not difficult to synthesize. Many of these are now also available commercially from Frinton Laboratories and the Syva Company. The secondary amine precursors of some of the small nitroxide molecules of the general classes I and II (Figure 1) are available from Frinton Laboratories and from Aldrich Chemical Company.

An interesting example of a potentially useful spin label drug is the spin label analog of digitoxigenin (Atsunobu Yoda, University of Wisconsin School of Medicine, personal communication). In this molecule the aglycone has been labeled at the 3 position by the method of Keana et al. (1967). Using a partially purified beef brain microsomal $(Na^+ + K^+)$-ATPase preparation, Yoda finds that the spin label digitoxigenin acts as an inhibitor. In preliminary experiments, the spin label inhibits the ATPase, but somewhat less effectively than digitoxigenin itself. The spin label digitoxigenin is probably a mixture of 3-α and 3-β stereoisomers, and this may increase the apparent inhibitory concentrations needed. The ATPase is normally membrane bound, and thus it may be possible to look at both the membrane-bound and the solubilized enzyme, provided that the binding is relatively specific.

Membrane-bound receptor sites can, in principle, be labeled by the synthesis of a spin label that contains in the molecule the chemical groups necessary for specificity of interaction with the receptor. Some possible approaches will be suggested by the examples mentioned on pp. 257–267. The geometry of the receptor site may be explored if a molecule known to bind specifically is spin labeled, and exhibits immobilization. Increasing the distance between the nitroxide and the binding site may serve as a spectroscopic ruler. When samples are optically opaque, spin labeling will be particularly useful in the titration of binding sites. If the receptor macromolecule contains unique reactive groups in or near the region of binding, these can be capitalized on in investigating possible conformational changes occurring during the binding of drugs. It is intriguing to speculate on the possibility of comparing conformational changes at or near the binding site when the receptor is solubilized with those changes occurring in the same receptor in intact tissues.

One of the more important needs of the spin labeling technique is the development of spin labels with increased specificity. In the past few years considerable progress has been made, and the next few years will undoubtedly see many more advances in this area. Not only can errors of interpretation arise from unrecognized nonspecific labeling, but such nonspecific binding obscures the effects associated with the fraction of labels that have bound in the intended position. The increased use of small computers to subtract out subcomponents of the ESR spectrum may be helpful in this sorting out of small effects that are partially obscured in a complex spectrum, but cannot substitute for development of spin labels with greater specificity.

Future labeling studies will take fuller advantage of the information regarding orientation, molecular motion, solvent effects, and nitroxide-nitroxide interactions. Some increase in sophistication in the technique can be expected (e.g., more use of computers and double resonance methods). However, the main trend will be to combine spin labeling with optical absorption, fluorescence, Raman, NMR, or other spectroscopic techniques in studies of biological problems at the molecular level.

ACKNOWLEDGMENTS

We are grateful for the technical assistance of Miss Dee Brightman, whose skill and persistence obtained the many spectra included in the figures. We are indebted to our colleagues Louis Libertini, Professor John Keana, and Professor Charles Klopfenstein for reading the manuscript and for their helpful suggestions. We thank Louis Libertini for the data for Figure 3 and the simulated spectra shown in Figure 17c, d, and Dr. Bruce Birrell for Figure 5. The patience of our colleagues in tolerating the heavy spectrometer use necessary in developing small computer applications and in collecting spectra for this chapter has been a real contribution. Finally, we wish to acknowledge support by U.S. Public Health Service grant CA 10337-03 from the National Cancer Institute. O. H. Griffith also acknowledges general support by the Alfred P. Sloan Foundation.

APPENDIX

The following are some useful references to the synthesis and applications of the nitroxide spin labels shown in Figure 1. Roman numerals designate the molecules, and the complete reference is listed in the References.

I, II, see Rozantsev (1970) for synthesis of a number of molecules in these two classes; III, Keana et al. (1967); IV, Rozantsev and Nieman (1964); Brière et al. (1965a); V, Briere et al. (1965b); VI, Rozantsev et al. (1965); VII, Lebedev and Kazarnovskii (1960); Rozantsev and Nieman (1964), Briere et al. (1965b); VIII, Rozantsev and Kokhanov (1966); IX, Tonomura et al. (1969), McConnell and McFarland (1970); X, Rassat and Rey (1967); XI, XII, XIII, XIV, Rosantsev and Krinitskaya (1965); XV, Rassat and Rey (1967); XVI, Krinitskaya et al. (1965); XVII, Rozantsev and Krinitskaya (1965); XVIII, McConnell and McFarland (1970); XIX, Hsia and Piette (1969a); XX, McConnell and McFarland (1970); XXI, Hoffman and Henderson (1961); XXII, Keith et al. (1968); XXIII, Griffith and McConnell (1966); XXIV, Ohnishi et al. (1966); XXV, Smith (1968); XXVI, Kosman et al. (1969); XXVII, XXVIII, Ogawa and McConnell (1967); XXIX, McConnell and Hamilton (1968); XXX, Hoffman et al. (1969); XXXI, Boeyens and McConnell (1966); XXXII, Griffith et al. (1967a); XXXIII, Berliner and McConnell (1966); XXXIV, Griffith et al. (1967b); XXXV, Griffith et al. (1967a); XXXVI, Hsia et al. (1969); XXXVII, Morrisett et al. (1969); XXXVIII, Hsia et al. (1969); XXXIX, Stryer and Griffith (1965); XL, XLI, XLII, Hsia and Piette (1969b); XLIII, XLIV, Hsia and Piette (1969a); XLV, Waggoner et al. (1967); XLVI, Roberts et al. (1969); XLVII, Weiner (1969); XLVIII, McConnell and McFarland (1970); XLIX, Kabat et al. (1970); L, Griffith and Waggoner (1969); LI, LII, LIII, Brière et al. (1965a); LIV, LV, LVI, Ferruti et al. (1970); LVII, LVIII, Keana et al. (1967); LIX, Rozantsev (1970);

LX, Rottschaefer (1970); LXI, Keana et al. (1967); LXII, Kosman et al. (1969); LXIII, Hubbell and McConnell (1969b); LXIV, Jost et al. (1971b); LXV, Hubbell and McConnell (1969a); LXVI, Rottschaefer (1970); LXVII, Jost et al. (1971b); LXVIII, Waggoner et al. (1969); LXIX, Hubbell and McConnell (1969a); LXX, Kosman et al. (1969); LXXI, Jost et al. (1971b); LXXII, Van (1970); LXXIII, Hubbell and McConnell (1969b); LXXIV, Hsia et al. (1970b); LXXV, Waggoner et al. (1968); LXXVI, Hubbell and McConnell (1969a); LXXVII, Keith et al. (1968).

REFERENCES

Alexandrov, I. V., A. N. Ivanova, N. N. Korst, A. V. Lazarev, A. I. Prikhozhenko, and V. B. Stryukov. 1970. The E.S.R. line shape for the iminoxyl radical in high viscosity media. Molec. Phys., 18:681-691.

Alger, R. S. 1968. Electron Paramagnetic Resonance: Techniques and Applications. New York, Wiley/Interscience.

Ayscough, P. B. 1967. Electron Spin Resonance in Chemistry. London, Methuen and Co.

Berliner, L. J., and H. M. McConnell. 1966. A spin-labeled substrate for α-chymotrypsin. Proc. Nat. Acad. Sci. U.S.A., 55:708-712.

Bersohn, M., and J. C. Baird. 1966. An Introduction to Electron Paramagnetic Resonance. New York, W. A. Benjamin, Inc.

Birrell, G. B., and O. H. Griffith. 1971. ESR study of X-irradiated long chain alcohols oriented in urea inclusion crystals. J. Phys. Chem. (in press).

———— A. A. Lai, and O. H. Griffith. 1971. ESR study of an acetylenic radical in two host crystals. X-irradiated methyl-2-nonynoate trapped in urea and perhydrotriphenylene inclusion crystals. J. Chem. Phys., 54:1630-1635.

Boeyens, J. C. A., and H. M. McConnell. 1966. Spin-labeled hemoglobin. Proc. Nat. Acad. Sci. U.S.A., 56:22-25.

Bolton, J. R., D. Borg, and H. Swartz, eds. 1971. Biological Applications of Electron Spin Resonance Spectroscopy. New York, Wiley/Interscience.

Brière, R., R.-M. Dupeyre, H. Lemaire, C. Morat, A. Rassat, and P. Rey. 1965a. Nitroxydes XVII: biradicaux stables du type nitroxyde. Bull. Soc. Chim. France, 1965:3290-3297.

———— H. Lemaire, and A. Rassat. 1965b. Nitroxydes XV: Synthèse et étude de radicaux libres stables piperidiniques et pyrrolidinique. Bull. Soc. Chim. France, 1965:3273-3283.

Butler, K. W., H. Dugas, I. C. P. Smith, and H. Schneider. 1970. Cation-induced organization changes in a lipid bilayer model membrane. Biochem. Biophys. Res. Commun., 40:770-776.

Calvin, M., H. H. Wang, G. Entine, D. Gill, P. Ferruti, M. A. Harpold, and M. P. Klein. 1969. Biradical spin labeling for nerve membranes. Proc. Nat. Acad. Sci. U.S.A., 63:1-8.

Carrington, A., and G. R. Luckhurst. 1964. The electron resonance spectra of free radicals dissolved in liquid crystals. Molec. Phys., 8:401-402.

———— and A. D. McLachlan. 1967. Introduction to Magnetic Resonance. New York, Harper and Row.

Chestnut, D. B., and W. D. Phillips. 1961. EPR studies of spin correlation in some ion radical salts. J. Chem. Phys., 35:1002-1012.

Commoner, B., J. Townsend, and G. E. Pake. 1954. Free radicals in biological materials. Nature (London), 174:689-691.

Corker, G. A., M. P. Klein, and M. Calvin. 1966. Chemical trapping of a primary quantum conversion product in photosynthesis. Proc. Nat. Acad. Sci. U.S.A., 56:1365-1369.

Corvaja, C., G. Giacometti, K. D. Kopple, and Ziauddin. 1970. Electron spin resonance studies of nitroxide radicals and biradicals in nematic solvents. J. Amer. Chem. Soc., 92:3919-3924.

Ehrenberg, A., B. G. Malmstrom, and T. Vaangard, eds. 1967. Magnetic Resonance in Biological Systems. Oxford and New York, Pergamon Press.

Falle, H. R., G. R. Luckhurst, H. Lemaire, Y. Marechal, A. Rassat, and P. Rey. 1966. The electron resonance of ground state triplets in liquid crystal solutions. Molec. Phys., 11:49-56.

Feher, G. 1970. Electron Paramagnetic Resonance with Applications to Selected Problems in Biology (Les Houches Lectures, 1969). New York, Gordon and Breach.

Ferruti, P., D. Gill, M. A. Harpold, and M. P. Klein. 1969. ESR of spin-labeled nematogenlike probes dissolved in nematic liquid crystals. J. Chem. Phys., 50:4545-4550.

_____ D. Gill, M. P. Klein, H. H. Wang, G. Entine, and M. Calvin. 1970. Synthesis of mono-, di-, and polynitroxides. Classification of electron spin resonance spectra of flexible dinitroxides dissolved in liquids and glasses. J. Amer. Chem. Soc., 92:3704-3713.

Forrester, A. R., J. M. Hay, and R. H. Thomson. 1968. Organic Chemistry of Stable Free Radicals. pp. 180-246. New York, Academic Press.

Glarum, S. H., and J. H. Marshall. 1966. ESR of the perinaphthenyl radical in a liquid crystal. J. Chem. Phys., 44:2884-2890.

_____ and J. H. Marshall. 1967. Spin exchange in nitroxide biradicals. J. Chem. Phys., 47:1374-1378.

Griffith, O. H. 1964. Electron spin resonance and molecular motion of the $RCH_2CHCOOR$ radicals in X-irradiated ester-urea inclusion compounds. J. Chem. Phys., 41:1093-1105.

_____ J. F. W. Keana, D. L. Noall, and J. L. Ivey. 1967a. Nitroxide mixed carboxylic-carbonic acid anhydrides. A new class of versatile spin labels. Biochim. Biophys. Acta, 148:583-585.

_____ J. F. W. Keana, S. Rottschaefer, and T. A. Warlick. 1967b. Preparation and magnetic resonance of nitroxide polymers. J. Amer. Chem. Soc., 89:5072.

_____ L. J. Libertini, and G. B. Birrell. 1971. Lipid spin labels in membrane physics. J. Phys. Chem. (in press)

_____ and H. M. McConnell. 1962. Electron spin resonance of X-irradiated organic inclusion compounds. Proc. Nat. Acad. Sci. U.S.A., 48:1877-1880.

_____ and H. M. McConnell. 1966. A nitroxide-maleimide spin label. Proc. Nat. Acad. Sci. U.S.A., 55:8-11.

_____ and A. S. Waggoner. 1969. Nitroxide free radicals: Spin labels for probing biomolecular structure. Accounts Chem. Res., 2:17-24.

Hamilton, C. L., and H. M. McConnell. 1968. Spin labels. In Rich A., and N. Davidson, eds., Structural Chemistry and Molecular Biology, 115-149. San Francisco, W. H. Freeman.

Hirota, N., and S. I. Weissman. 1964. Electronic interaction in ketyl radicals. J. Amer. Chem. Soc., 86:2538-2545.

Ho, C., J. J. Baldassare, and S. Charache. 1970. Electron paramagnetic resonance studies of spin-labeled hemoglobins and their implications to the nature of cooperative oxygen binding to hemoglobin. Proc. Nat. Acad. Sci. U.S.A., 66:722-729.

Hoffman, A. K., and A. T. Henderson. 1961. A new stable free radical: Di-t-butylnitroxide. J. Amer. Chem. Soc., 83:4671-4672.

Hoffman, B. M., P. Schofield, and A. Rich. 1969. Spin-labeled transfer RNA. Proc. Nat. Acad. Sci. U.S.A., 62:1195-1202.

Hsia, J. C., D. J. Kosman, and L. H. Piette. 1969. Organophosphate spin-label studies of inhibited esterases, α-chymotrypsin and cholinesterase. Biochem. Biophys. Res. Commun., 36:75-78.

_____ and L. H. Piette. 1969a. Spin-labeling as a general method in studying antibody active site. Arch. Biochem. Biophys., 129:296-307.

_____ and L. H. Piette. 1969b. Spin-labeled hapten studies of structure heterogeneity and cross-reactivity of the antibody active site. Arch. Biochem. Biophys., 132:466-469.

_____ H. Schneider, and I. C. P. Smith. 1970a. Spin label studies of oriented phospholipids: Egg lecithin. Biochim. Biophys. Acta, 202:399-402.

_____ H. Schneider, and I. C. P. Smith. 1970b. A spin label study of the effects of cholesterol in liposomes. Chem. Phys. Lipids, 4:238-242.

Hubbell, W. L., and H. M. McConnell. 1968. Spin-label studies of the excitable membranes of nerve and muscle. Proc. Nat. Acad. Sci. U.S.A., 61:12-16.

_____ and H. M. McConnell. 1969a. Motion of steroid spin labels in membranes. Proc. Nat. Acad. Sci. U.S.A., 63:16-22.

_____ and H. M. McConnell. 1969b. Orientation and motion of amphiphilic spin labels in membranes. Proc. Nat. Acad. Sci. U.S.A., 64:20-27.

Hudson, A., and G. R. Luckhurst. 1969. The electron resonance line shapes of radicals in solution. Chem. Rev., 69:191-225.

Hutchison, C. A., Jr., and B. W. Mangum. 1961. Paramagnetic resonance absorption in naphthalene in its phosphorescent state. J. Chem. Phys., 34:908-922.

Ingram, D. J. E. 1969. Biological and Biochemical Applications of Electron Spin Resonance. New York, Plenum Press.

Itzkowitz, M. S. 1967. Monte Carlo simulation of the effects of molecular motion on the EPR spectrum of nitroxide free radicals. J. Chem. Phys., 46:3048-4056.

Jardetsky, O., and C. D. Jardetsky. 1962. Introduction to magnetic resonance spectroscopy methods and biochemical applications. In Glick, D., ed., Methods of Biochemical Analysis, vol. 9:235-410. New York, John Wiley and Sons.

Jost, P. C., U. Brooks, and O. H. Griffith. 1971a. Lipid structures in spin labeled membranes and model membranes: The effect of osmium tetroxide. (in preparation)

_____ L. J. Libertini, V. Hebert, and O. H. Griffith. 1971b. Lipid spin labels in lecithin multilayers. A study of motion along fatty acid chains. J. Molec. Biol., 59:77-98.

_____ A. S. Waggoner, and O. H. Griffith. 1971c. Spin labeling and membrane structure. In Rothfield, L., ed. Structure and Function of Biological Membranes, New York, Academic Press, Inc., pp. 84-144.

Kabat, D., B. Hoffman, and A. Rich. 1970. Synthesis and characterization of a spin-labeled aminoacyl transfer ribonucleic acid. Biopolymers, 9:95-101.

Kawamura, T., S. Matsunami, and T. Yonezawa. 1967. Solvent effects on the g-value of di-t-butyl nitric oxide. Bull. Chem. Soc. Japan, 40:1111-1115.

Keana, J. F. W., S. B. Keana, and D. Beetham. 1967. A new versatile ketone spin label. J. Amer. Chem. Soc., 89:3055.

Keith, A. D., A. S. Waggoner, and O. H. Griffith. 1968. Spin-labeled mitochondrial lipids in *Neurospora crassa*. Proc. Nat. Acad. Sci. U.S.A., 61:819-826.

Klein, M. P., and G. W. Barton, Jr. 1963. Enhancement of signal-to-noise ratio by continuous averaging: Application to magnetic resonance. Rev. Sci. Instrum., 34:754-759.

Kosman, D. J., J. C. Hsia, and L. H. Piette. 1969. ESR probing of macromolecules: function and operation of structural units within the active site of α-chymotrypsin. Arch. Biochem. Biophys., 133:29-37.

Krinitskaya, L. A., E. G. Rozantsev, and M. B. Neiman. 1965. Izv. Akad. Nauk SSSR, Ser. Khim., 1965:115 (cited in Rozantsev, 1970).

Lai, A. A., G. B. Birrell, and O. H. Griffith. 1970. Electron spin resonance study of X-irradiated single crystals of di-n-butyl oxalate-urea and di-n-butyl malonate-urea inclusion compounds. J. Chem. Phys., 53:4399-4400.

Landgraf, W. C., and G. Inesi. 1969. ATP dependent conformational change in "spin labeled" sarcoplasmic reticulum. Arch. Biochem. Biophys., 130:111-118.

Lebedev, O. L., and S. N. Kazarnovskii. 1960. Catalytic oxidation of aliphatic amines with hydrogen peroxide. Zhur. Obschchei Khim., 30:1631-1635.

Leute, R., E. F. Ullman, A. Goldsten, and L. A. Herzenberg. 1971. A rapid new immunoassay technique (FRAT): Determination of morphine by electron spin resonance spectroscopy. Submitted to Science.

Levine, Y. K., and M. H. F. Wilkins. 1971. The structure of oriented lipid bilayers. Nature (London), 230:69-72.

Libertini, L. J., and O. H. Griffith. 1970. Orientation dependence of the electron spin resonance spectrum of di-t-butyl nitroxide. J. Chem. Phys., 53:1359-1367.

———— A. S. Waggoner, P. C. Jost, and O. H. Griffith. 1969. Orientation of lipid spin labels in lecithin multilayers. Proc. Nat. Acad. Sci. U.S.A., 64:13-19.

Luckhurst, G. R. 1966. The structure of Coppinger's radical and its orientation within a cluster of a liquid crystal. Molec. Phys., 11:205-211.

———— and G. F. Pedulli. 1970. Interpretation of biradical electron resonance spectra. J. Amer. Chem. Soc., 92:4738-4739.

McConnell, H. M., W. Deal, and R. T. Ogata. 1969. Spin-labeled hemoglobin derivatives in solution, polycrystalline suspensions, and single crystals. Biochemistry (Washington), 8:2580-2585.

———— and C. L. Hamilton. 1968. Spin-labeled hemoglobin derivatives in solution and in single crystals. Proc. Nat. Acad. Sci. U.S.A., 60:776-781.

———— C. Heller, T. Cole, and R. W. Fessenden. 1960. Radiation damage in organic crystals. I. $CH(COOH)_2$ in malonic acid. J. Amer. Chem. Soc., 82:766-775.

———— and B. G. McFarland. 1970. Physics and chemistry of spin labels. Quart. Rev. Biophys., 3:91-136.

Mildvan, A. S., L. Waber, J. J. Villafranca, and H. Weiner. 1970. Studies of dehydrogenase mechanisms using ADP-tetramethylpiperidine-1-oxy (ADP-R•), a paramagnetic analog of NAD. (Gren Symposium on Structure and Function of Oxidation-Reduction Enzymes, Stockholm, August, 1970.)

———— and H. Weiner. 1969a. Interaction of a spin-labeled analog of nicotinamide-adenine dinucleotide with alcohol dehydrogenase. II. Protein relaxation rate and electron paramagnetic resonance studies of binary and ternary complexes. Biochemistry (Washington), 8:552-562.

———— and H. Weiner. 1969b. Interaction of a spin-labeled analogue of nicotinamide adenine dinucleotide with alcohol dehydrogenase. III. Thermodynamic, kinetic and structural properties of ternary complexes as determined by nuclear magnetic resonance. J. Biol. Chem. 244:2465-2475.

Morrisett, J. D., C. A. Broomfield and B. E. Hackley, Jr. 1969. A new spin label specific for the active site of serine enzymes. J. Biol. Chem., 244:5758-5761.

Ogawa, S., and H. M. McConnell. 1967. Spin-label study of hemoglobin conformations in solution. Proc. Nat. Acad. Sci. U.S.A., 58:19-26.

———— H. M. McConnell, and A. Horwitz. 1968. Overlapping conformation changes in spin-labeled hemoglobin. Proc. Nat. Acad. Sci. U.S.A., 61:401-405.

Ohnishi, S., J. C. A. Boeyens, and H. M. McConnell. 1966. Spin-labeled hemoglobin crystals. Proc. Nat. Acad. Sci. U.S.A., 56:809-813.

———— T. J. R. Cyr, and H. Fukushima. 1970. Biradical spin-labeled micelles. Bull. Chem. Soc. Japan, 43:673-676.

_____ and H. M. McConnell. 1965. Interaction of the radical ion of chlorpromazine with deoxyribonucleic acid. J. Amer. Chem. Soc., 87:2293.

Palmer, G. 1967. Electron paramagnetic resonance. *In* Estabrook, R. W., and M. E. Pullman, eds., Methods in Enzymology, vol. X:594-609. New York, Academic Press.

Poole, C. P., Jr. 1967. Electron Spin Resonance. New York, Wiley/Interscience.

Pooley, D., and D. H. Whiffen. 1961. Electron spin resonance of $(CO_2H)CH_2$ $-CH(CO_2H)$ in succinic acid. Molec. Phys., 4:81-86.

Rassat, A., and P. Rey. 1967. Preparation d'aminoacides radicalaires et de leurs sels complexes. Bull. Soc. Chim. France, 1967:815-817.

Roberts, G. C. K., J. Hannah, and O. Jardetsky. 1969. Noncovalent binding of a spin-labeled inhibitor to ribonuclease. Science, 165:504-506.

Robertson, J. D. 1966. Design principles of the unit membrane. *In* Wolstenholme, G. E. W., and M. O'Connor, eds., Principles of Biomolecular Organization, Ciba Foundation Symposium, 357-408. London, J. & A. Churchill Ltd.

Rottschaefer, S. 1970. Ph. D. thesis, University of Oregon.

Rozantsev, E. G. 1970. Free Nitroxyl Radicals, New York and London, Plenum Press.

_____ V. A. Golubev, and M. B. Nieman. 1965. Izv. Akad. Nauk SSSR, Ser. Khim., 1965, 391-393 (cited in Rozantsev, 1970).

_____ and Yu. V. Kokhanov. 1966. Izv. Akad. Nauk SSSR, Ser. Khim., 8:1477 (cited in Rozantsev, 1970).

_____ and L. A. Krinitskaya. 1965. Free iminoxyl radicals in the hydrogenated pyrrole series. Tetrahedron, 21:491-497.

_____ and M. B. Nieman. 1964. Organic radical reactions involving no free valence. Tetrahedron, 20:131-137.

Schofield, P., B. M. Hoffman, and A. Rich. 1970. Spin-labeling studies of aminoacyl transfer ribonucleic acid. Biochemistry (Washington), 9:2525-2533.

Seelig, J. 1970. Spin label studies of oriented smectic liquid crystals (A model system for bilayer membranes). J. Amer. Chem. Soc., 92:3881-3887.

Seidel, J. C., M. Chopek, and J. Gergely. 1970. Effect of nucleotides and pyrophosphate on spin labels bound to S_1 thiol groups of myosin. Biochemistry (Washington), 9:3265-3272.

Smith, I. C. P. 1968. A study of the conformational properties of bovine pancreatic ribonuclease A by electron paramagnetic resonance. Biochemistry (Washington), 7:745-757.

_____ 1971. The spin label method. *In* Bolton, J. R., D. Borg, and H. Schwartz, eds., Biological Applications of Electron Spin Resonance Spectroscopy. New York, Wiley/Interscience. (in press)

Stone, T. J., T. Buckman, P. L. Nordio, and H. M. McConnell. 1965. Spin-labeled biomolecules. Proc. Nat. Acad. Sci. U.S.A., 54:1010-1017.

Stryer, L., and O. H. Griffith. 1965. A spin-labeled hapten. Proc. Nat. Acad. Sci. U.S.A., 54:1785-1791.

Tonomura, Y., S. Watanabe, and M. Morales. 1969. Conformational changes in molecular control of muscle contraction. Biochemistry (Washington), 8:2171-2176.

Valentine, R. C., and N. M. Green. 1967. Electron microscopy of an antibody-hapten complex. J. Molec. Biol., 27:615-617.

Van, S. P. 1970. (unpublished) University of Oregon, Eugene, Oregon.

Waggoner, A. S., O. H. Griffith, and C. R. Christensen. 1967. Magnetic resonance of nitroxide probes in micelle-containing solutions. Proc. Nat. Acad. Sci. U.S.A., 57:1198-1205.

_____ A. D. Keith, and O. H. Griffith. 1968. Electron spin resonance of solubilized long-chain nitroxides. J. Phys. Chem., 72:4129-4132.

_____ T. J. Kingzett, S. Rottschaefer, O. H. Griffith, and A. D. Keith. 1969. A spin-labeled lipid for probing biological membranes. Chem. Phys. Lipids, 3:245-253.

Weaver, E. C., and H. P. Chon. 1966. Spin label studies in *Chlamydomonas*. Science, 153:301-303.

Weiner, H. 1969. Interaction of a spin-labeled analog of nicotinamide-adenine dinucleotide with alcohol dehydrogenase. I. Synthesis, kinetics, and electron paramagnetic resonance studies. Biochemistry (Washington), 8:526-533.

Wilmshurst, T. H. 1968. Electron Spin Resonance Spectrometers. New York, Plenum Press.

Chapter **8**

Scattered Light Measurement for Molecular Pharmacology

David N. Teller

Associate Research Scientist, Biochemistry, New York State Research Institute for Neurochemistry and Drug Addiction, Wards Island, New York, New York

INTRODUCTION

Some of the most pleasurable memories we retain of natural scenes are due to the effects of light-scattering. Sunsets, auroras, the colors of sea and sky, cloud forms, campfire smoke and the mist over mountain valleys, the softening colors of the desert at dusk, the harvest moon—all are seen, remembered and appreciated emotionally, because they were not observed as sharp line and point displays. These natural phenomena are all examples of light-scattering effects.

However, in the laboratory we are not as likely to sigh with pleasure when a protein solution is not crystal clear.

Useful Light-Scatter

The use and measurement of light-scattering (L.S.) has been fundamental to progress in certain areas of technology. Polymers, paints, fibers, and foods have been developed to display certain effects of L.S. to enhance salability. In other fields, such as long-distance radio communications, weather-mapping by radar, oceanographic studies, and much of modern astronomy, progress depends on measurements of the scatter of electromagnetic radiation, which is very closely related to L.S.

One hundred years ago, Tyndall and Rayleigh developed mathematical descriptions for physical processes of L.S. For the next three generations these developments were almost entirely devoted to the testing of theories concerning the nature of electromagnetic radiation and of devices (primarily optical) used in these studies. However, there were not enough trained investigators available to handle the mathematics and physical measurement problems associated with other L.S. phenomena until synthetic fiber, coating, and food-processing technology expanded in the 1930's. The requirements of aerial photography, penetrating radar, and sonar for small signal amplification, both optical and electronic, provided the technological environment during and after World War II for engineering advances that made modern biochemical L.S. measurement possible. Thus, although the theoretical foundation for L.S. measurement has been available for 100 years, the technique is still in a developmental stage.

Differences Between Scatter and Turbidity

Turbidity and L.S. are terms often interchanged but they are not the same. Before describing their mathematical relationship, and simplifying enormously, the difference may be ascribed to the relative intensity observed. A turbid solution can be thought of as absorbing a fraction of the light so that it does not reach the observer, whereas a scattering solution angularly displaces the incident light. The eye, which integrates light signals over a volume of space, is responsive to scattered light that an electronic photodetector might miss. By moving the photodetector to various distances from the illuminated solution, or by changing the angle between source, solution, and detector, one obtains varying intensities due to refraction and angular dispersion from surfaces, energy dissipation by collision with media, interference by refraction harmonics, and polarization effects. These phenomena can be described mathematically in terms relating to frequency, intensity, phase, and vibrational direction (polarization). Instruments are available that contain the detectors and optics necessary for these angular intensity measurements. However, for certain crude or semiquantitative measurements in experimental problems, a single aspect of the scattered light yields valuable data. In some instances, the observation contains an orbitary multiplicity of the vectors and scalars describing the entire L.S. process. For example, in bacteriological work, the relative growth of the microorganisms in the culture broth is first appreciated by the change in "opalescence" of the medium, long before it becomes turbid. The saturation of protein solutions with ammonium sulfate, crystallization of product from reaction media, immunological response in diffusion plates, suspending ability of surfactants, gel formation, and ultrafiltration all involve some aspects of L.S. measurement. However, most of these processes are allowed to develop into turbidimetric problems, with the loss of much information or time, because L.S. measurement procedures appear unduly difficult or complicated.

Theoretical Background and Terminology

TYNDALL reported in 1869 on the production of light-scattering by aerosols. This type of L.S. is commonly understood to be due to colloidal particles (from approximately 50 to 200 nm), which are smaller than the wavelength of incident light. However, the report of these effects stimulated Lord Rayleigh to publish a large body of theoretical work starting in 1871, which attempted the description of the physical processes involved in L.S.

RAYLEIGH scattering is produced by particles much smaller than the wavelength (λ) of incident light. It is usually attributed to particles whose size is less than $\lambda/20$. If the refractive indexes of particle and medium are close, each discontinuity represents a scattering source for the incident light. These secondary waves do not exactly cancel each other, so that a small amount of the incident light is directed outwards at various angles. A particle which is set into motion by the light will reemit the light with its plane of vibration (the polarization plane) parallel to the axis of the vibration of the particles. This is explained in more detail below.

RAMAN scatter is due to a shift in position by the centers of the molecules, whose electrons produced Rayleigh scatter. The atomic nuclei absorb a tiny fraction of the vibration of the incident light and, by converting it to vibrational energy, permit reemission at a changed frequency.

Therefore, one could arbitrarily divide L.S. phenomena into several theoretical groupings. *Inelastic scattering* produces a frequency shift from the incident to scattered light by molecular resonance (Raman scatter), and by fluorescence. Such a shift in frequency may also be caused by the Doppler effects of the motion of the particles, which may be caused by sonic effects (Brillouin scatter). Inelastic scattering is not covered in this section. Mooradian (1970) has written an excellent brief review of this area related to current laser technology, and Parker (1968) has described the relation of these effects to luminescence in general.

Multiple scattering, defined operationally as the repeated encounters by the particles in the light beam with the incident light, often occurs in situations where neither concentration nor volume can be changed (as in atmospheric and space studies). In the laboratory where small volumes and dilute solutions are available, multiple scattering may readily be identified by its concentration independence. This situation may be considered analogous to "infinitely-thick" radioisotopic preparations.

Single light-scattering is related to concentration by a derivation of the Beer-Lambert equations, described below, and has been described and defined for many media, including solids and gases. For a complete theoretical treatment, see Kerker (1969). Generally, simple L.S. is considered to be due to the single encounter of independent particles with the incident beam of light. The name of Lord Rayleigh is most often associated with this subdivision of L.S., although other notable scientists, Debye, Gans, Lorenz, and Smolochowski, for example, contributed vital theories relating this phenomenon to general electromagnetic field theory. Stacey (1956, 1961) has reviewed the subject of L.S. in relation to physical chemistry and to the measurement of molecular weights and sizes of protein molecules.

Calculations and Measurements Necessary for Full and Formal Description of Light-Scattering

In the simplest case, L.S. by small spherical particles with radii much less than λ, such as an ideal gas of low density, can be related to the theory of linear electric oscillators. The particle reradiates the energy received without changing frequency. The electron motion in the particle is forced by the frequency of the oscillating electric field of the incident light. Although this forcing frequency is not the same as the resonance frequency of the electrons, it does produce another series of harmonics by those electrons that vibrated in the plane of the forcing frequency. The light is scattered by these electrons in planes perpendicular to the electron's vibrational plane so that the scattered light is polarized relative to the incident light. The intensity of scattered light is proportional to the square of the amplitude, because oscillation velocity (at constant frequency and wavelength) increases as the amplitude increases, and the oscillating section of the particle has farther to go in unit time (Bull, 1964). Therefore, since (energy) is proportional to (velocity)^2, the intensity is proportional to (amplitude)^2.

Accurate data are required for the following parameters to describe L.S. by particles in solution or suspension:

(1) The intensity of scattered light (I_s) (or $[I_\theta]$ at various angles (θ) to the incident intensity $[I_0]$), in the presence and absence of scatterer; the distance of scatterer to detector (r), and the wavelength of light being scattered (λ);

(2) The chemical concentration (c) in grams per millimeter or the number of particles (N) per unit volume and the solution light path length (l);

(3) The refractive index of the solvent (n_0) and particles (n), the polarizability of the medium (α) in regard to the ease of displacement of particle electrons in that medium.

Of these parameters, (1) and (2) are incorporated into the experimental and instrumental design, but (3) is obtained indirectly and is described later.

These parameters can be related by various equations. For example it can be shown that

$$(I_\theta r^2/I_0) = 8\pi^4\alpha^2/\lambda^4 (1+\cos^2\theta) \tag{1}$$

in which the left hand term is called Rayleigh's ratio (R_θ), or reduced intensity observed at θ^0 angular displacement to the incident light (Zimm, 1948a,b).

The energy losses from I_0 to the medium by L.S. of particles are related to absorption losses in spectrophotometry by:

$$I = I_0 e^{-\tau l} \tag{2}$$

in which l is the transmission path length. The turbidity function, τ, can be equated to the relative intensities of all the scattered light beams, which are therefore the amount by which I_0 is diminished. R_θ and τ are related when no depolarization of I_s or interference with λ occurs between beams from the various scattering particles. One convenient form is:

$$\tau = 16\pi/3 (R_{90^\circ}) = (8\pi/3) R_\theta \tag{3}$$

For angles other than 90°, the angular dependence of $R_\theta = R_{90^\circ} (1+\cos^2\theta)$.

The amplitude of I_s is proportional to α^2, where α is the polarizability of the medium [see equation (1)]. However, the polarizability of a given medium is related to its optical dielectric constant, which in turn is equal to the square of the refractive index of the medium. In a single equation, therefore:

$$\alpha = (D - D_0)/4\pi N D_0 = (n^2 - n_0^2)/4\pi N n_0^2 \qquad (4)$$

where D_0 = the dielectric constant of the medium; D = the dielectric constant of the particles; N = the number of particles per unit volume; n = the refractive index of the particles in the medium; and n_0 = the refractive index of the medium (Bull, 1964). I_s and I_0 are therefore related to the refractive index increase due to the particles in the solution. This has produced the term, "specific refractive increment," where:

$$I_s = (dn/dc)^2 K I_0 \qquad (5)$$

in which dc is the concentration change, and K is a proportionality constant (Stacey, 1961). I_s is also proportional to the (volume)^2 of the particle and to $1/r^2$. However, I_s/I_0 is a dimensionless number and the proportionality between these two intensities, relating volume and distance, requires the reciprocal of a scalar to the fourth power. This scalar is the wavelength of light, λ, in equation (1).

If I is the light transmitted through a turbid solution, then since $I = I_0 e^{-\tau l}$:

$$\tau = 1/l[\ln(I_0/I)] = K'cM \qquad (6)$$

where K' is a new proportionality constant. Thus, as the molecular weight, M, of the particle increases, L.S. increases per mass unit. The turbidity can be so slight (except for particles larger than $1/20$th of λ) that I_s is more sensitive than I as a measure of c. Then, $K'c/\tau = 1/M$ = the reciprocal of the particle's molecular weight.

In practice, measurements of I_s are made at various angles to I_0, and, for particles with sizes less than $\lambda/20$ (less than approximately 200 angstrom units),

$$K'c/\tau = 1/M + 2K''c \qquad (7)$$

K'' derives from the osmotic pressure description of the solution, an interaction term often referred to as the "second virial," which accounts for the nonideality of the particles as independent units. K'' may be established empirically from osmotic pressure measurements or, more practically, with a known solution of a scattering substance, such as a suspension of colloidal silica (Ludox). Stacey (1961) has described the technical details of this and other procedures necessary for equipment and solution standardization. A graphic plot of $K'c/\tau$ versus c may yield a straight line with $1/M$ = y-intercept and slope = $2K''$. A straight line does not occur, however, when the scattering particles associate (among other reasons).

As the particles become larger, the number of individual refractive or reflective centers per particle increases. Some of these centers reflect towards I_0, some at right angles, and some scatter the light in a forward ($\theta = 180°$) direction. Since I_s varies with the angle of observation, marked departures (dissymmetries) occur from the original spherical distribution of I_s when M increases to a volume greater than 1/20 of the wavelength of the light *in the medium*. This may be measured by the ratio of $I_{45°}/I_{135°}$. Correction factors characteristic of rods, coils, or spheres can be compared to the dissymmetry ratio of the unknown. This in turn will partially correct M, the weight-average molecular weight. If the particles do not associate, M will be constant over a wide range of concentrations when tested by these procedures; see also Sadron and Daune (1962).

In addition, $K'c/\tau_\theta$ plotted versus $\sin^2(\theta/2) + K''c$ can be extrapolated to $\theta = 0$ or $c = 0$, K'' being used to spread out the graphic display. Ideally, both sets of extrapolations will meet at the intercept, $K'c/\tau_0$, when $c = 0$. Then $1/K'c\tau_0$ equals the molecular weight when I_0 is vertically polarized, and is equal to twice the molecular weight when I_0 is unpolarized. Such graphs, called Zimm plots (Zimm 1948a,b), have been used for the determination of molecular weights of aggregating macromolecules.

As the scattering particles become larger, more light is obscured, but forward scatter increases until $I_s(180°) = 0$ at a particle radius $= \lambda/4$. With still larger particles, I_s drops to zero at low values of θ, while $I_s(180°)$ begins to increase again. These maxima and minima in the L.S. envelope can be used to follow changes in particle size. However, if the particle population is heterogeneous, then the various size (volume) functions tend to cancel these reinforcement and interference effects and no maxima or minima occur. This is a test of polydispersity of the particle population. Finally, when τ approaches 0.2, multiple scattering begins to interfere with I_s over much of the angular dispersion, and more complex equations are necessary for description of L.S.

These are only the most fundamental relationships calculated in L.S. studies, and those familiar with the regular equation format will shudder at my oversimplifications and glosses. However, the purpose of this article is to stimulate rather than sedate; more detailed and thorough explanations of the physical measurements are available in Stacey (1956, 1961), Kerker (1969), and Tanford (1961). In the following sections some simple measurements of $I_s(\theta = 90°)$ are described which have been useful in molecular pharmacological studies.

INSTRUMENTATION

Effects of L.S. in Other Optical Measurements

SPECTROPHOTOMETRY. One of the more important uses of L.S. measurements has been in accurate color rendition for dye and paint effects on surfaces. In particular, scattered light from surfaces and yarns is the main subject of a comprehensive book on spectrophotometry by Stearns (1969). Extension of some of the industrial procedures may be useful for laboratory situations: "densitometry" of chromatograms and thin layer plates; analysis of powdered or pelleted formulations that are unstable in solution; preparation of solid standards for quality control; in forensic pharmacology and toxicology—the characterization of fabric stains and biological pigment deposits.

In contrast, turbidity in solutions for spectrophotometric analysis may prevent accuracy. In general, if the observed transmittancy of a solution changes due to variation in the distance to the detector, fluorescence or L.S. may be the source of error. Spectrophotometry of highly scattering solutions is treated elsewhere in this volume. (See also Cowles, 1965.) Latimer and Eubanks (1962) have shown how distorted absorption spectra of the biological suspension can be in simple spectrophotometers. Their report may be of particular value to those using optical measurements of drug effects on hemolysis and erythrocyte stability. However, Walstra (1965) took advantage of the same type of artifacts to determine the optical density of turbid milk fat at various wavelengths.

FLUOROMETRY.   Other spectroturbidimetric determinations related to pharmacological problems will be discussed later, but L.S. per se is not nearly as serious in a spectrophotometer cuvette as in spectrophotofluorometers. The difference in emphasis here between these two optical systems is due to the relative intensities of the observed light. While it may be common to use up to 90% of the incident intensity for spectrophotometry, it is rare that fluorescent quantum efficiency provides one tenth of that intensity for detection. The primary reason for the analytical sensitivity obtainable with fluorescence procedures—that "new" light appears in a "dark" portion of the spectrum—makes this system relatively more sensitive to L.S. effects (Parker, 1968, p. 418). Chen (1966) and Price et al. (1962) have reviewed the problem, and polarizers are usually used to reduce the effects of L.S. in fluorometry. The opposite problem, correction of L.S. intensity for a fluorescence component, can be solved by the methods of Tuzar and Kratochvil (1968).

Scattered light can be an insidious problem in titrations of proteins to measure changes of polarization of protein fluorescence. The excitation and emission wavelengths are close (280 to 300 nm, and 340 to 360 nm, respectively), and because many soluble proteins have low quantum efficiencies (requiring large slits, and therefore a wide spectral band width of activation frequencies), increases in L.S. due to titrant addition often cause the intensity of the "fluorescence" in the parallel mode to appear progressively increased. This is an easily observed artifact if full fluorescence spectra are recorded after each titrant addition. The more resolution of the fluorescence peak from that of the Rayleigh scatter peak in the parallel polarizer configuration is insufficient to prevent an apparent increase in polarization of protein fluorescence from being amplified, because the same scattering also reduces the intensity of excitation light for fluorescence in the horizontal electrical vector. (See also Aronson and Morales, 1969, p. 4518.) In addition, under less severe scattering conditions the optical apertures (resolution of excitation from emission) must be sufficiently discrete to prevent a "shoulder" in the emission display of excitation scatter from increasing the parallel vector intensity of fluorescence, even when the shoulder on the long wavelength side of the scatter peak is initially a small signal. Increases in polarization of fluorescence of protein-bound drugs and dyes are subject to the same artifact during titrations. In general, if (a), the fluorescence intensity observed with the electrical vector parallel to that of excitation appears to increase during a titration while (b), the intensity of fluorescence with the vector perpendicular to that of the polarized excitation remains relatively constant or decreases slightly after each titrant addition, then possible interference by increased L.S. is indicated. This problem is particularly acute if the titrant quenches or dilutes the protein fluorescence, so that any small scattering signal becomes a progressively larger component of the total emission, even when there is no change in the total L.S. during titration.

Two recent examples of this artifact in fluorescence polarization titrations of proteins, where the authors saw the original fluorescence emission spectra, are seen in Figure 5 of Teller et al. (1968), and Figure 3 of González-Rodríguez et al. (1970). In both cases, notation was made that this was an "apparent polarization." In the first case, it was noted that the large values for positive polarization of protein fluorescence were theoretically unverifiable as due solely to fluorescence effects, and it is now apparent that this was largely due to L.S. interference. In the second case, the changes in "fluorescence polarization" that may be free of L.S. artifacts occur at the very start of the titration, and show evidence for a small reproducible alteration in protein structure *prior* to the obscuring effects of the L.S. increase. In both cases, fortunately, the reports emphasize the effects of drugs in altering protein structure. The revised interpretation of a small part of the original data as due to L.S. changes reinforces this emphasis.

Use of a Spectrophotofluorometer for Simple Measurements of L.S. Solutions

As noted above, measurement of I_s ($\theta = 90°$) is a first step in many classical L.S. studies. This can be accomplished with common spectrophotofluorometers as well as with some filter fluorometers (Phillips and Elevitch, 1965) in which the fluorescence is viewed normally to the excitation light beam. A few refinements are useful, such as control of the cuvette temperature, of spectral band width (by filters), and the use of a polarizer in the incident beam to polarize completely the incident light. In many L.S. instruments, the incident beam is purposely *not* polarized since more than double intensity in the cuvette is achieved with randomly oriented light. However, fluorescence excitation beams are vertically polarized by vertical arc light sources, by prism dispersion, and, more importantly, by gratings with vertical rulings, as well as by refraction effects from the edges of narrow slits. Therefore, it may be more useful to polarize the incident light completely in most common spectrophotofluorometers rather than to assume its random nature.[1] In addition, many modifications may be made in existing instruments such as double-

---

[1] Film polarizers may be an inexpensive alternative for instruments lacking prism space. P. C. Schwartz and R. A. Passwater have described the efficiency and transmission characteristics of film polarizers; see Fluorescence News, Vol 4, Nos. 3 and 4, 1969, American Instrument Co.

beam spectrophotometers with commercially available accessories to adapt them for L.S. studies. However, the following sections describe several L.S. measurements performed with the Aminco-Bowman spectrophotofluorometer in essentially unmodified form.

Detection of Proteins and Subcellular Particles

There are numerous uses for simple L.S. detection when monitoring gel column effluents for protein components. Tappan (1966), among others, has described how a spectrophotometer can be used as a nephelometer for this purpose. However, the relatively greater sensitivity of the spectrophotofluorometer to L.S. will routinely permit detection of less than 1 μg protein per ml. The protein need not be fluorescent or monodisperse, and refractive index changes due to variations in elution solvent composition merely add slightly to a large signal. In the author's laboratory, a special ultramicro-flow-cell was constructed inexpensively from commercial quartz tubing so that the fluorescence spectrum of flowing solutions could be monitored. However, a large scatter signal is obtained when only a few particles move through the micro-tube because of the accidentally critical internal dimensions. The L.S. signal is diminished in intensity with larger-bore tubing. Rectangular and square continuous-flow microcuvettes are not as useful for L.S. measurements because of the large reflective surfaces relative to the volume illuminated.

The first use of this simple L.S. measuring system was for the detection of subcellular brain particles in sucrose density gradients after ultracentrifugation. A note on the construction of this flow cell and some results obtained with it has appeared (Teller and Denber, 1969). General Electric type 204 quartz tubing, 0.5 mm i.d. by 1.5 mm o.d., was bent into a "U"-shape so that one leg of the "U" would interrupt the intersection of excitation and fluorescence light paths in the cuvette holder of the Aminco-Bowman. The quartz tubing was cemented into an epoxy-putty block to hold it in position (although a cardboard-mounted prototype worked just as well, until it got wet). Teflon tubing connectors were swaged to the heated quartz. Tubing ends and the joints were encapsulated within the block of putty (Figure 1). A wooden lid was prepared for the cuvette compartment with tubing connections mounted in it, so that lid, tubing and micro flow cell formed a single, removable unit. A standard system was used for pumping the centrifuged gradient contents through the tubing. With this arrangement we have been able to detect and record the sedimentation position of less than 10 μg of particles in a 5 ml sucrose gradient.

The general preparation of subcellular particles from rat cortical gray matter provides 3 to 6 mg of protein in the band of nerve ending particles (NEPs). These are distributed in 3 to 5 ml of approximately molar sucrose (see Figure 2). For the usual protein assay with copper carbonate and Folin-phenol reagent, a final concentration of at least 20 μg per assay tube or 200 μg per ml is desirable. Therefore, a single rat brain NEP preparation perhaps may be diluted only fivefold for treatment in vitro with drugs for binding studies by subsequent gradient centrifugation.

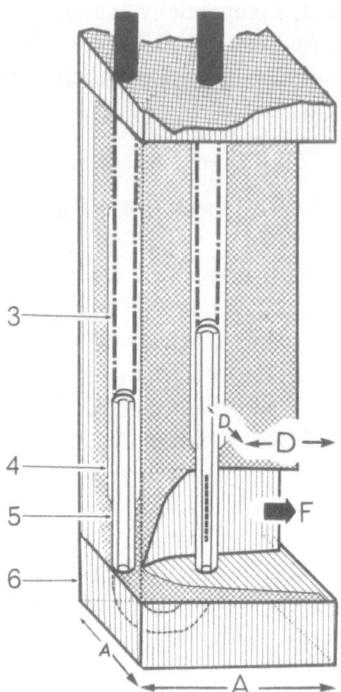

FIG. 1. Scale drawing of a micro pressure resistant flow cell for use in an Aminco-Bowman spectrophotofluorometer.

Dimensions: A=11.8 mm, D=5.9 mm. F is the direction of observing fluorescence, the broken line (— — — — —) is the excitation slit image on the quartz tube. The stainless steel hypodermic tubing (3), indicated by (—·—·), shown in the cut-away view (crosshatched surfaces), is connected to the quartz tube ends (5) by a sleeve of Teflon tubing (4) which is encapsulated in the epoxy putty block (6). Flow can be in either direction, and the author's unit withstood 250 p.s.i. with no leakage. The exact orientation of the optical section is critical and should be carefully adjusted before the casting sets. The entire unit can be dipped into India ink for a nonreflective surface coating, and the optical section of the quarts U-tube is wiped clean with a wet, cotton-tipped applicator stick. A hole drilled into the rear of the block (behind the excitation image position) permits measurements of absorbancy. (From Teller and Denber. 1969. *Fluorescence News*, 4(4):4-6. Courtesy of American Instrument Company.)

This restriction on dilution is required to provide an adequate protein concentration in the sucrose for accurate assays of the protein distribution in the gradient after centrifugation. However, the preparation of the NEPs is time consuming and it is useful to have a detection system for these particles that permits a greater number of experimental gradients to be analyzed rapidly, i.e., to provide data from additional NEP protein:drug combinations or with greater dilutions of protein. The measurement of the L.S. from the particles in the gradient elution profile satisfies these criteria, and the fractions containing these particles can be reproducibly sampled for drug content (see Figure 3).

Changes of NEP sedimentation rate and pattern that are due to the pharmacological effects of an experimental drug can be recorded accurately and with less

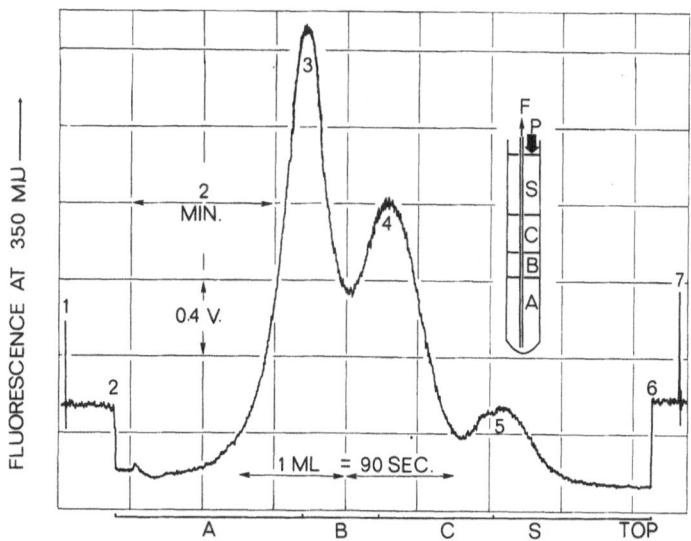

FIG. 2. Analysis of a sucrose density gradient containing subcellular fractions by fluorescence in a quartz U-tube pressure flow cell.

A Moseley 7001-A recorder was used to record the meter multiplier output (all records at 0.001 meter multiplier, 38 sensitivity, 1P-21 p.m. tube). The recorder was set to produce 1 inch Y displacement for each 0.2 v signal. The peristaltic pump (Buchler "Polystaltic") was adjusted to pump 1 ml in 90 seconds. Slit openings were 1/16, ρ, 1/32 in the excitation beam and 1/8, ρ, 3/16 in the emission path (ρ is a Glan-Thompson polarizer prism). The analyzing polarizer was perpendicular to the excitation polarizer. A 3/16-inch slit was used in front of the p.m. tube. The temperature was 20°C.

A suspension (S) of nerve ending particles in 0.8 M sucrose was layered over a discontinuous gradient consisting of 1.2 (A), 1.0 (B) and 0.9 M (C) sucrose that was filtered through charcoal and adjusted to pH 7.2 with Tris buffer. The total volume in the centrifuge tube was 4.9 ml. The tube was centrifuged in an SW-39 rotor at 100,000×g (average) for 75 min in a Beckman/Spinco L2 ultracentrifuge.

The tube contents were pumped at 42 p.s.i. as shown in the inset drawing (which is not to scale). Oil was pumped (P) over the tube contents that were forced up through a steel cannula (F). The 350 nm (mμ) fluorescence excited at 290 nm was recorded at 30 seconds per inch.

Legend for identifying numbers: (1) Pump switched on (electronic noise); (2) Residual air out of quartz U-tube; (3) Nerve ending particles, 1,2-1,0 M sucrose interface; (4) Nerve ending particles, 1.0-0.9 M sucrose interface; (5) Nerve-ending particles, 0.9-0.8 M sucrose interface; (6) Oil has displaced all tube contents (down to base of cannula); (7) Pump switched off. Elapsed time: 7 minutes. The top of peak (3) is distorted because it was redrawn. The pen went off scale and the recorder was switched to 0.5 v per inch until the signal dropped (see Fig. 3, for example).

This solution can not be monitored as easily by absorbancy measurement because of the intense turbidity (the tube contained 6.4 mg protein). The protein concentrations of peaks 3-5 were proportional to the height of the peak. (From Teller and Denber. 1969. *Fluorescence News*, 4(4):4-6. Courtesy of American Instrument Company.)

labor by L.S. than by the usual methods. The latter entails discrete sampling of collected (and pooled) drops, which necessarily must contain a high protein concentration, for chemical determination of the location of the particle band (s). In addition, one can detect reliably the release of small amounts of protein by the particles as they settled into the gradient. These fragments tell something about the stability of the particle population. Needless to say, solutions for L.S. determina-

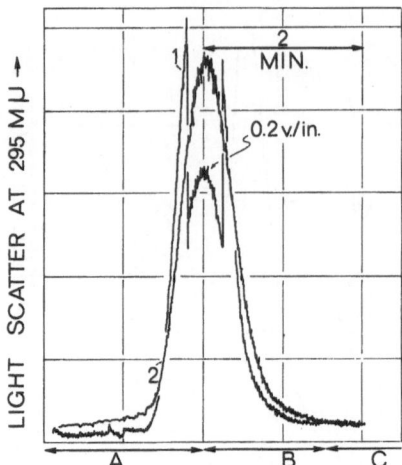

FIG. 3. Analysis of a density gradient containing nerve ending particles by light-scattering in a quartz U-tube pressure flow cell.

The middle portion of the fraction of 1 ml (peak 3, Fig. 2) containing 3.64 mg nerve ending particle protein was diluted with 0.25 M sucrose to produce 0.32 M. Two aliquots were centrifuged again, under the same conditions as noted in the legend to Figure 2. The tubes contained 200 and 100 μg protein. Only one faintly visible band appeared in the tubes after centrifugation, at the 1.2-1.0 M (A-B) interface.

The activation and emission polarizers and cams were set at 295 nm to provide the highest signal possible with a 100 μg per ml reference sample of diluted peak 3 (Fig. 2) in 1.1 M sucrose. Then the aliquots that had been centrifuged again in the density gradient were analyzed by their effects on L.S. For recording 1, the v per inch was set at 0.1 v (as contrasted with 0.2 v in Fig. 2). However, the faint band of particles in the gradient of tube 1, which originally contained 200 μg protein in the sample layer, produced so much scattering that the recorder was "folded" (0.2 v per inch) until the peak passed through. The L.S. of the bands of nerve ending particles from these two aliquots of peak 3 (Fig. 2) indicated 75 and 150 μg protein per ml, compared to the 100 μg per ml reference sample.

These findings indicate that: L.S. increases linearly with small concentrations of nerve ending particles (75 and 150 μg per ml); the procedure of sample handling is reproducible; the relative purity of the center fraction of peak 3 (Fig. 2) is 75%; and L.S. measurement is much more sensitive than fluorometry for this purpose. (From Teller and Denber. 1969. *Fluorescence News*, 4(4):4-6. Courtesy of American Instrument Company.)

tions must be free of large dust or lint particles. They may be clarified by centrifugation (Stacey, 1961) or by ultrafiltration.

Density gradients that contain microsomes, mitochondria, lysosomes, and other subcellular components can also be examined before and after various drug treatments by this method. In a similar way, commercial L.S. detectors are used in flow systems to measure air and water pollution, to record bacterial growth, and generally to monitor filtration processes as in beer-making.

Effects of Phenothiazines on Myosin-B

A valid objection was raised to some of the conclusions drawn in one of the reports cited before (see discussion, Teller et al., 1968), that certain changes in fluorescence parameters might have been due to the aggregation of the particles being titrated with phenothiazine drugs, rather than to change in protein structure. In a subsequent report, therefore, Levine et al. (1968) monitored the L.S. changes throughout the fluorometric titrations of myosin-B with these same drugs. By following L.S. changes at the critical activation wavelengths, the authors were able to show that there was no interference in the fluorescence polarization measurements. The effects of some phenothiazines were to decrease abruptly the observed polarization of myosin-B fluorescence. However, the scatter at the activation wavelength showed only small changes that were not enough to account for the fluorescence changes. Similarly, the possibility was ruled out that the alteration in fluorescence was due to aggregation, which would have greatly increased L.S. In this way, a particularly useful fluorescence titration technique was controlled by L.S. measurement of "artifact." These studies suggest that the phenothiazine drugs may act pharmacologically at very low concentrations by altering the conformation of proteins and subcellular particles.

Effects of Mescaline on Nerve Ending Particles

The weak fluorescence of mescaline in aqueous media, the low concentrations found in rat brains after a dose equivalent to that used clinically (10 mg per kg), and the lack of tight binding of this compound to subcellular particles (Denber, 1967; Denber and Teller, 1968) make the study of the effects of this psychotomimetic amine on brain particle structure difficult. However, the sedimentation pattern of NEPs (recorded by the apparatus described above) appeared to be changed after mescaline treatment in vivo (Teller and Denber, 1970). Not only was 5 to 15% less protein recovered in the NEP band of the gradients after mescaline injection (per rat brain), but the particles just below the original sample position appeared increased in number (Figure 4).

In gradients prepared from the brains of mescaline-treated rats there are indeed great numbers of vesicles, membrane fragments, and NEP debris, trapped within the myelin layer. This upper layer forms at the diffuse boundary formed when the original crude particulate fraction in 0.32 M sucrose is layered over the denser sucrose in the centrifuge tube. Those particles dense enough to settle into the gradient always leave some soluble protein and fragments in this uppermost gradient section. This can be seen in Figure 4 as a relative plateau at the end of the time sequence, when the top layer of the tube contents is finally pumped out through the micro flow cell. However, the preparation used for the experiment shown in Figure 4 had been purified by a previous gradient centrifugation and the myelin contamination was nil.

Gradients prepared from untreated rat brains do not show the fragments from the NEPs in the myelin layer to the same extent as those from mescaline-treated rats. Electron microscope photographs of the gradient bands clearly show this changed distribution of the subcellular material, and preliminary accounts of these findings have been presented (Denber and Teller, 1969, 1970). It appears that

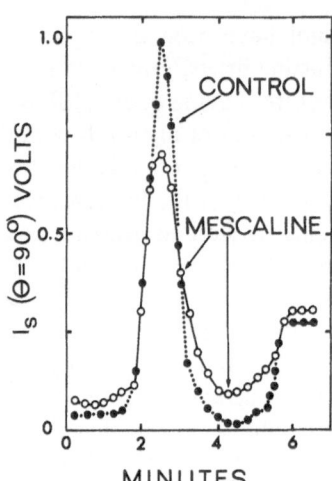

FIG. 4. L.S. profile at 430 nm of density gradients containing NEPs from brains of control and mescaline-treated rats.

The excitation grating was set at 430 nm, slit openings were 1/32, ρ, 1/64; 1/32, ρ, 1/32 on emission side. The NEPs prepared from untreated adult rat brain cortical grey matter (see peak 3, Fig. 2) were resuspended into 0.32 M sucrose at 1.5±0.05 (S.E.M.) mg protein per ml, and 0.6 ml was layered over a gradient containing 2 ml each of 0.8 and 1.2 M sucrose. Similarly, NEPs (1.5 mg protein per ml) prepared in the same way, from a rat that had received 10 mg per kg of mescaline hydrochloride, i.p., 30 min before the brain was removed, were layered over a second gradient. These were centrifuged for two hours at 50,000×g (average). The tube contents were pumped through the micro flow cell without disturbing the mitochondrial pellet. The flow rate was 0.6 ml per minute at 75 p.s.i.

The emission grating was set at 435 nm so that the first aliquots of 1.2 M sucrose, pumped from just above the mitochondrial pellet of the control tube, produced an 80% transmission reading on the meter of the photomultiplier tube amplifier. The recorder was then set at 200 mv per inch, equivalent to a theoretical 400% transmission per inch of y-axis displacement. The chart speed was 15 seconds per inch. The gradient containing the mescaline-treated rat NEPs was scanned 15 minutes later, having been refrigerated meanwhile.

This shows the broadening of the mescaline-NEPs band and the detection of particles from the NEPs remaining in the upper, less dense, 0.8 M sucrose (after about 3 to 5 minutes of flow). This does not occur to the same extent in the gradient from the control animals' NEP preparation. At the point on the L.S. profiles indicated by the *vertical* arrow under "MESCALINE," the control signal (●) was 42% transmission, while the L.S. from the mescaline-treated animal's gradient was 185% (O).

The gradient sections from 2 to 4 minutes after flow started were assayed for proteins. The control NEPs band contained 610±20 μg per ml; the mescaline NEPs contained less, 540±22 μg per ml. Note that in this optical configuration, L.S. is no longer proportional to protein when the scatter exceeds 250% transmission (125 mv). Nevertheless, the L.S. signal is more than two orders of magnitude greater than the fluorescence from the same type of suspension, and shows clear differences between experimental and control, particularly where the protein is too dilute to be assayed chemically.

mescaline injection causes a change in the relative stability of the NEP membrane, as had been postulated on the basis of more indirect evidence (Teller and Denber, 1968). This destabilization of the NEP membrane permits some of the synaptic contents to escape during the separation technique and these remain in the layers above the final NEP band. In addition, determination of norepinephrine per mg protein in the gradient layers indicates an additional release of this catecholamine by the NEPs from treated rat brains as the particles settle into the denser layers of sucrose during centrifugation. This is not observed with NEPs from control animals.

These findings come from studies in progress that were originally stimulated by the indirect evidence of the L.S. profile being changed in the density gradients from treated rats' brains. Attempts to duplicate this effect on the NEPs by mixture with mescaline in vitro are presently only partially successful, and considerable work remains. Nevertheless, had it not been for those L.S. measurements, it might have been much more difficult to postulate a "target" organelle for this hallucinogen.

Interaction of Various Drugs with Proteolipid in Chloroform, Methanol

The proteolipid was soluble in chloroform-methanol (4:1), and attempts to remove it to methanol alone or into aqueous phase only succeeded in denaturing it. Previously it had been shown to bind a variety of radioactive drugs, carrying them through Sephadex LH-20 columns. However, the scarcity (and cost) of radioactive drugs suitable for gel-filtration spurred interest in other methods for demonstrating drug-binding by this proteolipid. In the course of experiments using the Aminco-Bowman for fluorescence polarization measurements, De Robertis et al. (1969) noticed that, after addition of atropine sulfate, the L.S. peak in the fluorescence spectrum shot off scale, while the fluorescence of the solution appeared unchanged. This was exciting because the atropine was being added not as the test drug, but prior to measurements of changes in the polarization of protein fluorescence due to dimethyltubocurarine (DMTC). The latter compound seemed to produce small changes in the fluorescence polarization of the proteolipid, but these were difficult to see, and it was thought that atropine sulfate might produce an amplification of any DMTC effects.

Atropine sulfate markedly increased the L.S. by the proteolipid solution (see also ref. 13 in La Torre et al., 1970), apparently causing micellar aggregation. This ultimately produced a turbid suspension. Other drugs interfered with or accelerated this L.S. effect. It was decided to treat the data as though the proteolipid was an "enzyme," the atropine sulfate was a "substrate," and the resultant L.S. was the "E.S." complex in classical Michaelis-Menten enzyme kinetics. By the test of strong inference, these drugs could be shown to be "competitive" or "uncompetitive inhibitors" of the L.S. formation and, therefore, in contact with the proteolipid.

In common with many real enzymatic reactions, the proteolipid L.S. caused by atropine sulfate showed the following characteristics:

(1) the total L.S. after each aliquot of atropine sulfate was proportional to the concentration increment;
(2) the final L.S. (before turbidity appeared) was proportional to the concentration of proteolipid;
(3) the rate of initial L.S. development after each aliquot of atropine sulfate was proportional to the concentration increment;

(4) addition of a large concentration of another known "substrate," i.e., acetyl-choline, decreased the total intensity of the L.S. ("E.S." concentration was re-duced), but did not affect the rate of L.S. formation;

(5) addition of a known "inhibitor" decreased the rate of L.S. produced by atro-pine sulfate (Figure 5). Other "inhibitors" besides DMTC had less effect. Hexamethonium, succinylcholine, even chlorpromazine interfered with the production of L.S. (De Robertis et al., 1969).

The L.S. measurements were performed in a thermostatted Aminco-Bowman spectrophotofluorometer in standard cm² quartz cuvettes. Narrow slits were used with vertically polarized incident light (410 or 430 nm) to reduce reflection from the cuvette walls. The analyzing polarizer, at $\theta = 90°$ to I_0, was set with its electrical vector vertical (parallel to the excitation vector) and the monochromators were set at 410 or 430 nm, where the Xenon lamp, grating blaze, and 1P-21 or 1P-28 photo-multiplier sensitivity were greatest. Use of this spectral region also prevented any

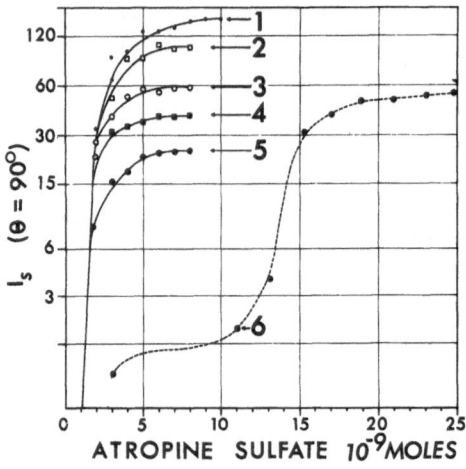

FIG. 5. Light-scattering produced by addition of atropine sulfate to proteolipid in chloroform and methanol (4:1).

Vertically polarized incident light at 410 nm (spectral bandwidth, 13.3 nm) was used to illuminate the cuvette in the Aminco-Bowman spectrophotofluorometer. L.S. intensity increase is recorded on the ordinate after subtracting the initial signal due to proteolipid or other drugs added before the atropine. The abscissa is the nanomoles of atropine sulfate added. Readings were made 40 to 100 seconds after addition of an aliquot of $10^{-3}M$ atropine sulfate. All com-ponents were in the same solvent mixture, 2.0 ml initial volume, at 8°C.

Curve 1 is the increase in L.S. with 8 µg proteolipid protein per ml from bovine cerebral cortex grey matter. Curves 2 and 3 are from cat cerebral cortex grey matter proteolipid at 10.6 and 5.3 µg protein per ml, respectively. Curves 4 and 5 are after 3 min incubation of replicate aliquots of cat proteolipid, at 5.3 µg protein per ml in 5×10^{-5} and $10^{-4}M$ acetylcholine. Curve 6 shows the very different effect of atropine sulfate in the presence of $5 \times 10^{-5}M$ DMTC on the cat proteolipid, also at 5.3 µg protein per ml.

Data are from previously unpublished experiments of October 1968, performed in collabo-ration with Prof. De Robertis and Dr. González-Rodríguez (Faculty of Medicine, Univ. Buenos Aires) during the author's visit. Subsequently, additional experimental data were published; see De Robertis et al. 1969.

possibility of absorption changes interfering with L.S. measurements, since at wavelengths below 360 nm solvent changes caused slight absorption artifacts. One other technical detail became crucial: cuvette cleaning. The usual nitric acid soaking of the cuvettes left a deposit in the corners that completely blocked any further L.S. reactions with new proteolipid solutions. The following less hazardous and more rapid cleaning procedure solved the problem: The cuvette was half filled with concentrated aqueous detergent and pure methanol was added. This procedure precipitated detergent onto the walls in an opaque layer. The deposit was immediately rinsed out with water followed by methanol, which then rapidly evaporated.

In this configuration the Aminco-Bowman was very sensitive to the turbidity that developed at the end of the L.S. titrations. In the author's laboratory these experiments were repeated in a Cary 14R spectrophotometer, using split cells as follows: Atropine sulfate was added to the reference cell chamber nearest to the detector at the concentrations used in the fluorescence cuvette and to both of the chambers of the split cell in the sample side of the Cary. In the other half of the reference cell the proteolipid was placed at a concentration equal to double that in the other two cuvettes. Using an expanded scale for optical density, and scanning from 300 to 1,000 nm, there was no change in absorption in the sample cell of the Cary (containing proteolipid *mixed* with atropine sulfate) until the L.S. stopped increasing in the parallel titration in the Aminco-Bowman. When the optical density in the Cary reached only 0.030 above the unmixed reference cell, the signal from the L.S. dropped by 8%. After this point was reached, additional atropine sulfate increased the optical density and further decreased the L.S. intensity in the fluorometer.

The rate of L.S. formation in the presence of various drugs was analyzed by Hill plots. In this method, the log of (L.S. increase per aliquot of atropine sulfate/ total L.S. achieved at the end of the titration) was plotted against the log of (atropine sulfate concentration after the aliquot was mixed in the cuvette). This method has recently been used by Levitzki and Koshland (1969) and compared to Michaelis-Menten and double-reciprocal graphs. In this type of graph, positive cooperativity between ligands is reflected by steeply positive slopes (Hill coefficient greater than 1). For the control reaction, without any other drug except atropine sulfate, the proteolipid L.S. produced a Hill coefficient of 3 to 3.5. In the presence of a strong inhibitor, such as DMTC, the coefficient was 8.6, while high concentrations of succinylcholine and hexamethonium (10^{-3} M) also gave values of 6.4 to 7.5, indicating a greater positive cooperativity of binding with the proteolipid than atropine sulfate, alone, showed. In contrast, acetyl choline produced a Hill coefficient of only 3.4 at 5×10^{-3} M, indicating that this concentration of the natural "substrate" was approximately equivalent in affinity to the proteolipid in the presence of atropine sulfate as the standard 1 to 2×10^{-6} M atropine sulfate was by itself. The drugs other than atropine sulfate often caused some small L.S. at the start of the titration, and since the various preparations of the proteolipid also showed slight initial differences, the concentrations and Hill coefficients were calculated at the point where the maximal L.S. occurred (De Robertis et al., 1969).

The aggregation and L.S. effect can also be produced by some other base-

sulfates; for example, mescaline hemisulfate. In addition, sulfates of eserine, strych-
nine, dibenzylamine, and amphetamine, but not those of aniline or betaine, produce
some L.S. with the proteolipid (De Robertis, personal communication; González-
Rodríguez et al., 1970). Neither the free bases themselves nor equivalent concentrations of sulfate or sulfuric ions caused the L.S. changes. Indeed, sulfuric acid,
at 1 to 5 microequivalents per ml, causes a reduction of any L.S. that resulted
from previous additions of atropine or mescaline sulfates. Conductometric titrations
of this proteolipid or the solvent alone with atropine sulfate showed that the
impedance of the solutions increased. This indicates that perhaps changes in electrostatic interactions are responsible for the initiation of the L.S. effect (González-
Rodríguez et al., 1970).

The L.S. reaction with atropine sulfate was fairly specific for the proteolipid
fraction that originally showed sensitive and tight binding capability for DMTC.
Other brain proteolipids responded with L.S. changes to the addition of atropine
sulfate, but much higher concentrations of the drug were necessary to initiate the
effect. Additional studies with a similar proteolipid preparation from the electric
organ of *Torpedo* and *Electrophorus* by La Torre et al. (1970), which does not
scatter light when atropine sulfate is added, show that the reaction of the brain
proteolipids is not universal. However, the possibility exists for studying other
proteolipids with suitable drugs by L.S. techniques. These materials are in mixed
solvents that are poorly defined, the chloroform absorbs strongly in the U.V., and
they are therefore not the ideal subjects for classical optical spectroscopic techniques. A thorough study of L.S. by bovine white matter proteolipid, by Zand
(1968), indicates solutions to some of these experimental problems when the
solvent composition can be specified exactly.

Other Molecular Associations, Micelle, and Aggregate Formation

Numerous other pharmacological studies of a complexity midway between
those for formal L.S. measurements of molecular weight and simple nephelometer
readings have been performed using L.S. techniques. Eye-lens protein response in
vitro to drugs and chemicals has been the subject of papers by Iwata and colleagues at Kyoto University (Iwata, 1964; Nakagaki et al., 1964, 1965). Tonomura
et al. (1967) studied the effects of synthetic ATP analogs in actomyosin systems to
clarify the role of the base, ribose, and triphosphate moieties.

In addition to investigations related to pharmacology by use of drugs or other
chemicals, a larger group of reports in biochemical and biophysical areas deals
with the nature of conformational changes in proteins and other macromolecules.
Denaturation of milk caseins (Dreizen et al., 1962), isoelectric aggregation of
ovalbumin (Tomimatsu, 1965), and ribonuclease (Rimai et al., 1970), salt polymerization of tropomyosin (Ooi et al., 1962), and renaturation of collagen (Kuhn
et al., 1964) illustrate the range of the use of L.S. techniques for studies of protein
solutions. Timasheff (1964) and Sadron (1966) reviewed some of the earlier

investigations using L.S. that were concerned with intramolecular forces and thermodynamics of interacting biological macromolecules in solution.

Conformational Changes of Subcellular Particles and Proteins

Perhaps the most challenging area for L.S. measurement is the study of conformational changes in subcellular particles relating to physiological function. Included here are conformational and allosteric effects due to ion and water flow, drugs, poisons, and substrate metabolism. The recent literature is abundant. Chance and Lee (1969) used nonspecific L.S. in conjunction with the fluorescent probe, 1,8-ANS, for lifetime kinetics of beef-heart mitochondrial membrane electron transport and energy coupling response to oligomycin, $SCN^-, I^-, Tris-NO_3^-$, perchlorate, and pentachlorophenol. Green et al. (1968) correlated the variation in L.S. due to mitochondrial inner membrane conformational changes with the electron microscopic structure. They conclude that conditions suited for generating or deenergizing the "energized-twisted" configuration shown in photographs produced marked effects on L.S. Respiratory inhibitors, uncouplers, and ADP all reversed L.S. changes occurring during the production of the "energized" configuration. This technique has been a powerful tool in the controversy concerning membrane structure during transport processes (Harris et al., 1969a,b).

Neurochemists and neuropharmacologists also have employed L.S. techniques with subcellular brain particles. Kamino and Inouye (1969) reviewed L.S. effects from rabbit brain microsomes in response to ionic and osmotic change, and Kamino (1969) reported the use of L.S. for studying the chemical dissection of the Na^+, K^+-dependent ATPase. Robinson (1967) also reviewed earlier studies. Keen and White (1970) described the osmometric behavior of NEPs in NaCl and their permeability to glucose, glycerol, thiourea, formamide, propylene glycol, and dimethyl sulfoxide. These organelles appear impermeable in vitro to Ca^{2+}, Mg^{2+}, PO_4^{2-}, SO_4^{2-}, and oxalate ions. L.S. measurements during these experiments defined the mean NEP osmotic volumes. Tasaki et al. (1968) recently studied whole nerve trunks of invertebrates using measurements of L.S., 1,8-ANS fluorescence, and birefringence. Changes in all of these parameters were associated with the electrogenic stimulation of the nerve.

In microbiology and botany, L.S. has been used to study transport and function of small biological particles. Bateman (1968) used *S. marcescens* and reviewed much of the recent literature relating to L.S., particularly multiple L.S., in bacteriological investigations. Wolf and Marcus (1969) showed that *Mycoplasma laidlawii* growth in liquid culture could be continuously followed with great savings in time and labor by using an L.S. method. This permits measurements of growth-rate differences during the growth course, rather than after the usual three-day wait for colony development, even in the presence of other scattering sources in the media, such as serum. A mechanized bacteria counter, described by Bowman et al (1968), operates by detecting L.S. *changes* in capillary tubes filled with semisolid media which have new or growing colonies.

In botanical physiology there are many reports of L.S. determinations. Packer (1962) employed chloroplast fragments, while Hind and Jagendorf (1965) used the entire organelle for photophosphorylation studies. Mukohata (1966) and Mukohata et al. (1966) investigated the effects of actinic irradiation on ion transport using L.S. from chloroplast suspensions. With this technique, Karlish and Avron (1969) demonstrated that Mg^{2+} binding produces the fall in steady-state L.S. that occurs during photophosphorylation. Bryant et al. (1969) have reviewed the theoretical and experimental problems associated with L.S. techniques in areas of study using yeast and chloroplast suspensions. These citations are only a few examples to show the range of subjects capable of study by L.S. techniques in fields that may be of interest to pharmacologists.

Scattered light has been used classically, as a means of gathering data on size and shape of macromolecules, and the literature is more abundant in this context. For example, there are the reports on helix-coil transitions. All of the following subjects were studied with L.S. techniques: RNA (Millar and Steiner, 1966), bovine serum albumin and creatine phosphotransferase (Friedberg and Ohman, 1963), and DNA (Eskin and Korotkina, 1965; Sharp and Bloomfield, 1968; Gruber and Schurz, 1969).

Other substances with heterogeneous or weak optical absorption have been investigated using L.S. Amylose and amylopectin (Banks et al., 1969), milk fat globules (Walstra, 1965), low density lipoproteins in serum (Stone and Thorp, 1966), and ultrasonically disrupted lecithin phospholipid micelles (Attwood and Saunders, 1965) are just a few examples.

POSSIBLE FUTURE APPLICATIONS FOR L.S. MEASUREMENTS IN MOLECULAR PHARMACOLOGY

Orientation of Solvent Molecules Around Drug-Treated Proteins

Some of the L.S. changes associated with drug-treated proteins, nucleic acids, and polysaccharides probably result from orientation changes in their electrostatic halo of water molecules and ions. This suggests that allosteric changes may be monitored by measurement of changes in n, the particle refractive index in the medium. Such changes, leading to variations in L.S., are more sensitive indicators than dye-probe or most other spectroscopic tools due to the relatively low concentrations of scattering particles required in L.S. methods. For example, in the proteolipid experiments, the usual protein concentration in the cuvette was only 4 to 30 μg per ml, while the atropine sulfate was added in microliter increments of millimolar stock solution. In contrast, at least 50 to 100 μg of protein per ml was required to measure the fluorescence of the proteolipid.

It would be helpful to know whether the solvent, in which the proteolipid is stable under refrigeration for more than eight months, duplicates the native electrostatic environment of the proteolipid in the cell membrane. A knowledge of the particular environment in vitro that permits duplication of the in vivo pharmacological reactivity may help to explain the functional cytoarchitecture of excitable membranes.

In the same manner, cooperative interactions between macromolecules that are based on the exclusion of intervening solvent may be studied conveniently by L.S. For example, Friedberg and Ohman (1963) demonstrated that dilute proteins in water-organic solvent mixtures underwent helix-coil transitions related to the relative solvent polarity prior to aggregation. As the concentration of protein increased, aggregation occurred more rapidly at increasing polarity.

Kinetic and Thermodynamic Studies

COMPLEX FORMATION IN EXTREMELY DILUTE SOLUTIONS. One of the advantages of L.S. measurements over many other spectroscopic methods is that high concentrations are unnecessary, particularly when aggregation or complex formation occurs. Millar and Steiner (1966) demonstrated that Mg^{2+} was involved with the helix-coil transitions of sRNA by showing a time-dependent aggregation which occurred in the presence of this ion in KCl-KOAc, and a reduced effect of Mg^{2+} in KCl alone. They concluded "that sRNA exists largely in associated form at 25° in $0.02M$ Mg^{2+} at concentrations >2 mg/ml." Such association not only interferes with other methods of molecular weight determination, but also is not easily detected by those methods. The degree of graphic aberration from the theoretical Zimm plot described above can be tested mathematically and corrected by alterations to the interaction term. A numeric expression of nonindependence of particles results, that can be tested experimentally to determine to what degree other solute or solvent parameters affect this same term. This is most conveniently performed by small calculator-computers with graphic display, and there are several of these now marketed. This L.S. technique may advance faster, now that the calculation tedium is avoidable. However, all of the above possible uses of L.S. measurements can be gathered into one general area, briefly discussed below.

UTILIZATION OF LIGANDS THAT ARE RELATIVELY INACTIVE OR COMPLEX OPTICALLY. Included here are substances of such complex composition that the usual spectroscopic or luminescence parameters are ill-defined. The effects of mescaline on NEPs and of atropine sulfate on proteolipid in mixed solvent are examples described before. Jerrard and Jennings (1966) used L.S. to study the effects of orienting electrical fields on macromolecules that were presumed to have either electronic anisotropies or permanent dipole moments. Bentonite, tobacco mosaic virus, poly-γ-benzyl-L-glutamate, and poly-L-proline were studied by analysis of Zimm plots obtained from data of L.S. with and without an electrical field. The results from poly-L-proline, for example, show that it consisted of flexible molecules with a permanent dipole moment.

The efficiency of energy transfer to ultrasonically irradiated lecithin solutions was followed by Attwood and Saunders (1965) with L.S. measurements during sonication. The asymmetrical aggregates were gradually broken down to symmetrical, stable particles with molecular weight ca. 2×10^6. Hind and Jagendorf (1965) followed L.S. change in response to flash irradiation of chloroplasts and discovered that the high-energy state in chloroplasts was not a simple kinetic form. Similarly, the L.S. measurements of Onishi et al. (1968) on myosin-ATP complexes indicate that the decrease in L.S. of actomyosin caused by ATP is one of the most rapid of the kinetic parameters in association or hydrolysis reactions with this macromolecule. Davis (1967) modified the Aminco-Bowman to provide a turbidimetric method for measuring platelet aggregation kinetics in a rotating Chandler tube of plastic. As the clot formed, increases in the L.S. and decreased transmission to the photomultiplier tube presented a continuous record of the reaction kinetics involved with thrombus formation in vitro.

In summary, although the formal expression of L.S. in mathematical and thermodynamic terms may be a formidable task, simplified L.S. measurements may be useful to identify interfering artifacts in other optical systems, to measure and record the association of dilute ligands, and to detect particles that are relatively inactive or complex, optically.

ACKNOWLEDGMENTS

The author is very grateful for the gracious hospitality of Dr. and Sra. Eduardo DeRobertis, Director, Instituto de Anatomía General y Embriología, Facultad de Medicina, Universidad de Buenos Aires, Argentina, during his visits while on leave from the New York State Department of Mental Hygiene. In addition, special thanks to Dr. José L. La Torre and his skilled associates for the many (seemingly endless) preparations of proteolipid. These investigations were supported in part by the New York State Department of Mental Hygiene and the Consejo Nacional de Investigaciones Científicas y Técnicas, Argentina.

REFERENCES

Aronson, J. F., and M. F. Morales. 1969. Polarization of tryptophan fluorescence in muscle. Biochemistry (Washington), 8: 4517-4522.

Attwood, D., and L. Saunders. 1965. A light-scattering study of ultrasonically irradiated lecithin sols. Biochim. Biophys. Acta, 98: 344-350.

Banks, W., C. T. Greenwood, and J. Sloss. 1969. Light-scattering studies on aqueous solutions of amylose and amylopectin. Carbohyd. Res., 11: 399-406.

Bateman, J. B. 1968. Osmotic responses and light scattering of bacteria. J. Colloid Interface Sci., 27: 458-474.

Bowman, R. L., P. Blume, and G. G. Vurek. 1968. Capillary-tube scanner for mechanized microbiology. Science, 158: 78-83.

Bryant, F. D., P. Latimer, and B. A. Seiber. 1969. Changes in total light scattering and absorption caused by changes in particle conformation. Test of theory. Arch. Biochem. Biophys., 135: 109-117.

Bull, H. B. 1964. An Introduction to Physical Biochemistry. New York, F. A. Davis.

Chance, B., and C.-P. Lee. 1969. Comparison of fluorescence probe and light-scattering readout of structural states of mitochondrial membrane fragments. Fed. Eur. Biochem. Soc. Lett., 4:181-184.

Chen, R. F. 1966. Reduction of light scatter in fluorometry by the use of horizontally polarized excitation. Anal. Biochem., 14:497-499.

Cowles, J. C. 1965. Theory of dual-wavelength spectrophotometry for turbid samples. J. Opt. Soc. Amer., 55:690-693.

Davis, R. B. 1967. Turbidimetric evaluation of platelet aggregation in the Chandler tube. Techn. Bull. Regist. Med. Techn., 37:127-131.

Denber, H. C. B. 1967. Intracellular localization of psychotomimetic and psychotropic drugs. Ph.D. Thesis, New York University.

_____ and D. N. Teller, 1968. Studies on mescaline XIX: A new theory concerning the nature of schizophrenia. Psychosomatics, 9:145-151.

_____ and D. N. Teller. 1969. Mescaline XXI: Subcellular localization in adult rats. The Pharmacologist, 11(2):291.

_____ and D. N. Teller. 1970. Subcellular localization of mescaline at the synapse. Arzneimittel-Forschung, 20:903-905.

DeRobertis, E., J. González-Rodríguez, and D. N. Teller. 1969. The interaction between atropine sulphate and a proteolipid from cerebral cortex studied by light scattering. Fed. Eur. Biochem. Soc. Lett., 4:4-8.

Dreizen, P., R. W. Nobel, and D. F. Waugh. 1962. 1962. Light-scattering studies of $\alpha_{s1,2}$-caseins. J. Amer. Chem. Soc., 84:4938-4943.

Eskin, V. E., and O. Z. Korotkina. 1965. Light scattering by solutions of native, denatured, and degraded DNA. Biofizika, 10:26-31.

Friedberg, F., and J. Ohman. 1963. Light-scattering measurements on proteins in water-organic solvent mixtures. Acta Chem. Scand., 17:1794-1796.

González-Rodríguez, J., J. L. La Torre, and E. DeRobertis. 1970. The interaction between atropine sulfate and a proteolipid from cerebral cortex studied by polarization of fluorescence. Molec. Pharmacol., 6:122-127.

Green, D. E., J. Asai, R. A. Harris, and J. T. Penniston. 1968. Conformational basis of energy transformations in membrane systems. III. Configurational changes in the mitochondrial inner membrane induced by changes in functional states. Arch. Biochem. Biophys., 125:684-705.

Gruber, E., and J. Schurz. 1969. Light-scattering measurements with native DNA. Monatsh. Chem., 100:419-426.

Harris, R. A., M. A. Asbell, J. Asai, W. W. Jolly, and D. E. Green. 1969a. Conformational basis of energy transduction in membrane systems. V. Measurement of configuration changes by light scattering. Arch. Biochem. Biophys., 132:545-560.

_____ M. A. Asbell, and D. E. Green. 1969b. Correlation between light-scattering changes and the energy state of phosphorylating submitochondrial particles. Arch. Biochem. Biophys., 131:316-318.

Hind, G., and A. T. Jagendorf. 1965. Light scattering changes associated with the production of a possible intermediate in photophosphorylation. J. Biol. Chem., 240:3195-3201.

Iwata, S. 1964. Biophysicochemical studies on phenoxazone compounds. VI. Precipitation titration of soluble protein in lens cortex by light scattering method. Yakugaku Zasshi, 84:435-440.

Jerrard, H. G., and B. R. Jennings. 1966. Light scattering by macromolecular solutions subjected to electric fields. Amer. Chem. Soc., Div. Polymer Chem., Preprints, 7:1184-1186.

Kamino, K. 1969. Light-scattering studies on rabbit brain microsomes. II. Effects of ATP chelation of Mg^{2+} on microsomal contraction. Biochim. Biophys. Acta, 183:48-57.

_____ and A. Inouye. 1969. Light-scattering studies on rabbit brain microsomes. I. Evidence for osmotic behavior. Biochim. Biophys. Acta, 183:36-47.

Karlish, S. J. D., and M. Avron. 1969. Effect of phosphorylating conditions on photo-induced changes in light scattering. Photosynthetica, 3:79-82.

Keen, P., and T. D. White. 1970. A light-scattering technique for the study of the permeability of rat brain synaptosomes *in vitro*. J. Neurochem., 17:565-571.

Kerker, M. 1969. The Scattering of Light and Other Electromagnetic Radiation. New York, Academic Press.

Kuhn, K., J. Engel, B. Zimmerman, and W. Grassmann. 1964. Renaturation of collagen. III. Reorganization of native collagen molecules from completely separated units. Arch. Biochem. Biophys., 105:387-403.

Latimer, P., and C. A. H. Eubanks. 1962. Absorption spectrophotometry of turbid suspensions: A method of correcting for large systematic distortions. Arch. Biochem. Biophys., 98:274-285.

La Torre, J. L., G. S. Lunt, and E. DeRobertis. 1970. Isolation of a cholinergic proteolipid receptor from electric tissue. Proc. Nat. Acad. Sci. U.S.A., 65:716-720.

Levine, R. J. C., D. N. Teller, and H. C. B. Denber. 1968. Binding of chlorpromazine and thioproperazine *in vitro*. III. Fluorometric measurement of changes in *Limulus polyphemus* (horseshoe crab) myosin-B structure and enzyme activity after treatment with phenothiazine drugs. Molec. Pharmacol., 4:435-444.

Levitzki, A., and D. E. Koshland, Jr. 1969. Negative cooperativity in regulatory enzymes. Proc. Nat. Acad. Sci. U.S.A., 62:1121-1128.

Millar, D. B., and R. F. Steiner. 1966. The effect of environment on the structure and helix-coil transition of soluble ribonucleic acid. Biochemistry (Washington), 5:2289-2301.

Mooradian, A. 1970. Laser Raman spectroscopy. Science, 169:20-25.

Mukohata, Y. 1966. Biophysical studies on subcellular particles. III. On the light scattering pattern of spinach chloroplast suspension. Ann. Rep. Biol. Works Fac. Sci. Osaka Univ., 14:121-134.

_____ M. Mitsudo, and T. Isemura. 1966. Biophysical studies on subcellular particles. II. Reduction of the amount of accumulated protons and the light scattering response of spinach chloroplasts by alkaline solution. Ann. Rep. Biol. Works Fac. Sci. Osaka Univ., 14:107-119.

Nakagaki, M., N. Koga, and S. Iwata. 1964. Light scattering titration of lens proteins. Chem. Pharm. Bull. (Tokyo), 12:848-850.

_____ N. Koga, and S. Iwata. 1965. Effects of catalin and its analogous phenoxazone compounds on lens proteins. Nippon Ganka Gakkai Zasshi, 69:1489-1496.

Onishi, H., H. Nakamura, and Y. Tonomura. 1968. Pre-steady state of the myosin-adenosine triphosphate system. VII. Kinetic studies on the decrease in light-scattering of actomyosin induced by ATP. J. Biochem. (Tokyo), 64:769-784.

Ooi, T., K. Mihashi, and H. Kobayashi. 1962. The polymerization of tropomyosin. Arch. Biochem. Biophys., 98:1-11.

Packer, L. 1962. Light-scattering changes correlated with photosynthetic phosphorylation in chloroplast fragments. Biochem. Biophys. Res. Commun., 9:355-360.

Parker, C. A. 1968. Photoluminescence of Solutions. New York, Elsevier.

Phillips, R. E., and F. R. Elevitch. 1965. Protein-monitoring columns. Traces, 4:45. (Published by G. K. Turner Assoc.)

Price, J. M., M. Kaihara, and H. K. Howerton. 1962. Influence of scattering on fluorescence spectra of dilute solutions obtained with the Aminco-Bowman spectrophotofluorometer. Appl. Optics, 1:521-533.

Rimai, L., J. T. Hickmott Jr., T. Cole, and E. B. Carew. 1970. Quasi-elastic light scattering by diffusional fluctuations in RNase solutions. Biophys. J., 10:20-37.

Robinson, J. D. 1967. Structural changes in microsomal suspensions. V. Interactions with nucleotides. Arch. Biochem. Biophys., 118:649-658.

Sadron, C. 1966. Configuration of macromolecules in solution. Methods of Study. I. Macromolecules. Acta Haemat. (Basel), 36:63-88.

_____ and M. Daune. 1962. Determination of mass, form and dimensions of large particles in solution. *In* Florkin, M., and E. H. Stotz, eds., Comprehensive Biochemistry, Vol. 3, 265-310. New York, Elsevier.

Sharp, P., and V. A. Bloomfield. 1968. Light-scattering from worm-like chains with excluded volume effects. Biopolymers, 6:1201-1211.

Stacey, K. A. 1956. Light-Scattering in Physical Chemistry. London, Butterworth.

_____ 1961. The use of light-scattering for the measurement of the molecular weight and size of proteins. *In* Alexander, P., and R. J. Block, eds., A Laboratory Manual of Analytical Methods of Protein Chemistry, Vol. 3, 246-275. Oxford and New York, Pergamon Press.

Stearns, E. I. 1969. The Practice of Absorption Spectrophotometry. New York, Wiley/Interscience.

Stone, M. C., and J. M. Thorp. 1966. A new technique for the investigation of the low-density lipoproteins in health and disease. Clin. Chim. Acta, 14:812-830.

Tanford, C. 1961. *In* Physical Chemistry of Macromolecules, 275-316. New York, John Wiley & Sons.

Tappan, D. V. 1966. A light scattering technique for measuring protein concentration. Anal. Biochem., 14:171-182.

Tasaki, I., A. Watanabe, R. Sandlin, and L. Carnay. 1968. Changes in fluorescence, turbidity, and birefringence associated with nerve excitation. Proc. Nat. Acad. Sci. U.S.A., 61:883-888.

Teller, D. N., and H. C. B. Denber. 1968. Defining schizophrenia with the techniques of molecular biology. Dis. Nerv. Syst., 29:93-112.

_____ and H. C. B. Denber. 1969. Increasing the utility of spectrophotofluorometers with inexpensive accessories. II. Macro and microflow cuvettes (cells). Fluorescence News, 4(4):4-6.

_____ and H. C. B. Denber. 1970. Mescaline and phenothiazines: Recent studies on subcellular localization and effects upon membranes. *In* Lajtha, A., ed., Protein Metabolism of the Nervous System, 685-697. New York, Plenum Press.

_____ R. Levine, and H. C. B. Denber. 1968. Binding of chlorpromazine and thioproperazine, in vitro. II. Fluorometric measurement of stoichiometry and alteration of protein structure. Agressologie, 9:167-187.

Timasheff, S. N. 1964. Light and small-angle X-ray scattering and biological macromolecules. J. Chem. Educ., 41:314-320.

Tomimatsu, Y. 1965. A light-scattering study of the aggregation of ovalbumin near its isoelectric pH. Biochim. Biophys. Acta, 94:525-534.

Tonomura, Y., K. Imamura, M. Ikehara, H. Uno, and F. Harada. 1967. Interaction between synthetic ATP analogs and actomyosin systems. IV. J. Biochem. (Tokyo), 61:460-472.

Tuzar, Z., and P. Kratochvil. 1968. Light scattering. XIX. Correction for fluorescence. Coll. Czech. Chem. Commun., 33:3381-3383.

Walstra, P. 1965. Light scattering by milk fat globules. Netherlands Milk Dairy J., 19:93-109.

Wolf, J. P., and L. Marcus. 1969. Rapid determination by light scattering of growth parameters of *Mycoplasma laidawii* in liquid media. Appl. Microbiol., 18:4-7.

Zand, R. 1968. Solution properties and structure of brain proteolipids. Biopolymers, 6:939-953.

Zimm, B. H. 1948a. The scattering of light and the radical distribution function of high polymer solutions. J. Chem. Phys., 16:1093-1099.

_____ 1948b. Apparatus and methods for measurement and interpretation of the angular variation of light scattering. J. Chem. Phys., 16:1099-1116.

Chapter **9**

The Spectrophotometric Measurement of Turbid Suspensions of Cytochromes Associated with Drug Metabolism[1]

Ronald W. Estabrook,[2] Julian Peterson, Jeffrey Baron, and Alfred Hildebrandt[3]

Department of Biochemistry, University of Texas (Southwestern) Medical School at Dallas, Dallas, Texas

INTRODUCTION

Optical spectrophotometry, a technique of high precision and wide application, has a significant role in biomedical research. In general pharmacologists have restricted the use of spectrophotometry to the characterization of substrates or products. In addition, the kinetics of a reaction which involves modification of a chromophoric group during the time course of a reaction can be studied by spectrophotometric techniques. A multitude of commercial instruments are available for these types of studies, and such instruments frequently incorporate simplicity of design and operation permitting their routine application in the laboratory. However, most commercial spectrophotometers are limited to the study of the spectral properties of pigments present in nonturbid solutions. Frequently, extension of these methods to turbid suspensions is unsuccessful because of limitations imposed by the geometry of design of the instrument and the low sensitivity of the system for detecting transmitted light.

[1] Supported in part by U.S.P.H.S. Grants 1 P11 GM 16488 and AM13366 and a Grant (I-405) from the Robert A. Welch Research Foundation, Houston, Texas.
[2] The Virginia Lazenby O'Hara Professor of Biochemistry
[3] Institut für Klinische Pharmakologie
der Freien Universität Berlin
1 Berlin 45 (GERMANY)

Over 20 years ago the development of rapid and sensitive spectrophotometric techniques for the measurement of spectral changes in turbid suspensions was pioneered by Britton Chance and his collaborators (Chance, 1947 and 1957; Yang, 1954; Yang and Legallais, 1954). Employing the principle of difference spectrophotometry, Chance demonstrated (Chance, 1952; Chance and Williams, 1956) the application of optical spectrophotometry to the quantitative study of hemoprotein reduction and oxidation as catalyzed by turbid, particulate membrane fragments or subcellular organelles. Of particular interest to the pharmacologist is the use of difference spectrophotometry to assess the rate and locus of alteration of cellular respiration by pharmacologically active compounds.

In recent years the recognition (Klingenberg, 1958; Omura and Sato, 1964; Estabrook et al., 1963; Cooper et al., 1965) of a unique hemoprotein, cytochrome P-450, bound to the membrane structure of the endoplasmic reticulum has extended the interests of pharmacologists to the application of spectrophotometry of turbid suspensions. The quantitative measurement of cytochrome P-450 content has often been used as an indicator of the liver's capacity to metabolize drugs oxidatively. The definition of the function of cytochrome P-450 holds the promise of a better understanding of the molecular mechanisms controlling the effectiveness of many drugs in humans. The present article will summarize the basic principles and illustrate the application of spectrophotometry to the study of membrane-bound cytochrome pigments functional during drug metabolism.

PRINCIPLES OF SPECTROPHOTOMETRIC MEASUREMENTS OF TURBID SUSPENSIONS

The Wavelength Scanning or Split-Beam Spectrophotometer

The electronic measurement of the percent of light transmitted or absorbed by a sample as a function of specific wavelengths of light is referred to as *optical spectrophotometry*. The amount of incident light that is absorbed by a sample is usually expressed in terms of *absorbance* (A) or *optical density* (O.D.) units, since the absorbance of a pigment is generally a linear function of the concentration of the absorbing species (Packer, 1967; Mellon, 1950). The *absorbance* of a pigment is defined as log (I_0/I) where I_0 is the energy of the incident light impinging on a sample, and I is the energy of the transmitted light as detected by a photomultiplier. The absorbance of a given pigment at any specified wavelength should follow Beer's law, $A = lc\varepsilon$, where A is the absorbance of the solution, l is the length of the light path, usually 1.0 cm, c is the concentration of the absorbing species, and ε is a constant which is referred to as the *absorptivity* or *extinction coefficient* of the pigment (Mahler and Cordes, 1966).

A schematic drawing of an idealized spectrophotometer (Beckman Instruments Instruction Manual, 1954) is shown in Figure 1. The simplest instruments have a light source, such as a tungsten lamp for the visible region of the spectrum (350 mμ to 800 mμ), or a hydrogen (or deuterium) lamp for the ultraviolet por-

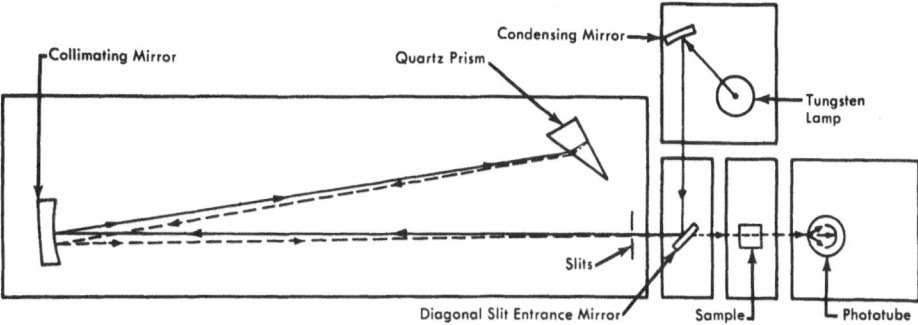

FIG. 1. Diagram of the Model DU Spectrophotometer Optical System, manufactured by Beckman Instruments, Inc. A tungsten or deuterium lamp serves as the light source. The light beam is first focused by the condensing mirror adjacent to the lamp and is then directed to the half-silvered slit entrance mirror where it is deflected into the monochromator. The light beam is reflected by a collimating mirror to a quartz prism, where it is refracted. The wavelength selector adjusts the position of the prism so that the desired wavelength of light is obtained. From the prism, the light beam is directed back to the collimating mirror, which reflects the desired wavelength of light onto the exit slit. The light beam passes through the exit slit to the sample cuvette and then to the phototube. As the transmitted light beam strikes the phototube there is an increase in phototube current, which can be amplified and registered on a meter or directed to a recorder. (From *Operating Instruction Manual for the Model DU Spectrophotometer*, 1954. Courtesy of Beckman Instruments, Inc.)

tion (220 mμ to 400 mμ) of the spectrum. A monochromator containing either a moveable prism or a diffraction grating[1] is used to disperse the light and permits the selection of the desired wavelength of light. A phototube or photomultiplier is used to detect the intensity of the transmitted light, and an analyzer circuit consisting of an amplifier (frequently coupled to a recorder) is employed to measure and record voltage changes arising from current changes in the photomultiplier. These voltage changes are proportional to the percent of light transmitted by the sample. With this type of instrument the procedure for determining the absorbance of a sample is quite straightforward. An opaque shutter is first inserted into the light beam of the monochromator and the voltage or current output of the analyzer circuit is made equal to zero percent transmission using a negative compensating voltage to equalize the dark current. A reference sample, devoid of an absorbing pigment, is then placed in the light beam and the output of the photomultiplier is adjusted by means of a variable resistor to a predetermined voltage equated with 100% transmittance. When the sample containing a chromophoric group is inserted into the light path, the percent transmittance of the sample can be recorded by determining the change in voltage or current output of the phototube or the photomultiplier. The monochromator can be adjusted to a new wavelength and the process repeated to determine the absorption spectrum of the sample. The

---

[1] The primary difference between a prism and a diffraction grating as used for the diffraction of light is that a diffraction grating gives a linear dispersion of light and a prism gives a logarithmic dispersion. Thus, changing the wavelength setting of a monochromator employing a diffraction grating does not require a change of the slit setting in order to maintain the same effective half-band width (purity) of the incident light beam (I_o).

values of percent transmittance then can be converted to absorbance units by the general formula:

$$A = \log\frac{100}{\text{percent transmittance}}$$

The advent of recording spectrophotometers with logarithmic amplifiers for conversion of percent transmittance to absorbance has made the determination of absorption spectra considerably easier. A diagrammatic outline (Hitachi Perkin-Elmer, 1968) of one type of commercially available recording spectrophotometer is shown in Figure 2. This instrument measures the absorbance of a sample with respect to a reference solution and is referred to as a *ratio recording spectrophotometer*. Although this type of instrument was designed principally for use with non-turbid solutions, a minor modification of the sample cell holder to alter the geometry of the system will permit the recording of absorption spectra of turbid suspensions.

The schematic diagram presented in Figure 3 shows another type of commercially available instrument (American Instrument Company, 1968) specifically designed for the study of turbid suspensions. This instrument is the Aminco-Chance dual wavelength and split-beam spectrophotometer and is described in greatest detail here because it is the type of instrument most frequently used in the authors' laboratory. Other commercial instruments[2] are available that will perform similar functions. This type of spectrophotometer generally utilizes a high intensity light source consisting of a tungsten-iodide filament in a quartz envelope. The light is divided at its source into two beams by a metal plate containing an optical attenuator. The light beams of equal intensity are focused on the entrance slit of the monochromator and then impinge on a collimating mirror, which focuses them on the two halves of a diffraction grating. In the Aminco-Chance instrument, the gratings can be locked together for recording light absorbance as a function of wavelength, or they can function independently for dual wavelength spectrophotometry (see below). The dispersed light from the diffraction gratings is focused by a telescope mirror onto the exit slit of the monochromator. Mechanical movement of the diffraction gratings permits the selection of the desired wavelength of light. The nonparallel beams of monochromatic light transmitted through the exit slit are chopped by a beam alternator, which permits the light to strike two front-surfaced mirrors. The reflected light is focused at the center of each of the two cuvettes. The beam alternator can simply be an oscillating mirror (Chance, 1957), which causes the beam to swing back and forth over the sample and reference cuvettes, or as shown in Figure 3, a sectored circle driven by a synchronous motor at 60 Hz. In this case, the beam alternator permits first the sample beam and then the reference beam to be transmitted to the front-surfaced mirrors and then to the respective cuvettes under examination. The light transmitted through the sample

---

[2] Comparable instruments are the Shimadzu Multipurpose Recording Spectrophotometer, MPS-50L; the Hitachi Perkin-Elmer Model 356 Two-Wavelength Double Beam Spectrophotometer; the Unicam SP-800 Spectrophotometer; and the Phoenix Double Beam Spectrophotometer.

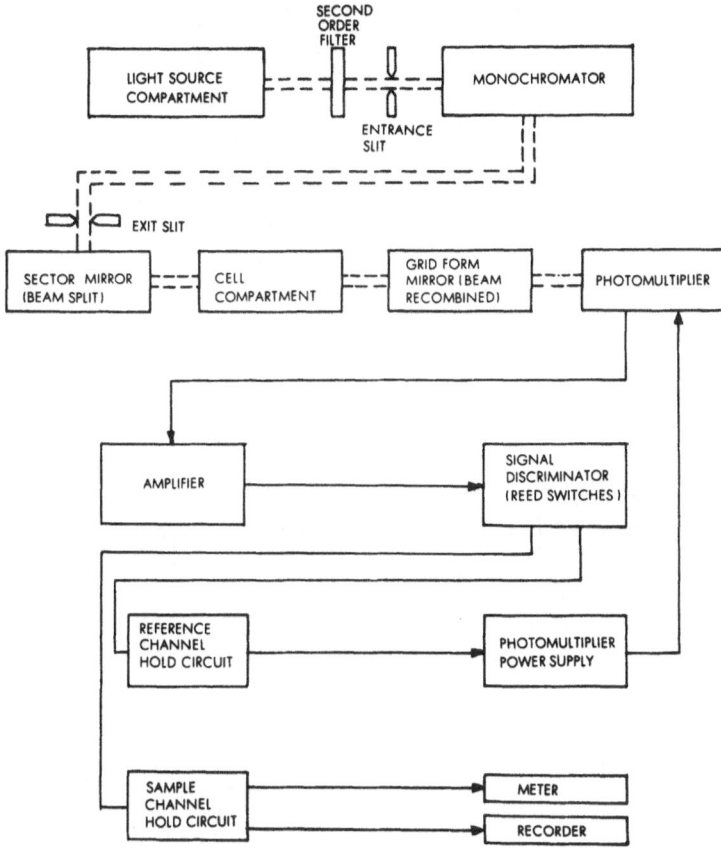

FIG. 2. A block diagram for the Model 124 Hitachi Perkin-Elmer Recording Spectrophotometer. The light source compartment contains a tungsten lamp and a deuterium lamp, either of which can serve as the light source. Second-order radiation is eliminated by a second-order filter, which automatically rotates into the light beam at wavelengths greater than 600 mμ. The light beam emitted from the lamp is focused onto the entrance slit and passes into the monochromator to the collimating mirror. The collimating mirror directs the light beam to a diffraction grating, which disperses the light beam to produce a spectrum, a portion of which is focused by the collimating mirror onto the exit slit. Upon emerging from the exit slit, the light beam is directed to a rotating mirror, which alternately passes and reflects the sample and reference beams into the sample compartment. As each beam leaves the sample compartment it is recombined by a mirror, which has alternate areas of transmitting quartz and reflecting aluminum. The recombined beams are then reflected to the photomultiplier where they generate electrical signals proportional to the intensity of the sample beam and reference beam alternately. These electrical signals are amplified and directed either as transmittance signals or as linear absorbance signals to the signal discriminator, which is directly connected to the rotating sector mirror. The signal discriminator mechanically separates the sample signal from the reference signal, and the separated signals are directed to their appropriate hold circuits where the pulses are converted into continuous DC signals. The reference signal is then transmitted to the photomultiplier power supply, where it is compared to a fixed voltage level. This results in changes in the voltage to the photomultiplier which either increase or decrease the photomultiplier sensitivity so that the reference signal remains at a constant level. The signal from the sample hold circuits is directed to both the meter and the recorder output jack where it indicates the ratio of sample-to-reference transmission directly. (From *Operating Directions for the Model 124 Double-Beam Grating Spectrophotometer*, 1968. Courtesy of the Hitachi Perkin-Elmer Company.)

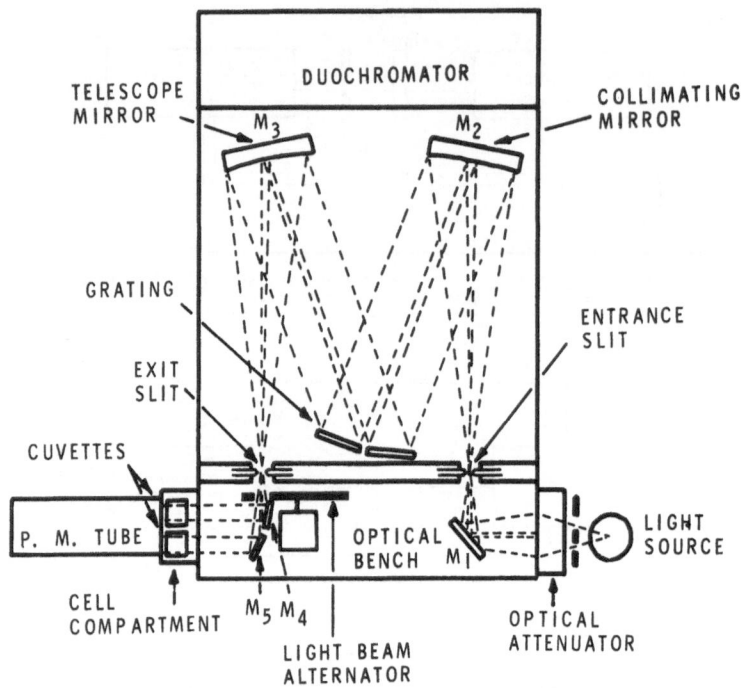

FIG. 3. Diagram of the duochromator optical configuration of the Aminco-Chance Instrument in the split-beam mode. Light from a quartz tungsten-iodide source is divided by a metal plate into two beams of light, the intensities of which are equalized by a manual optical attenuator. The two light beams are reflected from mirror M_1 and are focused onto the entrance slit of the duochromator. The beams impinge on a concave collimating mirror (M_2) and are then dispersed by the two diffraction gratings, which are locked together in the split-beam mode so that they function as a single diffraction grating. The two beams of dispersed light are then focused onto the exit slit by a concave telescope mirror (M_3). Since the diffraction gratings can rotate about a vertical axis, the light dispersed from their surfaces can be rotated so that only the desired wavelengths are focused on the exit slit. As the nonparallel beams of monochromatic light emerge from the exit slit they are chopped by a light beam alternator, which alternately passes light through the reference and sample cells after focusing by two front-surfaced mirrors (M_4 and M_5). A lens at the exit slit focuses the images of the gratings at the center of the cells. As light transmitted through the two cells impinges on the large end-on photomultiplier, an AC signal is generated. The signal is amplified and separated into reference and sample signals by an electrical chopper in the demodulator. The reference signal is then compared to a stable voltage and the difference is used to control the voltage to the photomultiplier by means of a dynode feedback system. This permits the scanning of an entire wavelength range at constant sensitivity. (From *Operating instrument manual for the Aminco-Chance Dual Wavelength/Split-Beam Recording Spectrophotometer*, 1968. Courtesy of the American Instrument Company.)

and reference cuvettes then impinges on the front surface of an end-on photomultiplier tube for the detection of the amount of light transmitted through each cuvette.

Figure 4 shows two possible arrangements of the sample and reference cuvettes relative to the light detector. In the conventional spectrophotometer, such as the one illustrated in Figure 2, the distance from the cuvettes to the photomultiplier precludes the use of highly turbid samples, which scatter light because a large amount of transmitted light is lost due to the small solid angle of scattered light

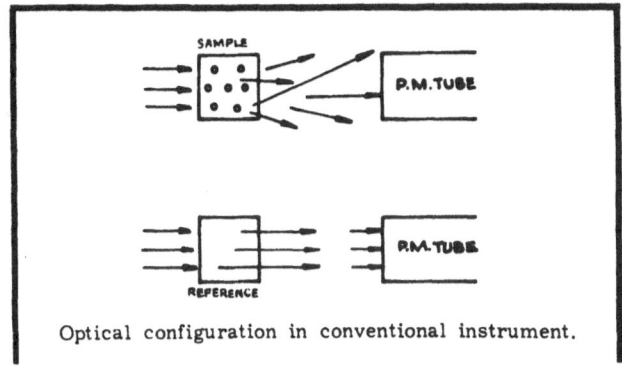

Optical configuration in conventional instrument.

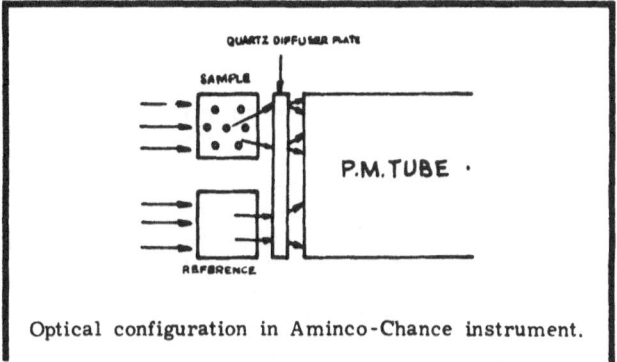

Optical configuration in Aminco-Chance instrument.

FIG. 4. Diagrams of the optical configuration of a conventional spectrophotometer and of an Aminco-Chance spectrophotometer. In a conventional instrument the photomultiplier tube is positioned between 5 and 25 cm from the reference and sample cells. Since turbid samples scatter light in a random fashion, a large portion of the transmitted light that is scattered fails to reach the photomultiplier, and the resulting spectra are poorly defined. The optical configuration in the Aminco-Chance spectrophotometer enhances the collection of scattered light by using a single end-on photomultiplier that has a large photosensitive area. In this instrument the photomultiplier is positioned less than 1 cm from both the sample and reference cells. In addition, a quartz diffuser plate is positioned between the photomultiplier and cells in order to ensure the even distribution of light over the photocathode of the photomultiplier. (From *Operating Instruction Manual for the Aminco-Chance Dual Wavelength/Split-Beam Recording Spectrophotometer*, 1968. Courtesy of the American Instrument Company.)

observed by the photomultiplier. This problem can be partially overcome by altering the geometry of the system, i.e., by moving the photomultiplier as close as possible to the cuvettes, as shown in Figure 4. In this case the solid angle of scattered light subtended by the photomultiplier is much greater. In addition, the ability to detect the scattered-transmitted light is further enhanced by increasing the size of the photosurface by using "end-on" photomultipliers. The ultimate in detecting scattered-transmitted light involves the use of "integrating spheres" (Palmer, 1967) containing the sample under examination.

For conventional spectrophotometric experiments the contents of the reference cuvette are generally clear, colorless solutions such as water or buffer. In this case the resulting absorption spectrum of the contents of the sample cuvette is referred

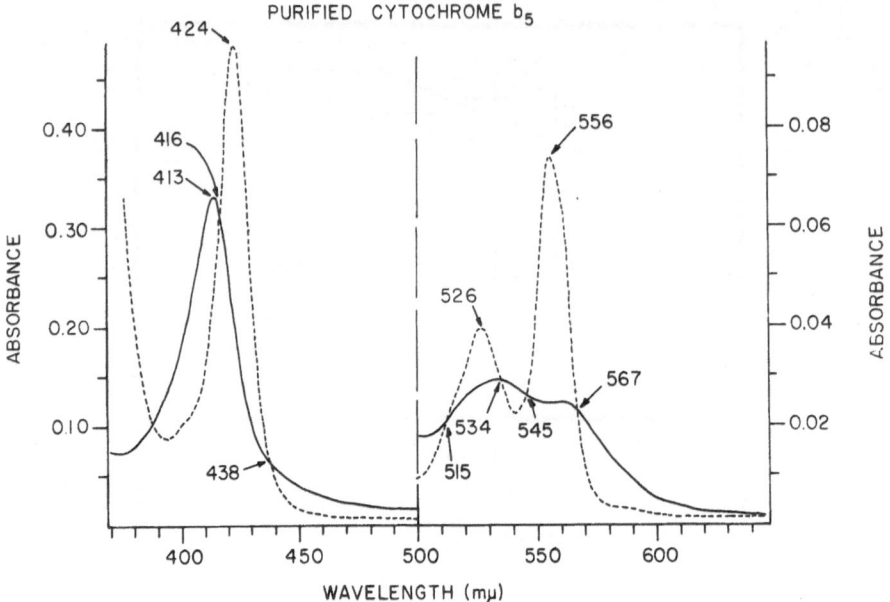

FIG. 5. Absolute absorption spectra of oxidized and reduced cytochrome b_5 purified from calf liver. Cytochrome b_5 was isolated and purified from calf liver microsomes according to the method of Strittmatter and Velick (Strittmatter and Velick, 1956; Strittmatter, 1960). Both the reference and sample cuvettes contained 0.1 M potassium phosphate buffer, pH 7.5. In addition, the sample cuvette contained 2.9 mμmoles of the purified cytochrome b_5 per ml. The solid line curve represents the absolute absorption spectrum of oxidized cytochrome b_5. The dashed line curve represents the absolute absorption spectrum of cytochrome b_5 obtained upon reduction with DPNH (200 μM final concentration) in the presence of a catalytic concentration of DPNH-cytochrome b_5 reductase.

to as an *absolute absorption spectrum*. Alternatively the reference cuvette may contain one form of an absorbing species, e.g., an oxidized hemoprotein, while the sample cuvette may contain another form of the same compound, e.g., a reduced hemoprotein. In this instance a *difference spectrum* is obtained—the spectrum is the result of the electronic compensation when the absorbance of the contents of the reference cuvette is subtracted from the absorbance of the contents of the sample cuvette. Difference spectrophotometry can compensate for loss of light due to scattering of the transmitted light beams by turbid suspensions. However, difference spectrophotometry restricts the investigator to the study of only those pigments undergoing a spectral perturbation by a reactant chemical species. *The technique of difference spectrophotometry does not provide any information about the initial state of the chromophore in the reference cuvette.* This restriction is frequently overlooked and may lead to a misinterpretation of the spectral changes under study. If the basic assumption concerning the initial state of the pigment under study is not tested in order to determine its validity, confusion and erroneous hypotheses are generated.

Difference spectrophotometry has the further advantage that electronic amplification permits scale expansion for better resolution and detection of small

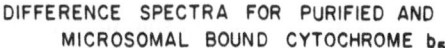

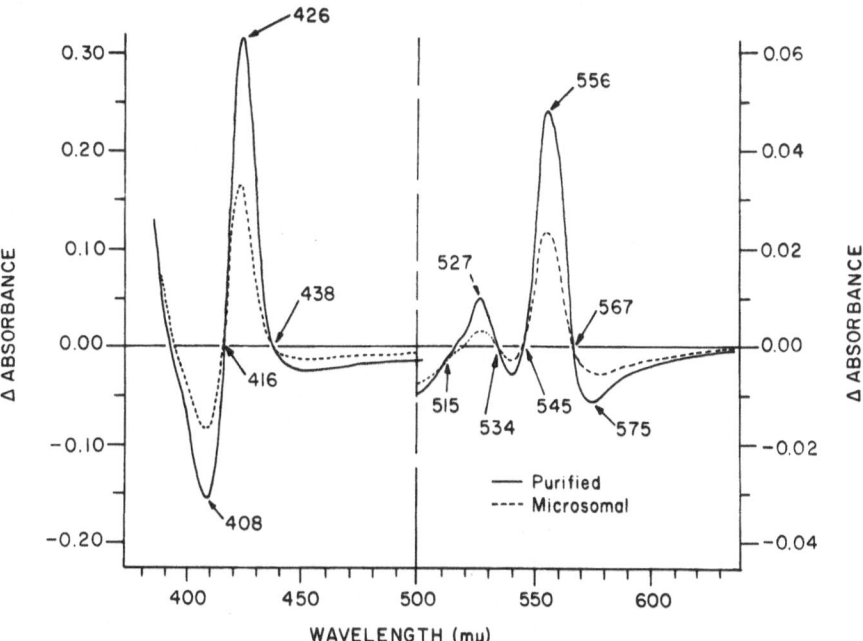

FIG. 6. The difference spectra of reduced minus oxidized purified and membrane-bound cyto-chrome b_5. The sample of purified cytochrome b_5 employed was the same as that shown in Figure 5. The sample and reference cuvettes contained 2.9 mμmoles of purified cytochrome b_5 per ml in 0.1 M potassium phosphate buffer, pH 7.5, and a catalytic concentration of DPNH-cytochrome b_5 reductase. After establishing a baseline of equal light absorbance, DPNH, at a final concentration of 200 μM was added to the sample cuvette, and a difference spectrum of reduced minus oxidized purified cytochrome b_5 was recorded (solid line). To obtain the differ-ence spectrum of membrane bound cytochrome b_5, rat liver microsomes were suspended in 0.1 M potassium phosphate buffer, pH 7.4. Both sample and reference cuvettes contained 2 mg of microsomal protein per ml (1.5 mμmoles cytochrome b_5 per ml). After establishing a baseline of equal light absorbance, DPNH (final concentration of 200 μM was added to the sample cuvette and the difference spectrum was recorded (dashed line).

absorbance changes in the presence of a large initial absorbance. The investigator must always remember, however, that studies of turbid suspensions by difference spectrophotometry have the implicit assumption that *no change in the light scattering properties of the contents of the reference or sample cuvettes occurs during the time of the measurement.* A change in light scattering properties can frequently be confused with a change in the spectral properties of a pigment under examination, and precautions must be taken to insure that spectral artifacts do not arise as a consequence of this type of change in the properties of the system under investigation.

The principle of difference spectrophotometry is illustrated by the spectra presented in Figures 5 and 6. In this study cytochrome b_5 was isolated and purified (Strittmatter and Velick, 1956; Strittmatter, 1960) from liver microsomes and the spectral properties of the pigment in its soluble form were compared to those observed when cytochrome b_5 is bound to the microsomal membrane. Isolated cytochrome b_5 was incubated with a catalytic (below the level of spectral detection) amount of the purified flavoprotein, DPNH-cytochrome b_5 reductase (Strittmatter and Velick, 1957). The absolute absorption spectrum (Figure 5) of the oxidized pigment was recorded using buffer in the reference cuvette. A major absorption band with a maximum at 413 mμ is observed in the Soret region[3] of the spectrum. Two additional rather broad absorption bands with maxima at about 530 and 565 mμ are observed in the visible region of the spectrum. The addition of a small aliquot of DPNH to the contents of the sample cuvette results in a reduction of cytochrome b_5 with the concomitant appearance of the absorption spectrum shown by the dashed lines. This change in the spectral properties of the cytochrome reflects a modification in the electron density distribution associated with the resonance conjugation of the porphyrin ring, resulting from a change in the electronic valence of the iron atom. In general the spectrum of reduced hemoproteins reveals an increase in the associated extinction coefficients at absorption band maxima, e.g., at 424, 526, and 556 mμ for cytochrome b_5. Of primary interest is the presence of isosbestic points at 416, 438, 515, 534, 545, and 567 mμ. An *isosbestic point signifies a wavelength at which there is equal light absorbance, i.e., the same extinction coefficient occurs at the isosbestic point for two forms of a pigment under study.* Examination of the two spectra presented in Figure 5 reveals that at different wavelengths either an *increase* or a *decrease* in light absorbance can occur during the transition from oxidized to reduced cytochrome b_5.

In order to examine the spectral properties of cytochrome b_5 by difference spectrophotometry an experiment similar to that described in Figure 5 was repeated using the isolated and purified soluble pigment (Figure 6). In this case a solution containing an equal concentration of oxidized cytochrome b_5 was placed in *both* the reference and sample cuvettes. Since identical solutions are present in both cuvettes the difference in light absorbance should be zero at all wavelengths examined. In difference spectrophotometry it is always necessary to determine a baseline of equal light absorbance before initiating an experiment. Frequently because of nonuniformity in the response of the photoactive surface of the photomultiplier this baseline does not appear as a perfectly straight line, indicating zero difference in light absorbance between the two cuvettes. Adjustment of the optical focus of the instrument as well as rotation of the photomultiplier should correct the deviation of the baseline from zero at high sensitivity. Moreover, any remaining distortion of the baseline can be corrected by either electronic compensation with a series of potentiometers associated with the recorder or by mechanical calculation when redrawing spectra for presentation in publications.

Addition of a source of reducing equivalents, DPNH, to the contents of the sample cuvette containing a catalytic amount of DPNH-cytochrome b_5 reductase

[3] The Soret region of the spectrum is named for the French radiologist J. L. Soret who discovered the absorption band of hemoglobin exhibiting a maximum at about 420 mμ. The Soret region is generally considered to be at the limit of the visible spectrum contiguous with the near ultraviolet portion of the spectrum.

results in the reduction of cytochrome b_5 with an associated change in the spectral characteristics of the pigment (compare Figure 5). The *difference spectrum* shown in Figure 6 by the solid line curve is the resultant of the absorbance of reduced cytochrome b_5 present in the sample cuvette *minus* the absorbance of oxidized cytochrome b_5 present in the reference cuvette. Comparison of this *difference spectrum* with the *absolute absorption spectra* illustrated in Figure 5 reveals the types of information obtainable by the two methods. The accuracy of the method is shown by the loci of the isosbestic points in the difference spectrum. *It should be noted that conclusions regarding the absolute absorption spectrum of a pigment cannot, in general, be made from difference spectra.* For example, the maximum of the Soret band of reduced cytochrome b_5 is displaced to 426 mμ in the difference spectrum because of the changes in absorbance of the oxidized pigment in this region of the spectrum. When a turbid suspension of rat liver microsomes is examined (Figure 6, dashed line) in the same way by difference spectrophotometry, the spectral characteristics of membrane-bound cytochrome b_5 conform very well to those observed with the isolated and purified pigment.

An attempt to examine the spectral properties of a turbid suspension of microsomes by *absolute absorption spectrophotometry* reveals the magnitude of increase in sensitivity obtainable by difference spectrophotometry for detection of pigment changes. For the experiment presented in Figure 7 rat liver microsomes were diluted in a buffer mixture and the absolute absorption spectra were recorded using *only* a clear solution of buffer in the reference cuvette. A large nondescript absorption is observed that increases in magnitude as the ultraviolet region of the spectrum is approached. Superimposed on this absorption due to turbidity are the absorption bands of the pigments present in liver microsomes. Attempts to increase the sensitivity of response of the spectrophotometer are limited by the concomitant amplification of the background absorbance due to turbidity. Changes in the oxidation-reduction state of the pigments by addition of the chemical reductant, sodium dithionite, in the presence or absence of carbon monoxide reveal in the visible spectrum barely discernible changes in the absorbance properties of the cytochromes. Spectral changes can be quantitated in the Soret region of the spectrum, but this is again often confused and distorted by the nonlinear contribution of the large amount of light scattering.

It is necessary to reemphasize that a major drawback associated with the use of difference spectrophotometry as a research method is the interpretation of the observed difference spectrum with respect to the original absorption spectral properties of the pigment under examination. *Difference spectrophotometry tells the experimenter nothing about the contents of chromophores in the reference cuvette. The only interpretation which can justifiably be made is that the addition of a reagent to the contents of the sample cuvette caused a change in light absorption with respect to the contents of the reference cuvette.*

Using a specially designed spectrophotometer and the techniques described above, small changes in absorbance can be measured over a large background absorbance that can result from the presence of a high concentration of another unchanging chromophore or turbidity present in the sample. If the sample is turbid

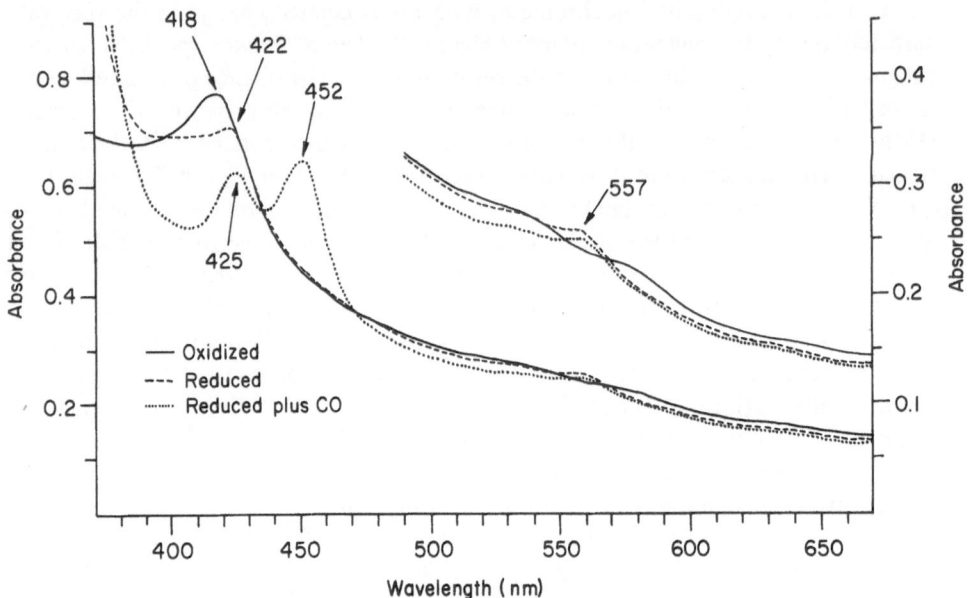

FIG. 7. The absolute absorption spectra of pigments of hepatic microsomes. Hepatic micro-somes from phenobarbital-treated rats (40 mg phenobarbital/kg i.p. for 4 days) were suspended to a concentration of 1 mg protein per ml in 0.1 M potassium phosphate buffer. The absolute absorption spectrum of the oxidized pigments of hepatic microsomes is represented by the solid line. A few crystals of sodium dithionite were then added to the sample cuvette and the absolute absorption spectrum of the reduced pigments of microsomes was recorded (dashed line). The sample cuvette was then gassed with carbon monoxide for 30 sec and the absolute absorption spectrum of the reduced cytochrome P-450—carbon monoxide complex and reduced cytochrome b_5 were recorded (dotted line). The absorbance values on the right ordinate of the figure apply only to the upper spectra in the visible region.

or highly dispersing, the amount of light transmitted will be a function of the absorbance of the pigments present plus the amount of light dispersed by the turbidity of the sample. The dispersion of light caused by turbidity of the material present in the sample cuvette can be compensated for by making the contents of the reference cuvette equally highly dispersing and then measuring the difference in light transmitted between the sample and reference cuvettes due to additions to the sample cuvette. Using a ratio-recording spectrophotometer such as described here, an absorbance change of 0.001 absorbance unit can be easily measured over a background absorbance of 3 to 4 absorbance units. Examples of spectra obtained using such techniques will be described later in this chapter.

Dual Wavelength Spectrophotometry

Dual wavelength spectrophotometry is generally used for the evaluation of the kinetics of change of a pigment that undergoes a modification in its absorption spectrum as a function of time. In practice a sample is examined initially by difference spectrophotometry as illustrated in the previous section. For dual wavelength spectrophotometry a sample wavelength is selected at or close to the maximal absorbance change of the component being examined, and a reference wavelength is selected at or near an isosbestic point. The reference wavelength is chosen as close as possible to the sample wavelength so that nonspecific absorbance changes due to changes in light scattering will be minimized. The necessary criteria for the proper selection of a wavelength pair is that the wavelengths chosen reflect absorbance changes only of the pigment of interest.

Adaptation of commercial spectrophotometers from the wavelength scanning split-beam mode to a dual wavelength configuration is generally achieved by merely disengaging the diffraction gratings so that they may be adjusted independently and by adjusting the focusing mirrors for the light beams such that the beams impinge on a single sample cuvette. The changes in the path of the light beams in the Aminco-Chance instrument are shown in Figure 8 for the two possible configurations most frequently employed. This figure illustrates the fundamental differences between the split-beam and the dual wavelength modes for this type of instrument. In the split-beam mode two light beams of the same wavelength and equal light

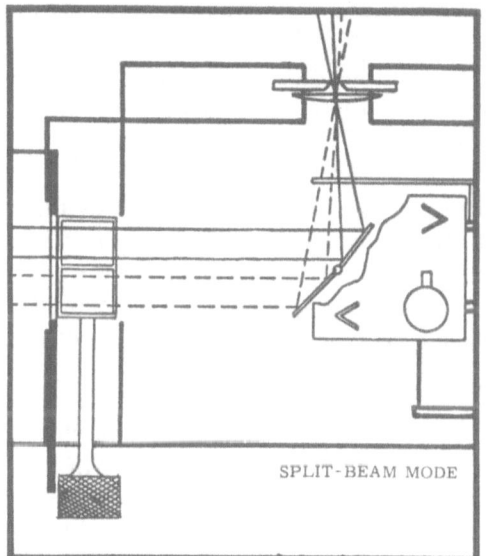 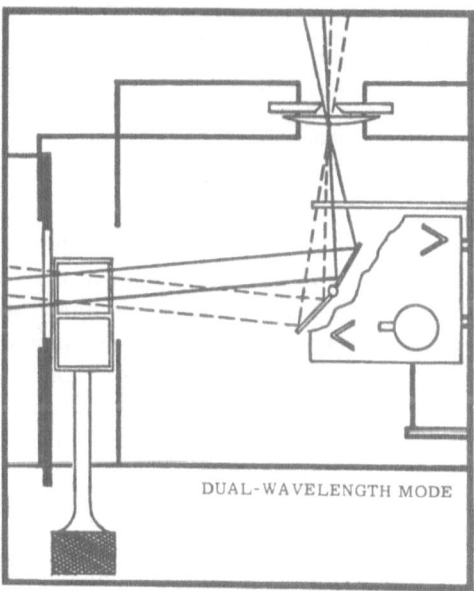

SPLIT-BEAM MODE

DUAL-WAVELENGTH MODE

FIG. 8. The light paths for the Aminco-Chance spectrophotometer when adjusted to the split-beam mode and dual wavelength mode. The split-beam configuration is indicated on the left side of the figure. The light beams passing through the sample and reference cuvettes are indicated by dashed and solid lines respectively. The configuration for the dual-wavelength mode is shown on the right side of the figure. In this case both light beams are focused by the adjustable mirrors to cross in the center of a single cuvette. The split-beam mode is used when recording difference spectra so that the two light beams are identical in wavelength. In the dual wavelength mode the two light beams are adjusted to different wavelength as discussed in the text. (From *Operating Instruction Manual for the Aminco-Chance Dual Wavelength/Split-Beam Recording Spectrometer*, 1968. Courtesy of the American Instrument Company.)

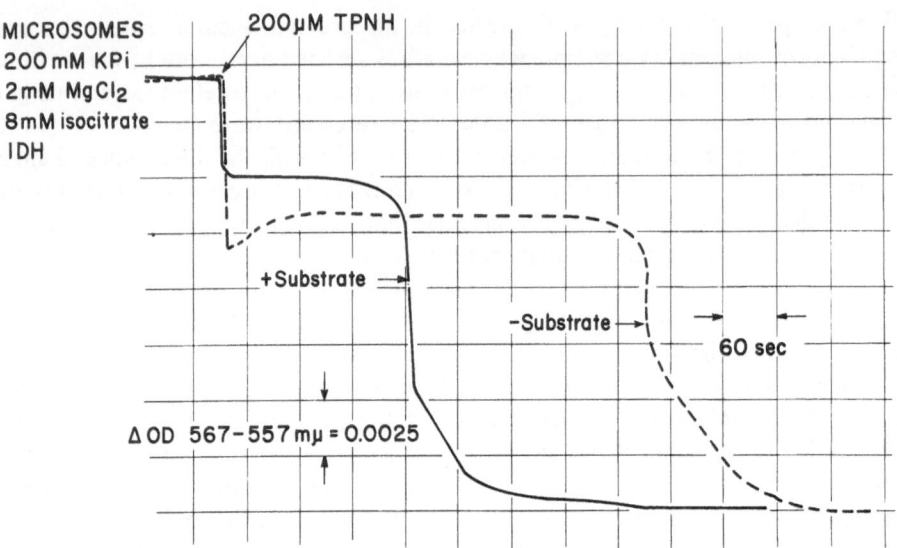

FIG. 9. The dual wavelength measurement of the steady-state reduction of cytochrome b_5 by TPNH using rat liver microsomes. Rat liver microsomes were suspended to a final concentration of 2 mg protein per ml in 7.0 ml of a buffer mixture containing 200 mM potassium phosphate buffer, pH 7.5, 2 mM MgCl$_2$, 8 mM sodium isocitrate, and excess isocitrate dehydrogenase. The absorbance changes resulting from the addition of 200 μM TPNH were recorded at 557 relative to 567 mμ. The solid line represents the results obtained in the absence of ethylmorphine. (From Hildebrandt and Estabrook. 1971. *Arch. Biochem. Biophys.*, in press.)

intensity are focused on *two cuvettes* and the difference in light transmitted by the contents of the *two cuvettes* is determined. In this configuration each cuvette is alternately flashed every 60th of a second with its corresponding light beam from the diffraction grating. In the dual wavelength mode a *single cuvette* is employed and the two light beams of different wavelengths alternately impinge on the contents of this single cuvette every 60th of a second.

An example of the use of the dual wavelength mode for assessing the kinetic transitions associated with cytochrome b_5 reduction in liver microsomes is illustrated in Figure 9. The kinetics of cytochrome b_5 reduction and the assessment of its extent of reduction during the steady state was followed by measuring the change in absorbance at 557 mμ relative to the isosbestic point at 567 mμ (Figure 6). For this experiment a sample of microsomes was diluted in an appropriate buffer and the cuvette was placed in the instrument. The intensity of the two light beams was equalized by the optical attenuator. Addition of reducing equivalents in the form of TPNH causes an increase in absorbance at 557 mμ, which is indicated by a downward deflection of the recorder tracing. The steady state of cytochrome b_5 reduction was established immediately and maintained for three to eight minutes depending on the presence or absence of a hydroxylatable substrate. Upon attainment of anaerobiosis a further change in absorbance was observed, as indicated by the subsequent downward deflection of the recorder tracing. In the case of cytochrome b_5 it is possible to select either of the isosbestic points at 545 or 567 mμ as indicated in Figure 6. However, when following the oxidation-reduction state of cytochrome b_5 during drug metabolism, as illustrated in Figure 9, the isosbestic point at 567 mμ is preferred since there is minimal interference from spectral changes associated with the reduction of cytochrome P-450 and the formation of the oxygenated state (Estabrook et al., 1971) of reduced cytochrome P-450. For these studies the reference light beam is used to monitor and compensate for any possible changes in the light scattering properties of the suspension while the sample light beam is used to measure changes in absorbance of the pigment of interest. The absorbance changes in the reference beam due to any changes in light scattering are automatically subtracted electronically from the absorbance changes observed at the sample wavelength. The resultant absorbance change is therefore attributable only to changes in the absorbing properties of the pigment under study, such as cytochrome b_5. Using techniques such as this the kinetics of oxidation or reduction of the various cytochromes and flavins functional during microsomal electron transport reactions can be measured.

Frequently, it is desirable to determine the initial rate of reaction of a pigment for better definition of the kinetics of interaction of the components under study. If the reaction is slow it may be recorded with a normal paper chart recorder that has a response time of about one second. For faster reactions special techniques are required both to mix the components of the reaction and to record the resultant absorbance changes. The application of rapid mixing techniques will be described below.

For the experiment described in Figure 9, the reaction was initiated by the addition of a small aliquot of TPNH with a glass stirring rod. Under optimal conditions the length of time required to mix a reagent manually into the 3 ml contents of a cuvette using this technique is about two to three seconds. There is available commercially[4] a plunger-type mixing device which will permit the addition of reagents in times approaching one half second. For faster mixing it is necessary to employ a manual or air driven syringe flow apparatus where mixing times as rapid as 3 milliseconds can be obtained.

It should be emphasized that the addition of reagents to a sample in the cuvette should be in the smallest volume possible. The techniques of dual wavelength spectrophotometry or split-beam spectrophotometry are extremely sensitive in detecting small spectral changes. The addition of 30 μl of a reagent to 3 ml results in a 1% dilution of the suspension. If not taken into account, this dilution may cause large spectral artifacts. Therefore, in practice, additions of only 15 μl to 20 μl are considered reasonable. Adequate controls should be carried out by adding an equal volume of buffer to the sample to assess the influence of dilution on the reaction solution.

---

[4] Special anaerobic cuvettes constructed with ports for gassing samples and containing a sealed plunger for addition of reactants is available from the American Instrument Company, Silver Spring, Maryland.

APPLICATION OF THE WAVELENGTH SCANNING, SPLIT-BEAM METHOD OF SPECTROPHOTOMETRY

Identification of Microsomal Pigments

The recognition that the cytochrome pigments that function in oxidative drug metabolism are bound to microsomal membranes (Brodie et al., 1955) presents unique problems which limit the investigator's ability to evaluate fully the spectral properties of the pigments of interest. A series of procedures has been developed in this laboratory which has been successfully applied to the identification and quantitation of these cytochrome pigments present in microsomes, thereby permitting a definition of their role in the oxidative degradation of xenobiotics.

As a general procedure microsomes are isolated from the liver (Schenkman et al., 1967) or any other organ of an animal and a sample of these microsomes is diluted to 6 ml in an appropriate buffer mixture (0.1 M potassium phosphate buffer or 50 mM tris-chloride buffer, pH 7.4 to 8.0) to a final protein concentration of approximately 1 to 2 mg per ml. The diluted microsomal suspension is then divided equally into two precisely matched cuvettes (i.e., identical light path) and placed in a spectrophotometer, such as the Aminco-Chance instrument, adjusted to the split-beam mode. The uniformity of the sample is first determined by recording the quality of the baseline of equal light absorbance as a function of wavelength. As indicated earlier, this baseline is frequently not a straight line, since small changes in the response of the nonuniform surface area of the photomultiplier are always present. The cuvettes are generally placed in the optical path with their frosted rather than their clear faces in the light beams. This insures a more uniform scattering of light through the sample, thereby giving a better statistical representation of the contents of the cuvettes. Further, in studies of this type a slit width as narrow as possible should be used in order to insure maximal spectral resolution of the pigments under study. Frequently a decision must be made as to the magnitude of the slit width, the photomultiplier dynode voltage, and the dilution of the sample in order to obtain optimal spectral response. If the baseline is grossly distorted the sample and the reference cuvettes should be transposed in the cuvette holder to determine whether the poor baseline is a consequence of poorly matched cuvettes rather than improper mixing of the sample. If the baseline is still distorted, realignment of the optical paths or rotation of the photomultiplier should be attempted, as described above.

After establishment of a baseline of essentially equal light absorbance between the sample and reference cuvettes, a small aliquot of DPNH (10 μl of a 60 mM solution) is added to the contents of the sample cuvette resulting in a spectral change attributable to the reduction of cytochrome b_5 (Figures 6 and 10). During the steady state in the presence of oxygen but in the absence of an added hydroxylatable substrate, the reduction of cytochrome b_5 is nearly complete (Hildebrant and Estabrook, 1971). The concentration of cytochrome b_5 in the microsomal prepara-

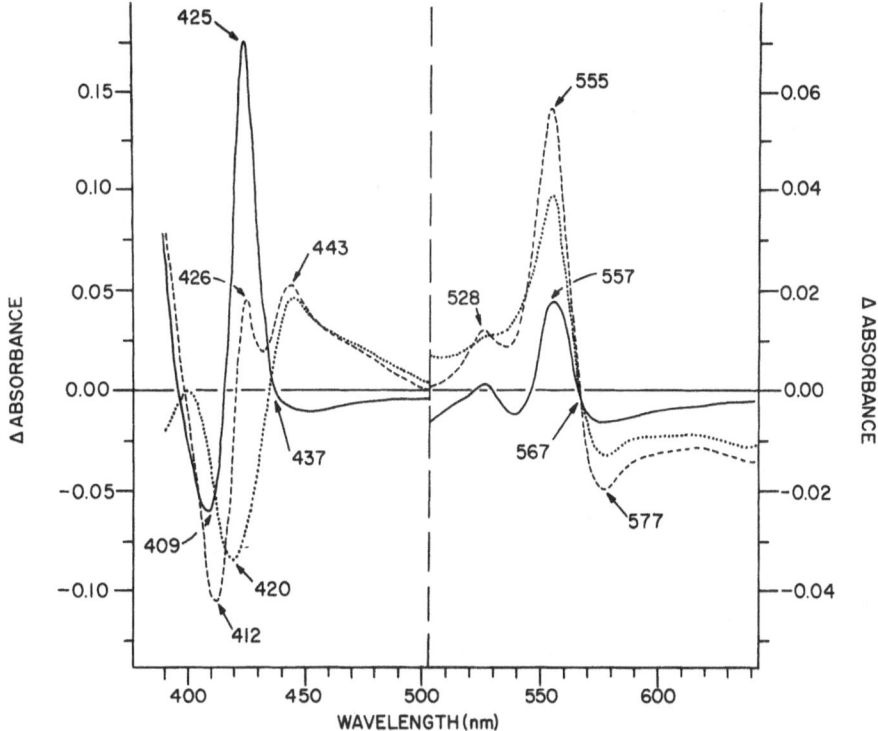

FIG. 10. The spectral properties of liver microsomal pigments as determined by difference spectrophotometry. Rat liver microsomes (15 mg of protein) were diluted to a final volume of 6.0 ml with 0.1 M potassium phosphate buffer, pH 7.4, and divided equally between the sample and reference cuvettes. After establishment of a baseline of equal light absorbance, the difference spectrum of reduced minus oxidized cytochrome b_5 was recorded after the addition of 10 μl of a 60 mM solution of DPNH to the sample cuvette. This is indicated by the solid line. A few crystals of solid $Na_2S_2O_4$ were then added to the contents of the sample cuvette in order to reduce other microsomal pigments, and the difference spectrum was recorded (dashed line). The change in absorbance attributable to the reduction of cytochrome P-450 is shown by the dotted line. This difference spectrum was obtained by adding 10 μl of 60 mM DPNH to the contents of the reference cuvette.

tion can be determined using the millimolar extinction coefficients of 20 (Klingenberg, 1958) or 185 (Omura and Sato, 1964) for the change in absorbance at 557 minus 575 mμ or 424 minus 409 mμ, respectively. As shown in Figure 10 the subsequent addition of a few crystals of fresh sodium dithionite ($Na_2S_2O_4$) results in a further spectral change attributable to the reduction of cytochrome P-450 in the sample cuvette. It is most important that *fresh* $Na_2S_2O_4$ be used for these experiments since exposure of powdered $Na_2S_2O_4$ to air and moisture results in its decomposition to an inactive form. The extent of decomposition of $Na_2S_2O_4$ can be assessed by carefully smelling the powdered compound, and if a strong pungent odor of bisulfite is apparent the sample of $Na_2S_2O_4$ should be discarded. Furthermore, the interaction of $Na_2S_2O_4$ with the oxygen dissolved in the buffer medium frequently results in the formation of hydrogen peroxide (H_2O_2), which can destroy some of the heme compounds present. Inadequate buffering capacity in the reaction mixture can result in the acidification of the sample on addition of $Na_2S_2O_4$ with the subsequent formation of colloidal sulfur.

It is apparent from the spectral data of Figure 10 that the addition of $Na_2S_2O_4$ does not give a true measure of the cytochrome b_5 content, since the resultant spectral changes represent the combined spectral contributions of reduced cytochrome b_5 and cytochrome P-450. The extent of the spectral change associated with the reduction of cytochrome P-450 can be directly determined (Figure 10) by adding an aliquot of DPNH to the contents of the reference cuvette. In this way one compensates for the spectral contribution of reduced cytochrome b_5. The unusual spectral properties of reduced and oxidized cytochrome P-450 results in an atypical hemoprotein difference spectrum in the Soret region of the spectrum. It is, therefore, most convenient to assess the content of cytochrome P-450 by measuring the magnitude of the absorbance change in the presence of the ligand carbon monoxide.

Cytochrome P-450 was first recognized and characterized (Klingenberg, 1958; Omura and Sato, 1962) by the presence of an absorption band with a maximum at about 450 mμ when a sample of microsomes was treated with a reducing agent plus carbon monoxide. The magnitude of this absorbance change observed at 450 mμ relative to 490 mμ does vary slightly depending on the type of experiment

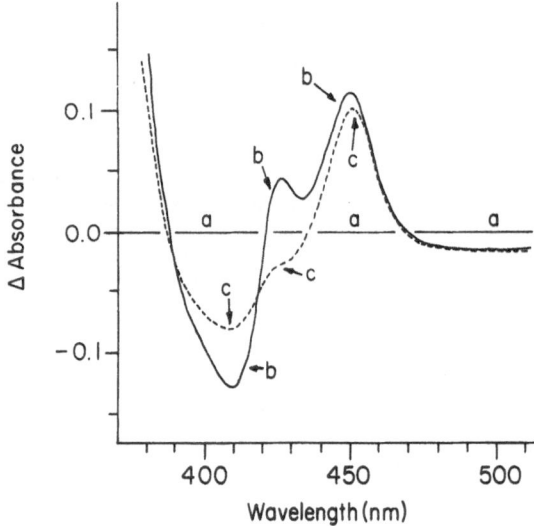

FIG. 11. The effect of the order of addition of reactants on the difference spectrum of the carbon monoxide-complex of reduced cytochrome P-450. Hepatic microsomes from phenobarbital-treated rats were diluted to 2 mg protein per ml in 0.1 M potassium phosphate buffer, pH 7.4. The suspension was divided equally into two cuvettes and a baseline of equal light absorbance recorded (curve a). The contents of the sample cuvette were then gassed with carbon monoxide for 3 min. A few crystals of $Na_2S_2O_4$ were added to the sample cuvette and the resulting difference spectrum of reduced cytochrome b_5 plus the CO-complex of reduced cytochrome P-450 was recorded (curve b). A few crystals of $Na_2S_2O_4$ were then added to the contents of the reference cuvette to reduce cytochrome b_5 and cytochrome P-450, and the resulting difference spectrum of the carbon monoxide reacting reduced pigments of the microsomal suspension was obtained (curve c).

performed. For the experiment shown in Figure 11, a sample of liver microsomes is diluted in a buffer mixture and divided equally into two cuvettes for the establishment of a baseline of equal light absorbance. The sample cuvette is removed from the spectrophotometer and its contents gassed for three minutes with carbon monoxide.[5] The sample is placed back in the spectrophotometer and a baseline is recorded again to determine the extent of hemoglobin contamination (see below). The subsequent addition of the chemical reductant $Na_2S_2O_4$ to the contents of the sample cuvette results in a difference spectrum which is the composite of reduced cytochrome b_5 *plus* the CO-complex of reduced cytochrome P-450. The subsequent addition of $Na_2S_2O_4$ to the contents of the reference cuvette (which has not been gassed with CO) decreases the magnitude of the absorption band at 450 mμ due to the negative contribution of reduced cytochrome P-450 in the reference cuvette. In a like manner the absorbance change at 425 mμ is also attenuated (Fig. 11) by compensating for the contribution of reduced cytochrome b_5 to the difference spectrum. The millimolar extinction coefficients employed in quantitatively evaluating the content of cytochrome P-450 are 100 when measuring the CO-complex of reduced cytochrome P-450 minus oxidized cytochrome P-450 (solid line curve, Figure 11) or 91 (Omura and Sato, 1964) when measuring the absorbance difference of the CO-complex or reduced cytochrome P-450 minus reduced cytochrome P-450 (dashed line curve, Figure 11). In both cases the wavelength 490 mμ is generally accepted as a reference wavelength for computation of the concentration of cytochrome P-450.

Interference by Hemoglobin

The isolation of microsomes free of hemoglobin contamination can be easily accomplished by using perfused livers and incorporating a washing step with dilute KCl (0.15 *M*) in the final preparation of the microsomal fractions. The extent of hemoglobin contamination should be routinely assessed by determining the extent of spectral change occurring on treatment of the dilute microsomal suspension with CO in the absence of any reductant. The spectral change associated with the conversion of oxyhemoglobin to carbonmonoxyhemoglobin can be readily detected by evaluating the magnitude of the spectral change at 430 mμ relative to 418 mμ (see Figure 12). The accurate spectrophotometric study of microsomal pigments can be accomplished only if the amount of hemoglobin contamination in the sample is below the level of spectral detection.

Studies of biopsy samples require the spectral examination of crude homogenates from unperfused tissues. Such studies can be successfully accomplished if appropriate precautions are taken to account for the possible spectral interference arising from hemoglobin. The following procedure has been routinely used (Raj and Estabrook, 1971) in this laboratory for evaluating the cytochrome P-450

---

[5] Commercial carbon monoxide may contain traces of impurities as well as oxygen and should be scrubbed by passing the gas through Fieser's solution (0.1 g of 2-anthraquinone sulfonic acid [sodium salt], 1.0 g of sodium dithionite [$Na_2S_2O_4$] dissolved in 100 ml of 0.1N NaOH), and distilled water. The rate of gas flow should be slow enough to avoid any loss of volume by evaporation from the sample. Since protein solutions frequently foam when bubbled with gases, a trace of Antifoam is added to the sample on the tip of a glass stirring rod.

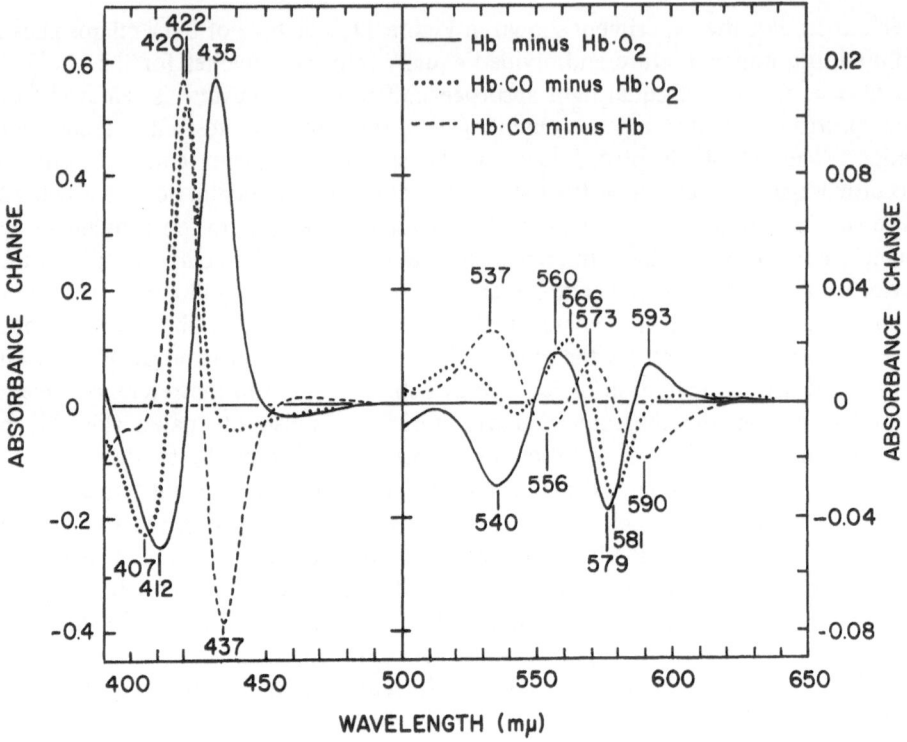

FIG. 12. The difference spectra obtained for various derivatives of hemoglobin. An aliquot of lysed, rat red blood cells was diluted in 0.1 M potassium phosphate buffer, pH 7.4, and gassed with oxygen for 10 minutes. The solution of oxyhemoglobin was divided equally into two cuvettes and a baseline of equal light absorbance recorded. A few crystals of $Na_2S_2O_4$ were added to the contents of the sample cuvette, and the difference spectrum of reduced hemoglobin minus oxyhemoglobin was recorded (solid line). The contents of the sample cuvette were then gassed with CO for 3 minutes and the difference spectrum of carbonmonoxyhemoglobin minus oxy-hemoglobin was recorded (dotted line). After addition of a few crystals of $Na_2S_2O_4$ to the contents of the reference cuvette, the difference spectrum of carbonmonoxyhemoglobin minus reduced hemoglobin was recorded (dashed line).

content of human liver samples that contain large and varying amounts of hemoglobin.

A small aliquot of liver (10 mg to 200 mg wet weight) is homogenized with a Potter-Elvehjem homogenizer using a minimal volume (approximately 1 ml) of 0.1 M potassium phosphate buffer, pH 7.4. The homogenized sample is chilled in ice and further disrupted by treatment with ultrasound (20 kHz for 20 to 60 seconds using a Branson sonifier with a microtip adaptor). The clarified sample of homogenate is then filtered through two layers of coarse cheese cloth to remove any residual undispersed connective tissue. An aliquot of this suspension is then diluted to 6 ml in 0.1 M potassium phosphate buffer, pH 7.4, and the sample is gassed for five minutes with carbon monoxide. In this manner the oxyhemoglobin in the sample is converted to carbonmonoxyhemoglobin. The CO-gassed sample is then divided equally into two cuvettes and a baseline of equal light absorbance

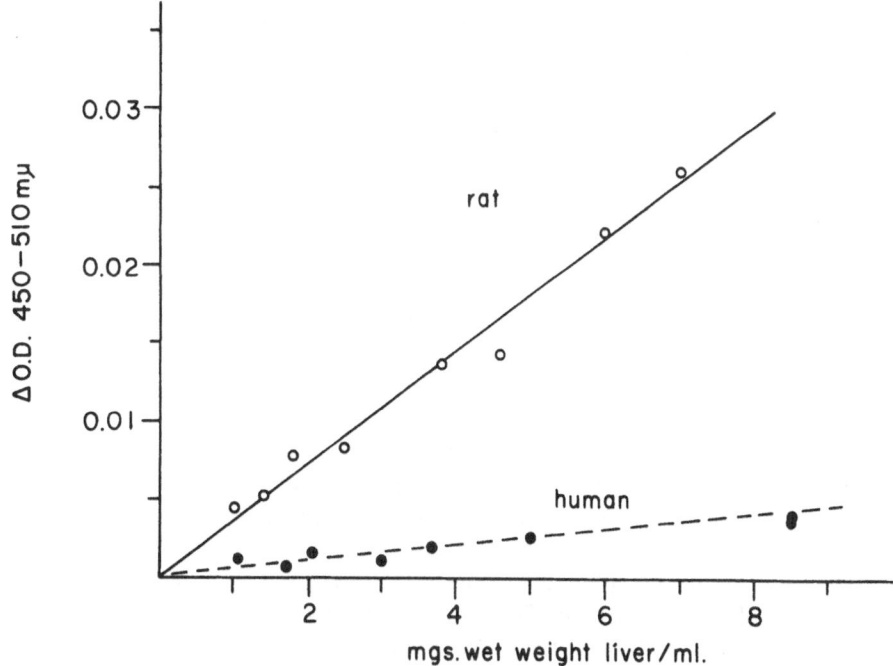

FIG. 13. The determination of the cytochrome P-450 content using homogenates from small samples of livers. Hepatic homogenates from biopsy samples were prepared as described in the text, and aliquots of these suspensions were diluted to 6.0 ml in 0.1 M potassium phosphate buffer, pH 7.4. The diluted suspensions were gassed for 3 minutes with carbon monoxide and divided equally into two cuvettes. After establishing a baseline of equal light absorbance, a few crystals of $Na_2S_2O_4$ were added to the contents of the sample cuvette and the difference spectra were recorded. The absorbance change at 450 mμ (the maximum of the CO-complex of reduced cytochrome P-450) relative to the isosbestic point at 510 mμ is indicated on the left ordinate. The isosbestic point was determined to be 510 mμ in crude liver homogenates rather than 490 mμ because of the contribution of flavoproteins to the difference spectrum.

is recorded. The spectral range that can be successfully examined is generally restricted, i.e., from about 430 mμ to greater than 520 mμ, since excessively high concentrations of carbonmonoxyhemoglobin present in the sample and reference cuvettes frequently absorb so much of the incident light that the dynode feedback circuit for the photomultiplier is overloaded, resulting in inaccurate spectra. Since absorbance changes occurring at wavelengths below 430 mμ cannot be accurately measured in the presence of hemoglobin without the possibility of gross spectrophotometric errors, the concentration of cytochrome b_5 cannot be accurately determined in crude homogenates by this method.

After establishing a baseline of equal light absorbance for the diluted homogenate, a few crystals of fresh $Na_2S_2O_4$ are added to the contents of the sample cuvette. This results in the reduction of cytochrome P-450 and other pigments present in the homogenate. A well-defined absorption band associated with the CO-complex of reduced cytochrome P-450 should be discernible, and calculations of cytochrome P-450 content can be carried out as described above using the millimolar extinction coefficient of 100 for the difference in absorbance at 450 minus 510 mμ. The application of this method to samples of rat and human liver is illustrated in Figure 13. It is apparent that reliable results can be obtained with as little as 10 mg wet weight of tissue.

Interference from Mitochondrial Pigments

In addition to hemoglobin, interference in the accurate determination of cytochrome P-450 can arise from the spectral contribution of mitochondrial pigments, particularly cytochrome oxidase. The magnitude of this interference is illustrated in Figure 14, where various ratios of isolated liver microsomes have been mixed with submitochondrial particles prepared from heart muscle. For these studies the procedure outlined in the previous section was employed, i.e., the diluted samples were first gassed with carbon monoxide and the mixture was divided equally between two cuvettes with the subsequent addition of Na$_2$S$_2$O$_4$ to the contents of only the sample cuvette. A marked perturbation of the spectrum of the carbon monoxide complex of reduced cytochrome P-450 occurs when the concentration of cytochrome P-450 (contributed by the microsomal fraction) equals the concentration of cytochrome oxidase (contributed by the submito-

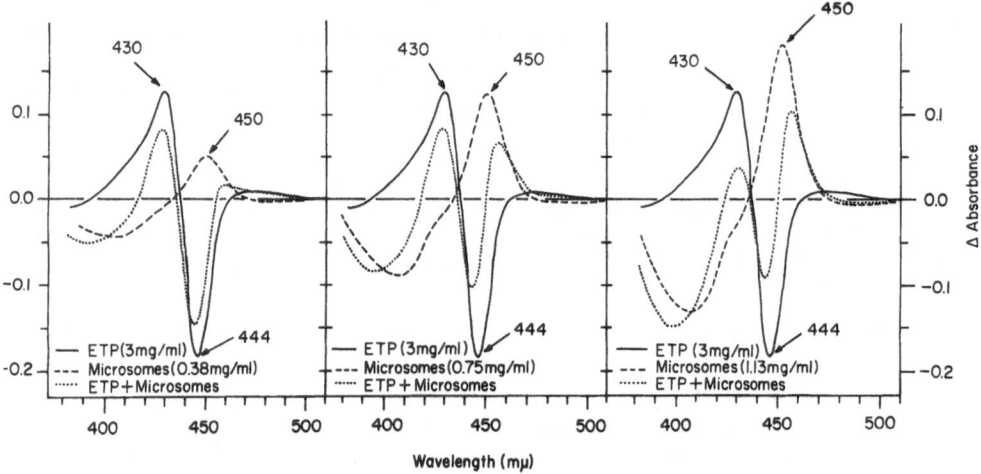

FIG. 14. The influence of mitochondrial cytochrome oxidase on the spectral determination of cytochrome P-450. Various ratios of rat liver microsomes and submitochondrial particles from heart muscle (ETP) were diluted in 0.1 M potassium phosphate buffer, pH 7.4, as indicated. In addition, the spectral properties of the pigments of microsomes and ETP were recorded independently. For these spectra the pigments of the diluted suspensions were reduced by the addition of a few crystals of Na$_2$S$_2$O$_4$ and a baseline of equal light absorbance recorded. The contents of the sample cuvette were gassed for 3 minutes with CO and the resulting difference spectrum recorded. The solid line represents the difference spectrum of the CO-complex of reduced cytochrome oxidase minus reduced cytochrome oxidase. The dashed line represents the spectral properties of the CO-complex of reduced cytochrome P-450, as described in Figure 11. The dotted line curve represents the difference spectrum obtained in the presence of ETP and various concentrations of microsomes, as indicated.

chondrial fraction). This perturbation results principally from the spectral changes occurring during the formation of the carbon monoxide complex of reduced cyto-chrome oxidase. In these studies one observes that the apparent absorption maximum for the carbon monoxide complex of reduced cytochrome P-450 undergoes a bathochromic shift; the magnitude of this displacement depends on the ratio of cytochrome oxidase to cytochrome P-450. There is a concomitant diminution of the absorbance change at about 450 mμ leading to an underestimation of the cytochrome P-450 concentration. Thus, it is apparent from this type of study that the observation of a carbon monoxide complex of reduced cytochrome P-450 exhibiting an absorption maximum in the region of 455 mμ or 460 mμ must be critically examined (Jakobsson et al., 1970) in order to evaluate the spectral contributions from other pigments such as cytochrome oxidase. An estimation of the cytochrome P-450 content can be made, however, by measuring the absorbance change at 460 mμ (an isosbestic point for the CO-complex of reduced cytochrome oxidase) relative to 490 mμ using a millimolar extinction coefficient of 52 (Kowal et al., 1970).

Undoubtedly many other factors can contribute to the erroneous estimation of cytochrome P-450 concentration in crude preparations of tissues. At this time one can only *estimate* the concentration of cytochrome P-450 because of the inherent inaccuracy in the methodology.

Spectral Properties of Microsomal Pigments in Liver Slices

One of the primary goals in studying cytochrome reduction and oxidation is to relate observations made in vitro to metabolic events occurring in vivo. The high concentration of the microsomal cytochromes in liver affords an excellent opportunity to evaluate the influence of the cellular milieu on drug oxidation reactions occurring concomitant with overall cellular metabolism. The technique of difference spectrophotometry described above has been extended (Estabrook et al., 1970) to the study of liver slices.

Livers of young rats are perfused in situ with an isotonic sodium chloride solution to remove as much hemoglobin as possible. The perfused liver is excised and slices 0.3 mm to 0.5 mm thick are made with a Stadie-Riggs tissue slicer, and the thin slices of liver are mounted in specially designed cuvettes of the type illustrated in Figure 15. The sealed cuvettes have exit and entrance ports allowing for the superfusion of the slices with reaction media. For these experiments two slices are selected having approximately the same thickness and uniformity of texture. The portion of the mounted slice in the light beam is determined by carefully masking the translucent portions of the cuvettes with black tape so that only the desired portion of the slice is irradiated. As in conventional difference spectrophotometry, a baseline of equal light absorbance is established after the slices are equilibrated with an oxygenated buffer, such as Hanks medium. Replacement of the oxygenated medium superfusing the slice in the sample cuvette with a nitrogen equilibrated medium containing sodium succinate results (Figure 16) in

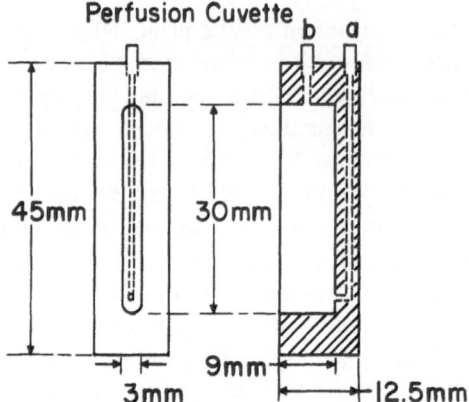

FIG. 15. Diagram of the special cuvette employed for spectral studies of liver slices. Cuvettes are constructed of Plexiglas with channels permitting the entrance (a) and exit (b) of the super-fusing medium. Slices of liver are mounted in the optical path and the cell is sealed and masked with black tape, as described in the text. (From Estabrook et al., 1970. *Advances Enzyme Regulat.*, 8:121-130.)

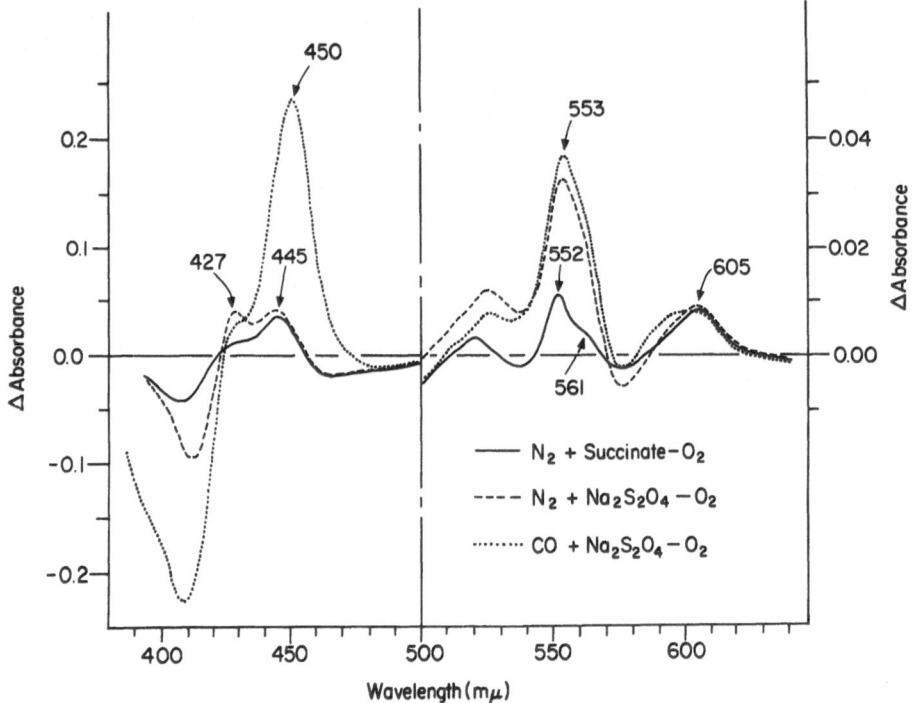

FIG. 16. Spectral changes observed with liver slices. Slices of liver (about 0.4 mm thick) from phenobarbital-treated male rats were mounted in specially designed cuvettes (see Fig. 15) and were superfused with oxygenated Hanks solution. After equilibration, a baseline of equal light absorbance was recorded. As described in the text, the superfusion medium passing through the sample cuvette was then replaced with nitrogen- or carbon monoxide-equilibrated Hanks solution supplemented with either sodium succinate or sodium dithionite. The spectral changes observed using these various conditions are indicated on the figure. (From Estabrook, et al. 1970. *Advances Enzyme Regulat.*, 8:121-130.)

a spectral change associated with the reduction of the mitochondrial cytochromes. The addition of sodium isocitrate plus TPN$^+$ or the chemical reductant Na$_2$S$_2$O$_4$ to the superfusion medium in the sample cuvette results in an additional spectral change attributable to the reduction of the cytochromes associated with the endoplasmic reticulum. This is most readily demonstrated by equilibrating the superfusion medium passing through the sample cuvette with carbon monoxide, as shown in Figure 16. Using this technique it is possible to measure directly cytochrome P-450 reduction in the intact cell under a variety of metabolic conditions. Furthermore, it is also possible to evaluate the extent of drug interaction with cytochrome P-450 (see below) and measure the presence or absence of cellular permeability restrictions on the movement of drugs across the cell membrane.

The spectral changes observed in slices of liver permit the quantitative measurement of cytochrome content in the intact liver cell. Assuming a density of 1.1 grams per ml, the exact thickness of the slice can be determined from its weight and area. These observations reveal (Estabrook et al., 1970) that cytochrome P-450 is the predominant cytochrome in liver and presumably accounts for a significant portion of the respiratory activity occurring in the liver.

Spectral Properties of Microsomal Cytochromes Cooled to the Temperature of Liquid Nitrogen

The application of low temperature spectrophotometric methods to the study of cytochromes has provided (Estabrook, 1961) much necessary information required for the identification and definition of cytochrome function. The low temperature spectrophotometric method has four primary advantages over conventional room temperature spectrophotometry. Firstly, by use of an appropriate solvent such as glycerol-water mixtures, it is possible to record absolute absorption spectra of rather turbid microsomal suspensions. This is accomplished by producing a large background turbidity in both the sample and reference cuvettes. This turbidity is associated with devitrification of the glycerol-water mixture (Keilin and Hartree, 1949) on warming from liquid nitrogen temperature to approximately $-80°C$. Secondly, a profound enhancement of the apparent extinction coefficient occurs in the devitrified state. This is presumed to be a consequence of effectively increasing the light path through the sample due to multiple internal reflections from the microcrystalline state of the solvent. This enhancement can be as great as 10- to 20-fold, thereby increasing the sensitivity of the spectrophotometric method and permitting the use of a significantly more dilute sample. Thirdly, absorption bands are markedly sharpened at liquid nitrogen temperature allowing for the spectral resolution of overlapping absorption bands. These spectra frequently reveal the existence of absorption maxima that are sequestered or fused at room temperature. The low temperature spectrophotometric technique also permits the trapping and stabilization of the steady state of reduction of cytochromes (Chance and Spencer, 1959). The ability to quench a reaction immediately by lowering the temperature holds great potential for the further examination

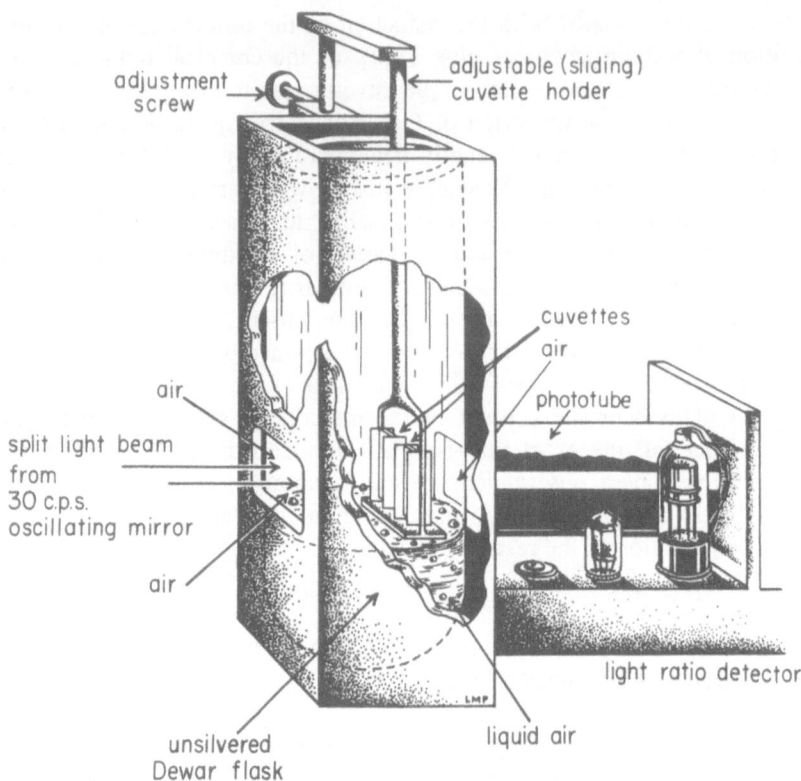

FIG. 17. Attachment for determining the spectral properties of pigments cooled to the temperature of liquid nitrogen. The light path of this attachment runs from left to right. The level of liquid nitrogen is maintained no higher than the base of the cuvettes, although the cuvettes may be immersed in the liquid nitrogen to provide for rapid freezing. The Dewar flask is unsilvered and approximately 3 inches (7.2 cm) in diameter; it is not provided with optically flat surfaces. (From Estabrook 1956. *J. Biol. Chem.*, 223:781-794.)

of unstable intermediates that are only fleetingly transient during the time course of drug metabolism at room temperature.

The accessory employed for the recording of absorption spectra of samples cooled to liquid nitrogen temperature is a rather simple arrangement composed of an unsilvered Dewar flask which replaces the normal cell compartment. Many varieties of the original design (Figure 17) are commercially available and are readily adapted for use with wavelength scanning recording spectrophotometers.

In order to determine the absolute absorption spectrum of the pigments in a sample of microsomes, the microsomal suspension is diluted in a buffer mixture, such as 0.1 M potassium phosphate buffer, pH 7.4, and glycerol is added so that the final reaction mixture contains 50% glycerol by volume[6]. If reduced pyridine

[6] An alternate technique for the preparation of samples for low temperature spectrophotometry has been described by Wilson (1967). Glycerol is replaced by sucrose (1.0 M final concentration). In this technique, the sucrose solution freezes directly to the devitrified state at the temperature of liquid nitrogen.

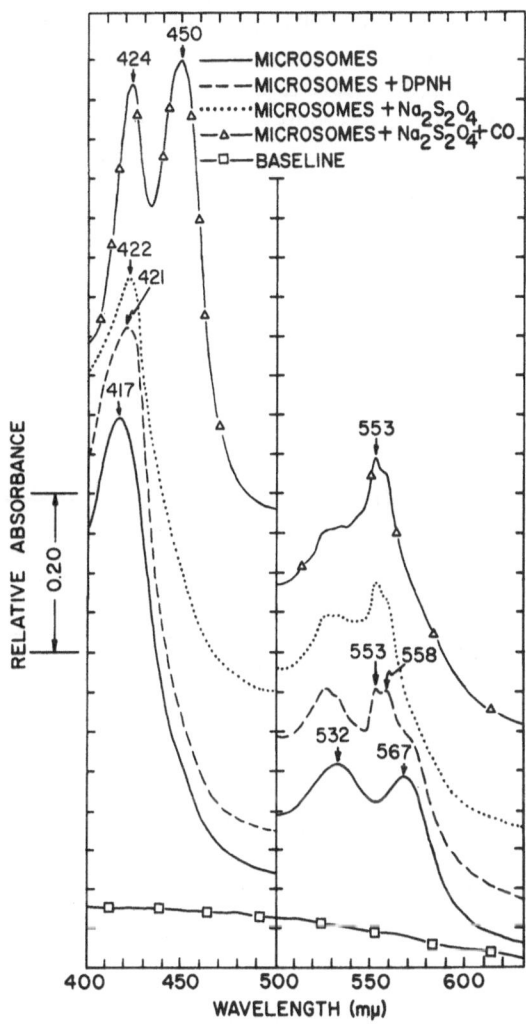

FIG. 18. The low temperature absolute absorption spectra of liver microsomes. Microsomes were prepared from phenobarbital-treated rats and spectra recorded as described in the text using a glycerol-buffer mixture without microsomes in the reference cuvette. The absorption spectra presented in the figure are displaced on the vertical axis for clarity and the absorbance of a given sample is not "absolute" because of the large background absorbance of the devitrified glycerol-buffer mixture. The microsomal suspension was diluted with 0.1 M potassium phosphate buffer, pH 7.4, and after the addition of reactants, was made 50% by volume in glycerol. The Soret region of the spectrum was recorded with a final concentration of 1.5 mg of protein per ml and the visible region with 3.0 mg of protein per ml. Symbols: the absolute absorption spectra of the pigments of microsomes in the absence of added reactants (—); DPNH (200 μM) treated microsomes (- - - - -); $Na_2S_2O_4$-treated microsomes (. . . .); and CO-gassed $Na_2S_2O_4$-treated microsomes (—△—); the baseline with the glycerol-buffer mixture in both sample and reference cuvettes (—□—).

nucleotides or $Na_2S_2O_4$ are to be added to the sample, it is necessary that these reductants be added *prior* to dilution of the sample with glycerol. The glycerol-containing sample is then placed in the sample cuvette, while a buffer mixture (without microsomes) containing 50% glycerol by volume is placed in the reference cuvette. The cuvettes are plunged into liquid nitrogen in the Dewar flask, where the samples rapidly freeze to a clear plastic-like state. Removal of the cuvettes from the liquid nitrogen permits gradual warming, and a marked change in the transmittance characteristics of the cuvette contents can be observed at a temperature of approximately $-80°C$. The appearance of the contents of the

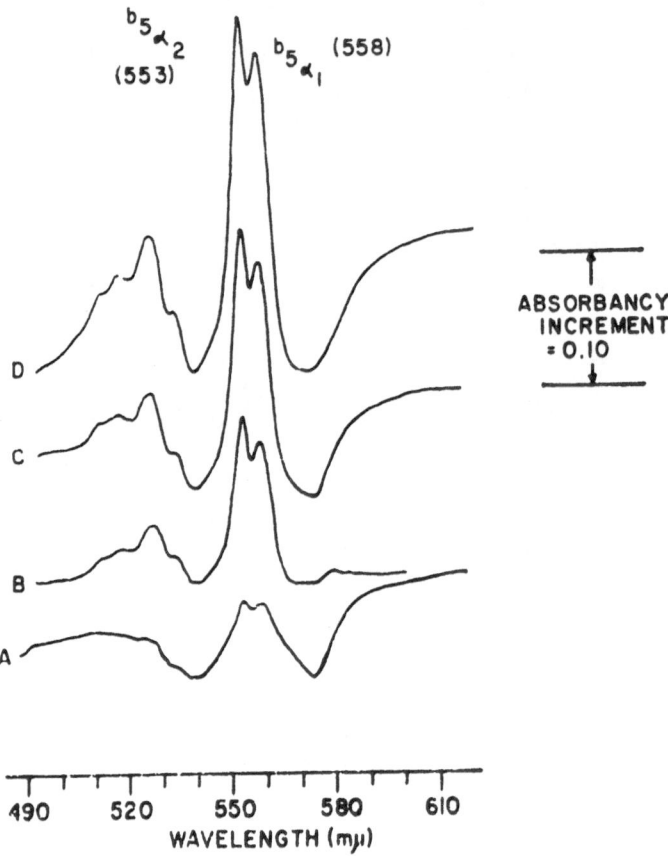

FIG. 19. Low-temperature trapped steady state for reduced cytochrome b_5 of liver microsomes. Rat liver microsomes were suspended in 0.1 *M* potassium phosphate buffer, *p*H 7.4, and were divided equally into two cuvettes of the low temperature accessory. An aliquot of DPNH was then added to the contents of the sample cuvette and the contents of the cuvettes were rapidly cooled by plunging them into liquid nitrogen. The difference spectra were recorded when DPNH sufficient to reduce 27% (curve A), 54% (curve B), and 81% (curve C) of the cytochrome b_5 was added. Curve D represents the difference spectrum obtained when a large excess of DPNH was added to the contents of the sample cuvette. The optical path of the cuvettes was 3 mm. (From Estabrook. 1961. *In* Falk and Morton, eds., *Hematin Enzymes*. Courtesy of Pergamon Press.)

cuvettes gradually changes to a milky opalescence when observed by reflected light. When observed by transmitted light, this transition in physical state, associated with the devitrification of the glycerol-water mixture, appears like an orange-red sunset on a hazy evening. After maximal development of the milky white devitrified state, the cuvettes are again plunged into liquid nitrogen and the microcrystalline state is stabilized. The cuvettes are then raised to just above the level of the liquid nitrogen into the light beams and absolute absorption spectra are recorded in a manner similar to that described in the earlier sections.

The absolute absorption spectra of the pigments of rat liver microsomes at liquid nitrogen temperature are depicted in Figure 18. When microsomes to which sodium dithionite has been added are gassed with carbon monoxide prior to freezing, an absorption band is seen at 450 mμ, corresponding to the absorption band of the CO-complex of reduced cytochrome P-450 observed in spectra obtained at room temperature. Of significance is the splitting of the α-absorption band of reduced cytochrome b_5 into two distinct absorption bands with maxima at 553 and 558 mμ. The absolute absorption spectra of the oxidized pigments of liver microsomes as observed at liquid nitrogen temperature are interesting but at the present time uninterpretable.

When the low temperature method is used for measuring the "trapped steady state" of reduction of the microsomal cytochromes, it is not desirable to include glycerol in the reaction mixture. For this type of experiment the protocol is similar to that described above for standard room temperature difference spectrophotometry. Spectra obtained using the "low temperature trapped steady state technique" are illustrated in Figure 19. An aliquot of liver microsomes is suspended in a buffer mixture (in the absence of glycerol) and a portion of the diluted suspension is added to the reference cuvette. DPNH is added to the remainder of the sample and a portion is *immediately* removed and placed into the sample cuvette. The contents of the two cuvettes are rapidly frozen by plunging into liquid nitrogen. Since glycerol is not present in the reaction mixture, devitrification will not occur; therefore, it is not necessary to warm the sample. In this case, the cooled cuvettes are merely raised to just above the level of the liquid nitrogen and into the path of the light beams and a difference spectrum is recorded. It is apparent from studies of the type presented in Figure 19 that the two absorption bands at 553 and 558 mμ, which are associated with reduced cytochrome b_5, appear simultaneously, suggesting that they are associated with a common pigment.

The "Apparent Absolute Absorption Spectra" of Induced Microsomal Pigments

Treatment of animals with a variety of drugs and carcinogens results in an enhancement of the liver's ability (Conney, 1967) to metabolize oxidatively a number of compounds. Associated with this increase in activity is the induction (Remmer et al., 1967 and 1968) of microsomal hemoproteins. One method of assessing the spectral properties of these induced pigments is a modified difference spectrophotometric technique which permits the recording of an "apparent absolute absorption spectrum." The interpretation of the results obtained by this method has been challenged by Mannering (1971). The basis for this disagreement concerns our assumption that an additive rather than a substitutive change in pigment composition occurs in liver microsomes during the inductive process. The fate of the cytochrome type originally present relative to those induced remains unanswered. The fact that interpretable spectra (Hildebrandt et al., 1968) can be obtained using the method of Kinoshita and Horie (1967) is encouraging and suggests that the method may be a valid measurement of pigment changes.

The method of "apparent absolute absorption spectrophotometry" first developed by Kinoshita and Horie (1967) has yielded results which serve as the basis of assigning the "low spin" and "high spin" states of cytochrome P-450 (Hildebrandt et al., 1968). Implicit in the use of this method is the assumption that the spectral contribution of the pigments present in microsomes prepared from livers of untreated animals can be subtracted from similar pigments present in microsomes prepared from livers of treated animals. In addition, the spectral properties of cytochrome b_5 must be assumed to be the same in both types of liver microsomes. Further, it must be assumed that the induction process does not modify or alter the spectral characteristics of the pigments originally present in microsomes. Thus the spectral changes measured must be considered only as the "absorption spectra" of those additional pigments present in microsomes from induced animals and *not* as a measure of the absolute absorption spectrum of *all* the pigments

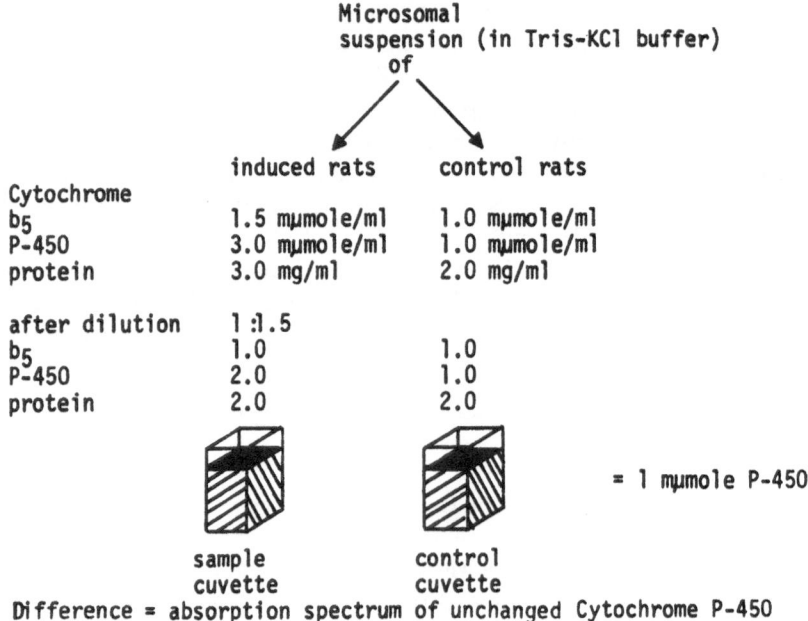

FIG. 20. An example of the experimental protocol for the determination of the "apparent absolute absorption spectrum" of pigments of liver microsomes induced by phenobarbital.

present in the microsomal preparation. For this reason spectra obtained by the method of Kinoshita and Horie (1967) are termed *"apparent absolute absorption spectra."*

In order to determine the "apparent absolute absorption spectrum," each sample of microsomes is initially examined by difference spectrophotometry to determine the content of cytochrome b_5 as described above (pp. 318-319). The "apparent absolute absorption spectrum" can then be recorded for the pigments induced by treatment of the experimental animals. This comparison is illustrated by the hypothetical experimental protocol shown in Figure 20. Samples of the two types of liver microsomes (i.e., from normal animals and treated animals) are diluted in a buffer so that they contain an equal concentration of cytochrome b_5. A portion of the diluted microsomes from normal animals is placed in the reference cuvette, while a portion of the diluted microsomes from treated animals is placed

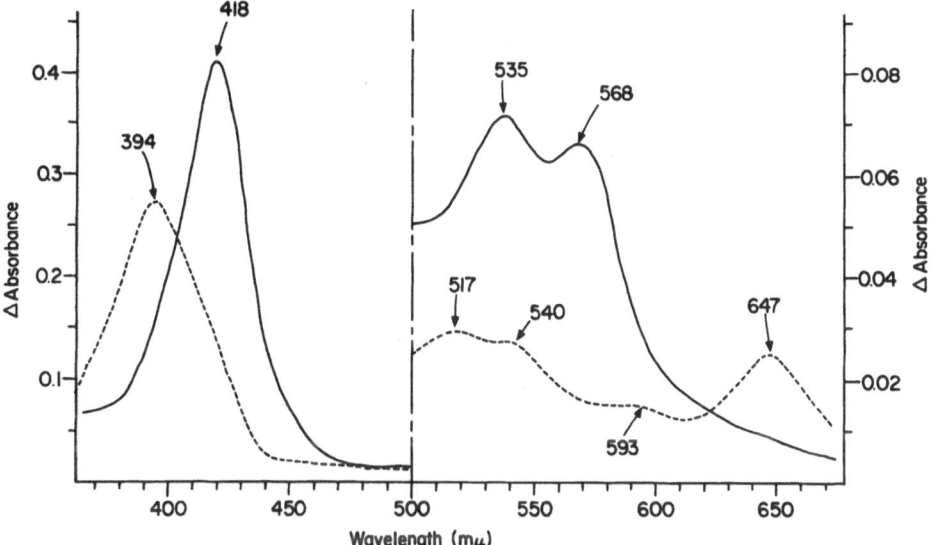

FIG. 21. Comparison of the absorption spectra of the oxidized hemoprotein of liver microsomes induced by treatment of rabbits with 3-methylcholanthrene or phenobarbital. Microsomes from livers of control, phenobarbital (PB)- or 3-methylcholanthrene (3-MC)-treated rabbits were examined spectrophotometrically in order to determine the content of cytochrome b_5 using the procedure described by Omura and Sato (1964). The spectrum of the additional pigment associated with microsomes from PB-treated rabbits (solid line) was determined by recording the spectral difference between a cuvette containing liver microsomes from PB-treated rabbits (2.2 mg protein per ml, 0.73 mμmoles cytochrome b_5 per mg, 2.92 mμmoles hemin per mg) minus a cuvette containing liver microsomes from a saline control rabbit (3.0 mg protein per ml, 0.51 mμmoles cytochrome b_5 per mg, 1.44 mμmoles hemin per mg). The additional pigment associated with microsomes from 3-MC-treated rabbits (dashed line) was determined in a similar manner by recording the spectral difference between a cuvette containing liver microsomes from 3-MC-treated rabbits (3.0 mg protein per ml, 0.79 mμmoles cytochrome b_5 per mg, 2.5 mμmoles hemin per mg) minus a cuvette containing liver microsomes from a corn oil treated rabbit (3.0 mg protein per ml, 0.78 mμmoles cytochrome b_5 per mg, 1.6 mμmoles hemin per mg). Microsomes were diluted in 50 mM tris-chloride buffer, pH 7.5, containing 15 mM KCl to the protein concentrations indicated. Temperature, 25°C. (From Hildebrandt et al. 1968. *Biochem. Biophys. Res. Commun.* 30:607-612.)

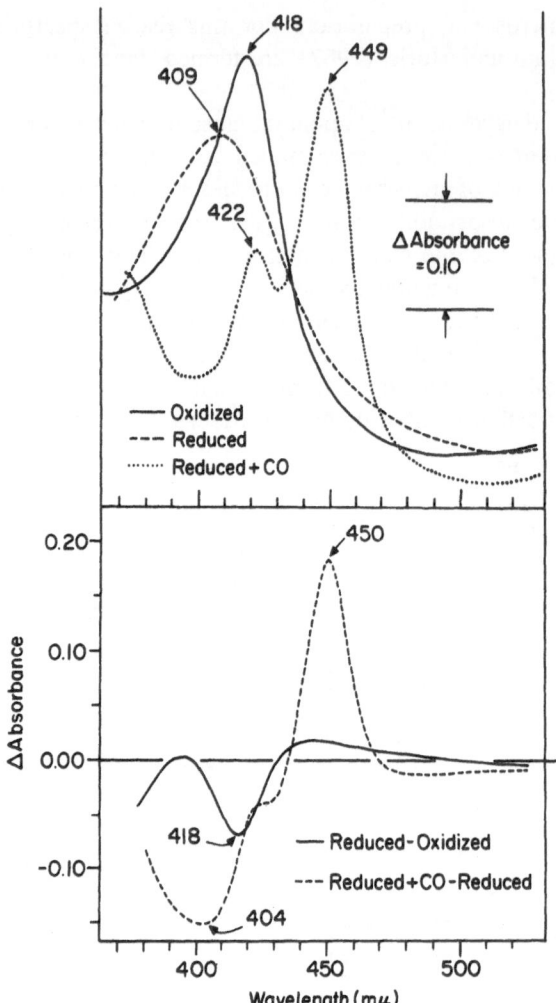

FIG. 22. The "apparent absolute absorption spectrum" of the oxidized, reduced, and carbon monoxide treated reduced hemoprotein induced in rat liver microsomes. Experiments were carried out as described in Figure 21 using an appropriate dilution of liver microsomes from phenobarbital-treated rats in the sample cuvette and a dilution of microsomes from livers of normal rats containing an equivalent concentration of cytochrome b_5 in the reference cuvette. The "apparent absolute absorption spectrum" of the oxidized pigment is shown by the solid line. A few crystals of $Na_2S_2O_4$ were added to the contents of *both* the sample and reference cuvette and the spectrum of the reduced hemoprotein was recorded (dashed line). The contents of *both* the sample and reference cuvettes were gassed with CO for 3 minutes and the spectrum of the CO-complex of the reduced hemoprotein recorded (dotted line).

in the sample cuvette. Since the concentration of cytochrome b_5 is equal in both the sample and reference cuvettes, it will not contribute to the spectral changes observed. The success of this method rests on the assumption that the spectral contribution of pigments present in the reference cuvette can be legitimately subtracted from the spectra of the same pigments present in the sample cuvette.

The application of this spectrophotometric method is shown by the experiment described in Figure 21, in which microsomes prepared from animals treated with either phenobarbital or 3-methylcholanthrene are compared to those from untreated animals. The presence of two spectrally distinct types of cytochrome P-450 is obvious. As seen in Figure 22, this method can also be used to obtain the "apparent absolute absorption spectra" of reduced cytochrome P-450 as well as its CO-complex. However, in contrast to the standard protocol of difference spectrophotometry, it is necessary to add the reactants, such as $Na_2S_2O_4$ and CO, to the contents of both the sample and reference cuvettes.

Similarly, samples can be examined at the temperature of liquid nitrogen by the technique of "apparent absolute absorption spectrophotometry." These low temperature spectra have been useful in the assignment of the high and low spin states of microsomal cytochrome P-450 (Hildebrandt et al., 1968). Further interpretation of the results obtained by these methods awaits a better understanding of the chemistry of cytochrome P-450.

Rapid Repetitive Scanning Difference Spectrophotometry

The discussion of difference spectrophotometry presented in the earlier sections did not consider transient spectral species of the microsomal electron transport system that might arise during the steady state. These intermediates can be detected by use of a modified split-beam spectrophotometer that permits continuous repetitive scanning of a limited portion of the spectrum. The X-Y recorder of the Aminco-Chance instrument is modified by the introduction of microswitches and solenoid actuators. The spectral range to be examined is controlled by contact microswitches, mounted on the recorder, which are activated by the pen bar of the X-Y recorder. The impulse from the microswitches raises or lowers the pen and drives a solenoid plunger which pushes either the forward or the reverse drive buttons of the recorder. Figure 23 shows the results obtained using this technique in which the wavelength range 375 to 475 mμ was scanned every 25 seconds. In this experiment liver microsomes were diluted in a reaction mixture containing hexobarbital and a TPNH-generating system. The sample and reference cuvettes were placed in the instrument in the same manner as described above for standard difference spectrophotometry. The repetitive scanning attachment was activated and a baseline of nearly equal light absorbance was recorded. After three scans of the baseline, TPNH was added to the contents of the sample cuvette and spectral transitions indicating the presence of an oxygenated form of reduced cytochrome P-450 (Estabrook et al., 1971) were observed. A further spectral transition occurred as anaerobiosis was attained by the contents of the sample cuvette. To aid in interpreting the multitude of spectra obtained, a strip chart recorder was run in parallel with the X-Y recorder so that each individual spectrum was recorded. The versatility of this method and the type of new information it yields cannot be overemphasized. It is hoped that this simple adaptation will be a standard accessory for commercial instruments in the near future.

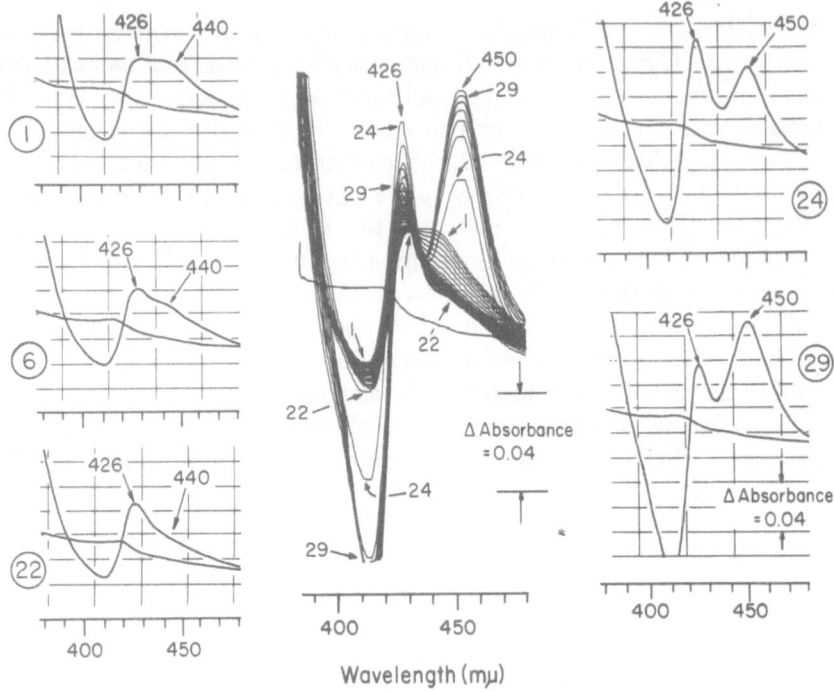

FIG. 23. Repetitive scanning of difference spectra of hepatic microsomal pigments in the presence of hexobarbital. Rat liver microsomes from phenobarbital-treated rats were diluted to a protein concentration of 2 mg per ml in a buffer mixture containing 50 mM tris-chloride buffer, pH 7.4, 150 mM KCl, 10 mM MgCl$_2$, 10 mM nicotinamide, 7 mM sodium isocitrate, 2 mM hexobarbital, and excess isocitrate dehydrogenase. The suspension of diluted microsomes was divided equally between two cuvettes, and a baseline of essentially equal light absorbance was recorded. TPNH (200 μM final concentration) was then added to the contents of the sample cuvette, and the difference spectra were continuously recorded using an Aminco-Chance spectrophotometer modified for repetitive scanning. A Varian strip chart recorder was run in parallel with the X-Y recorder and individual spectral curves recorded as shown. The individual difference spectra for scans 1, 6, 22, 24, and 26 are illustrated in order to aid in resolving the multitude of tracings obtained during the repetitive scan experiment.

APPLICATION OF THE DUAL WAVELENGTH SPECTROPHOTOMETRIC METHOD

Measurement of Slow Spectral Transitions

Recording spectral transitions at a fixed wavelength as a function of time permits the evaluation of the kinetics of a reaction and the influence of various factors on the steady state. However, the turbidity of particulate suspensions imposes a number of limitations on the study of the kinetics of spectral transitions. As discussed earlier (pp. 314-317), it is best to measure a spectral change at an absorption band maximum relative to a nearby isosbestic point. If light scattering changes occur during the time course of the reaction and if the reference wavelength is far removed from the sample wavelength (i.e. greater than 50 mμ), significant errors can be introduced. A severe limitation is imposed on the type of experiment performed due to the relatively slow response time of the amplifier circuit associated

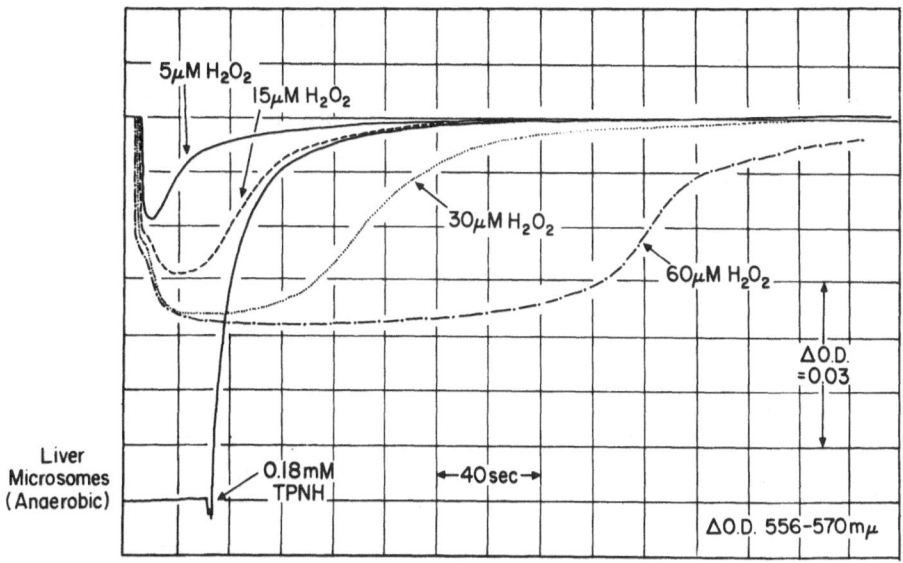

FIG. 24. The effect of varying concentrations of oxygen on the oxidation of reduced cytochrome P-450 of liver microsomes. Rat liver microsomes were diluted in a tris-chloride buffer mixture containing heart muscle submitochondrial particles, sodium succinate, nicotinamide, catalase, sodium isocitrate, and isocitrate dehydrogenase. After the sample became anaerobic (about 10 minutes) an aliquot of TPNH was added and the reduction of cytochrome b_5 and cytochrome P-450 was measured at 556 minus 570 mμ. The effect of adding varying concentrations of hydrogen peroxide on the oxidation of cytochrome P-450 is shown by the superimposed traces in the upper part of the figure. (From Estabrook et al. 1968. Hoppe-Seyler Z. Physiol. Chem., 349:1605-1608.)

with a conventional recorder (1 to 2 sec). By suitably modifying the amplifier circuit for the photomultiplier signals, it is possible to record very rapid spectral changes of turbid suspensions (see below) utilizing an oscilloscope.

An example of the dual wavelength method in which the wavelength pair 556 minus 570 mμ was used to monitor the oxidation or reduction of cytochrome P-450, is illustrated in Figure 24. Liver microsomes, suspended in a buffer medium containing a TPNH-generating system as well as a catalytic amount of submitochondrial particles and catalase, were placed in an anaerobic cuvette equipped with a plunger. After gassing the sample with argon for about five minutes, sodium succinate was added to the contents of the cuvette and the reaction mixture permitted to attain anaerobiosis. The cuvette containing the anaerobic sample was then placed in the spectrophotometer and the intensity of the light beam transmitted at 556 mμ was equalized to the intensity of the light beam transmitted at 570 mμ. On adding TPNH to the anaerobic sample, an immediate increase in absorbance was observed at 556 mμ relative to 570 mμ. This transition is associated with the reduction of cytochrome b_5 and cytochrome P-450. After the anaerobic steady state of reduced cytochrome b_5 and cytochrome P-450 was attained, a small aliquot of H_2O_2 was introduced into the sample by means of the plunger. This resulted in a rapid decrease in absorbance due to the oxidation of reduced cytochrome P-450 by the oxygen generated from H_2O_2 by catalase. As shown in Figure 24, the oxidized state of cytochrome P-450 is transiently present and the lifetime of the oxidized state is dependent on the concentration of H_2O_2 added to the reaction mixture. The time scale used in this experiment is excellent for demonstrating the cycles of oxidation and reduction associated with the functioning of cytochrome P-450, although little or no information can be gained about the initial rate of oxygen interaction with reduced cytochrome P-450.

One of the more important assays of cytochrome P-450 function in drug metabolism is the measurement of the rate of enzymic reduction of cytochrome P-450. The rate of reduction of cytochrome P-450 is determined in the presence of carbon monoxide so that the large increase in absorbance associated with the formation of the CO-complex of reduced cytochrome P-450 can be measured at 450 mμ. The results obtained from this type of measurement are interesting since it has been observed that the kinetics of reduction are complex, i.e., they do not conform to a simple first order reaction (Diehl et al., 1970). Also, it has been shown by Gigon et al. (1968) that the presence of certain hydroxylatable substrates markedly affects the rate of cytochrome P-450 reduction. For studies of this type it is imperative that oxygen be completely removed from the reaction medium. This is accomplished by using an anaerobic cuvette and by gassing the sample of diluted microsomes with carbon monoxide for about five minutes. After gassing the sample with carbon monoxide, the cuvette is sealed and placed in the spectrophotometer with the measuring wavelength at 450 mμ and the reference wavelength at 490 mμ. As shown in Figure 25, the addition of TPNH causes a rapid increase in absorbance at 450 mμ relative to 490 mμ. The use of a rapid time scale for recording the absorbance changes reveals the limitation imposed by the mixing of TPNH with

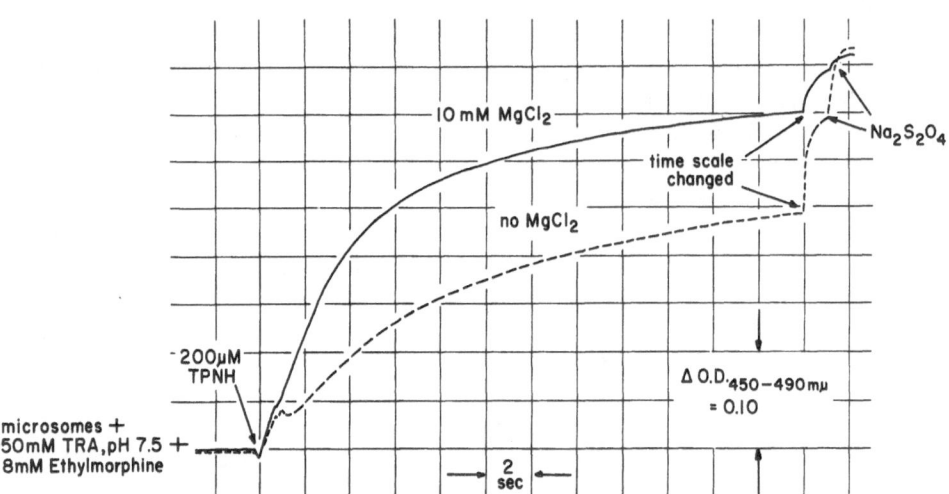

FIG. 25. The kinetic measurement of cytochrome P-450 reduction in the presence of carbon monoxide. Rat liver microsomes were diluted in 50 mM triethanolamine buffer (TRA), pH 7.5, containing 8 mM ethylmorphine. Magnesium chloride was added where indicated. After gassing the samples for 5 minutes with CO in an anaerobic cuvette, the reaction was initiated by the addition of TPNH (200 μM final concentration) with the plunger of the anaerobic cuvette. The increase of absorbance for the wavelength pair 450 minus 490 mμ was determined.

the cuvette contents. The interruption of the kinetic tracing for the first second is attributable to this mixing artifact. Thus, the time of response of the measurement is dictated by the speed of mixing the reactants. The development of rapid mixing attachments which can be incorporated with dual wavelength spectrophotometers has greatly extended the usable time for such kinetic studies.

Measurement of Rapid Spectral Changes

The development of rapid mixing techniques, in particular as applied to the spectrophotometric measurement of biological samples, has been summarized in several reviews (Chance et al., 1964; Gibson, 1969). The application of this technique to the study of pharmacologically interesting reactions is only now gaining favor, and it can be predicted that greater interest in this area will develop in the near future (see also Chapter 10).

The schematic drawing presented in Figure 26 (American Instrument Com-

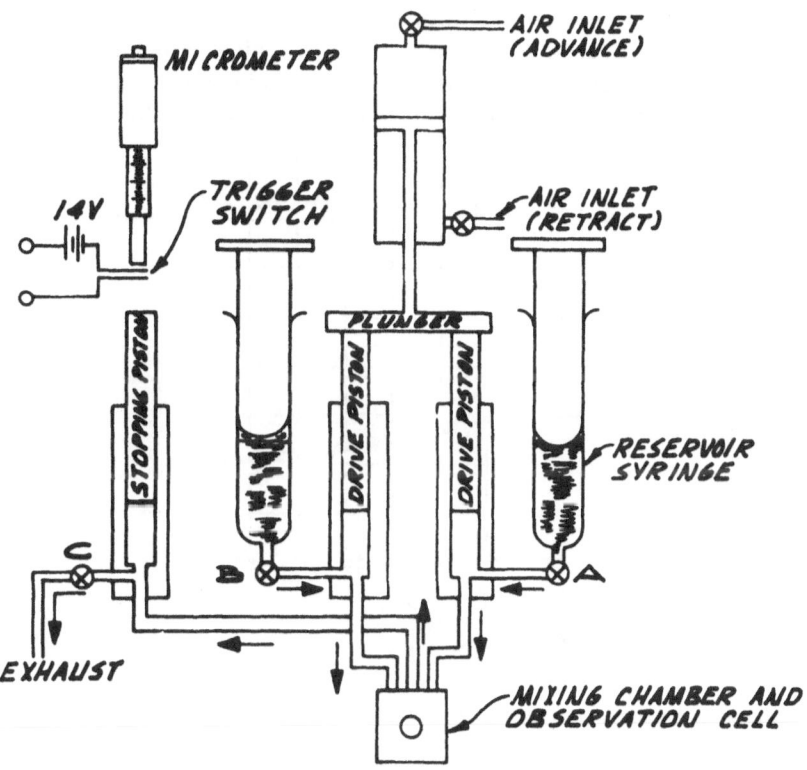

FIG. 26. A schematic representation of the Aminco-Morrow stopped flow apparatus. The diluted suspension of microsomes is placed in the reservoir syringe *A* and a solution of the reactant in reservoir syringe *B*. The two solutions are displaced by the drive pistons into the mixing chamber, which is mounted in the light beams of the spectrophotometer. (From *Operating Instruction Manual for the Aminco-Morrow Stopped Flow Apparatus,* 1970. Courtesy of the American Instrument Company.)

pany, 1970) represents one type of instrument that can be employed for the spectro-photometric evaluation of rapid reaction kinetics. For this method the sample to be examined is placed in one of the driving syringes of the apparatus while a solution of the compound initiating the reaction is placed in the second driving syringe. The contents of the driving syringes are discharged by manual or air pressure displacement of the syringe plungers, so that the syringe contents interact in a mixing chamber. The design of suitable mixing chambers provides for the complete mixing of the reactants without introducing artifacts resulting from cavitation or birefringence patterns. The Aminco-Morrow apparatus used in the authors' laboratory incorporates the mixing chamber into the spectrophotometer in place of the normal cuvette. With such an apparatus, spectral changes which occur slower than 3 milliseconds can be readily measured. The restrictions imposed by turbid suspensions, discussed in the early parts of this chapter, must also be considered in experiments involving rapid mixing techniques.

The composite tracing in Figure 27 demonstrates the application of the rapid mixing technique to the measurement of the combination of CO with reduced cytochrome P-450 of rat liver microsomes. The microsomes were suspended in buffer and the pigments reduced by the addition of sodium dithionite. This anaerobic suspension was placed in one syringe of the rapid mixing apparatus, and a solution of buffer (without microsomes) containing sodium dithionite, which had

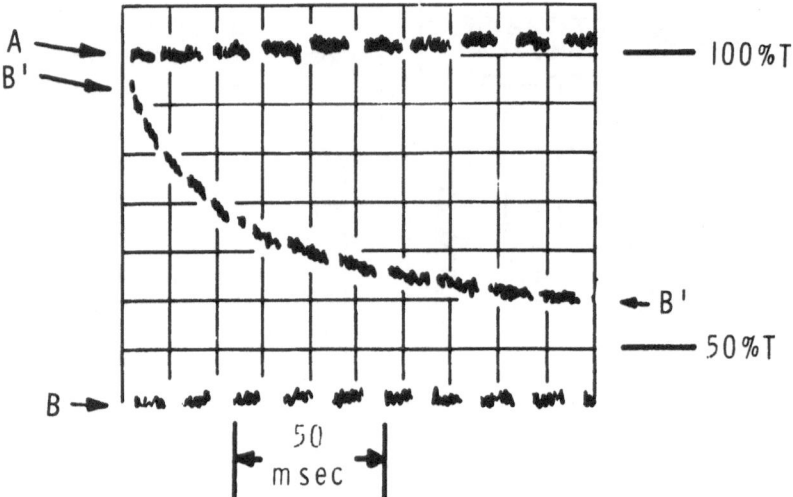

FIG. 27. The rapid kinetic measurement of the rate of CO combination with reduced cytochrome P-450. As described in the text, a sample of liver microsomes from phenobarbital-treated rats was diluted to 4 mg per ml in 0.1 M potassium phosphate buffer, pH 7.4, and a few crystals of $Na_2S_2O_4$ were added. The anaerobic sample was placed in one syringe of the stopped-flow apparatus (cf. Fig. 26). A solution of 0.1 M potassium phosphate buffer, pH 7.4, containing $Na_2S_2O_4$ was gassed with CO for 10 minutes and placed in the other syringe. At zero time, the contents of the two syringes were mixed and the changes in percent of transmission at 490 mμ (A) and 450 mμ (B') were determined. At the conclusion of the reaction the extent of the reaction as measured at 450 mμ was determined (B). The experiment was repeated and the results superimposed on the oscilloscope tracing.

been gassed for about five minutes with carbon monoxide, was placed in the other syringe. At zero time, the contents of the two syringes were mixed, and the reaction of CO with reduced cytochrome P-450 was followed at 450 mμ and 490 mμ. In this experiment the light beam alternator was operating, and absorbance changes at 490 mμ were monitored to insure that no significant change in the light scattering properties of the sample occurred. Since the light beam alternator was employed, the photomultiplier observed two signals of about 8 milliseconds duration every 16.7 milliseconds. The experiment was repeated twice and the results superimposed permitting the more complete evaluation of the kinetic tracing. As illustrated in Figure 27 the time resolution is increased by a factor of nearly 100, as compared to the results obtained using the dual wavelength spectrophotometric method described above. Use of this technique will allow a better delineation of pigment function associated with oxidative drug metabolism.

SPECIAL PROBLEMS: SPECTRAL MEASUREMENTS OF SUBSTRATE INTERACTION WITH CYTOCHROME P-450

The recognition that cytochrome P-450 functions as the terminal oxidase in many drug oxidation reactions led to studies on the interaction between drugs and the pigments of liver microsomes. Following the observation of Narasimhulu et al. (1965) that spectral changes occur when steroid substrates are added to adrenocortical microsomes, Remmer et al. (1966) and Imai and Sato (1966) reported comparable spectral changes when certain drug substrates were added to liver

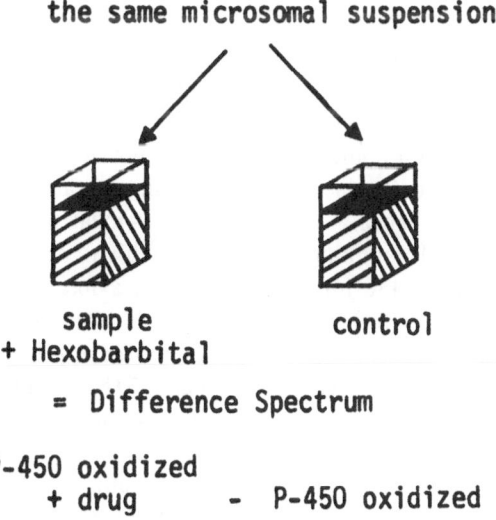

FIG. 28. The experimental protocol employed when determining the difference spectrum resulting from drug (hexobarbital) interaction with microsomal cytochrome P-450.

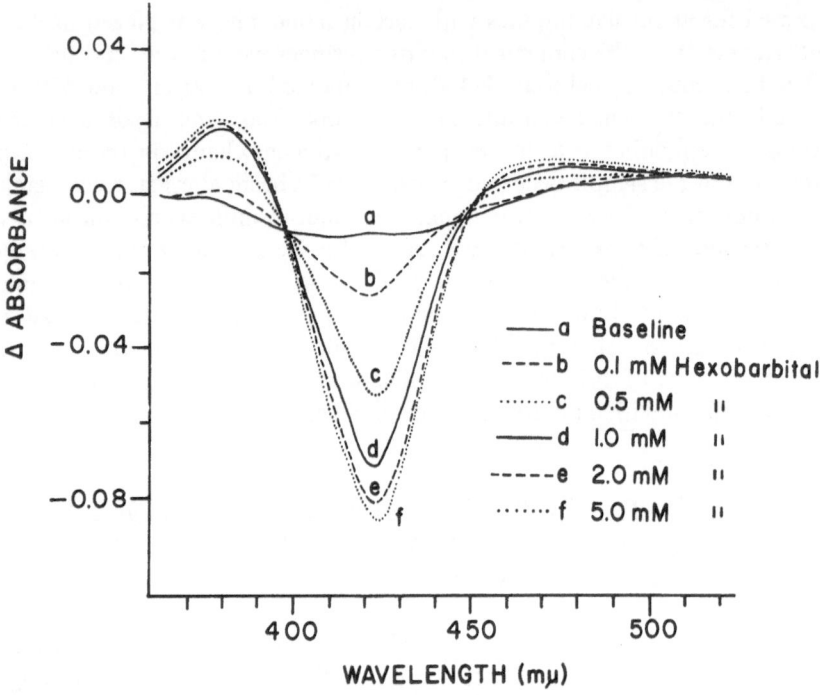

FIG. 29. Spectral changes associated with the interaction of hexobarbital with microsomal cyto-chrome P-450. A sample of rat liver microsomes was diluted to 1 mg protein per ml in 50 m*M* tris-chloride buffer, *p*H 7.4, containing 150 m*M* KCl. The diluted sample was divided equally into two cuvettes and a baseline of nearly equal light absorbance was recorded (curve *a*). Varying concentrations of a hexobarbital solution were added to the contents of the sample cuvette and the difference spectrum was recorded. The data presented are the composite of a number of experiments using a fresh sample of diluted microsomes for each experiment.

microsomal suspensions. It was observed that substrates produced either of two different types of spectral changes and that these substrates could be divided into two general classes of compounds: Type I compounds are those which interact with cytochrome P-450 to give a loss of absorbance at about 420 mμ concomitant with an increase in absorbance at about 385 mμ as measured by difference spectro-photometry; and Type II compounds are those which cause the appearance of an absorption band at about 430 mμ associated with a loss of absorbance at 395 to 405 mμ. The study of spectral changes that result from the interaction of a sub-strate molecule with cytochrome P-450 is simply an application of the difference spectrophotometric method described on page 318, as indicated schematically in Figure 28. An example of the type of results obtained is shown in Figure 29. For this experiment a sample of liver microsomes was suspended in a suitable buffer and divided equally into two cuvettes and a baseline of equal light absorbance established. Then a small aliquot of a solution of substrate, such as hexobarbital (a Type I substrate) is added to the contents of the sample cuvette and the difference spectrum is recorded. As the concentration of hexobarbital in the sample cuvette is increased, the changes in absorbance increase. The fact that isosbestic points are maintained near 400 and 445 mμ during the titration experiment is evidence that only one type of spectral change is occurring and that no significant artifacts arise from a modification of the light scattering properties of the suspension. It is imperative that the volume changes of the contents in the cuvettes be minimal, generally no larger than 15 to 20 μl. Furthermore, it is necessary to demonstrate that identical spectral results are obtained when either multiple additions of a dilute solution of a substrate or a single addition of a more concentrated solution of the substrate is made to another sample of microsomes, e.g., the spectral change observed after five additions of 3 μl aliquots of a 0.2 M solution of hexobarbital should be the same as that observed after addition of a single 5 μl aliquot of a 0.6 M solution of hexobarbital. This type of spectral titration can also be carried out using a spectrophotometer in the dual wavelength configuration by measuring the decrease in absorbance at 420 mμ relative to an isosbestic point or to the maximum at 385 mμ. Since the magnitude of the spectral change is frequently rather small, it is best to confirm the results obtained using the dual wavelength type of experiment by repeating the experiment using the split-beam difference spectrophotometric method.

The magnitude of the spectral change resulting from substrate interaction with oxidized cytochrome P-450 is dependent not only on the concentration of substrate but also on the concentration of cytochrome P-450 in the microsomal suspension. This is illustrated by the series of experiments presented in Figure 30, in which aminopyrine was added to varying concentrations of liver microsomes. The rela-

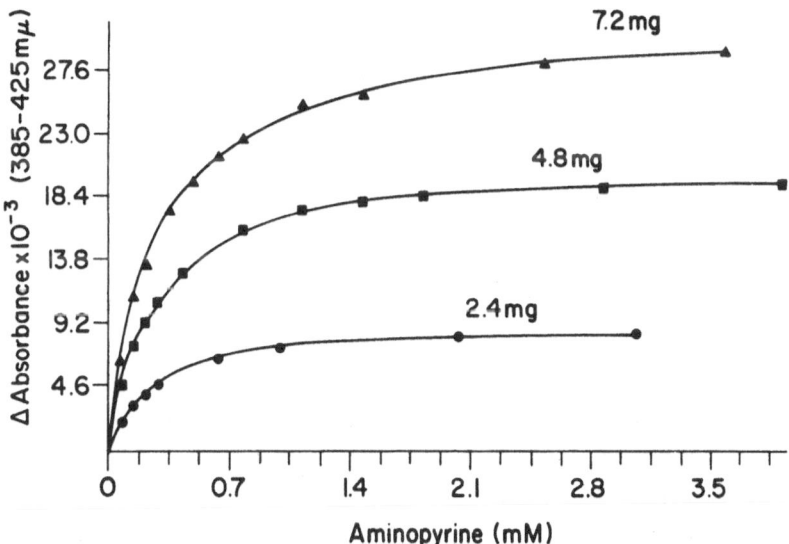

FIG. 30. The effect of varying concentrations of aminopyrine on the magnitude of the spectral change observed with different concentrations of liver microsomes. Rat liver microsomes prepared from phenobarbital-treated animals were diluted in a buffer mixture containing 50 mM tris-chloride, pH 7.4, and 150 mM KCl to the protein concentrations indicated. Varying concentrations of aminopyrine were added to the sample cuvette, and the magnitude of the spectral change at 385 mμ relative to that at 425 mμ was determined.

tionship form of Lineweaver-Burke (Mahler and Cordes, 1966) enables one to determine (Figure 31) a binding constant, K_s, *defined as the concentration of reactant that results in a spectral change of 50% of the theoretical maximal spectral change obtainable.* By definition, K_s is independent of protein concentration and, therefore, if the measured K_s varies with protein concentration, it is only an "apparent K_s." The interpretation of this constant is still unknown, although there are suggestions (Schenkman et al., 1967) that it is related to the affinity of the overall metabolic reaction for some substrates.

As indicated above, the evaluation of the spectral change observed on addition of a substrate to oxidized cytochrome P-450 is the subject of much speculation. This is undoubtedly a consequence of the impurity of the system and the possible heterogeneity of cytochrome P-450. This is readily apparent when comparing the results obtained using liver microsomes with results obtained (Peterson, 1971) employing the isolated purified cytochrome P-450 of the bacterium *Pseudomonas putida.*

Studies of substrate binding to cytochrome P-450 of liver microsomes using the technique of *apparent absolute absorption spectrophotometry* described above (pp. 331-335) show, as illustrated in Figure 32, that on addition of hexobarbital

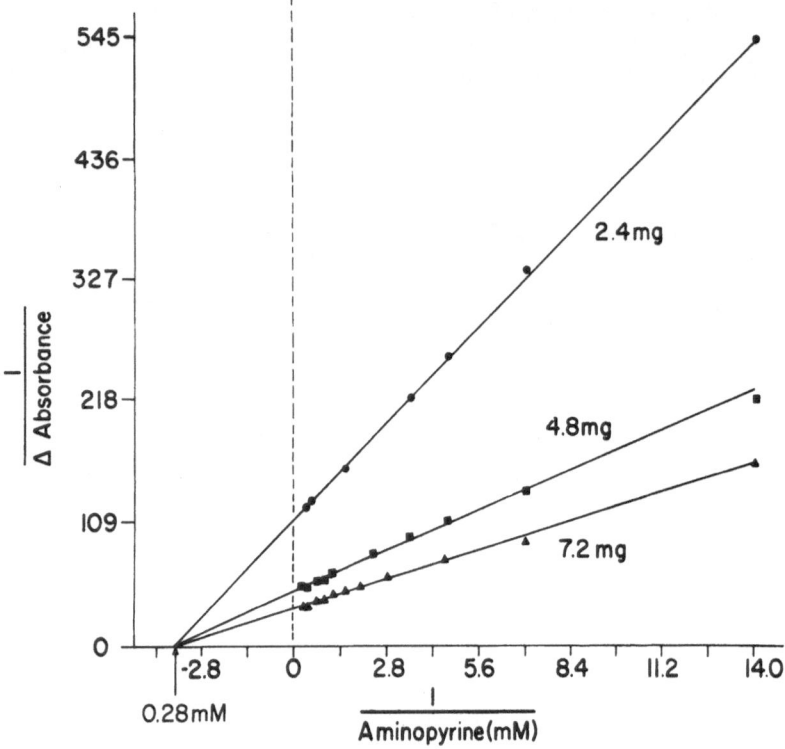

FIG. 31. Graphic determination of the spectral binding constant, K_s. The data presented in Figure 30 have been plotted in the reciprocal form of Lineweaver and Burk. The value of K_s can be readily determined from the reciprocal of the negative intercept with the abscissa.

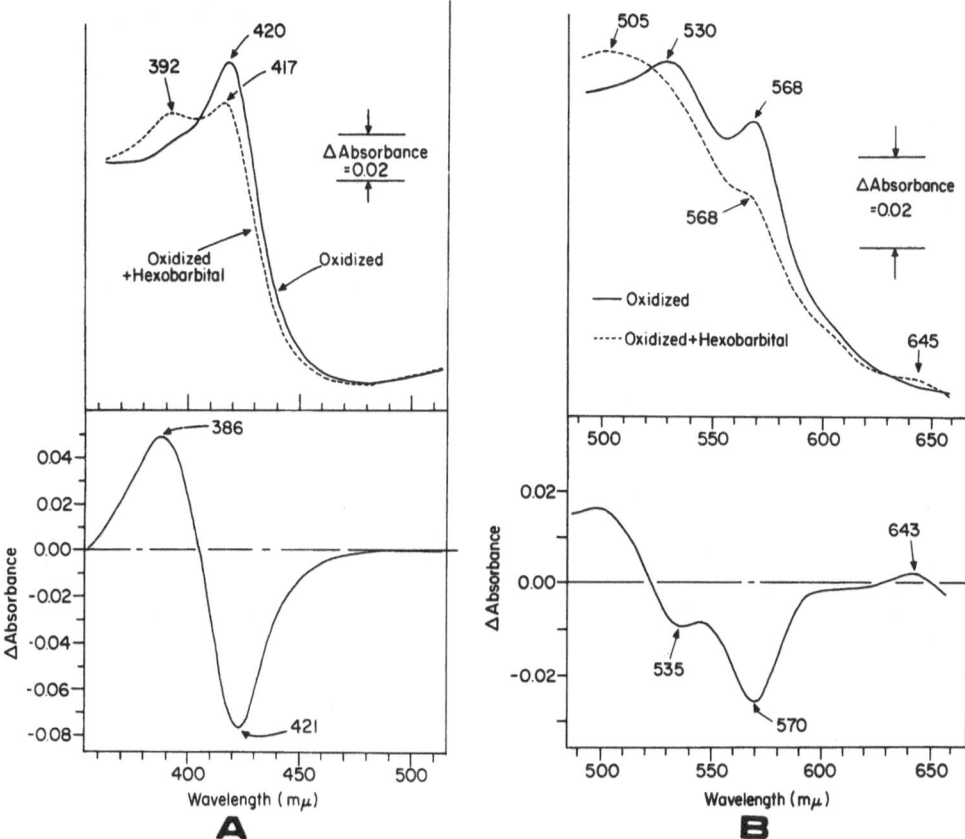

FIG. 32. The "apparent absolute absorption spectra" of cytochrome P-450 in the presence and absence of hexobarbital. A series of spectral studies were carried out as described in Figure 22 employing liver microsomes from phenobarbital-treated rats and from control rats. The solid line represents the spectrum of cytochrome P-450 induced by phenobarbital in the absence of hexobarbital, while the dashed line is the spectrum in the presence of hexobarbital. The changes in the difference spectrum observed on addition of hexobarbital to liver microsomes is shown in the lower portions of the figure. The concentration of protein used was approximately four times greater for the spectral studies in the visible region (B) than for the studies in the Soret region (A) of the spectrum.

there is only a partial conversion of the spectral species of oxidized cytochrome P-450 with a maximum at 420 mμ to the form with an absorption maximum at about 388 mμ. The nature of the nonreactive form of cytochrome P-450 present in liver microsomes remains a mystery and a challenge for future investigations. In contrast, comparable studies with the isolated and purified cytochrome P-450 of bacteria (Peterson, 1971) reveals (Figure 33) an almost complete spectral transition on the addition of the substrate camphor to oxidized cytochrome P-450 from the form with an absorption band maximum at 418 mμ to the form with an absorption band maximum at 392 mμ.

The Type II class of substrates is typified by a compound such as aniline.

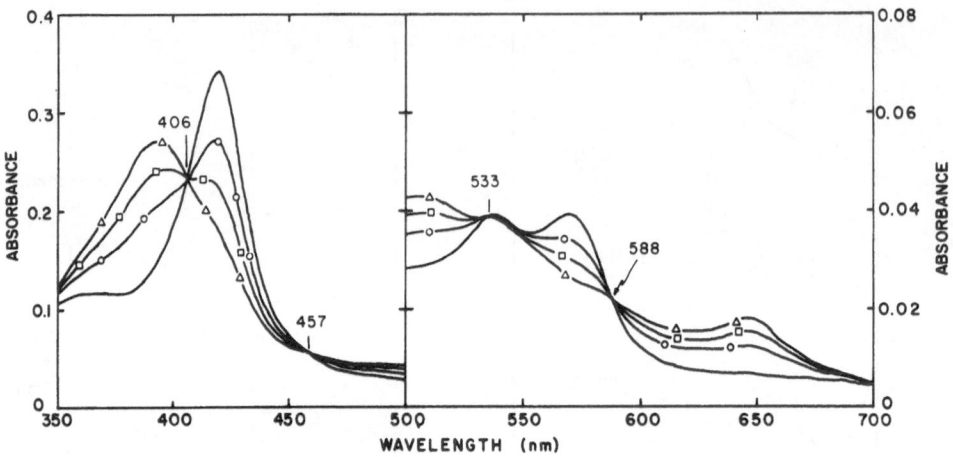

FIG. 33. Titration of camphor-free *P. putida* cytochrome P-450 with camphor. Camphor-free cytochrome P-450 was diluted to a final concentration of 3.3 μM in 50 mM tris-chloride buffer, pH 7.4, containing 0.1 M KCl. The reference cuvette contained buffer without cytochrome P-450. Aliquots of buffer containing camphor were added to the sample and reference cuvettes. The final concentration of camphor in each sample was: O (—); 2μM (—O—); 6μM (—□—); and 20.5 μM (—△—). (From Peterson. 1971. *Arch. Biochem. Biophys.*, in press.)

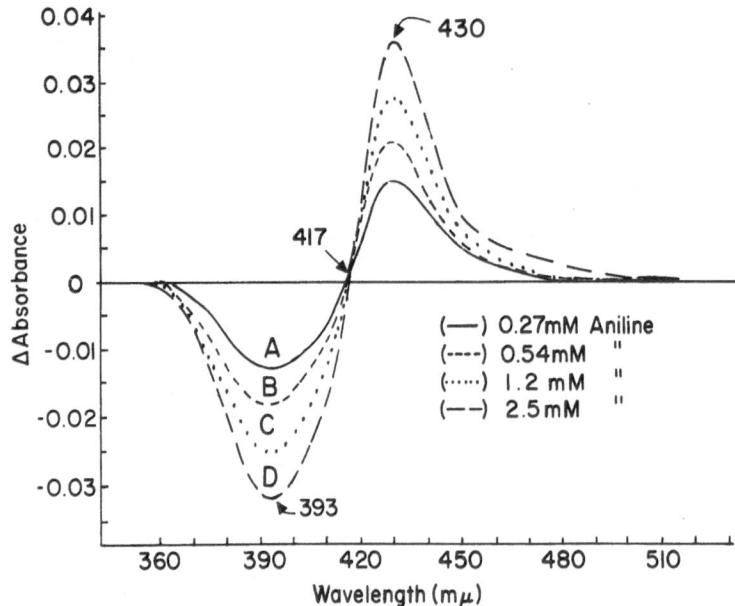

FIG. 34. The effect of various concentrations of aniline on the magnitude of the Type II spectral change. Liver microsomes from phenobarbital-treated rats were diluted in 50 mM tris-chloride buffer, pH 7.4, containing 150 mM KCl, and divided equally into two cuvettes. After establishment of a baseline of equal light absorbance, various concentrations of aniline were added to the sample cuvette as indicated. (From Schenkman et al. 1967. *Molec. Pharmacol.*, 3:113-123.)

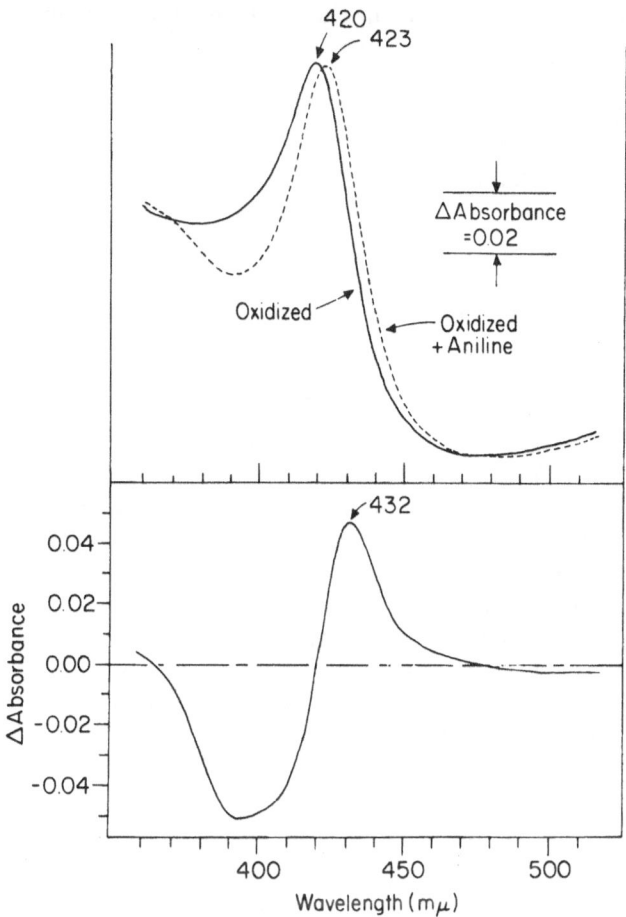

FIG. 35. The "apparent absolute absorption spectra" of cytochrome P-450 in the presence and absence of aniline. Spectral studies were carried out as described in Figure 22 by comparing liver microsomes from phenobarbital-treated rats with liver microsomes from control rats. The solid line represents the spectrum in the absence of aniline, while the dashed line represents the spectrum after 2.5 mM aniline (final concentration) was added to the contents of both the sample and reference cuvettes. The lower part of the figure demonstrates the difference spectrum obtained in the presence of aniline (cf. Fig. 34).

As illustrated in Figure 34, addition of small aliquots of an aniline solution results in progressive spectral changes that are dependent on the aniline concentration present in the reaction cuvette. In this instance a single isosbestic point at 417 mμ is observed. Again one may determine a spectral constant K_s and estimate the concentration of aniline required to give 50% of the maximal theoretical spectral change. The interpretation of how nitrogenous base substrates interact with cytochrome P-450 is even less clear since a variety of reactions can occur (i.e., co-ordinate covalent linkage of the nitrogen with the iron of the heme group). Applying the technique of *apparent absolute absorption spectrophotometry* to

measure the spectral changes occurring during the binding of aniline by cytochrome
P-450, one observes, as shown in Figure 35, that the spectral changes are markedly
different from those obtained when a Type I substrate such as hexobarbital is added
to liver microsomes (compare Figure 32). The further delineation of the chemistry
of cytochrome P-450 and the nature of its natural ligands will be required before a
more definitive interpretation of these spectral results can be made.

CONCLUSION

As indicated in this article, optical spectrophotometry can be an extremely
valuable technique in furthering our understanding of the series of events which
occur at the molecular level during oxidative drug metabolism. The membrane
association of pigments functional in drug metabolism imposes a number of restrictions on the approaches and interpretations that are possible when employing
conventional spectrophotometric methods. Difference spectrophotometry of turbid
suspensions is an extremely powerful method which can be used to circumvent in
part these limitations. However, the sensitivity of this technique may be a disadvantage since it may mislead the investigator into a series of pitfalls resulting
in artifacts and spurious conclusions. Extreme care and a variety of approaches
should be taken in order to insure the validity of any spectral observation. It is
hoped that the present article will give some insight into the types of studies
possible and the results that might be expected. In writing an article of this type
it is frightening to consider the many things that have been left unsaid, but it is
hoped that any investigator who undertakes a series of rapid and sensitive spectrophotometric experiments will use prudence in designing his experiments and
interpretating his results. Publication of bad experiments will incur the displeasure
of one's colleagues and will constitute an abuse of a method which holds great
promise for furthering our understanding of the reactions associated with drug
metabolism.

REFERENCES

American Instrument Company. 1968. Operating Instruction Manual for the Aminco-
Chance Dual Wavelength/Split-Beam Recording Spectrophotometer.
_____ 1970. Operating Instruction Manual for the Aminco-Morrow Stopped-Flow
Apparatus.
Beckman Instruments, Inc. 1954. Operating Instruction Manual for Model DU Spectrophotometer.
Brodie, B. B., J. Axelrod, J. R. Cooper, L. Gaudette, B. N. LaDu, C. Mitoma, and
S. Udenfriend. 1955. Detoxication of drugs and other foreign compounds by liver
microsomes. Science, 121:603-604.
Chance, B. 1947. Stable spectrophotometry of small density changes. Rev. Sci. Instrum.,
18:601-609.
_____ 1952. Spectra and reaction kinetics of respiratory pigments of homogenized
and intact cells. Nature (London), 169:215-221.
_____ 1957. Techniques for the assay of the respiratory enzymes. In Colowick, S. P.,
and N. O. Kaplan, eds., Methods in Enzymology, Vol. 4, 273-329. New York,
Academic Press.

_____ R. H. Eisenhardt, Q. H. Gibson, and K. K. Lonberg-Holm, eds. 1964. Rapid Mixing and Sampling Techniques in Biochemistry. New York, Academic Press.

_____ and E. L. Spencer. 1959. Stabilization of "steady states" of cytochromes at liquid nitrogen temperatures. Discuss. Faraday Soc., 27:200-205.

_____ and G. R. Williams. 1956. The respiratory chain and oxidative phosphorylation. Advances Enzym., 17:65-134.

Conney, A. H. 1967. Pharmacological implications of microsomal enzyme induction. Pharmacol. Rev., 19:317-366.

Cooper, D. Y., S. Levin, S. Narasimhulu, O. Rosenthal, and R. W. Estabrook. 1965. Photochemical action spectrum of the terminal oxidase of mixed function oxidase systems. Science, 147:400-402.

Diehl, H., J. Schädlin, and V. Ullrich. 1970. Studies on the kinetics of cytochrome P-450 reduction in rat liver microsomes. Hoppe-Seyler Z. Physiol. Chem., 351:1359-1371.

Estabrook, R. W. 1956. The low temperature spectra of hemoproteins. I. Apparatus and its application to a study of cytochrome c. J. Biol. Chem., 223:781-794.

_____ 1961. Spectrophotometric studies of cytochromes cooled in liquid nitrogen. In Falk, J. E., R. Lemberg, and R. K. Morton, eds., Hematin Enzymes, pp. 436-457. Oxford and New York, Pergamon Press.

_____ D. Y. Cooper, and O. Rosenthal. 1963. The light reversible carbon monoxide inhibition of steroid C-21 hydroxylase system of the adrenal cortex. Biochem. Z., 338:741-755.

_____ A. Hildebrandt, J. Baron, K. J. Netter, and K. Leibman. 1971. A new spectral intermediate associated with cytochrome P-450 function in liver microsomes. Biochem. Biophys. Res. Commun., 42:132-139.

_____ A. G. Hildebrandt, and V. Ullrich. 1968. Oxygen interaction with cytochrome P-450. Hoppe-Seyler Z. Physiol. Chem., 349:1605-1608.

_____ A. Shigematsu, and J. B. Schenkman. 1970. The contribution of the microsomal electron transport pathway to the oxidative metabolism of liver. Advances Enzyme Regulat., 8:121-130.

Gibson, Q. H. 1969. Rapid mixing: stopped flow. In Kustin, K., ed., Methods in Enzymology, Vol. 16, 187-228. New York, Academic Press.

Gigon, P. L., T. E. Gram, and J. R. Gillette. 1968. Effect of drug substrates on the reduction of hepatic microsomal cytochrome P-450 by NADPH. Biochem. Biophys. Res. Commun., 31:558-562.

Hildebrandt, A. G., and R. W. Estabrook, 1969. Spectrophotometric studies of cytochrome P-450 of liver microsomes after induction with phenobarbital and 3-methylcholanthrene. In Gillette, J. R., A. H. Conney, G. J. Cosmides, R. W. Estabrook, J. R. Fouts, and G. J. Mannering, eds., Microsomes and Drug Oxidations, pp. 341-349. New York, Academic Press.

_____ and R. W. Estabrook, 1971. Evidence for the participation of cytochrome b_5 in hepatic microsomal mixed function oxidation reactions. Arch. Biochem. Biophys. (in press)

_____ H. Remmer, and R. W. Estabrook. 1968. Cytochrome P-450 in liver microsomes. One pigment or many? Biochem. Biophys. Res. Commun., 30:607-612.

Hitachi Perkin-Elmer Company. 1968. Operating Directions for the Model 124 Double-Beam Grating Spectrophotometer.

Imai, Y., and R. Sato. 1966. Substrate interaction with hydroxylase system in liver microsomes. Biochem. Biophys. Res. Commun., 22:620-628.

Jakobsson, S., H. Thor, and S. Orrenius. 1970. Fatty acid inducible cytochrome P-454 of rat kidney cortex microsomes. Biochem. Biophys. Res. Commun., 39:1073-1080.

Keilin, D., and E. F. Hartree. 1949. Effect of low temperature on the absorption spectra of hemoproteins; with observations on the absorption spectrum of oxygen. Nature (London), 164:254-257.

Kinoshita, T., and S. Horie. 1967. Studies on P-450. III. On the absorption spectrum of

P-450 in rabbit liver microsomes. J. Biochem. (Tokyo), 61:26-34.

Klingenberg, M. 1958. Pigments of rat liver microsomes. Arch. Biochem. Biophys., 75:376-386.

Kowal, J. E., E. R. Simpson, and R. W. Estabrook. 1970. Adrenal cells in tissue culture. V. On the specificity of the stimulation of 11β-hydroxylation by adrenocorticotropin. J. Biol. Chem., 245:2438-2443.

Mahler, H. R., and E. H. Cordes. 1966. Biological Chemistry. New York, Harper and Row.

Mannering, G. J. 1971. Properties of cytochrome P-450 as affected by environmental factors: Quantitative changes due to the administration of polycyclic hydrocarbons. Metabolism, 2:228-245.

Mellon, M. G., ed. 1950. Analytical Absorption Spectroscopy. New York, John Wiley and Sons.

Narasimhulu, S., D. Y. Cooper, and O. Rosenthal. 1965. Spectrophotometric properties of a triton clarified steroid 21-hydroxylase system of adrenocortical microsomes. Life Sci., 4:2101-2107.

Omura, T., and R. Sato. 1962. A new cytochrome in liver microsomes. J. Biol. Chem., 237:PC1375-1376.

———— and R. Sato, 1964. The carbon monoxide-binding pigment of liver microsomes. J. Biol. Chem., 239:2370-2385.

Packer, L. 1967. Experiments in Cell Physiology, pp. 62-70. New York, Academic Press.

Palmer, G. 1967. Diffuse reflectance spectrophotometry. *In* Estabrook, R. W., and M. E. Pullman, eds., Methods in Enzymology, Vol. 10, 583-594. New York, Academic Press.

Peterson, J. A. 1971. Camphor binding by *Pseudomonas putida* cytochrome P-450. Arch. Biochem. Biophys. (in press)

Raj, P. P., and R. W. Estabrook. 1971. Quantitative measurement of cytochrome P-450 content in biopsy samples and homogenates of mammalian liver. (in preparation)

Remmer, H., R. W. Estabrook, J. B. Schenkman, and H. Greim. 1968. Induction of microsomal liver enzymes. *In* Hodgson, E., ed., Enzymatic Oxidation of Toxicants, pp. 65-85. Raleigh, North Carolina State University Press.

———— H. Greim, J. B. Schenkman, and R. W. Estabrook. 1967. Methods for the evaluation of hepatic microsomal mixed function oxidase levels and cytochrome P-450. *In* Estabrook, R. W., and M. E. Pullman, eds., Methods in Enzymology, Vol. 10, pp. 703-708. New York, Academic Press.

———— J. Schenkman, R. W. Estabrook, H. Sasame, J. Gillette, S. Narasimhulu, D. Y. Cooper, and O. Rosenthal. 1966. Drug interaction with hepatic microsomal cytochrome. Molec. Pharmacol., 2:187-190.

Schenkman, J. B., H. Remmer, and R. W. Estabrook. 1967. Spectral studies of drug interactions with hepatic microsomal cytochrome. Molec. Pharmacol., 3:113-123.

Strittmatter, P. 1960. The nature of the heme binding in microsomal cytochrome b_5. J. Biol. Chem., 235:2492-2497.

———— and S. F. Velick. 1956. The isolation and properties of microsomal cytochrome. J. Biol. Chem., 221:253-264.

———— and S. F. Velick. 1957. The purification and properties of microsomal cytochrome reductase. J. Biol. Chem., 228:785-799.

Wilson, D. F. 1967. Effect of temperature on the spectral properties of some ferrocytochromes. Arch. Biochem. Biophys., 121:757-768.

Yang, C. C. 1954. A rapid and sensitive recording spectrophotometer for the visible and ultraviolet region. II. Electronic circuits. Rev. Sci. Instrum., 25:807-813.

———— and V. Legallais. 1954. A rapid and sensitive recording spectrophotometer for the visible and ultraviolet region. I. Description and performance. Rev. Sci. Instrum., 25:801-807.

Chapter **10**

Fast Reactions–Flow and Relaxation Methods

Palmer W. Taylor

Division of Pharmacology, Department of Medicine, University of California, San Diego, La Jolla, California

INTRODUCTION

Over the past 50 years the measurable time range for chemical kinetics has been extended by approximately eight orders of magnitude. The application of flow methods to reacting systems by Hartridge and Roughton (1923) shortened the mixing time for reactants to the millisecond range. In the past two decades the development of chemical relaxation techniques by Eigen and his colleagues (Eigen, 1954) has completely eliminated the mixing-time barrier, allowing reactions taking place within times of 10^{-7} sec to be examined. Thus, the time range between conventional measurements (2 to 3 sec) and spectroscopic measurements (10^{-8} to 10^{-9} sec) is presently accessible to kinetic experimentation. The above developments have permitted investigation of elementary kinetic processes, thereby greatly enhancing our understanding of reaction mechanisms. Widespread application of rapid reaction methods to biological systems has occurred only within the past decade.

Consider the reactions (1) and (2), which represent the enzymic conversion of substrate to product and the formation of an inhibitor complex, respectively:

$$E + S \rightleftarrows ES \rightleftarrows E + P \tag{1}$$

$$E + I \rightleftarrows EI \tag{2}$$

In the case of reaction (1), the continuous generation of P or disappearance of S, accompanying the repeated turnover of E to ES and back to E, may be followed over a specified time interval. From steady-state kinetics with S in excess, overall reaction kinetics may be measured, and limitations on the rates of individual steps often estimated even though formation and dissociation of ES are likely to be extremely fast processes. However, if kinetic constants for individual steps are desired, or if dissociation of the complex does not give rise to a new chemical species as in reaction (2), then it is probable that techniques applicable to short time intervals must be employed to measure the rate of complex formation.

Formation of a complex without subsequent alteration of the covalent structure of the combining ligand is fundamental to drug disposition and binding studies as well as drug-receptor relationships. Rapid reaction methods for investigating small molecule-macromolecule interactions, thus, have a potentially wide-range application in pharmacology. Measurement of individual kinetic parameters of complex formation has the distinct advantage over equilibrium affinity determinations in that ionizing groups or structural changes affecting the reactivity of the free macromolecule may be correlated with the association process. Likewise, dissociation kinetics may be correlated with the structure and reactivity of the ligand-macromolecule complex. Moreover, kinetics provide an important operational test of mechanism, and to understand reaction mechanism in detail the time sequence of formation and dissociation of transient reaction intermediates must be known.

Of the fast reaction methods, stopped-flow and temperature-jump relaxation probably show the widest applicability to future pharmacology research and will be the two primary subjects of this chapter. Finally, some specific studies applying fast reaction methods to biological systems will be considered in order to point out the potential information obtainable from this kind of approach. From this short survey of methods and applications it is hoped that the reader can gain an impression of the possibilities and limitations of each technique and the types of reaction systems amenable to investigation. The experimental methods and underlying theory of fast reactions have been the subject of numerous reviews and books (Roughton and Chance, 1963; Eigen and de Maeyer, 1963; Caldin, 1964; Czerlinski, 1964; Kustin et al., 1965; Czerlinski, 1966; Hammes, 1966). In addition, various reviews have dealt specifically with the application of these methods to biological systems (Eigen and Hammes, 1963; Gibson, 1966; Hammes, 1968; Eigen, 1968); and a recent issue of *Advances in Enzymology* (Kustin, 1970) is devoted entirely to fast reactions. These sources should be consulted when a more intensive examination of a particular area is desired.

The basic principles of the flow and relaxation (equilibrium perturbation) methods greatly differ; consequently each will be considered separately. Certain spectroscopic and electrochemical methods may also be employed to yield kinetic information on fast reactions. This situation arises when a physical process with a finite lifetime depends on the chemical state of the species. Magnetic resonance and fluorescence spectroscopy are examples of such methods, and these areas are the subject of separate chapters in this volume.

FLOW AND STOPPED-FLOW METHODS

Basic Principles

In a properly designed mixing chamber two reactant solutions may be efficiently mixed within 1 to 2 msec. If flow through this chamber is made continuous, subsequent progress of the reaction may be followed at variable distances from the point of mixing. This simple scheme enabled Hartridge and Roughton (1923) to examine kinetically the reaction of hemoglobin with oxygen and carbon monoxide. It is not difficult to achieve flow rates approaching 10 meters/sec; therefore a distance of 1 cm between the mixing and observation sites would correspond to an elapsed time of 10^{-3} sec. Observation can also be made at a fixed distance from the mixing site with variation of the flow rate, and this is the basis of the accelerated-flow techniques developed by Chance (1940) for studying catalase- and peroxidase-catalyzed reactions. A second alternative to this is an arrangement of mixing chambers in series where the two mixed reactants are allowed to react with a third substance at a prescribed distance along the flow tube. The third reactant is a "quenching" agent, which fixes the reaction at a stage dependent on the transit time between the first and second mixing chambers (Roughton, 1934). Rapid flow quenching techniques are extremely useful for trapping transient intermediates in cases where slow methods of detection must be employed (e.g., separation and analysis of the substance). This technique has been applied to observe rates of production or decomposition of transient reaction intermediates in enzyme catalysis (Gutfreund, 1969).

Although continuous-flow techniques do not place drastic limitations on detector response times, they do require large volumes of reactants, making them impractical for many biological systems. The stopped-flow method, however, largely circumvents this problem. In this modification, flow and mixing of reactants is initiated and then suddenly arrested so that the mixed solution comes to rest within 1 msec. The mixing chamber and point of observation are positioned closely together, the only limitation being the completeness of mixing at the observation point. Observation is usually made during and after cessation of flow, thus providing a measure of the complete course of the reaction. During flow, if the reactant transit time between the mixing and observation points is considerably less than the reaction time, a signal from the mixed, but unreacted, substances is initially observed. For stopped-flow, a rapidly responding detection system must be employed, and the detector response is usually applied to a cathode-ray oscilloscope.

Experimental Method

An apparatus developed by Gibson and Milnes (1964) has been the prototype of most of the stopped-flow instrumentation now in use for biological studies, and

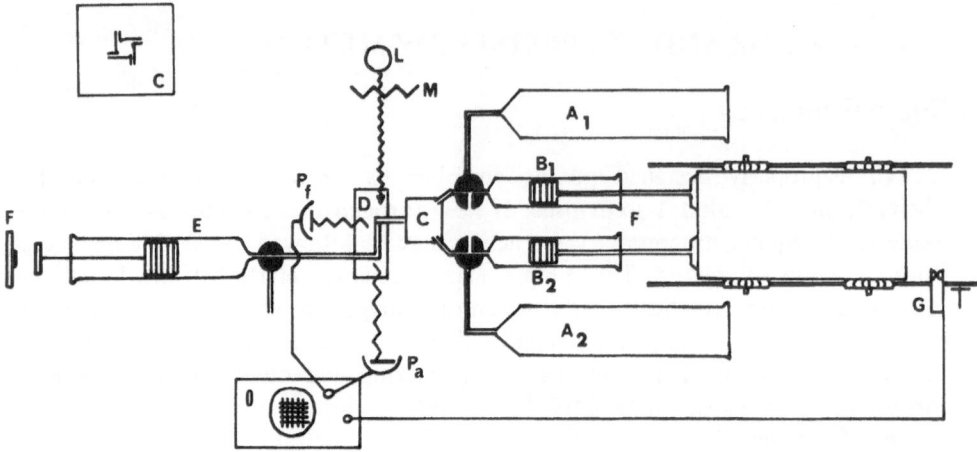

FIG. 1. Diagram of a stopped-flow apparatus patterned closely after that of Gibson and Milnes (1964). A_1, A_2, reactant reservoirs; B_1, B_2, drive syringes; C, 4-channel mixing chamber (see insert); D, observation window; E, collection syringe; F, stopping pins; G, trigger; L, light source; M, monochromator; P_A, photomultiplier (and monochromator) positioned for absorption; P_F, photomultiplier (and monochromator) positioned for fluorescence; O, oscilloscope. The observation cell is in a 90° plane with respect to the drive system.

is illustrated in Figure 1. Many of the components have similar specifications to those used in the continuous flow system. Reactant solutions are contained in 0.2 to 2.0 ml syringes, usually of ceramic plunger and glass barrel type, which are driven simultaneously. In most instrumentation this is done manually or hydraulically, but more recent modifications have employed an air-pressure system (Berger et al., 1968). The syringe-drive system is connected by three-way valves to the reactant reservoirs and mixing chamber. Satisfactory mixing can be obtained with four to eight jets of 0.5 mm diameter, which enter a 2-mm common chamber tangentially. It is desirable to achieve a high degree of turbulence without the onset of cavitation. To minimize the dead time, the observation point should be within 1 to 2 cm from the mixing chamber. Flow is usually led into a collection syringe which comes against a seating, thereby arresting flow. Alternatively, flow may be arrested by having the syringe-drive system meet an external stop. As the collection syringe imparts a slight resistance to flow, it tends to reduce inertia and pulsing effects. This syringe also enables one to sample the reaction mixture for pH or other measurements. Temperature of the system should be carefully controlled, since temperature differentials between the drive system and observation chamber can create time-dependent optical artifacts.

Precision and time limitations of the apparatus are highly dependent on the design of the flow and mixing system. The two drive syringes should experience equal resistance to flow. The fluid stopping time, completeness of mixing, flow rate, and the distance between the observation and mixing sites will be the primary factors affecting the resolution or dead time of the flow apparatus. Clearly, this time should be small relative to the reaction time. Various operational tests of mixing efficiency based on an optical or thermal measurement of known rates of reactions have been devised (Roughton and Chance, 1963; Chance, 1940). The proceedings of a symposium on rapid mixing give a detailed discussion of the design and performance of various mixing systems (Chance et al., 1964).

Although the common means of detection is spectrophotometric, other procedures such as conductivity (Sirs, 1958), glass electrode (Sirs, 1958; Rossi-Bernardi and Berger, 1968), thermal (Berger and Stoddart, 1964), and electron paramagnetic resonance (EPR) (Borg, 1964), all show experimental promise. However, limitations on the response or recording times currently restrict glass electrode and EPR to continuous flow methods. Both absorption and fluorescence spectrometry have been widely employed to monitor small molecule-macromolecule interactions, and often the optical system can be modified to accommodate either means of detection. The versatility and sensitivity of optical detection systems approach those used in the equilibrium methods. For instance, dual-wavelength recording (De Sa and Gibson, 1966) and fluorescence polarization (Gibson et al.,

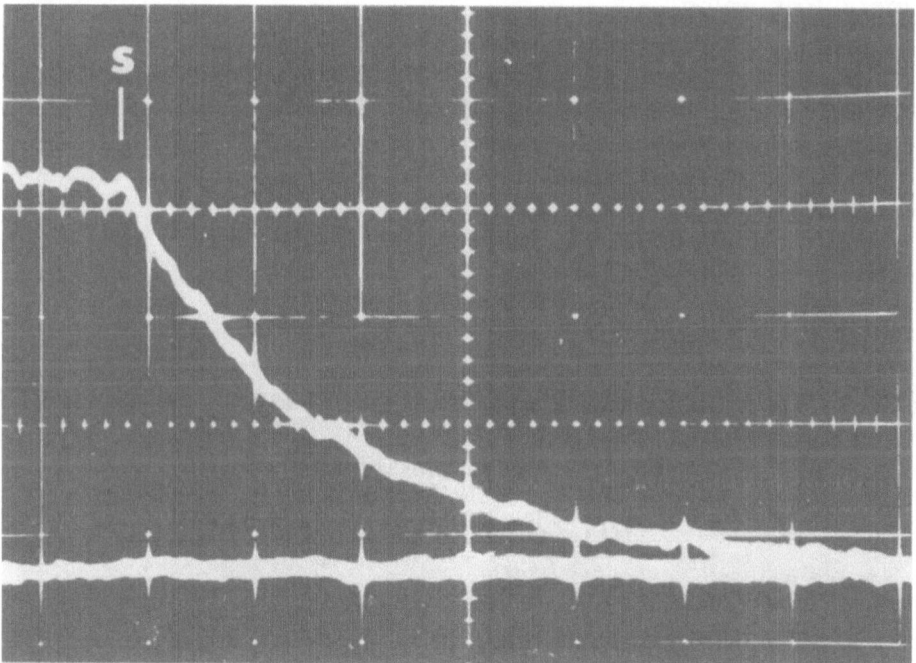

FIG. 2. Oscilloscope trace recording changes in enzyme fluorescence with time for the reaction between 0.625 μM human carbonic anhydrase C and 14.0 μM p-nitrobenzene sulfonamide. The oscilloscope was triggered with the initiation of flow so that the time dependence of fluorescence is monitored during and after flow. Stoppage of flow occurs at S. Fluorescence was measured by excitation at 290 mμ with emission at 345 mμ. The difference in fluorescence signal is a consequence of quenching of protein-tryptophan fluorescence associated with complex formation. Each large horizontal increment corresponds to 50 msec while the vertical increments represent a signal difference of ~100mV. (From Taylor et al. 1970. *Biochemistry* [*Washington*], 9:2638.)

1966) have been coupled with stopped-flow. Absorption spectrometry has employed optical paths between 0.2 and 2.0 cm (Gibson and Milnes, 1964), and a path length of 1.0 mm was used for fluorescence measurements in the presence of absorbing substances that reduce the intensity of the excitation radiation (Taylor et al., 1970a). A micro-stopped-flow apparatus employing volumes of ~0.1 ml has been developed (Strittmatter, 1964).

Photomultiplier signals are displayed on an oscilloscope whose beam may be triggered by the initiation or stopping of flow (Figure 2). Photomultiplier shot noise is reduced by a series of loading capacitances whose time constants of attenuation must be calibrated and made sufficiently short to preclude interference with the time dependence of the observed reaction (<0.1 of the reaction $t_{1/2}$). Photographic recordings of oscilloscope traces are usually made; however, a recent innovation has been the application of computer data collection with analog to digital conversion of the photomultiplier output (De Sa and Gibson, 1969).

Kinetic Principles

The simplest equation describing reversible ligand-macromolecule interactions is given by the bimolecular-unimolecular reversible reaction:

$$E + I \underset{k_{-1}}{\overset{k_1}{\rightleftarrows}} EI \tag{2}$$

Then,
$$-\frac{d(E)}{dt} = \frac{d(EI)}{dt} = k_1(E)(I) - k_{-1}(E)I \tag{3}$$

It is most convenient to examine association as a pseudo-first-order process with one reactant, e.g., I, in excess. In this case, the observable parameter is the disappearance of E or the appearance of EI. Since I is essentially constant,

$$-\frac{d(E)}{dt} = \frac{d(EI)}{dt} = k_1'(E) - k_{-1}(EI) \tag{4}$$

where $k_1' = k_1(I_0)$. This equation may be rearranged and integrated to give:

$$\ln\left(\frac{E_0 - \bar{E}}{E - \bar{E}}\right) = (k_1' + k_{-1})t = [k_1(I_0) + k_{-1}]t \tag{5}$$

where E_0 and $\bar{E}$ are the initial and equilibrium concentrations of E (cf. Frost and Pearson, 1961). The approach to equilibrium has an effective rate constant equal to the sum of the rate constants in the forward and reverse directions. Since the logarithmic quantity is dimensionless, any measure of the difference from the equilibrium concentration, such as vertical distances in Figure 2, may be directly substituted for $E - \bar{E}$. Furthermore, with the first-order equation it is not necessary to determine E_0 to evaluate the rate. A plot of $\ln(E - \bar{E})$ against time yields $k_1(I_0) + k_{-1}$. If pseudo-first-order conditions are maintained over a range of concentrations of I_0, both k_1 and k_{-1} can be determined from the apparent association rate.

Under some conditions it may be advantageous to employ equal concentrations of reactants, since this may yield a larger signal difference or a slower apparent reaction velocity. If $E_0 = I_0$, the rate expression for equation (2) integrates to:

$$\ln\left[\frac{(E_0)^2 - F(\bar{E})^2}{(E_0)^2(1-F)}\right] = k_1\left(\frac{(E_0)^2 - (\bar{E})^2}{E_0}\right)t \tag{6}$$

where F, the fractional approach to equilibrium, equals $\dfrac{E_0 - E}{E_0 - \bar{E}}$. F, being dimensionless, can be measured from the respective vertical distances on the oscilloscope trace. In contrast to the first-order case, this equation requires us to know the initial and equilibrium concentrations of E and their respective detection signals for the evaluation of k_1. Also, k_{-1} can not be determined directly. If observation is made along the length of the flow tube rather than transverse to it, second-order conditions may present an additional complication, since the relative extent of completion of the reaction will be dependent on the distance along the flow tube. The magnitude of this error can be estimated by dividing the optical path into a series of sections and calculating the rate from summation of the individual sections.

The time required for mixing still represents the major limitation on the resolution time for the stopped-flow method, and is usually in the region of 3 msec. More recent adaptations using air-pressure-driven syringes and a zero-displacement stopping valve have reduced this time to ~ 0.2 msec (Berger et al., 1968); but, owing to the very high pressures required for enhanced flow velocities, it cannot be expected that resolution times of the flow methods can be appreciably lowered. If we accept a reaction half-time of 3 msec as a lower limit, reaction rates with a first-order rate constant greater than 200 sec^{-1} cannot be followed easily by flow techniques. The more sensitive detection methods permit the use of reactant concentrations as low as 10^{-7} M. Provided that the affinity of the complex is strong, bimolecular rate constants approaching the diffusion limitation of 10^9 M^{-1} sec^{-1} may be followed. Thus, for reaction (2) it is primarily the magnitude of the dissociation rate constant, k_{-1}, which determines whether stopped-flow methods can be used for the particular system under consideration.

Because of the limitation on resolution times, most stopped-flow studies of bimolecular association are carried out with relatively low concentrations of reactants. Suppose that formation of the complex, $(EI)_2$, is preceded by formation of a less stable intermediate, $(EI)_1$, as follows:

$$E + I \underset{k_{-1}}{\overset{k_1}{\rightleftarrows}} (EI)_1 \underset{k_{-2}}{\overset{k_2}{\rightleftarrows}} (EI)_2 \tag{7}$$

If the concentration product, $(E \cdot I)$, is low, $k_1(E \cdot I) < k_{-1}(EI)_1 + k_2(EI)_2$, the bimolecular step is rate limiting, and detectable concentrations of $(EI)_1$ do not build up during the course of the reaction. It is for this reason that flow methods often do not detect individual steps in a sequential reaction involving an initial bimolecular collision.

Flow methods, however, do not restrict one to conditions close to the equilibrium state. Thus, as a general rule, considerably larger detection signals can be obtained with these techniques.

RELAXATION METHODS

Basic Principles

Chemical relaxation methods, which were introduced and developed by Eigen and coworkers as a means for investigating chemical kinetics, have already contributed substantially to our understanding of ligand-macromolecule associations and enzyme catalysis (Hammes, 1968; Eigen, 1968). The relaxation principle is based on sudden perturbation of a system in reversible equilibrium by alteration of some external parameter such as temperature or pressure. The transient approach of the system to a new equilibrium is then monitored. The extent of perturbation defines the difference between the initial and final thermodynamic equilibrium states. The time dependence of re-equilibration can be related to the rate constants of the reaction. This method may be contrasted with the flow techniques in that mixing is avoided and the reacting species are always close to their equilibrium state. A wider range of resolution times, varying between 10^{-8} and 1 second, can potentially be attained with these methods. The procedure may involve a single pulse of energy shifting the equilibrium, or the perturbation may be periodic such as equilibrium displacement by ultrasonic waves. In the latter case, phase relationships between the external parameter and the response of the system are followed. Unfortunately, periodic displacement methods require very high concentrations of substance under investigation and have yet to be generally applied to biological macromolecules; thus we shall consider only single-step perturbations.

Kinetic Principles

Perturbation of the equilibrium is intentionally kept small so that differential equations describing the rate processes may be linearized. The variables are deviations in concentration from an appropriate reference value, usually the final equilibrium concentration. Let us again consider the simple bimolecular-unimolecular reversible reaction:

$$E + I \underset{k_{-1}}{\overset{k_1}{\rightleftarrows}} EI \tag{2}$$

   Assume that this system is initially at equilibrium with concentrations E_0, I_0, and EI_0. Following perturbation, the system will adjust itself to a new equilibrium with concentrations $\bar{E}$, $\bar{I}$, and $\bar{EI}$. At time t, the concentrations differ from the final equilibrium concentration by an amount x, so that

$$x = E - \bar{E} = I - \bar{I} = \bar{EI} - EI \tag{8}$$

The rate of approach to equilibrium is

$$-\frac{dx}{dt} = k_1 (E)(I) - k_{-1}(EI) \tag{9}$$

and

$$k_1(\bar{E})(\bar{I}) = k_{-1}(\bar{EI}) \tag{10}$$

If (8) and then (10) are substituted into (9),

$$-\frac{dx}{dt} = k_1(\bar{E}+x)(\bar{I}+x) - (\bar{EI}-x)$$

$$= k_1(\bar{E}+\bar{I})x + k_1 x^2 + k_{-1}x \tag{11}$$

Restricting ourselves to small perturbations, $x \ll \bar{E}$, $\bar{I}$, we may neglect the second order term so that

$$\frac{dx}{dt}\left(\frac{1}{x}\right) = k_1(\bar{E}+\bar{I}) + k_{-1} = k_{exptl} \tag{12}$$

We now have a simple first-order approach to equilibrium with apparent rate constant, k_{exptl}. Integration of the above equation yields

$$\frac{x}{x_0} = e^{-k_{exptl}t} \tag{13}$$

where x_0 is the difference from the final equilibrium state immediately after perturbation. It is convenient to define a time constant, τ, the relaxation time, as the reciprocal of the first-order rate constant, k_{exptl}. If τ is substituted into equation (13), $\frac{x}{x_0} = \frac{1}{e} \simeq 0.37$. Therefore, the relaxation time is the time required for the concentration difference from equilibrium to be reduced to $\frac{1}{e}$ of its original value. The half-time of the reaction, $t_{1/2}$, is related to τ by

$$\frac{t_{1/2}}{\tau} = k_{exptl}t_{1/2} = \ln 2 = 0.693 \tag{14}$$

Irrespective of the molecularity of the reaction, provided perturbations are kept small, only first-order equations are involved in the relaxation treatment. Moreover, the observed relaxation times will be independent of both the perturbation and means of detection.

For equation (2), k_1 and k_{-1} may be evaluated by determining τ at a series of different equilibrium concentrations. However, with a simple reversible unimolecular reaction, the relaxation experiment does not allow a unique evaluation of the two rate constants since the forward and reverse rates cannot be measured independently as can often be done with the flow methods.

Consecutive Reactions

As illustrated with single-step reactions above, if perturbations are kept small, relaxation spectra of complex reactions may also be described by a series of linear differential equations which take the form:

$$F(t) = \sum_n A_n e^{-\frac{t}{\tau_n}} \qquad (15)$$

where the A_n's are constants which must be specifically evaluated according to a given mechanism (Eigen and de Maeyer, 1963; Guillain and Thusius, 1970). Each of n steps, thus, may be characterized by a time constant, τ_n.

Consider the two step interaction between a ligand and macromolecule as shown below:

$$
\begin{array}{ccc}
k_1 & & k_2 \\
E + I \rightleftharpoons (EI)_1 & \rightleftharpoons & (EI)_2 \\
k_{-1} & & k_{-2} \\
\tau_1 & & \tau_2
\end{array}
\qquad (7)
$$

When $(I) >> (E)$, steady state assumptions yield

$$k_{exptl} = \frac{k_1 k_2 (I_o) + k_{-1} k_{-2}}{k_{-1} + k_2} \qquad (16)$$

These assumptions usually do not allow a unique determination of individual rate constants. However, owing to the short resolution times of the relaxation experiment, the concentration of reactants, E and I, may be sufficiently large to cause appreciable concentrations of $(EI)_1$ to be present during the course of the reaction. Under these conditions the steady state assumption becomes invalidated, but it is likely that discrete steps of interconversion between species will be directly observed. Thus, for equation (7) two relaxation times may be found and the four rate constants evaluated. A good example of this is the interaction of the competitive inhibitor, proflavin, with chymotrypsin (Havsteen, 1967). This reaction obeys the reaction scheme shown above where binding of the inhibitor is followed by a unimolecular isomerization of the complex. Plots of $\left(\dfrac{1}{\tau_1}+\dfrac{1}{\tau_2}\right)$ and $\left(\dfrac{1}{\tau_1}\cdot\dfrac{1}{\tau_2}\right)$ against the sum of concentration of reactants, $(\bar{E}+\bar{I})$, yield the four rate constants.[1]

Individual relaxation times for a multiple-step system are given by a sum of rate constants each of which must be multiplied by a fractional equilibration factor involving the preceding equilibrated steps. Consequently, expressions for each relaxation time will also contain kinetic or equilibrium constants from the coupled faster steps of the reaction scheme.

Since the differential rate equations are linearized, individual rate constants and the sequence of primary steps in more complex reaction schemes may be determined. A number of mathematical treatments employing matrix algebra have been applied to analyzing relaxation spectra of multistep systems (Eigen and de Maeyer, 1963; Castellan, 1963; Hammes and Schimmel, 1966; 1967; Eigen, 1968). In practice, in order to resolve individual rate constants for a complex process, at least a four- to fivefold separation should exist between relaxation times, and signal amplitudes of elementary relaxation steps should not greatly differ. Accuracy of measurement of relaxation times is a critical limiting factor in detailing the formal mechanism of complex reactions. For sequential and cyclic reaction schemes, the relationship between $\left(\dfrac{1}{\tau_n}\right)$ and concentration represents the essential means for discerning between alternative reaction pathways. Unfortunately, the concentration range where adequate signals may be obtained is often limited; thus, insufficient information may preclude an unambiguous description of the reaction pathway.

Transient methods which detect the presence of changing concentrations of intermediate species are required in order to establish the formal reaction path for reactions in which binding steps are accompanied by first-order isomerization processes. In ligand-macromolecule interactions as many as three discrete relaxation times have been experimentally observed (Kirschner et al., 1966) (Figure 3). Temperature-jump relaxation studies have been successfully used for distinguishing between proposed models accounting for cooperative binding or allosteric behavior. For the allosteric enzymes, glyceraldehyde-3-phosphate dehydrogenase (Kirschner et al., 1966; Eigen, 1968) and aspartate transcarbamylase (Eckfeldt et al., 1970), relaxation spectra are consistent with the Monod model (Monod, Wyman, and Changeux, 1965) for coenzyme or modifier binding to the oligomeric proteins. Moreover, these investigations both indicate a concerted mechanism of isomerization of protomers with an "all or none" transition between the two states of the oligomeric enzyme.

Analysis of detection signal amplitudes resulting from equilibrium perturbation not only yields information on intensive variables characterizing the equilibrium state (such as reaction enthalpy, ΔH), but also constitutes an important means for

---

[1] The characteristic equation describing the relaxation times and rate constants is solved by determinants where the reciprocal relaxation times are the eigen values (c.f. Havsteen, 1967).

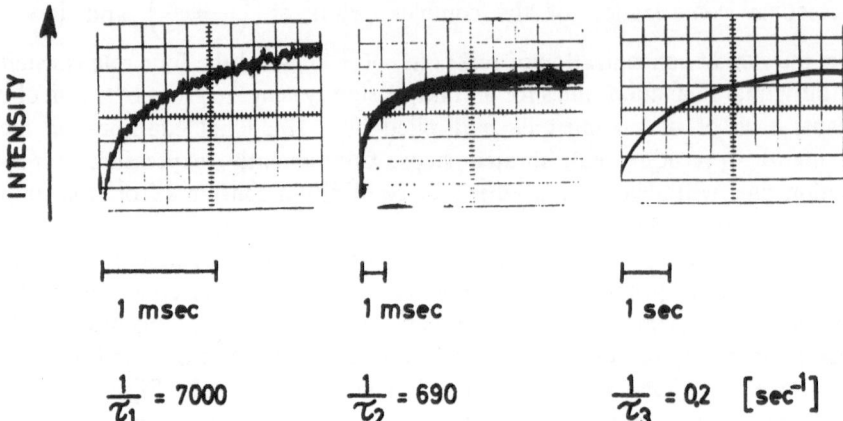

FIG. 3. Temperature-jump relaxation spectra for the cooperative binding of NAD to yeast glyceraldehyde-3-phosphate dehydrogenase; the enzyme and NAD concentrations are 1.43 $\times 10^{-4} M$ and $6 \times 10^{-4} M$, respectively. (From Kirschner et al. 1966. *Proc. Nat. Acad. Sci. U.S.A.*, 56:1663.)

confirming a formal reaction sequence deduced from temporal measurements. In multistep reaction systems the relationship between signal amplitude and reactant concentration is dependent on the relative rates and respective order of coupled steps (Eigen and de Maeyer, 1963; Guillain and Thusius, 1970).

Conditions for achieving optimal signal amplitudes can be predicted from the affinity of the complex and reactant concentrations. Consider the bimolecular association

$$E + I \underset{k_{-1}}{\overset{k_1}{\rightleftharpoons}} EI; \text{ where } \bar{E} = \bar{I} \tag{2}$$

If α is the degree of dissociation and E_T is the total enzyme or inhibitor concentration,

$$\alpha = \frac{\bar{E}}{E_T} = \frac{\bar{I}}{E_T} \text{ and } K = \frac{\alpha^2 E_T}{1 - \alpha} \tag{17}$$

then

$$\left(\frac{\partial \alpha}{\partial T}\right) = \frac{\left(\dfrac{\partial K}{\partial T}\right)}{\left(\dfrac{\partial K}{\partial \alpha}\right)} \tag{18}$$

then
$$\left(\frac{\partial \alpha}{\partial T}\right) = \frac{\dfrac{\Delta H \cdot K}{RT^2}}{\dfrac{\alpha E_T \ (2-\alpha)}{(1-\alpha)}} \tag{19}$$

$$= \frac{\Delta H}{RT^2}\left[\frac{1-\alpha}{2-\alpha}\right]\alpha$$

A maximal change in $\left(\dfrac{\partial \alpha}{\partial t}\right)$, thus, can be effected when $\alpha = 0.58$; that is, where the concentrations of species on both sides of the reaction are nearly equal. Consequently, low sensitivity of detection may preclude relaxation experiments on high affinity complexes where α only becomes appreciable at low concentration.

The term, Γ_c, is used to denote the relationship between the change in equilibrium function and the concentration variable (Eigen and de Maeyer, 1963). In this case,

$$\Gamma_c = E_T\Gamma\alpha = E_T\left(\frac{\alpha(1-\alpha)}{2-\alpha}\right) \tag{20}$$

Relationships between concentration changes and signal amplitudes depend on the method of detection. With fluorescence the relative change in concentration $\left(\dfrac{dE}{E}\right)$ is proportional to the relative difference in signal intensity $\left(\dfrac{dI}{I}\right)$; whereas, in absorption spectrometry, the absolute concentration change (dE) is proportional to $\left(\dfrac{dI}{I}\right)$. In practice, the signal-to-noise ratio determines the sensitivity of the method. Instrumental noise is primarily photomultiplier shot noise produced from the illumination background. Eigen and de Maeyer (1963) and Czerlinski (1966) give a detailed discussion of the instrumental and external factors which can optimize this ratio.

Temperature-Jump Relaxation

Temperature-jump (Joule heating) is, by far, the simplest and most widely used application of relaxation methods to biological systems. Actual temperature changes are small, 5° to 10°C, and this technique can be applied to any system whose equilibrium is sensitive to temperature. The magnitude of the shift in equilibrium constant can be predicted from the van't Hoff law:

$$\left(\frac{\partial \ln K_{eq}}{\partial T}\right)_P = \frac{\Delta H}{RT^2} \tag{21}$$

and reaction enthalpies, ΔH, are easily determined experimentally. Thus, for a reaction with a typical ΔH of 12 kcal, a temperature jump of 10° causes a twofold change in the equilibrium constant. In cases where ΔH is small, the system may be perturbed by coupling the reaction under investigation to a second, faster, reaction possessing a greater ΔH. The second reaction may cause a concentration jump which perturbs the reaction of interest. As an example, suppose that the buffer system possesses a large heat of ionization and the reaction of interest involves proton liberation or uptake. A temperature jump shifts the pH which, in turn, causes relaxation step to occur in the pH-dependent reaction of interest. This represents an important means by which a concentration-jump is attainable without resorting to the slower mixing process.

The usual method of detection is spectrophotometric. In pH-dependent equilibria a chemical indicator may be introduced into the system to facilitate detection. Care must be taken to ensure that indicator and buffer equilibria are established more rapidly than the equilibria under investigation.

Experimental Method

Sudden temperature jumps are achieved by charging a capacitor to high voltage and then discharging the stored electrical energy through the reaction mixture. The electrode-containing sample cell is connected across the capacitor by activation of a spark gap (Figure 4). Although selection of instrumental parameters is largely based on the system under investigation, we should briefly consider some of the essential factors. Temperature-jumps of 10° or less usually give adequate sensitivity without affecting linearization of the differential equations. The dissipated energy required to effect a temperature rise is proportional to the mass and specific heat of the sample between the electrodes. To minimize the required energy, sample sizes should be kept small; however, additional criteria must be kept in mind when selecting a suitable volume: (1) sensitivity of detection is proportional to the optical path length, and (2) short interelectrode spaces often lead to convection, temperature nonuniformity, and surface electrode reactants interfering with observation. Typical sample cells have volumes between 0.2 to 1.0 ml, optical paths of 0.5 to 2 cm, and at least a 5-mm spacing between electrodes.

Dissipation of power to the sample is equal to

$$\frac{V_0{}^2}{R} - e^{-\frac{2t}{RC}} \qquad (22)$$

where V_0 is the initial voltage in the capacitor of capacitance, C, and R is the solution resistance. The heating time constant is $\frac{1}{2} RC$. Since this determines the resolution time of the instrument, shortest temperature rise times are found with low capacitance and solution resistance. To lower solution resistance an inert supporting electrolyte at a concentration of 0.1 to 0.2 M is employed. The energy stored in a capacitor is equal to $\frac{1}{2} CV$. Therefore, high potential and low capacitance favor

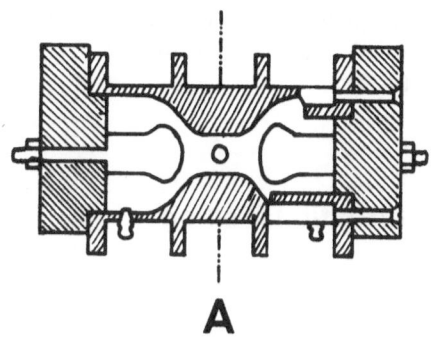

A

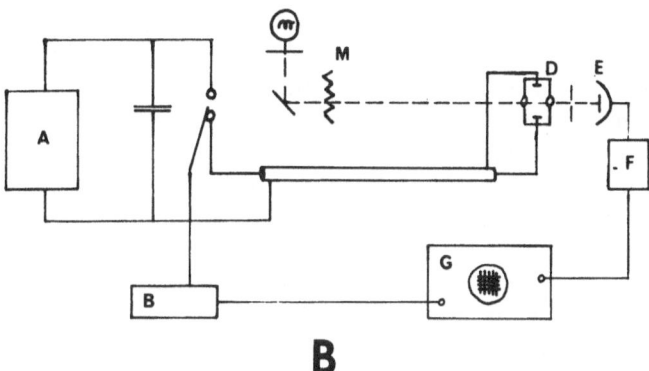

B

FIG. 4. *A.* Temperature-jump sample cell. Sample loading occurs from the ports of the top, and the optical path is perpendicular to the page. (From Eigen and de Maeyer. 1963. *In* Weissberger, ed., *Technique in Organic Chemistry Vol. VIII Part II,* p. 971. Courtesy of Wiley/Interscience.) *B.* Schematic diagram of a temperature-jump apparatus. A, voltage supply; B, trigger; C, spark gap; D, sample cell; E, photomultiplier; F, pre-amp; G, oscilloscope. (From Eigen and de Maeyer. 1963. *In* Weissberger, ed., *Technique in Organic Chemistry Vol. VIII, Part II,* p. 978. Courtesy of Wiley/Interscience.)

short temperature rise times; however, a high potential discharge may severely affect photomultiplier stability. Ordinarily the charge is stored in a 0.2 to 1 μF capacitor at a potential of 2 to 50 kV. This produces temperature rise times in the vicinity of 20 μsec. For shorter rise times discharge through the cell may be terminated by activation of a second spark-gap circuit which by-passes the cell, thereby drawing off the excess capacitance (Eigen and de Maeyer, 1963; Bewick et al., 1965). Thus, the time of discharge through the cell is controlled by the interval between activation of the two spark gaps. Under optimal conditions current resolution times of temperature jump approach 1 to 2 μsec. Optical perturbations resulting from temperature inhomogeneities limit the duration of time in which a "slow" reaction can be followed, usually in the range of 0.1 to 1 sec. This arises from heat flow through the electrodes, causing eventual convection. A discussion of the capabilities of various instrumental designs may be found in the book by Czerlinski (1966).

Nonequilibrium Perturbation Methods

The system being perturbed need not be in true thermodynamic equilibrium, but the net change in concentration of reactants over the time interval of interest must be less than that arising from the relaxation steps being examined. It is therefore possible to obtain meaningful relaxation spectra on stationary-state concentrations of transient reactants. This approach is extremely useful for investigating fast intermediate steps when the overall equilibrium is shifted far in one direction. Of particular importance is its application to enzymic reactions where rapid and nearly complete conversion to product is observed. Thus, if the net reaction takes place in milliseconds or seconds, relaxation times measured in the microsecond range should be uninfluenced by the overall conversion of substrate to product. Perturbations on transient reactants can be carried out through combination of rapid mixing and relaxation techniques; in fact, coupled stopped-flow–temperature-jump instrumentation has been in use for a number of years (Eigen and de Maeyer, 1963; Erman and Hammes, 1966a). Perhaps the most extensive use of this technique are the studies of Hammes and his collaborators on ribonuclease-substrate interactions (cf. del Rosario and Hammes, 1970). The stopping syringe is used to trigger the temperature-jump. By using appropriate time-delay circuits the temperature-jump may be applied from 10 msec to seconds after the mixing of reactants.

APPLICATIONS

Ligand-Macromolecule Complex Formation

Fast reaction techniques have found their primary use in biochemistry in the study of small molecule-macromolecule interactions. As various drug-macromolecule complexes reach a state of sufficient purity, both flow and relaxation techniques will offer an essential means for understanding the specificity and mechanism of complex formation. In Table 1 the kinetic parameters and methods employed to obtain these data are tabulated for a series of ligand-macromolecule complexes. It is not intended for this to represent a comprehensive listing of all of the fast-reaction studies of complex formation, but it should serve to illustrate the methods and detection systems in common use and the range of experimental rate constants observed.

The maximum rate at which complexes can form is limited by diffusion-controlled encounter between reactants. Owing to relative sizes of the ligand and macromolecule, the ligand will diffuse more rapidly, so that the macromolecule can be regarded as being effectively immobile. If it is assumed that the ligand and its site of interaction have similar dimensions, this encounter rate constant can be calculated to be $2 \times 10^9 \ M^{-1} \ sec^{-1}$ (Alberty and Hammes, 1958). These considerations are based on radial diffusion of the ligand to a site on the outer surface of the macromolecule. This collision rate will clearly be influenced by a variety of factors which include the geometry of the combining site, orientation for effective collision, and the charge relationship between combining reactants. Various treatments of the quantitative influence of these factors have been given (Debye, 1942; Alberty and Hammes, 1958; Burgen, 1966). They may also be examined experimentally through either structural variation of the ligand and macromolecule or by changing solvent or external parameters, such as ionic strength or temperature.

For association of the complexes in Table 1 many of the values approach the diffusion limitation but none, as expected, exceed this value. The fact that even the fastest rate constants are slightly less than the theoretical diffusion limitation probably reflects geometric limitations on access to the combining site and rigid orientation requirements for binding. Rates substantially below $10^8 \ M^{-1} \ sec^{-1}$ indicate an activation barrier in the actual association process. An additional test for diffusion control of the association rate comes from the enthalpy of the association process. For a diffusion-controlled reaction this value should be equivalent to diffusion in water (2.5 to 4 kcal/mole).

Structure-Affinity Relationships

A kinetic approach to complex formation presents an additional dimension to interpretation of structure-activity or structure-affinity relationships. Different physical parameters may control the apparent rates of the association and dissociation processes, and the equilibrium affinity represents a composite measure of the energetics of both processes. An example of modification of ligand structure selectively affecting association or dissociation can be observed with a series of ring substituted aromatic sulfonamides and human carbonic anhydrase (Figure 5). Substituent variation on the aromatic ring affected the rate of association (k_1) to a greater extent than dissociation (k_{-1}). However, if a substituent was placed *ortho* to the sulfonamido moiety, a selective increase in k_{-1} was observed when compared with the unsubstituted congener. This effect was characteristic for only the C isozyme, since human carbonic anhydrase B did not exhibit an enhanced dissociation rate with *ortho* substitution (Taylor et al., 1970a). In the series of hapten-antibody complexes, where the association rates approach that of a diffusion-controlled reaction, differences in hapten affinity are largely a consequence of dissociation rate variation (Table 1).

TABLE 1

Kinetic Parameters and Methods for Studies on Ligand-Macromolecule Complexes

Reaction	k_1 ($M^{-1}sec^{-1}$)[b]	k_{-1} (sec^{-1})[b]	Method	Detection	Reference
Antibody (γ-globulin) with:					
2-(2,4-dinitrophenylazo)-1-naphthol-3,6-disulfonic acid	8×10^7	1.4	stopped-flow	fluorescence	Day et al. (1963)
2,4-dinitrophenyl lysine	8×10^7	1.0			
2,4-dinitrophenylaminocaproate	1×10^8	1.1			
1-naphthol-4-[4-(4' azobenzene-azo) phenylarsonic acid]	2×10^7	50	T-jump	visible	Froese et al. (1962)
4,5-dihydroxy-3-(p-nitrophenylazo) 2,7-naphthalene disulfonic acid	1.8×10^8	7.6×10^2	T-jump	visible	Froese and Sehon (1965)
Aspartate transcarbamylase[a] with Br-CTP	1.17×10^6	513	T-jump	UV	Eckfeldt et al. (1970)
Carbonic anhydrase with various sulfonamides	5.5×10^4 to 1.13×10^7	0.033 to 2.71	stopped-flow	fluorescence	Taylor et al. (1970)
Chymotrypsin with proflavin[a]	1.14×10^8	2.2×10^3	T-jump	visible	Havsteen (1967)
Cytochrome C with					
Fe(CN)$_6$ $^{4-}$	2.0×10^4	—	T-jump	visible	Brandt et al. (1966)
Fe(CN)$_6$ $^{3-}$	8.4×10^6	—			
DNA with					
Actinomycin C[a]	1.5×10^4	0.25	stopped-flow	visible	Müller and Crothers (1968)
Actinomine V[a]	3.0×10^6	40	stopped-flow	visible	
Proflavin[a]	1.0×10^7	3×10^3	T-jump	visible	Li and Crothers (1968)
Horseradish peroxidase with					
fluoride	2×10^6	4.6×10^2	T-jump	visible	Dunford and Alberty (1967)
cyanide	1.2×10^5	0.32	stopped-flow	visible	Ellis and Dunford (1968)
Hemoglobin with					
O$_2$[a]	2.7×10^6	22	T-jump	visible	Brunori and Schuster (1969)
haptoglobin[a]	4×10^6	—	stopped flow	fluorescence	Nagel and Gibson (1967)
Lactoglobulin with bromophenol blue	1.2×10^6	1.5×10^3	T-jump	visible	Colen (1970)
Lactoperoxidase with cyanide	1.05×10^6	36	T-jump	visible	Dolman et al. (1968)

Liver Alcohol dehydrogenase with					
NADH	1.7×10^7	3.4	stopped-flow	fluorescence	Theorell et al. (1967)
deamino NADH	1.3×10^6	2.6	stopped-flow		Geraci and Gibson (1967)
reduced 3-acetylpyridine adenine dinucleotide	5.6×10^6	34.8	stopped-flow	visible	Shore (1969)
Lysozyme with					
di N-acetylglucosamine[a]	4.6×10^6	950	T-jump	visible	Chipman and Schimmel (1968)
tri N-acetylglucosamine[a]	4.4×10^6	28	T-jump	visible	Holler et al. (1969)
hexa N-acetylglucosamine[a]		3.5	stopped-flow	fluorescene	Holler et al. (1970)
Malate dehydrogenase with					
NADH[a]	5×10^8	5×10^1	T-jump	fluorescence	Czerlinski and Schreck (1963)
Myoglobin with					
cyanide	2×10^2	1.2×10^{-4}	stopped-flow	visible	Ver Ploeg and Alberty (1968)
imidazole	3.3×10^2	4.3	T-jump	visible	Diven, and Alberty (1965)
benzimidazole	5.1×10^2	8	T-jump		
azide	2.8×10^5	4	T-jump	visible	Goldsack et al. (1965)
cyanate	2.5×10^4	44	T-jump		
hydrogen sulfide	2.9×10^1	63	T-jump	visible	Goldsack et al. (1966)
oxygen	1.9×10^7	11	T-jump	visible	Brunori and Schuster (1969)
Ribonuclease with					
cytidyl 3',5'-cytidine[a]	1.4×10^7	7×10^3	T-jump	visible	Erman and Hammes (1966b)
cytidine 2',3'-cyclic phosphate[a]	5×10^7	$1-2 \times 10^4$	T-jump	visible	Erman and Hammes (1966c)
cytidine 3'-phosphate[a]	6×10^7	4×10^3	T-jump	UV and visible	Cathou and Hammes (1965)
cytidine 2'-phosphate[a]	1×10^7	3×10^3	T-jump	visible	Hammes (1968)
uridine 3'-phosphate[a]	6.1×10^7	1.1×10^4	T-jump	UV and visible	Hammes and Walz (1969)
uridine 2',3'-phosphate[a]	1.1×10^7	2.1×10^4	T-jump	visible	del Rosario and Hammes (1970)
tRNA with					
ethidium bromide[a]	2.3×10^6	15	T-jump	visible	Bittman (1969)
Serum albumin (bovine) with					
1-naphthol-4-[4-(4'-azobenzene-azo)-phenylarsonic acid]	2.1×10^6	35	T-jump	visible	Froese et al. (1962)
1-naphthol-2 sulfonic acid-4-[4-(4'-azo-benzene-azo)-phenylarsonic acid]	3.6×10^5	2.5	T-jump	visible	Froese et al. (1962)
Trypsin with					
benzamidine	2.9×10^7	6×10^2	T-jump	visible (competition reaction)	Gullian and Thusius (1970)
proflavin	7.6×10^7	9.5×10^3	T-jump	visible	
Tryptophan synthetase[a] with tryptophan	2.8×10^6	3.7×10^3	T-jump	visible	Faeder and Hammes (1970)

[a]Multiphasic kinetics observed (two or more steps).

[b]Apparent rate constants (in cases where the pH-profile of the kinetics has been examined, the maximum rate has been selected).

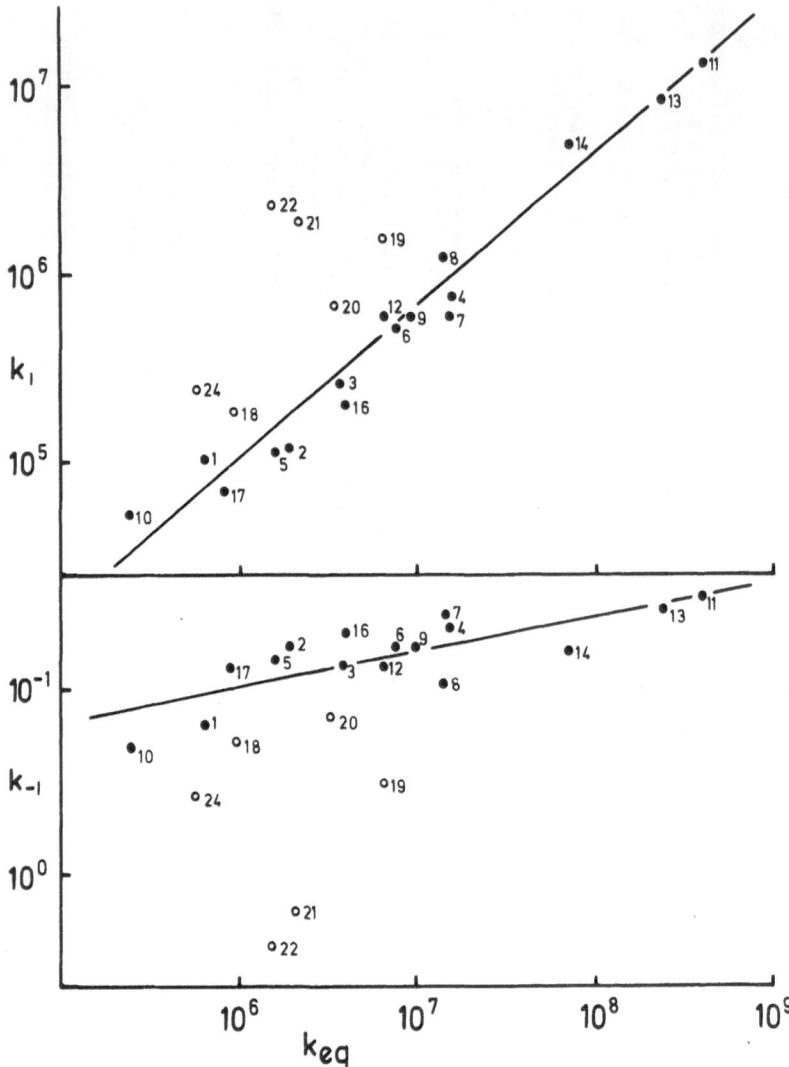

FIG. 5. *Top.* Relationship between the rate constant of complex formation and the affinity of the complex K_{eq} for various aromatic sulfonamides and human carbonic anhydrase C. *Bottom.* Relationship between the dissociation rate of the complex and K_{eq}: (o), *ortho*-substituted sulfonamides; (●) non-*ortho*-substituted. The diagonal lines have slopes of 0.83 and 0.18 respectively and were calculated from a least-squares analysis by considering only the non-*ortho*-substituted sulfonamides. (From Taylor et al. 1970. *Biochemistry* [*Washington*], 7:2638.)

pH Dependence of Complex Formation

A knowledge of the *pH* dependence of complex formation is essential for understanding the reaction path of ligand association. This can best be illustrated by considering the following three examples.

(1) MYOGLOBIN. The three-dimensional structure of this protein is known (Stryer et al., 1964), and kinetic findings have been correlated with structure in order to identify probable ionizing groups influencing complex formation. Ligands binding to this metalloprotein occupy a single coordinate position with a six-coordinate ferric ion. From an analysis of the pH-dependence of complex formation, Alberty and coworkers (Diven et al., 1965; Goldsack et al., 1965, 1966) have proposed the following scheme for ligand-myoglobin association:

$$\underset{k_{-1}}{\overset{k_1}{\rightleftarrows}}$$

$$H_2Mb + HL \quad \underset{k_{-1}}{\overset{k_1}{\rightleftarrows}} \quad H_2MbHL \tag{23}$$

$$K_A \; \updownarrow$$

$$HMb + HL \quad \underset{k_{-2}}{\overset{k_2}{\rightleftarrows}} \quad HMbHL \tag{24}$$

$$K_B \; \updownarrow$$

$$Mb + HL \quad \underset{k_{-3}}{\overset{k_3}{\rightleftarrows}} \quad MbHL \tag{25}$$

$$K_L \; \updownarrow$$

$$H_2Mb + L \quad \underset{k_{-4}}{\overset{k_4}{\rightleftarrows}} \quad H_2MbL \tag{26}$$

$$K_A \; \updownarrow$$

$$HMb + L \quad \underset{k_{-5}}{\overset{k_5}{\rightleftarrows}} \quad HMbL \tag{27}$$

$$K_B \; \updownarrow$$

$$Mb + L \quad \underset{k_{-6}}{\overset{k_6}{\rightleftarrows}} \quad MbL \tag{28}$$

The observed pH-dependences of association and dissociation differ considerably, and a kinetic investigation of complex formation is required to identify the species in the various protonation states involved in complex formation. Thus far, only association has been analyzed in detail for the various ligands (Table 2), and the data can be well fitted to an assignment of $pK_A = 4.7$ and $pK_B = 5.7$. From the x-ray structure it has been suggested that the groups involved are propionic acid and histidine residues in the vicinity of the iron. When the kinetic constants are resolved according to the proposed mechanism, there is little variation in the association rate constants for the ligands attacking as anionic species (Table 2). Thus, differences in apparent affinity for these ligands are largely a consequence of the respective K_L and dissociation rate variation, a behavior that is typical for most metal-coordination complexes (Eigen and Wilkens, 1965).

(2) CARBONIC ANHYDRASE. Carbonic anhydrase is also a metal-

TABLE 2

Bimolecular Rate Constants $(M^{-1}sec^{-1})$ for the Association of Ligands with Metmyoglobin[a]

Rate Constant	Ligand			
	HN$_3$	HOCN	H$_2$S	HCN
k_1	$\leqslant 10^2$	$\leqslant 10^2$	$\leqslant 10^2$	30
k_2	$\leqslant 10^2$	$\leqslant 10^2$	$\leqslant 10^2$	30
k_3	$\leqslant 10^2$	$\leqslant 10^2$	$\leqslant 10^2$	30
k_4	8.5×10^5	1.1×10^5	7.9×10^6	1×10^6
k_5	3.6×10^4	1.5×10^3	2.4×10^5	8×10^4
k_6	2.5×10^3	2.7×10^2	3.2×10^3	2×10^3

[a] Data from Diven et al. 1965; Goldsack et al. 1965, 1966.

loenzyme, and aromatic sulfonamides and many monovalent anions appear to bind within or close to the coordination sphere of the metal (Fridborg et al., 1967). The pH-dependence of ligand association is consistent with the following scheme (Taylor et al., 1970a,b):

$$[HCA]^+ + Anion^- \underset{k_{-a}}{\overset{k_a}{\rightleftarrows}} Anion{\cdot}HCA \qquad (29)$$

$$K_E \updownarrow$$

$$[CA] + RSO_2NH_2 \underset{k_{-s}}{\overset{k_s}{\rightleftarrows}} RSO_2NH{\cdot}HCA$$
$$+$$
$$H^+ \quad K_S$$
$$RSO_2NH^- + H^+$$

Cobalt may be substituted for the single zinc atom in carbonic anhydrase with the retention of similar catalytic and inhibitor binding properties (Lindskog, 1963). The spectra arising from the Co(II) d-d transitions demonstrate a H$^+$-dependent equilibrium between two coordination forms of the enzyme represented above by K_E. The pH dependence of this equilibrium varies with the particular human carbonic anhydrase isozyme: isozyme C, $pK_E = 6.5$; isozyme B, $pK_E = 7.3$ and carboxymethylated B, $pK_E = 9.1$. A similar pH dependence of sulfonamide complex formation is observed for the Zn and Co(II) enzymes, and the pH dependence of sulfonamide association rates correlates closely with the Co(II) spectral pH dependence. Thus the metal coordination structure of the "non-liganded" enzyme and the ionization equilibrium of the sulfonamide proton, K_S, govern the pH dependence of association of these inhibitors. Combination between the anionic sulfonamide species, RSO$_2$NH$^-$, and [HCA]$^+$ will yield a pH dependence of association identical with the reaction path designated by k_s. Monovalent anions, such as CN$^-$, SCN$^-$, Cl$^-$, and CH$_3$COO$^-$, combine with the [HCA]$^+$ species; however, this pathway involving the sulfonamido anion can be ruled out mainly on the basis of an improbably high bimolecular rate constant, $\geqslant 10^{10}\ M^{-1}$ sec^{-1}. This exceeds the theoretical rate limitation on encounter controlled reactions and is considerably greater than any observed ligand-macromolecule association rates (cf. Table 1). Since ultraviolet difference spectroscopy has indicated that the deprotonated sulfonamido anion (RSO_2NH^-) is the species in the stable complex (King and Burgen, 1970), a mechanism has been proposed where the sulfonamide combines as a neutral species with subsequent transfer of the sulfonamido proton to a site on the enzyme (Taylor et al., 1970b). This obligate proton transfer may provide an explanation for the vast difference in affinity for carbonic anhydrase between the structurally similar sulfonamides and sulfonic acids.

A unique Co(II) d-d spectrum is generated for the carbonic anhydrase-sulfonamide complex which is pH-insensitive, thus indicating that with ligand binding the coordination state of the enzyme becomes fixed. Correspondingly, dissociation rates of the sulfonamide complexes are pH-invariant.

(3) CYTOCHROME-C. A third example in which a kinetic analysis of pH-dependence has been informative in establishing a probable reaction mechanism is the oxidation-reduction of cytochrome-C (Brandt et al., 1966). Temperature-jump studies have shown no pH-dependence for the observed rate constants of the redox reaction:

$$\text{Cyt-C}^{III} + \text{Fe(CN)}_6^{4-} \rightleftharpoons \text{Cyt-C}^{II} + \text{Fe(CN)}_6^{3-} \tag{30}$$

However, both the spectroscopic equilibrium constant for the overall reaction and the redox potential are pH-dependent. This behavior can be interpreted by assuming that ferricytochrome exists in at least two isomeric forms, one of which can be converted to the ferrocytochrome. The equilibrium between isomeric forms is pH-dependent and adjusts itself slowly relative to the electron transfer process. Confirmation of this interpretation comes from stopped-flow studies that indicate that a pH-dependent isomerization of cytochrome-C occurs with a slow half-life of several seconds. Thus, kinetic constants and the pH-dependence of the ratio of inactive to active forms can be evaluated and the mechanism written as follows:

$$
\begin{array}{l}
\text{H}^+ \\
+ \\
[\text{Cyt-C}^{III}]_i \\
\updownarrow \qquad\qquad\qquad\qquad k_r \\
[\text{Cyt-C}^{III}]_a + \text{Fe(CN)}_6^{4-} \underset{k_0}{\rightleftharpoons} [\text{Cyt-C}^{II}] + \text{Fe(CN)}_6^{3-} \qquad (31)
\end{array}
$$

The actual electron transfer process is pH-independent. Here, as with the other two systems, detailed kinetic measurements are required to delineate the elementary steps, their pH-dependence, and participating isomeric forms of the macromolecule.

In enzyme catalysis more elaborate mechanisms must be proposed when the species involved in each elementary step are considered. Ribonuclease, for example, has three ionizing groups which appear to influence substrate binding, and two isomeric states of each respective complex can be shown to exist (Hammes and Walz, 1969; del Rosario and Hammes, 1970). The pK of the influential ionizing groups cannot be expected to be the same in the isomeric states of the free enzyme and its complexes. All of these features must be taken into account in detailing a reaction scheme consistent with the experimental data. The minimal mechanism for ribonuclease catalysis developed from the pH-dependences of five observed relaxation times and the steady-state rate constants involves the consideration of 24 enzyme or enzyme-substrate species (Hammes and Walz, 1969).

Other Applications

Various macromolecular isomerizations or conformational changes have also recently been examined by fast-reaction techniques. Kinetic investigations of reversible or irreversible transitions induced thermally (Pohl, 1969; Spatz and Crothers, 1969) or by external agents (Polet and Steinhardt, 1969; Schechter et al., 1970) allow one to investigate the dynamics and energetics of cooperative *intramolecular* interactions such as protein folding and unfolding.

Use of fast-reaction techniques, however, has largely been restricted to relatively pure systems, primarily proteins and nucleic acids. Purity of the preparation will continue to be a limiting factor, since rapidly responding, sensitive and direct detection must be employed. Nevertheless, in some instances fast-reaction methods have been extended to more heterogeneous systems with favorable results. For certain membrane systems, kinetics of interaction of fluorescence probes and the kinetics of local anaesthetic-induced perturbation of membrane structure have been examined by flow techniques (Chance et al., 1969). With such complex processes a kinetic approach can yield important information regarding accessibility of combining sites and transitions in membrane structure. Stopped-flow (Sha' Afi et al., 1967) and more recently temperature-jump methods (Owen et al., 1970) have been employed in the investigation of water fluxes in red cells and red cell ghosts under osmotic gradients. Scattered white light has been used for detection with an optical arrangement similar to that employed for fluorescence.

PROGNOSIS

From the applications briefly discussed here, it can be seen that fast-reaction techniques can potentially provide a great deal of detailed information on dynamic aspects and the elementary steps of drug-macromolecule interactions. The rapid development in the application of these techniques to biological systems can be attributed to: (1) advances in instrumentation, much of which is now available commercially; (2) many biological problems that have progressed to a state where detailed kinetic studies on the isolated systems will provide valuable information on mechanism. The increasing body of knowledge on macromolecular structure has yielded complementary information necessary for mechanistic interpretations of the kinetic data.

To understand specificity of drug interactions on a molecular basis, the dynamic behavior of reaction between the small molecule and its complementary site of binding must be examined. From this approach essential details on the sequence of elementary steps and the role of ligand-induced or stabilized conformational changes in complex formation can be learned. This, in turn, should be coupled with structural information on the spatial relationships of interacting sites. It is this kind of approach that should prove most valuable to the correlation of chemical structure with biological activity.

ACKNOWLEDGMENTS

I am grateful to Professor A. S. V. Burgen, Medical Research Council, Molecular Pharmacology Unit, Cambridge, England, and Dr. E. Grell, Max Planck Institut für Physikalische Chemie, Göttingen, Germany, for helpful discussions and suggestions. This manuscript was largely prepared during the tenure of an NIH fellowship in Cambridge, England.

REFERENCES

Alberty, R. A., and G. G. Hammes. 1958. Application of the theory of diffusion controlled reactions to enzyme kinetics. J. Phys. Chem., 62:154-159.

Bewick A., M. Fleischman, J. N. Middleton, and L. Wynne-Jones. 1965. Examination of proton transfer reactions by temperature jump and electrochemical methods. Discuss. Faraday Soc., 39:149-158.

Berger, R. L., B. Balko, W. Borcherdt, and W. Friauf. 1968. High speed optical stopped-flow apparatus. Rev. Sci. Instrum., 39:486-493.

———— and L. C. Stoddart. 1964. A thermal stopped-flow apparatus. In Chance, B., R. H. Eisenhardt, Q. H. Gibson, and K. K. Lonberg-Holm, eds., Rapid Mixing and Sampling Techniques in Biochemistry. New York, Academic Press.

Bittman, R. 1969. Studies on the binding of ethidium bromide to transfer ribonucleic acid: Absorption, fluorescence, ultracentrifugation and kinetic investigations. J. Molec. Biol., 46:251-258.

Borg, D. C. 1964. Continuous flow methods adapted to EPR apparatuses. In Chance, B., R. H. Eisenhardt, Q. H. Gibson, and K. K. Lonberg-Holm, eds., Rapid Mixing and Sampling Techniques in Biochemistry, 135-149. New York, Academic Press.

Brandt, K. G., P. C. Parks, G. Czerlinski, and G. P. Hess. 1966. On the elucidation of the pH-dependence of the oxidation-reduction potential of cytochrome C at alkaline pH. J. Biol. Chem., 241:4180-4185.

Brunori, M., and T. M. Schuster. 1969. Kinetic studies of ligand binding to hemoglobin and its isolated subunits by the temperature-jump relaxation method. J. Biol. Chem., 244:4046-4053.

Burgen, A. S. V. 1966. The drug-receptor complex. J. Pharm. Pharmacol., 17:137-149.

Caldin, E. F. 1964. Fast Reactions in Solution. Oxford, Blackwell.

Castellan, G. W. 1963. Calculation of the spectrum of chemical relaxation times for a general reaction mechanism. Ber. Bunsenges. Physik. Chem., 67:898-908.

Cathou, R. E., and G. G. Hammes. 1965. Relaxation spectra of ribonuclease III. Further investigation of the interaction of ribonuclease and cytidine-3'-phosphate. J. Amer. Chem. Soc., 87:4674-4680.

Chance, B. 1940. The accelerated flow method for rapid reactions. J. Franklin Inst., 229:737-766.

———— A. Azzi, L. Mela, G. Radda, and H. Vainio. 1969. Local anaesthetic induced changes of a membrane bound fluorochrome. Fed. Eur. Biochem. Soc. Letters, 3:10-13.

————R. H. Eisenhardt, Q. H. Gibson, and K. K. Lonberg-Holm, eds. 1964. Rapid Mixing and Sampling Techniques in Biochemistry. New York, Academic Press.

Chipman, D. M., and P. R. Schimmel. 1968. Dynamics of lysozyme-saccharide interactions. J. Biol. Chem., 293:3771-3774.

Colen, A. H. 1970. Temperature jump studies of the binding of bromophenol blue to β-lactoglobulin in the vicinity of the N→R transition. J. Biol. Chem., 245:738-745.

Czerlinski, G. 1964. Application of chemical relaxation to biochemical systems. J. Theor. Biol., 7:435-484.

———— 1966. Chemical Relaxation. An Introduction to the Theory and Application of Stepwise Perturbation. New York, Marcel Dekker.

———— and G. Schreck. 1963. Chemical relaxation of the reaction of malate dehydrogenase with reduced nicotinamide adenine dinucleotide determined by fluorescence detection. Biochemistry (Washington), 3:89-100.

Day, L. A., J. M. Sturtevant, and S. J. Singer. 1963. The kinetics of the reactions between antibodies to the 2,4-dinitrophenyl group and specific haptens. Ann. N.Y. Acad. Sci., 103(2):611-625.

Debye, P. 1942. Reaction rates in ionic solutions. Trans. Amer. Electrochem. Soc., 82:265-272.

del Rosario, E. J., and G. G. Hammes. 1970. Relaxation spectra of ribonuclease, VII. The interaction of ribonuclease with uridine 2',3'-cyclic phosphate. J. Amer. Chem. Soc., 92:1750-1753.

De Sa, R. J., and Q. H. Gibson. 1966. Dual beam stopped flow spectrophotometer utilizing modulated xenon arcs. Rev. Sci. Instrum., 37:900-906.

———— and Q. H. Gibson. 1969. A practical automatic data acquisition system for stopped-flow spectrometry. Computers Biomed. Res., 2:494-505.

Diven, W. F., D. E. Goldsack, and R. A. Alberty. 1965. Temperature jump kinetic studies of the binding of imidazole by sperm whale metmyoglobin. J. Biol. Chem., 240:2437-2441.

Dolman, D., H. B. Dunford, D. M. Chowdhury, and M. Morrison. 1968. Kinetics of cyanide binding by lactoperoxidase. Biochemistry (Washington), 7:3991-3996.

Dunford, H. B., and R. A. Alberty. 1967. The kinetics of fluoride binding by ferric horseradish peroxidase. Biochemistry (Washington), 6:447-451.

Eckfeldt, J., G. G. Hammes, and S. C. Mohr. 1970. Relaxation spectra of aspartate transcarbamylase I. Interaction of 5-bromocytidine triphosphate with native enzyme and regulatory subunit. Biochemistry (Washington), 9:3353-3362.

Eigen, M. 1954. Methods for investigation of ionic reactions in aqueous solutions with half-times as short as 10^{-9} sec. Discuss. Faraday Soc., 17:194-204.

———— 1968. New looks and outlooks on physical enzymology. Quart. Rev. Biophys., 1:3-23.

———— and L. de Maeyer. 1963. Relaxation methods. In Weissberger, A., ed., Techniques of Organic Chemistry, Vol. VIII, Part II, 895-1051. New York, Wiley/Interscience.

———— and G. G. Hammes. 1963. Elementary steps in enzyme reactions. Advances Enzym., 25:1-38.

———— and R. G. Wilkens. 1965. The kinetics and mechanism of formation of metal complexes. Advances Chem. Series, 49:55-80.

Ellis, W. D., and H. B. Dunford. 1968. The kinetics of cyanide and fluoride binding by ferric horseradish peroxidase. Biochemistry (Washington), 7:2054-2062.

Erman, J. E., and G. G. Hammes. 1966a. Versatile stopped flow temperature jump apparatus. Rev. Sci. Instrum., 37:746-750.

———— and G. G. Hammes. 1966b. Relaxation spectra of ribonuclease. IV. The interaction of ribonuclease with cytidine 2':3'-cyclic phosphate. J. Amer. Chem. Soc., 88:5607-5613.

———— and G. G. Hammes, 1966c. Relaxation spectra of ribonuclease. V. The interaction of ribonuclease with cytidylyl-3':5'-cytidine. J. Amer. Chem. Soc., 88:5614-5617.

Faeder, E. J., and G. G. Hammes. 1970. Kinetic studies of tryptophan synthetase. Interaction of substrate with the B subunit. Biochemistry (Washington), 9:4043-4049.

Fridborg, K., K. K. Kannan, A. Liljas, J. Lundin, B. Strandberg, R. Strandberg, B. Tilander, and G. Wiren. 1967. Crystal structure of human erythrocyte carbonic anhydrase C. J. Molec. Biol., 25:505-515.

Froese, A., and A. H. Sehon. 1965. Kinetic and equilibrium studies of the reaction between anti-p-nitrophenyl antibodies and a homologous hapten. Immunochemistry, 2:135-143.

———— A. H. Sehon, and M. Eigen. 1962. Kinetic studies of protein-dye and antibody-hapten interactions with the temperature jump method. Canad. J. Chem., 40:1786-1797.

Frost, A. A., and R. G. Pearson. 1961. Kinetics and Mechanism, 2nd ed. New York, John Wiley & Sons.

Geraci, G., and Q. H. Gibson. 1967. The reaction of liver alcohol dehydrogenase with reduced diphosphopyridine nucleotide. J. Biol. Chem., 242:4275-4278.

Gibson, Q. H. 1966. Application of rapid reaction techniques to biological oxidations. Ann. Rev. Biochem., 35:435-456.

———— J. W. Hastings, G. Weber, W. Duane, and J. Massa. 1966. The interaction of flavin mononucleotide with an enzymic system from *Photobacterium fischeri*. *In* Slater, E. C., ed., Flavins and Flavoproteins, 358-366. Amsterdam, Elsevier.

———— and L. Milnes. 1964. Apparatus for rapid and sensitive spectrophotometry. Biochem. J., 91:161-171.

Goldsack, D. E., W. S. Eberlein, and R. A. Alberty. 1965. Temperature jump studies of sperm whale metmyoglobin. II. J. Biol. Chem., 240:4312-4315.

———— W. S. Eberlein, and R. A. Alberty, 1966. Temperature jump studies of sperm whale metmyoglobin. III. J. Biol. Chem., 240:2653-2660.

Guillain, F., and D. Thusius. 1970. The use of proflavin as an indicator in temperature-jump studies of the binding of a competitive inhibitor to trypsin. J. Amer. Chem. Soc., 92:5534-5536.

Gutfreund, H. 1969. Rapid mixing: continuous flow. Meth. Enzym., 16:229-249.

Hammes, G. G. 1966. Very fast reactions in solution. Science, 151:1507-1511.

———— 1968. Relaxation spectrometry of biological systems. Advances Protein Chem., 23:1-43.

———— and P. R. Schimmel. 1966. Chemical relaxation spectra: Calculation of relaxation times for complex mechanisms. J. Phys. Chem., 70:2319-2324.

———— and P. R. Schimmel. 1967. Relaxation spectra of enzymatic reactions. J. Phys. Chem., 71:917-923.

———— and F. G. Walz, Jr. 1969. Relaxation spectra of ribonuclease. VI. The interaction of ribonuclease with uridine 3'-monophosphate. J. Amer. Chem. Soc., 87:7179-7186.

Hartridge, H., and F. J. W. Roughton. 1923. A method of measuring the velocity of very rapid chemical reactions. Proc. Roy. Soc. London, A104:376-394.

Havsteen, B. H. 1967. The kinetics of the two step interaction of chymotrypsin with proflavin. J. Biol. Chem., 242:769-771.

Holler, E., J. Rupley, and G. P. Hess. 1969. Kinetics of lysozyme-substrate interactions. Biochem. Biophys. Res. Commun., 37:423-429.

————— J. Rupley, and G. P. Hess. 1970. Kinetics of lysozyme-substrate interactions. Biochem. Biophys. Res. Commun., 40:166-170.

King, R. W., and A. S. V. Burgen. 1970. Sulphonamide complexes of human carbonic anhydrases—ultraviolet difference spectroscopy. Biochim. Biophys. Acta, 207:278-285.

Kirschner, K., M. Eigen, R. Bittman, and B. Voigt. 1966. The binding of nicotinamide-adenine dinucleotide to yeast-D-glyceraldehyde-3-phosphate dehydrogenase: Temperature-jump relaxation studies on the mechanism of an allosteric enzyme. Proc. Nat. Acad. Sci. U.S.A., 56:1661-1667.

Kustin, K., ed. 1970. Fast Reactions. Meth. Enzym., 16.

————— D. Shear, and D. Kleitman. 1965. Theory of relaxation spectra; the kinetics of coupled chemical reactions. J. Theor. Biol., 9:186-211.

Li, H. J., and D. M. Crothers. 1968. Relaxation studies of the proflavin-DNA complex: The kinetics of an intercalation reaction. J. Molec. Biol., 39:461-477.

Lindskog, S. 1963. Effects of pH and inhibitions on some properties related to metal binding in bovine carbonic anhydrase. J. Biol. Chem., 238:945-951.

Monod, J., J. Wyman, and J. P. Changeux. 1965. On the nature of allosteric transitions, a plausible model. J. Molec. Biol., 12:88-118.

Müller, W., and D. M. Crothers. 1968. Studies of the binding of actinomycin and related compounds to DNA. J. Molec. Biol., 35:251-290.

Nagel, R. L., and Q. H. Gibson. 1967. Kinetics and mechanism of complex formation between hemoglobin and haptoglobin. J. Biol. Chem., 242:3428-3434.

Owen, J. D., B. C. Bennion, L. P. Holmes, E. M. Eyring, M. W. Berg, and J. L. Lords. 1970. Temperature jump relaxations in aqueous saline suspensions of human erythrocytes. Biochim. Biophys. Acta, 203:77-82.

Pohl, F. M. 1969. On the kinetics of structure transition I of some pancreatic proteins. Fed. Eur. Biochem. Soc. Letters, 3:60-63.

Polet, H., and J. Steinhardt. 1969. Sequential stages in the acid denaturation of horse and human ferrihemoglobins. Biochemistry (Washington), 8:857-864.

Rossi-Bernardi, L., and R. L. Berger. 1968. The rapid measurement of pH by the glass electrode. J. Biol. Chem., 248:1297-1302.

Roughton, F. J. W. 1934. The kinetics of hemoglobin. Proc. Roy. Soc. (London), B 115:495-503.

————— and B. Chance. 1963. Fast reactions. *In* Weissberger, A., ed., Techniques of Organic Chemistry. Vol. 8, Part II:704-792. New York, Wiley/Interscience.

Schechter, A. N., R. F. Chen, and C. B. Anfinsen. 1970. Kinetics of folding of *Staphylococcus* nuclease. Science, 167:886-887.

Sha' Afi, R. I., G. T. Rich, V. W. Sidel, W. Bossert, and A. K. Soloman. 1967. The effect of the unstirred layer on human red cell water permeability. J. Gen. Physiol., 50:377-390.

Shore, J. D. 1969. The rates of binding of reduced nicotinamide-adenine dinucleotide analogs to liver alcohol dehydrogenase. Biochemistry (Washington), 8:1588-1590.

Sirs, J. A. 1958. Electrometric stopped flow measurements of rapid reactions in solution. Trans. Faraday Soc., 54:20-212.

Spatz, H., and D. M. Crothers. 1969. The rate of DNA unwinding. J. Molec. Biol., 42:191-219.

Strittmatter, P. 1964. Simple, micro stopped-flow apparatus. *In* Chance, B., R. H. Eisenhardt, Q. H. Gibson, and K. K. Lonberg-Holm, eds., Rapid Mixing and Sampling Techniques in Biochemistry, 71-85. New York, Academic Press.

Stryer, L., J. C. Kendrew, and H. C. Watson. 1964. The mode of attachment of the azide ion to sperm whale metmyoglobin. J. Molec. Biol., 8:96-104.

Taylor, P. W., R. W. King, and A. S. V. Burgen. 1970a. Kinetics of complex formation between human carbonic anhydrases and aromatic sulfonamides. Biochemistry (Washington), 9:2638-2645.

_____ R. W. King, and A. S. V. Burgen. 1970b. The influence of pH of the kinetics of complex formation between aromatic sulfonamides and human carbonic anhydrase. Biochemistry (Washington), 9:3894-3902.

Theorell, H., A. Ehrenberg, and C. de Zalenski. 1967. The binding of NADH to liver alcohol dehydrogenase: A two step reaction. Biochem. Biophys. Res. Commun., 27:309-314.

Ver Ploeg, D. A., and R. A. Alberty. 1968. Kinetics of binding of cyanide to sperm whale metmyoglobin. J. Biol. Chem., 243:435-440.

Chapter **11**

X-Ray Diffraction

S. H. Kim

Department of Biology, Massachusetts Institute of Technology, Cambridge, Massachusetts

and

Colin F. Chignell

Laboratory of Chemical Pharmacology, National Heart and Lung Institute, National Institutes of Health, Bethesda, Maryland

INTRODUCTION

For Those Who ...

The first three sections (Kim) of this chapter are intended for those who are interested only in understanding the minimal basic concepts of x-ray crystallography and the use of the technique to determine the three-dimensional structure of a molecule. The final section (Chignell) deals with the x-ray crystallography of some drugs and other pharmacologically important compounds.

In order to understand any phenomenon at a molecular level, the three-dimensional structure of the molecules involved must be known. X-ray diffraction is the most powerful tool for the determination of molecular structure. The use of x-ray diffraction to determine three-dimensional structure can be divided into two categories: one dealing with large molecules such as proteins and nucleic acids; the other, with small or intermediate sized molecules. The impact of "large molecule crystallography" on molecular biology has been well demonstrated by the structure determinations of such macromolecules as deoxyribonucleic acid, myoglobin, hemoglobin, lysozyme, ribonuclease, and others. However, the high operational expense and long man-hours required for such a project put large molecule crystallography out of the reach of a vast majority of research workers. Besides its operational difficulties, the theory and techniques of large molecule crystallography have not been developed to the point where noncrystallographers can apply the technique on their work within a short period of learning time. A good review of large molecule crystallography has been written by Holmes and Blow (1966).

What is the situation in "small molecule crystallography?" Can one find the three-dimensional structure of a small molecule containing, say, 50 to 100 atoms (not counting hydrogens) within a few months without knowing the details of theory and methods? The answer is yes, most of the time. This chapter deals with the category of small molecule crystallography.

Structure of a Small Molecule Can Be Found by Following a "Catalogued Procedure"

During the last decade, the theories and techniques of crystallography have been developed greatly. The instruments have been automated to such an extent that a system can be set up in which the decision-making steps during structure determination are few. This leaves the preparation of a "right" compound and the growing of single crystals of it as the most critical and important steps in the whole process.

It should be noted, of course, that it is necessary to have a consulting crystallographer to set up such a system and to aid at a few critical steps. Nevertheless, it should be possible by following a catalogued procedure to find the three-dimensional structure of any compound of interest. This type of approach has been very successfully demonstrated in a number of laboratories; the Rapid Organic Structure Analysis Project at the California Institute of Technology is a good example. The hardware of this system is an automated data collection device and a high-speed, large-core memory computer, both of which are commercially available. A recent review of the technological advances in these two areas has been written by Hamilton (1970).

An attempt is made here to present the diffraction phenomena by means of illustrations and analogies, keeping to a minimum the number of mathematical expressions, since these are often very indirect in revealing the relationship between the diffraction pattern and the diffracting structure. In the latter part of the article, the structure determination process is divided into five steps. The essence of each step will be discussed so that the reader can get some basic ideas about each one.

For a more detailed discussion of the practical aspects of x-ray crystallography the reader is referred to books by Stout and Jensen (1968) and Buerger (1960).

THEORY

X-Ray Behaves Like Light

If one sends a parallel beam of light through a hole, the light is diffracted by the hole and produces an optical diffraction pattern as shown in Figure 1H. When

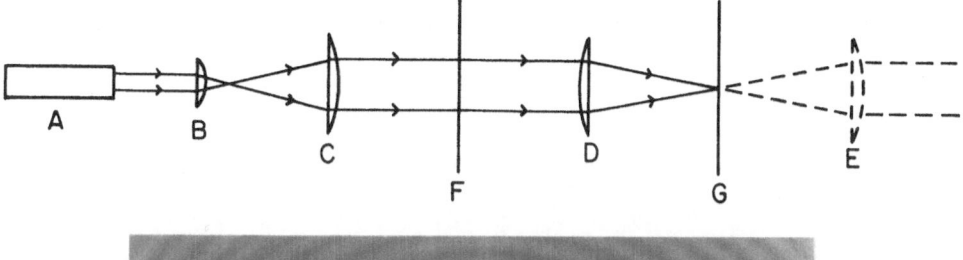

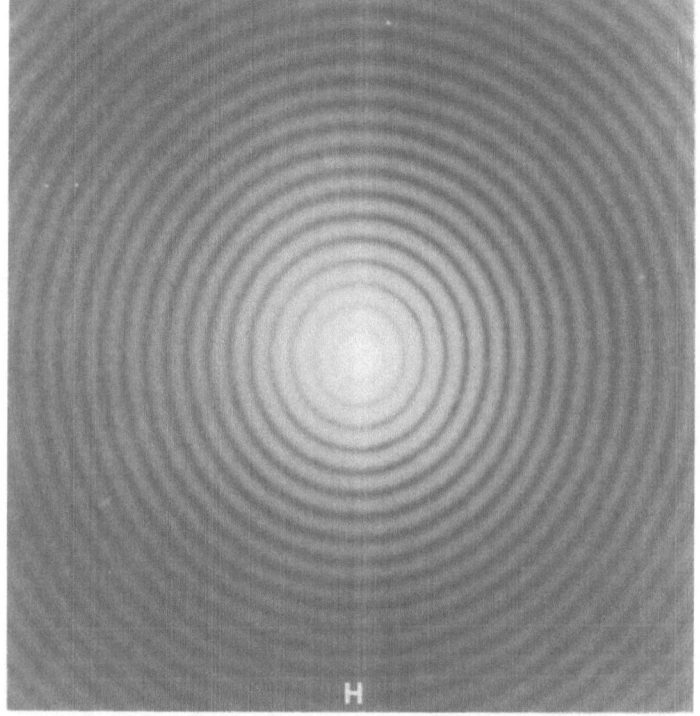

FIG. 1. Schematic drawing of an optical diffraction apparatus. (A) laser as a light source; (B), (C), (D), (E) lenses; (F) object; (G) plane where diffraction pattern is recorded. (H) The diffraction pattern from a small hole. (Photo courtesy of Dr. H. Slator.)

one hole is replaced by six holes as shown in Figure 2a, the diffraction pattern becomes more complex (Figure 2A). When one repeats this with six holes systematically arranged in a two-dimensional array (Figure 2f), the optical diffraction pattern will be F (Figure 2).

Now let us imagine that everything is reduced in size so that each hole is now the size of an atom, which is about one Angstrom in diameter, and the distance between the holes is a few Angstroms. The wavelength of the light is also reduced to a few Angstroms, making it in the x-ray range. If one sends the parallel x-rays through this hypothetical two-dimensional crystal (which is now equivalent to a two-dimensional array of a molecule with six atoms), one will get basically the same diffraction pattern as F in Figure 2.

The same analogy can be extended to the three-dimensional crystal.

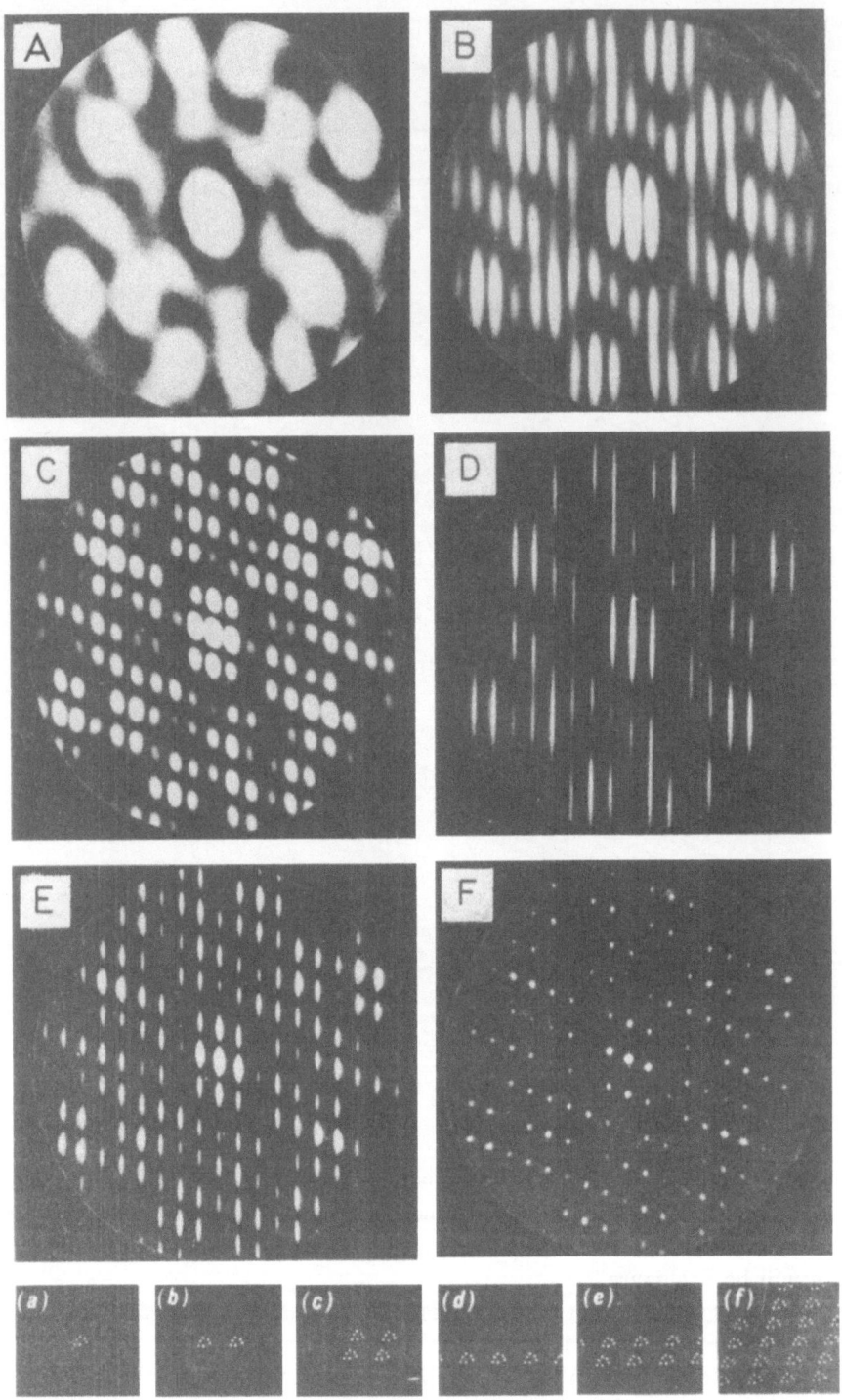

FIG. 2. (A), (B), (C), (D), (E), and (F) are optical diffraction patterns from the objects (a), (b), (c), (d), (e), and (f), all of which contain the same motif of six holes. (From Taylor and Lipson. 1965. *Optical Transforms*. Courtesy of Bell and Sons, Ltd.)

There Is No "X-Ray Lens" to Resynthesize a Diffraction Pattern Into a Diffracting Object

In Figure 1, if the photographic film, G, is removed and another lens is set further to the right, the optical diffraction pattern will continue to travel as shown in dotted lines. It will go through the lens and then form an image which is exactly the same as the object from which the diffraction occurred, i.e., a hole.

Unfortunately, there is no lens for the x-ray that does a similar job. And this is where the heart of x-ray crystallography lies, i.e., to find a mathematical "lens" which will perform the same operation as the optical lens and resynthesize the optical diffraction.

Mathematical Expressions for X-Ray Diffraction and Resynthesis

In Figure 3d and e, and Figure 2f, where the six-atom motif is the same but its lattice buildup is different, the three resultant diffraction patterns are different (Figure 3D and E; Figure 2F). From the symmetry and geometry of the diffraction pattern, one can find the symmetry and geometry by which the single motif is repeated and arranged in a crystal. Furthermore, the intensity of each dot in the diffraction pattern contains information about the relative locations of atoms in a molecule which make up a single crystal. These dots are called reflections and each occupies a unique position, so that each reflection can be identified by the vector $\mathbf{S}$ away from the origin (center of the diffraction pattern). The intensity (brightness) of a reflection in this case is proportional to the square of a complex quantity called the structure factor ($\mathbf{F}$). Thus if $I(\mathbf{S})$ is the intensity of a reflection which can be identified by a vector $\mathbf{S}$, and $\mathbf{F}(\mathbf{S})$ is the corresponding structure factor, then

$$I(\mathbf{S}) \propto |\mathbf{F}(\mathbf{S})|^2 \tag{1}$$

In equation (1) $\mathbf{F}(\mathbf{S})$ is a complex number with a magnitude of $|\mathbf{F}(\mathbf{S})|$ and a phase ϕ such that

$$\mathbf{F}(\mathbf{S}) = |\mathbf{F}(\mathbf{S})|\exp(i\phi) \tag{2}$$

The electron density at any point within a molecule can be expressed as $\rho(\mathbf{R})$, where $\mathbf{R}$ is a vectorial quantity which defines the position of the point relative to an arbitrary origin. Thus $\rho(\mathbf{R})$ will have a large value when $\mathbf{R}$ coincides with an atom, but will be zero when $\mathbf{R}$ falls between atoms. If $\rho(\mathbf{R})$ is known for all points within a molecule, then it follows that the structure of the molecule will also be known.

The structure factor, $\mathbf{F}$, is related to the electron density, $\rho(\mathbf{R})$, within a molecule by the expression

$$\mathbf{F}(\mathbf{S}) = k_1 \int_{-\infty}^{\infty} \rho(\mathbf{R}) \exp[2\pi i \mathbf{R} \cdot \mathbf{S}] d\mathbf{R} \tag{3}$$

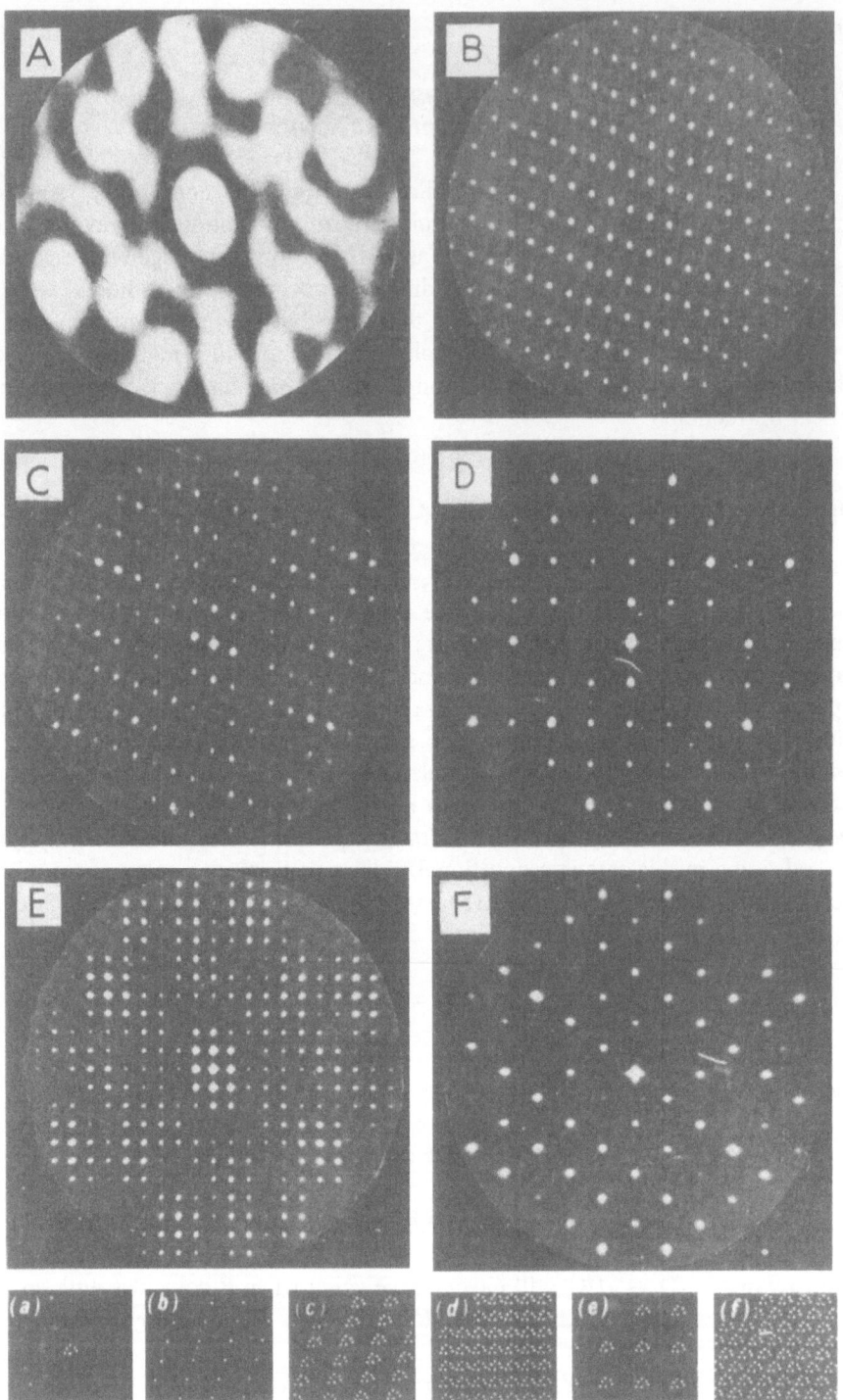

FIG. 3. (A), (B), (C), (D), (E), and (F) are optical diffraction patterns from the objects (a), (b), (c), (d), (e), and (f). (From Taylor and Lipson. 1965. *Optical Transforms*. Courtesy Bell and Sons, Ltd.)

$\rho(\mathbf{R})$ is a function that describes a diffracting object (Fig. 1F), while the absolute value of $|\mathbf{F}(\mathbf{S})|^2$ is a function that describes the diffracting pattern (Fig. 1G). In equation 3 the right-hand expression is known mathematically as the Fourier transform of the electron density. It can be shown that the inverse relation is

$$\rho(\mathbf{R}) = k_2 \int_{-\infty}^{\infty} \mathbf{F}(\mathbf{S}) \exp[-2\pi i \mathbf{R} \cdot \mathbf{S}] d\mathbf{S} \tag{4}$$

which is to say that the electron density is equal to the Fourier transform of the structure factors. Thus, the Fourier transform is the "mathematical lens" which is necessary to resynthesize the x-ray diffraction pattern. Since the diffraction pattern has intensities only at discrete positions, the integral in equation (3) can be replaced by the summation:

$$\rho(\mathbf{R}) = k_3 \Sigma_s \mathbf{F}(\mathbf{S}) \exp[-2\pi i \mathbf{R} \cdot \mathbf{S}] \tag{5}$$

What this expression says is that, if one knows the position, $\mathbf{S}$, and the structure factor, $\mathbf{F}$, of each reflection in a diffraction pattern, one can calculate electron density at all points $\mathbf{R}$, and therefore the position of each atom. Now the only problem is to find the structure factors, which are complex numbers, as can be seen from equation (3). The magnitude of structure factor can be calculated from equation (1): $|\mathbf{F}(\mathbf{S})| \propto \sqrt{I(\mathbf{S})}$, but the phases ($\phi$ in equation [2]) of structure factor are lost in the process of recording the intensities.

The finding of the phase for each structure factor is, therefore, the central problem of x-ray crystallography. This will be discussed in more detail later.

FIVE STEPS IN STRUCTURE DETERMINATION

In the following section the essence of each step will be discussed as simply as possible. The cyclic nature of the sequence of the steps is shown in Figure 4.

Preparation of Single Crystals

Single crystals are usually grown by one of the following ways:
(1) The slow evaporation of solvent in which the compound is dissolved.
(2) The diffusion of the vapor of a solvent in which the solute is less soluble into the solution.
(3) The diffusion of a second solvent in which the solute is less soluble into the solution.
(4) A slow change of temperature (usually cooling).
(5) Sublimation and condensation.

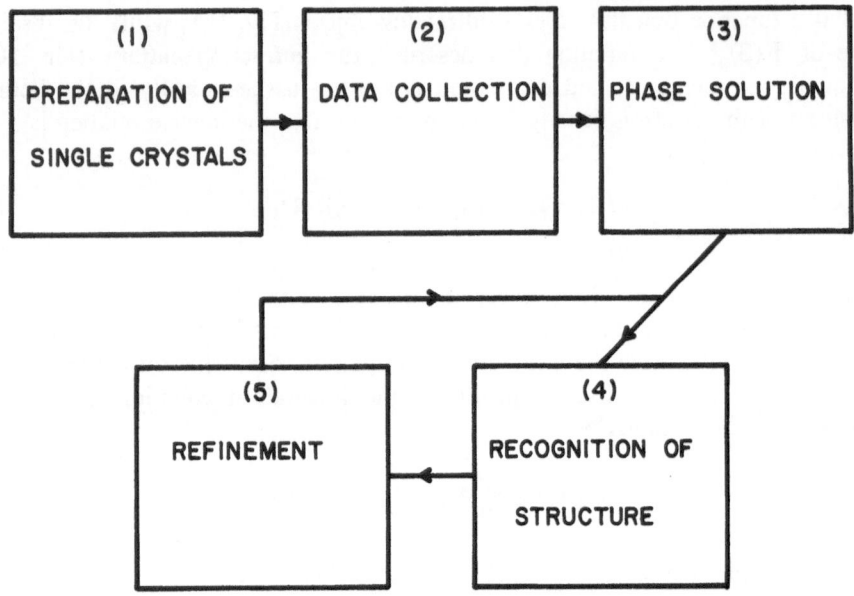

FIG. 4. A flow diagram showing the sequence of five steps in the structure determination.

(6) Mixing with a second compound which will form an insoluble complex with the starting compound.

Good single crystals are usually clear and have a definite geometrical shape such as a cube, prism, pyramid, or plate. However, the ultimate test for the quality of a single crystal is to expose it to an x-ray and examine the sharpness of each reflection. The optimal crystal size for x-ray diffraction study varies depending on the atomic species in the crystal, the x-ray, and the procedure by which the data are collected. A reasonable size is a cube of about 0.3 mm on the edge, which corresponds to about 0.04 mg for most organic compounds.

The most important point to be made here is that the crystal should be grown from the solution where the compound is in its "functional" conformation. Furthermore, it is very useful to introduce one or more electron-rich atoms such as bromine or iodine atoms into the molecule through a covalent, ionic, or coordination bond. The reason for this is that the heavy atoms allow one to use the *heavy-atom method*, a well established technique for solving the structure by a catalogued procedure. This method will be discussed later.

Collection of the Diffraction Data

When a single crystal is irradiated by a monochromatic x-ray, diffraction occurs; the discrete diffracted x-ray beams, called the reflections, radiate out from the crystal as schematically shown in Figure 5. The direction in which each diffracted beam emerges depends on the wavelength of x-ray, the orientation of the crystal

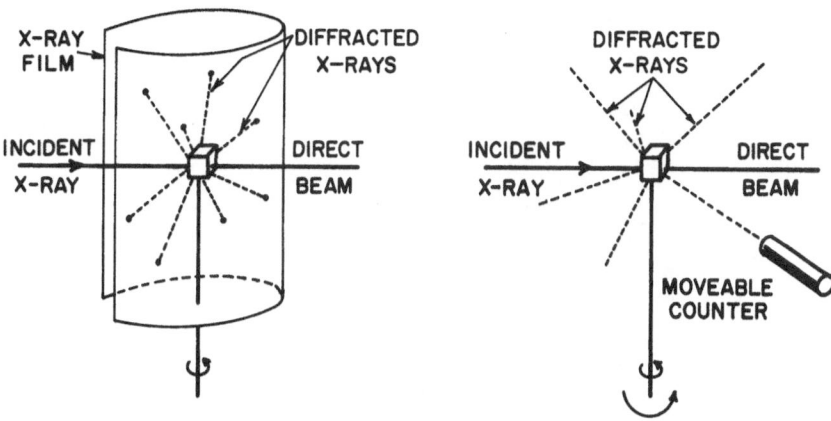

FIG. 5. Schematic drawing of diffraction data collection by photographic method (*left*) and counter method (*right*).

with respect to the incident beam, and the size and shape of the unit cell, the building block of the single crystal. The intensity of each reflection is a function of the species of atoms and their relative positions in the unit cell, that is to say, the three-dimensional structure, as expressed in equation (3).

The intensities of these reflections are usually recorded either on x-ray film or with a radiation counter, as schematically shown in Figure 5. The first is called the photographic method; the second, the counter method. Each method has advantages as well as disadvantages over the other.

PHOTOGRAPHIC METHOD.   This method had been the most common way of data collection until a few years ago, when the counter method became popular. The two most commonly used devices are the Weissenberg camera and the precession camera, as shown in Figure 6. These two cameras allow one to collect only some particular sets of reflections at a time, thereby making the identification (indexing) of each reflection easy. Sample photographs taken by these cameras are also shown in Figure 6. The blackening on the x-ray film by the diffracted x-radiation is measured by visual comparison with a series of calibrated standard intensities or by a photometric scanning followed by computer processing. One such scanner is shown in Figure 7. Although visual measurement has been most commonly used to date, electronic scanning will undoubtedly become more popular since it is quicker and requires the least amount of tedious manual work. Recently, there has been a resurgence of interest in the photographic method. Coupled with the electronic scanner and computer programs, the photographic method can be a faster way of collecting data than the counter method, especially for macromolecular crystals.

COUNTER METHOD.   This method has been the most popular one for the last few years. The accuracy of the data obtained by this method is usually higher than that obtained from the photographic method. The greatest disadvan-

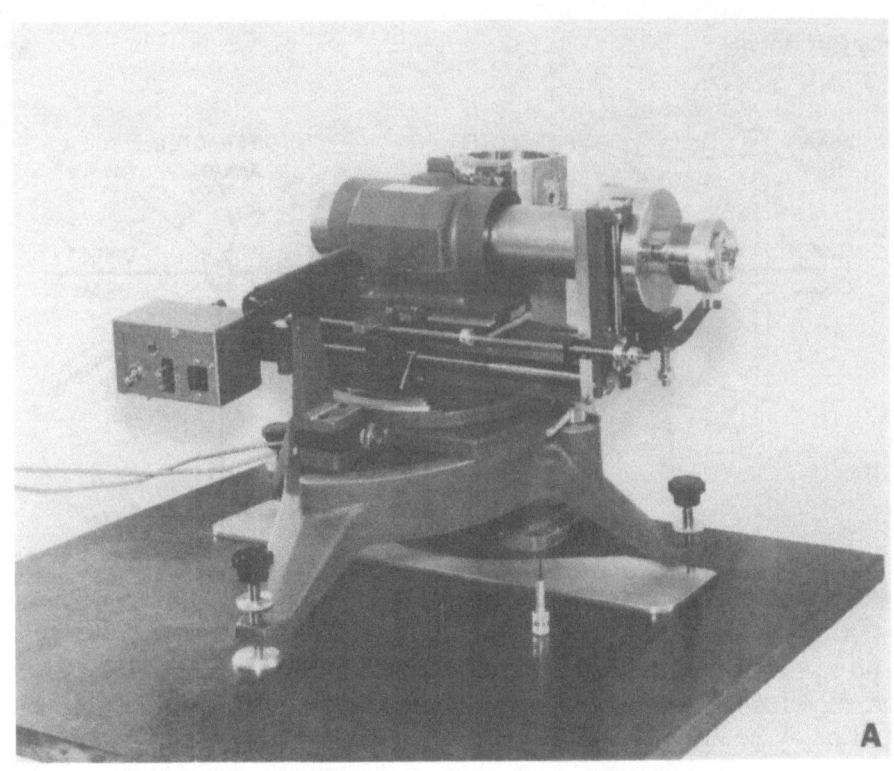

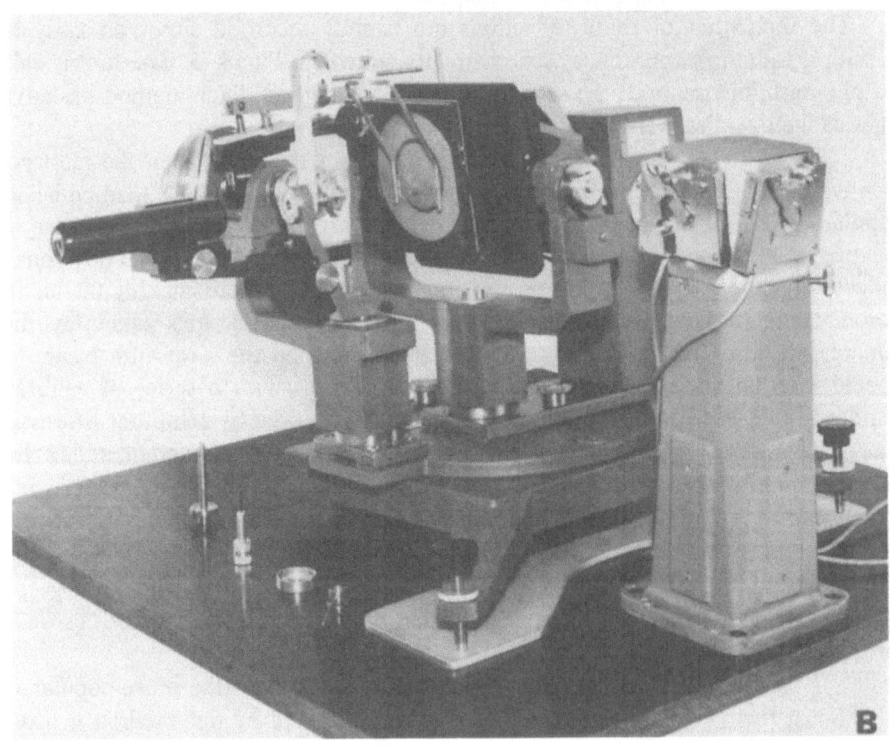

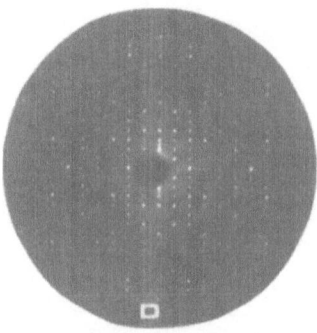

FIG. 6. Photographic cameras for the diffraction data collection. *A.* Weissenberg camera; *B.* Precession camera (Photos Courtesy of Charles Supper Co.); *C.* Negative of a diffraction photograph recorded using a Weissenberg Camera; *D.* Negative of a diffraction photograph recorded using a precession camera.

tage with this method is that the radiation counter can measure only one reflection at a time, even though many reflections appear at the same time. This becomes a serious problem when the crystal is unstable under x-radiation. However, if the crystal is stable, this method is still the best one for the crystal of a small molecule.

The point to be made here is that, in both methods, the automatic instruments and computer programs make data collection an automatic and routine operation. One such system for the counter method is shown in Figure 8.

Interpretation of Diffraction Data (Phase Solution)

The first two pieces of information which can be obtained from the diffraction pattern (especially from the precession photographs) are the space group (sym-

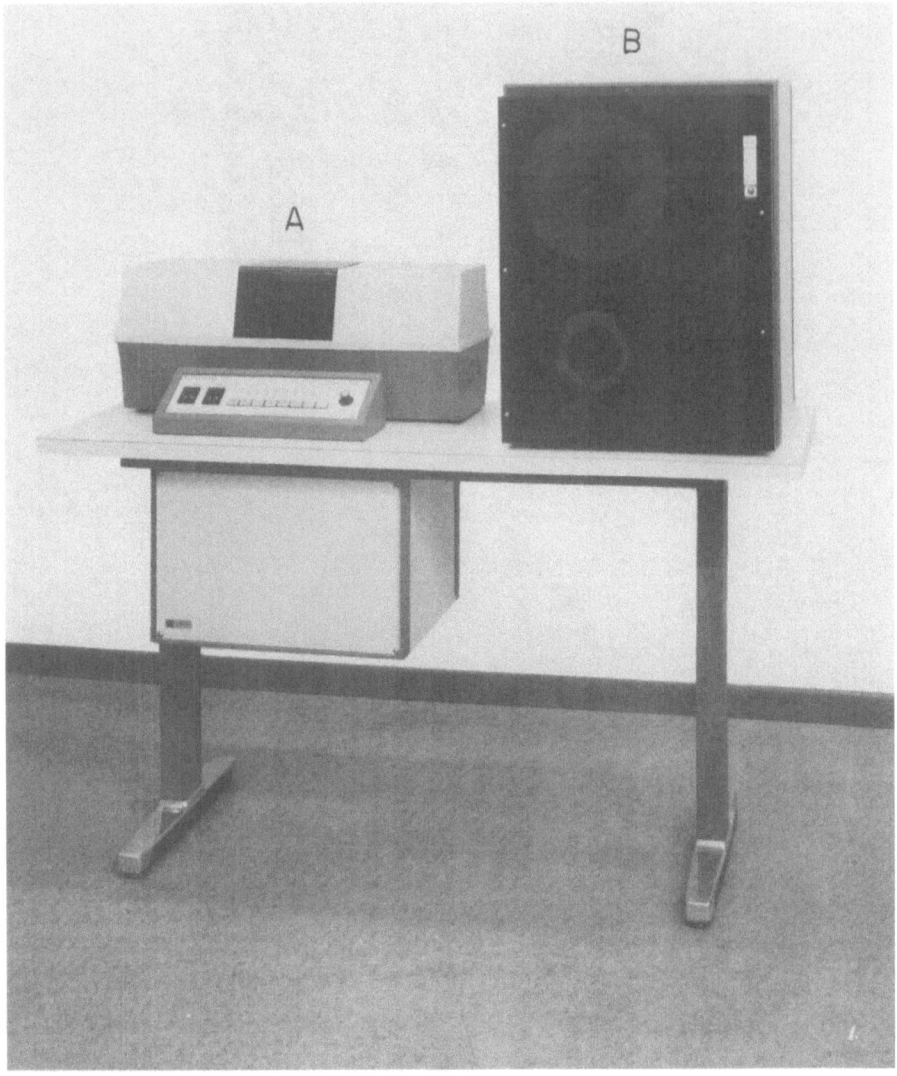

FIG. 7. One photometric scanning device commercially available. *A* contains a drum with a
window where a film will be placed, the illuminating and imaging optics and stepping device;
B magnetic tape drive; digitized optical densities are recorded on the magnetic tape. (Photo
Courtesy of Optronics International, Inc.)

metry with which each molecule is arranged in a crystal) and the unit cell (the
building block) of the crystal. From this information and the density, one can
determine the molecular weight (including hydration water) within 4% accuracy.
Once all the intensities have been measured either by the photographic method or
the counter method, the first interpretation available is the distribution of inter-

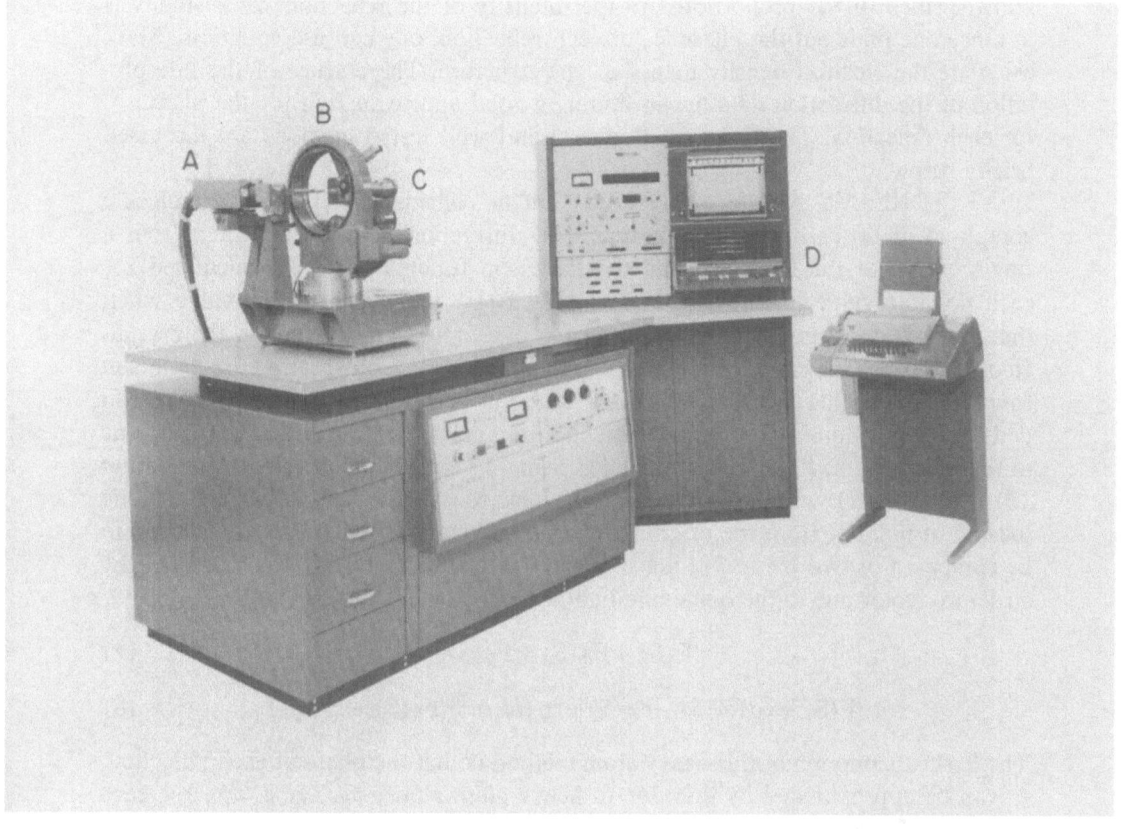

FIG. 8. An automatic diffractometer system. (A) X-ray source; (B) goniostat, which orients the crystal; (C) radiation counter; (D) small computer; (E) teletype to command the computer and to type out the result. (Photo Courtesy of Picker Corporation.)

atomic vectors in the structure. This is obtained by calculating Fourier transform of the intensities called Patterson function (**P**):

$$\mathbf{P}(\mathbf{U}) = k_4 \sum_{\mathbf{s}} I(\mathbf{S}) \exp[2\pi i \mathbf{U} \cdot \mathbf{S}] \tag{6}$$

Quantities appearing in equation (6) have been defined earlier. A large value of **P(U)** means that, in the crystal, there are many atomic pairs in which two atoms are separated by the vector **U**. **P(U)** will also have a big value when two heavy atoms (atoms with many electrons) are separated by the vector **U**. Although, in a few very simple cases, one can deduce the structure from the information about interatomic vectors, the Patterson function does not generally give enough information to find the whole structure. However, it supplies a very important clue about the structure.

As was pointed out earlier, the structure factor, **F(S)**, is a complex quantity with a magnitude $|F(S)|$ and a phase ϕ (equation 2). $|F|$ for each index (S) is known, since $|F|^2$ is proportional to the intensity of the reflection whose index is S. Once one finds out the phase, ϕ, of each reflection, one can use equation (5) to calculate the electron density map, i.e., the structure. The essence of the interpretation of the diffraction data lies in finding a good approximation for the phase, ϕ, for each reflection. The three most general and well tested methods are discussed briefly below.

HEAVY ATOM METHOD. Let us consider a hypothetical molecule composed of 80 carbons and 1 iodine. The diffraction data are collected from a single crystal of this molecule and the Patterson function $P(U)$ is calculated for each possible value of interatomic vector U. $P(U)$ will have a large value when the vector U corresponds to the vector from one iodine to the other in the crystal. In other words, one can identify the iodine-iodine vector by inspecting the Patterson function. From this *heavy atom vector* and the space group symmetry, one can deduce the position of the iodine atoms in a unit cell. Then the structure factor due to the heavy atom, F_H, can be calculated using an equation equivalent to equation (3), where $\rho(R)$ will now represent the electron density of iodine atom alone located at point R from the origin. Now one can consider each structure factor to be composed of two parts: F_H, the structure factor due to heavy atom; and F_L, the structure factor due to the remaining light atoms (carbons in this case):

$$F(S) = F_H(S) + F_L(S) \qquad (7)$$

$$|F(S)|\exp(i\phi_S) = |F_H(S)|\exp(i\phi_H) + |F_L(S)|\exp(i\phi_L) \qquad (8)$$

The basic assumption of this heavy atom method is that the phase of each reflection, ϕ, can be approximated by that due to heavy atom alone, ϕ_H, i.e., $\phi \approx \phi_H$ for each reflection. Now, one can calculate an approximate electron density map using equation (4), where $F(S)$ is replaced by $|F(S)|\exp(i\phi_H)$, i.e., $|F(S)|$ from the intensity and ϕ_H from the position of the iodine in the unit cell. If the iodine is "heavy enough," the resulting electron density map will reveal most of the structure. The heavy atom is considered heavy enough when (number of electrons in heavy atom)^2 $>1/2$ (sum of [number of electrons in light atoms]^2).

The heavy atom method has been programmed in such a way that the whole process of structure analysis becomes automatic except for a few decision-making steps.

SEARCH METHOD. Quite often, one knows the structure of part of the molecule, say the aromatic portion, and would like to find out the rest of the structure. A search is made by first calculating the interatomic vector set from the known structure and then moving this set around in Patterson function space (interatomic vectors calculated from the intensities of the reflections) in an attempt to find the best fit according to various criteria. A similar search can be made by calculating the intensities due to a known partial structure at various orientations and comparing them with the experimentally observed intensities. Once the orientation and location of a partial structure is known, one can treat it as a heavy atom and calculate the heavy atom phases that can be used to obtain the electron density map. This method has been less successful, in practice, than the heavy-atom method, even though there are many cases where it had definite advantages over the others.

DIRECT METHOD. The direct method is fundamentally different from the other two. The two previously mentioned methods involve, at the initial stage, the identification of a heavy atom (s) or a partial structure in the "real space," i.e., in the unit cell. The direct method, on the other hand, involves the identification of a set of reflections, which is related to one reflection by some relationship derived through a probability approach. The simplest form of this relation, for the centrosymmetric space group, is:

$$\text{sign } S[F(S)] \approx \text{sign } S[F(S')] \times \text{sign } S[F(S-S')] \qquad (9)$$

i.e., the sign of F, the structure factor, with index S is probably equal to the product of the sign of F with index S', and that of F with index $S-S'$. This method does not assume any knowledge about the structure. The degree of success with this method has been very high in recent years. It has proven its potential in solving structures of small- or medium-size molecules.

Computer programs for all three discussed methods are well developed, so that it requires only a few decision-making steps to apply these methods to solve a structure.

Recognition of the Structure

Once the approximate phase of each reflection has been determined by one of the methods mentioned earlier, one can calculate the first electron density map using equation (5). Examining the map, one finds places where electron densities are high. The centers of the high electron density areas correspond to the positions of atoms. The electron density at the center will be proportional to the atomic number, i.e., the number of electrons, of that particular atom. The first electron density map will reveal varying portions of the structure depending on how good the approximations of phases were. If they were not very good, the map will reveal only some portion of the molecule. This is the stage where a knowledge of the chemical structure becomes very helpful. Information on the conformation of a part of the molecule is also very helpful in recognizing that part of the molecule in the first electron density map.

Although part of structure recognition can be made automatic by computer programming, this is still the step that most requires human interaction—with the possible exception of the initial preparation of the crystal.

Refinement of the Structure

From the first electron density map, one tries to find as many atoms as possible. Based on these atoms, structure factors can be calculated for each reflection using an equation derived from equation (3). Now, the phases of these calculated structure factors will be better approximations than the initial phases, which were calculated solely from the position of a heavy atom or a known portion of the molecule. Using these new phases, one can calculate the second electron density map. This map will reveal more of the structure than the first map. This process can be repeated until the whole structure is revealed finally. At this point, the refinement of the position of each atom starts.

The most commonly used refinement procedure is the least-squares method. When the whole structure is revealed, one can calculate expected structure factors, $|F_{calc}|$, from the positions of atoms and compare them with the observed ones, $|F_{obs}|$. The position of each atom is shifted until the sum of $(|F_{obs} - F_{calc}|)^2$ over all the reflections becomes the minimum.

THE X-RAY CRYSTALLOGRAPHY OF SOME PHARMACOLOGICALLY IMPORTANT COMPOUNDS

X-ray crystallography can contribute in two major ways to structural studies involving pharmacologically active compounds. Firstly, this technique can be used to determine the chemical structure of natural products, synthetic drugs, and their metabolites. For example, the structure of the antibiotic penicillin was not established with certainty until the x-ray diffraction studies of Crowfoot et al. (1949). Although the interpretation of the x-ray crystallographic data obtained from penicillin was made easier by a prior knowledge of some of the chemistry of this antibiotic, it is nowadays possible to determine structure in the absence of any chemical data. Recently, Johnson et al. (1969) have shown that in one 19-minute run on an IBM 7094 computer it was possible to proceed directly from the raw

TABLE 1

Some Pharmacologically Important Compounds Whose Structure Has Been Determined by X-ray Crystallography

Compound	Reference
Penicillin	Crowfoot et al. (1949)
Muscarine iodide	Jellinek (1957)
Choline chloride	Senko and Templeton (1960)
Codeine hydrobromide	Kartha et al. (1962)
L-Cocaine hydrochloride	Gabe and Barnes (1963)
Ammonium barbiturate	Craven (1964)
Nicotine dihydroiodide	Koo and Kim (1965)
Acetylcholine bromide	Canepa et al. (1966)
Noradrenaline hydrochloride	Calrström and Bergin (1967)
Phenobarbital complex with 8-bromo-9-ethyladenine	Kim and Rich (1968)
Lactoyl choline	Chothia and Pauling (1968)
Valinomycin	Pinkerton et al. (1969)
Procaine and phenocaine complexes with bis-p-nitrophenylphosphate	Sax and Pletcher (1969)
L-(+)-acetyl-β-methylcholine iodide	Chothia and Pauling (1969a)
Acetyl-α-methylcholine	Chothia and Pauling (1969b)
Hyoscine hydrobromide	Pauling and Petcher (1969b)
Procaine hydrochloride	Beall et al. (1970)
Serotonin picrate	Bugg and Thewalt (1970)
Diphenylhydantoin and diazepam	Camerman and Camerman (1970)
Diethylstilbestrol	Weeks et al. (1970)
1,1-Dimethyl-4-phenylpiperazinium iodide	Chothia and Pauling (1970)
Actinomycin-D complex with deoxyguanosine	Sobell et al. (1971)

intensity data to a stereoscopic plot of the structure of fumaric acid $(C_4H_4O_4)$ without the intervention of a crystallographer! However, it should be emphasized that fumaric acid is a relatively simple organic molecule and that such rapid structural determination is the exception rather than the rule. Nevertheless, in the Rapid Organic Structure Analysis Project at the California Institute of Technology, it has been found possible to carry out a complete crystal structure determination so that results of chemical significance could be obtained in less than two weeks (Hamilton, 1970). Listed in Table 1 are several pharmacologically important compounds whose structures either have been or could have been solved semiautomatically by the procedure described in this chapter.

A second possible application of x-ray crystallography is to provide an accurate picture of the spatial arrangement of atoms in drug molecules. Using this technique, Kartha et al. (1962) have established the absolute configuration of codeine, while Carrel and coworkers (1970) have recently determined the absolute configuration of fluorocitrate, an inhibitor of the enzyme aconitase. Such information can then be used to construct models of tissue and enzyme receptor sites, which may in turn lead to the design of better drug molecules. Another good example of this kind of application is the recent determination of the structure of the local anesthetic procaine hydrochloride (Beall et al., 1970). Although it is well established that procaine and other local anesthetics block nerve conduction by interfering with the cross membrane movement of sodium and potassium ions, their precise site of action is unknown. Beall and coworkers (1970), noting the structural similarity between procaine (I) and the neurotransmitter acetylcholine (II),

$$H_2N - \bigcirc - \overset{\overset{\displaystyle O}{\|}}{C} - O - CH_2CH_2 \overset{\overset{\displaystyle C_2H_5}{|\oplus}}{\underset{\underset{\displaystyle H}{|}}{N}} - C_2H_5$$

(I)

$$CH_3 - \overset{\overset{\displaystyle O}{\|}}{C} - O - CH_2CH_2 \overset{\overset{\displaystyle CH_3}{|\oplus}}{\underset{\underset{\displaystyle CH_3}{|}}{N}} - CH_3$$

(II)

postulated that local anesthetics might compete with natural nerve transmission effectors for specific receptor sites in the above membrane. They therefore determined the three-dimensional structure of procaine hydrochloride (Figure 9) and compared it with the structure of acetylcholine bromide, which had been previously determined by Canepa et al. (1966). Their results showed (Table 2) that the related bond distances and angles of procaine and acetylcholine were the same within experimental error. The only major difference between the two molecules

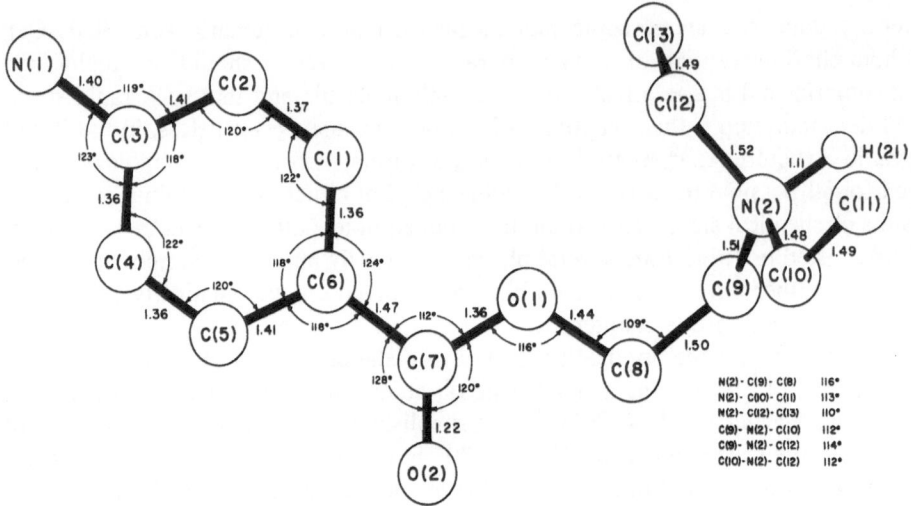

FIG. 9. Molecular dimensions of procaine hydrochloride. (From Beall et al. 1970. *Biochim. Biophys. Res. Commun.*, 39:329-334. Courtesy Academic Press, Inc.)

TABLE 2

Comparison of Selected Interatomic Distances Found in Compounds Related to Procaine Hydrochloride[a]

Compound	N(2) ... O(1)	C(12) ... O(1)
Procaine hydrochloride	3.07	3.00
Acetylcholine bromide[b]	3.29	3.02
Choline chloride[c]	3.26	3.07
Muscarine iodide[d]	3.07	2.87
Glycerylphosphorylcholin[e]	3.14	3.03
L-(+)-cis-2-5-Methyl-4-(R)-trimethylammonium-methyl-1-3-dioxolan iodide[f]	3.18	
Van der Waals' contact[g]	2.9	3.4

[a]From Beall, Herdklotz, and Sass. 1970. *Biochem. Biophys. Res. Commun.*, 39:329-334. Courtesy of Academic Press, Inc.

[b]Canepa et al. (1966).

[c]Senko and Templeton (1960).

[d]Jellinek (1957).

[e]Abrahamsson and Pascher (1966).

[f]Pauling and Petcher (1969a).

[g]Pauling (1960).

was that the C—O—C—C torsion angle was about 80° in acetylcholine, as compared to 172.8° in procaine. Nevertheless, in spite of this conformational difference, the relative position of the ether oxygen with respect to the quaternary ammonium group is quite similar in acetylcholine and procaine as well as in a variety of related substances (Table 2). The average N(2)...O(1) distance in these compounds was 3.17 Å, while the average C(12)...O(1) distance was 3.00 Å. Beall and coworkers (1970) suggested that the proximity of the ammonium nitrogen atom to the ether oxygen atom and the orientation of the ammonium substituents, relative to the ether oxygen, were important features for a good effector-receptor interaction.

Several complexes between drugs and other small molecules have been studied (Table 1). Sax and Pletcher (1969) have determined the structure of complexes between bis-*p*-nitrophenyl phosphate and procaine or phenacaine. They have suggested that the formation of a hydrogen-bonded complex between the drug and an acceptor group on the membrane is a feature in the action of local anesthetics. However, as Beall et al. (1970) have pointed out, in both procaine hydrochloride and in the complex, procaine bis-*p*-nitrophenyl phosphate, only the para amino and not the carbonyl group participates in the binding. Yet, replacing the amino group with an ethoxy group, which cannot act as a donor in a hydrogen bond, increases the local anesthetic ability of procaine severalfold (Galinsky et al., 1963). Obviously, much more work on the structural properties of local anesthetics is necessary before a clear picture of the nerve-blocking mechanism can be drawn.

Another interesting complex whose structure has been determined by means of x-ray crystallography is that formed between one molecule of phenobarbital and two molecules of 8-bromo-8-ethyl adenine (Kim and Rich, 1968). It was found that one of the adenine derivatives was hydrogen-bonded to the barbiturate, using the same bonds found between the adenine and thymine pair in the double-helical form of DNA. The suggestion by Kim and Rich (1968) that hydrogen-bonding between barbiturates and adenine derivatives is 'a general phenomenon, which may be related to the mode of action of barbiturates in biological systems, is of great interest since Smythies (1970) has recently postulated that receptor sites may be nucleoproteins.

REFERENCES

Abrahamsson, S., and I. Pascher. 1966. Crystal and molecular structure of L-α-glycerylphosphorylcholine. Acta Cryst., 21:79-87.

Beall, R., J. Herdklotz, and R. L. Sass. 1970. Molecular properties of local anesthetics: The crystal structure of procaine hydrochloride. Biochim. Biophys. Res. Commun., 39:329-334.

Buerger, M. J. 1960. Crystal Structure Analysis. New York, John Wiley and Sons.

Bugg, C. E., and U. Thewalt. 1970. Crystal structure of serotonin picrate, a donor-receptor complex. Science, 170:852-854.

Camerman, A., and N. Camerman. 1970. Diphenylhydantoin and diazepam: Molecular structure similarities and steric basis of anticonvulsant activity. Science, 168:1457-1458.

Canepa, F. G., P. Pauling, and H. Sörum. 1966. Structure of acetylcholine and other substrates of cholinergic systems. Nature (London), 210:907-909.

Carlström, D., and R. Bergin. 1967. The structure of the catecholamines. I. The crystal structure of noradrenaline hydrochloride. Acta Cryst., 23:313-319.

Carrell, H. L., J. P. Glusker, J. J. Villafranca, A. S. Mildvan, R. J. Dummel, and E. Kun. 1970. Fluorocitrate inhibition of aconitase: Relative configuration of inhibitory isomer by x-ray crystallography. Science, 170:1412-1414.

Chothia, C., and P. Pauling. 1968. Conformations of acetylcholine. Nature (London), 219:1156-1157.

_____ and P. Pauling. 1969a. The structure of the potent muscarinic against L-(+)-acetyl-β-acetyl-β-methylcholine iodide. J. Chem. Soc., Section D:627-7.

_____ and P. Pauling. 1969b. Two conformations of the cholinergic agonist acetyl-α-methylcholine. A new conformation of cholinergic molecules. J. Chem. Soc. Section D:746-747.

_____ and P. Pauling. 1970. The conformation of molecules at nicotinic nerve receptors. Proc. Nat. Acad. Sci. U.S.A., 65:477-488.

Craven, B. M. 1964. The crystal structure of ammonium barbiturate. Acta Cryst., 17:282-289.

Crowfoot, D., C. W. Bunn, B. W. Rogers-Low, and A. Turner-Jones. 1949. The x-ray crystallographic investigation of the structure of penicillin. _In_ Chemistry of Penicillin, Clarke, H. T., and J. R. Johnson, eds. Princeton, New Jersey, Princeton University Press.

Gabe, E. J., and W. H. Barnes. 1963. The crystal structure and molecular structure of _l_-cocaine hydrochloride. Acta Cryst., 16:796-801.

Galinsky, A. M., J. E. Gearien, A. J. Perkins, and S. V. Susina. 1963. Electronic effect of para-substituents on the local anesthetic activity of 2-diethylaminoethyl benzoate and related compounds. J. Med. Chem., 6:320-322.

Hamilton, W. C. 1970. The revolution in crystallography. Science, 169:133-141.

Holmes, R. C., and D. M. Blow. 1966. The Use of X-Ray Diffraction in the Study of Protein and Nucleic Acid Structure. New York, John Wiley and Sons.

Jellinek, F. 1957. The structure of muscarine. Acta Cryst., 10:277-280.

Johnson, Q., G. S. Smith, and E. Kahara. 1969. Automatic determination of crystal structure. Science, 164:1163-1164.

Kartha, G., F. R. Ahmed, and W. H. Barnes. 1962. Refinement of the crystal structure of codeine hydrobromide and establishment of the absolute configuration of the codeine molecule. Acta Cryst., 15:226-333.

Kim, S. H., and A. Rich. 1968. The structure of a crystalline complex containing one phenobarbital molecule and two adenine derivatives. Proc. Nat. Acad. Sci. U.S.A., 60:402-408.

Koo, C. H., and H. S. Kim. 1965. The crystal structure of nicotine dihydroiodide. Daeha Hwakak Hwojee, 9:134-141.

Pauling, L. 1960. The Nature of the Chemical Bond. Ithaca, New York, Cornell University Press.

Pauling, P., and T. J. Petcher. 1969a. The crystal structure of L-(+)-cis-2-(S)-methyl-d-(R)-trimethylammonium-methyl-1,3-dioxolan iodide. J. Chem. Soc., Section D:1258-1259.

_____ and T. J. Petcher. 1969b. The crystal structure of (-)-(S)-hyoscine hydrobromide. J. Chem. Soc., Section D:1001-1002.

Pinkerton, M., L. K. Steinrauf and P. Dawkins. 1969. The molecular structure and some transport properties of valinomycin. Biochem. Biophys. Res. Commun., 35:512-517.

Sax, M., and J. Pletcher. 1969. Local anesthetics: Significance of hydrogen bonding in mechanism of action. Science, 166:1546-1548.

Senko, M. E., and D. H. Templeton. 1960. Unit cells of choline halides and structure of choline chloride. Acta Cryst., 13:281-285.

Smythies, J. R. 1970. The chemical nature of the receptor site. Int. Rev. Neurobiol., 13:181-222.

Sobell, H. M., S. C. Jain, T. D. Sakore, and C. E. Nordman. 1971. Concerning the stereochemistry of actinomycin binding to DNA: an actinomycin-deoxyguanosine crystalline complex. Nature, in press.

Stout, G. H., and L. H. Jensen. 1968. X-ray Structure Determination—A Practical Guide. New York, Macmillan Company.

Taylor, C. A., and H. Lipson. 1965. Optical Transforms. Their Preparation and Application to X-ray Diffraction Problems. Ithaca, New York, Cornell University Press.

Weeks, C. M., A. Cooper, and D. Norton. 1970. Crystal and molecular structure of diethylstilbestrol. Acta Cryst., B26:429-33.

Chapter **12**

Applications of Mass Spectrometry to Pharmacological Problems

Catherine Fenselau

Department of Pharmacology and Experimental Therapeutics, The Johns Hopkins University School of Medicine, Baltimore, Maryland

INTRODUCTION

Mass spectrometry (MS) as a technique for obtaining analytical and structural information has proven to be of great value in a number of different areas of pharmacology. This chapter is a selective review, in which the utility of mass spectrometry in pharmacology will be discussed, examples will be cited of different kinds of applications, and limitations will be pointed out. Emphasis has been placed on pharmacology and clinical research at the expense of some aspects of biochemistry that do not bear directly on clinical disorders and their treatment. The reader is referred to a number of recent reviews for general applications in biochemistry (Van Lear and McLafferty, 1969; Milne, 1970; Das and Lederer, 1970; and Cooks and Johnson, 1971).

Although the principle of the instrument has been understood since the early part of the century, only in the last decade has commercial instrumentation become adequate to analyze involatile samples with polar functional groups and masses up to 1500. This capability has extended the usefulness of the technique into many new areas of chemistry and biochemistry. However, sample vapor pressure requirements and analyzer mass range remain the primary instrumental parameters limiting further expansion of biochemical and medical applications.

The principle of the instruments most commonly used in analyses of organic compounds can be stated as follows. Ionized molecules and a variety of ionized fragments are formed by some process, usually bombardment by electrons, then accelerated through an electrostatic potential, and separated in a magnetic field according to the ratio of their mass to charge. The equation

$$m/e = \frac{H^2 r^2}{2V}$$

shows the relation of the various parameters, where m = mass, e = charge, H = magnetic field, r = radius of deflection, and V = accelerating voltage. Instruments are usually constructed so that the great majority of ions formed carry only a single charge, i.e., $e = 1$. Thus the mass of the ion can be measured directly. Either the magnetic field or the accelerating potential is varied (scanned) to bring the entire collection of ions into the detector at a constant r. The spectrum is a recording of the mass to charge ratio of these ions and of their relative abundances.

INSTRUMENTATION

The mass spectrometer consists of four different components—an inlet system, an ionization chamber (source), an analyzer, and a detector. Each of these components is available in a variety of types based on different physical and electronic principles (Biemann, 1962; Roboz, 1968). A schematic diagram is presented in Figure 1 of one common kind of mass spectrometer, an instrument with electron impact ionization and a magnetic analyzer.

In the traditional inlet system, a gaseous sample flows from a reservoir through

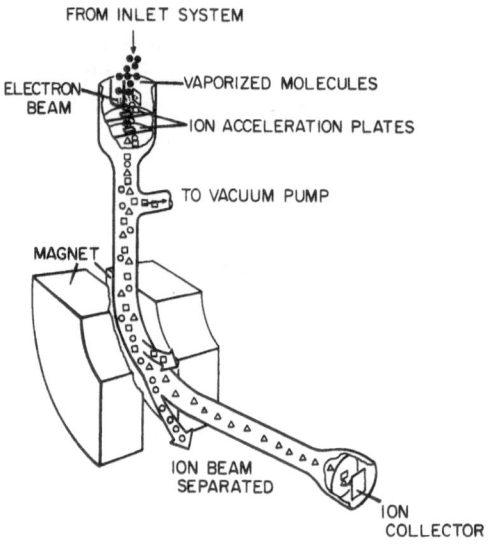

SINGLE FOCUSING MASS SPECTROMETER

FIG. 1. A single-focusing sector instrument with an electron impact source.

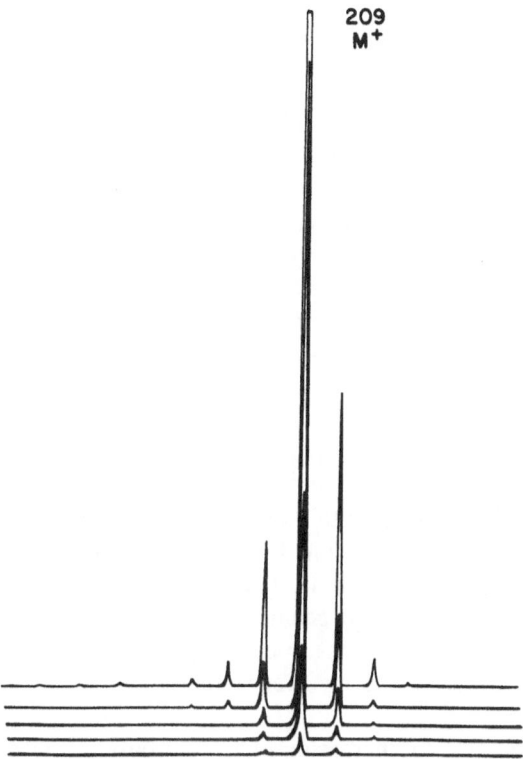

209
M⁺

FIG. 2. Oscillograph tracing of a portion of the spectrum of STP (2,5-dimethoxy-4-methylamphetamine).

a pinhole leak through several feet of tubing into the source. The most useful inlet systems for pharmacological samples are the gas chromatographic (discussed below) and the direct (or probe) inlet systems. In the latter the solid sample is advanced directly into the source, to within a few millimeters of the ionizing electron beam; omission of the leak minimizes the vapor pressure required to produce a suitable number of ionizing collisions. In addition, loss of sample by wall collision in the tubing is eliminated.

The most commonly used detector is a multistage electron multiplier. The spectrum is usually recorded on light sensitive paper using several galvanometers, suitably attenuated to record a sensitivity range of about 10,000. A portion of such an oscillograph tracing is reproduced in Figure 2. Data are usually presented in bar graph or tabular form with peak heights measured relative to that of the highest peak.

The choice of inlet system, source, analyzer, or detector best suited for a given analysis depends in large part on the nature of the sample, as well as on the kind of information desired.

In order to discuss instrumental requirements for pharmacological applications, the characteristics of the samples must be considered. Biochemical and clinical samples are often characterized by (1) the minute amounts available, (2) high levels of impurities, (3) thermal instability, (4) low vapor pressure resulting from high molecular weight and/or the polar chemical properties which make these samples water soluble, and (5) instability to the ionization process itself.

To deal with the first characteristic and successfully obtain information on small amounts of sample, micrograms or nanograms, an instrument with high sensitivity is required. This instrumental parameter is difficult for the manufacturers to specify and even more difficult for the customer to confirm.

Achievement of maximum sensitivity from an instrument requires consideration of a number of factors. Use of faster scanning rates reduces the time during which sample pressure must be maintained, and thus reduces the amount of sample required. Several laboratories report that signal to noise ratio and thus the effective sensitivity of their instruments is enhanced by averaging a number of scans (Biros, 1970; Markey et al., 1970). In this situation the data processing is best done by computer.

An alternative to scanning with a detector that records one ion at a time is to use a detector that records all the ions formed at the same time, integrating all the signals while the sample pressure lasts. This approach is currently available only in instruments with Mattauch Herzog geometry, which focus ions of all masses into a plane. A photoplate sensitive to ions is placed in the focal plane and the complete spectrum can be recorded additively over as long a period of time as is possible or desired.

A fourth approach to increasing the sensitivity of mass spectrometers or decreasing the requisite sample size is to monitor only a few peaks deemed necessary and sufficient by the investigator for identification of a compound. The instrument switches rapidly between several peaks preset by the operator, providing virtually continuous monitoring of these ions. This obviates the need for scanning a wide mass range, wasting many ions, and obtaining some superfluous information. This approach is not suitable for analysis of unknown materials, but is best used to confirm the presence of anticipated compounds (Hammar et al., 1968). The technique is available in a number of commercial instruments. When the mass spectrometer is used as a detector for a gas chromatograph, the technique of monitoring selected peaks (called mass fragmentography by some workers) can provide greater sensitivity than an electron capture detector (Hammar et al. 1968a). This comparison is made in Table 1. The last entry in the table is the sensitivity estimated

TABLE 1

Sensitivity of Gas Chromatographic Detectors[a]

Methods of Detection	Sensitivity (in grams)
Electron capture	10^{-9}
Mass spectrometer	
Mass fragmentography	10^{-12}
Total ion monitor	10^{-8}

[a]After Hammar, Holmstedt, and Ryhage. 1968. *Anal. Biochem.*, 25:532-548.

for the total ion monitor, which measures 10 to 20% of all the ions formed. This latter signal is usually not amplified through the electron multiplier, as the signal is when monitoring selected peaks or scanning complete spectra.

The second characteristic of biochemical and clinical samples, high levels of impurities, can be dealt with in the mass spectrometry laboratory in several ways. Most simply, differential heating of the inlet system may effect fractional vaporization and allow some separation of the mixture. Alternatively, the spectrum of the entire mixture may be recorded and attempts (preferably computerized) made to sort out peaks or spectra belonging to various components. This is most rigorously done in a high-resolution instrument where the mass of each ion may be measured to several decimal places (the generally accepted accuracy being ±0.003 atomic mass units). Measurement of the exact mass allows an empirical formula to be assigned to each ion, and makes the selection of various ions as decomposition products of a given compound in a mixture several orders of magnitude more reliable than assignments made from a low-resolution spectrum.

The approach to purification favored in most laboratories involves the use of a gas chromatograph as an inlet system. The critical feature of the interface of this coupled instrument is a device for separating carrier gas from sample. Separators or enrichers have been designed on several different principles (Watson, 1969). These separators, and indeed the entire interface, are a source of additional problems for the investigator, which include the efficiency of sample recovery during separation of the carrier gas, clogging of the separator, and also thermal degradation of the sample in passing through the interface. One recent development which may circumvent difficulties with separators is the combination of gas chromatographs with mass spectrometers that have chemical ionization sources (Vestal, 1970; Arsenault et al., 1970). In this tandem instrument methane may be used as both the carrier gas in the chromatograph and the ionizing gas in the mass spectrometer. Thus, the carrier gas need not be separated from the sample in the interface. In at least one report (Arsenault et al., 1970) retention times and separation observed using methane carrier gas were comparable to those observed using helium.

Since it is much more difficult to vaporize a compound for gas chromatography (GC) than for high vacuum mass spectral analysis, compounds that could be handled unmodified on a direct probe often must be chemically modified in order to be introduced through the gas chromatograph. It must be remembered that the preparation of derivatives—especially via the commonly used silylation procedures —usually introduces more artifacts or impurities into the mixture. The actual modification used depends, of course, on the class of compound being analyzed and is subject to the guidelines already well worked out in gas chromatography. Mention will be made of specific derivatives throughout the chapter.

Use of the proper derivatives may also provide solutions to the last three problems characteristic of pharmacological samples: thermal instability, low vapor pressure, and instability of the molecular ion after ionization. Thermal instability and low vapor pressure are often interlocking problems. Raising the source and inlet temperatures may facilitate sublimation; it may also promote pyrolysis. In general the direct probe is a superior inlet system for samples of low volatility and/or

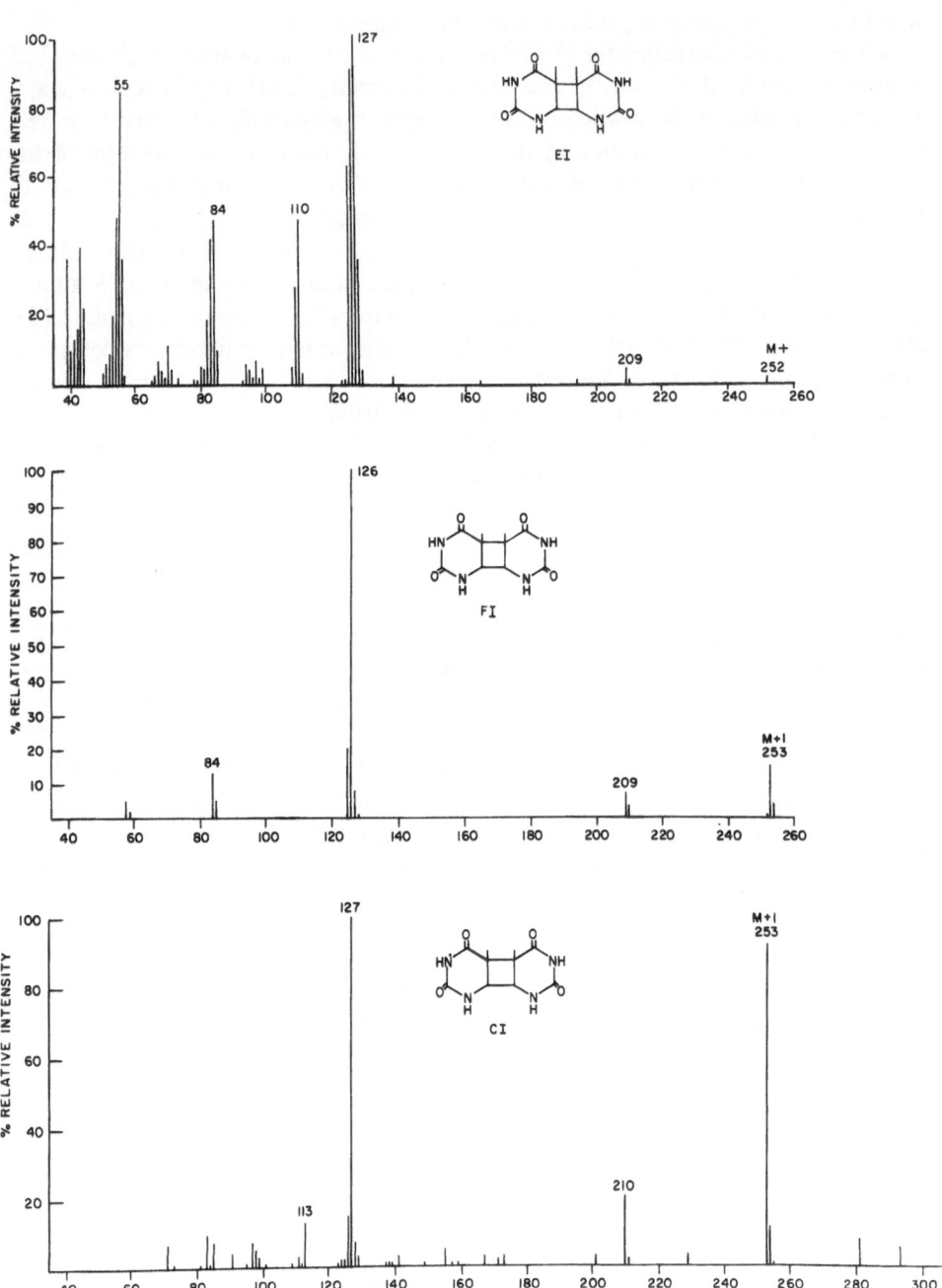

FIG. 3. Electron impact, field ionization, and chemical ionization mass spectra of *cis*, syn thymine photodimer.

thermal instability, because much less vapor pressure is required to produce an adequate number of ions. It has also been suggested that thermally unstable samples (T. A. Milne, 1969) and high polymers (Dole et al., 1968) could be put into the vapor phase in a sort of aerosol.

The sources and inlet systems of different instruments have quite different thermal characteristics, and in some instruments thermal energy will make noticeable contributions to postionization fragmentation processes, if not to preionization pyrolysis. Thus, more ions will fragment and the molecular ion peak, highly desirable for assigning molecular weights, can be diminished beyond recognition. If the molecular ion peak is too small to be unambiguous at the conventional 70 electron volt ionizing energy, ionizing energies below 20 eV may enhance its intensity by reducing fragmentation.

For some compounds field ionization (Beckey, 1969) or chemical ionization (Fales et al., 1969; Fales, 1971) may produce spectra containing larger molecular ion peaks. In field ionization an electron is removed from the molecule by a strong electric field (of the order of 10^8 volts per cm) with little or none of the vibrational and electronic excitation which accompanies electron impact ionization. In chemical ionization, methane (or some other gas) is introduced into the source at a relatively high pressure, about 1 Torr. An electron beam is used to ionize some of the molecules of methane. These undergo intermolecular reactions with neutral molecules, and a reproducible equilibrium of ions (48% CH_5^+, 40% $C_2H_5^+$ for methane at 1 Torr [Field and Munson, 1965]) is established. The analytical sample is introduced into the source and is ionized by proton transfer from, or hydride abstraction by, this plasma. As with field ionization, this process imparts much less excess energy to the molecular ion and leads to less fragmentation than the electron impact process.

The set of spectra (shown in Figure 3) of the major photodimer of thymine were obtained on three different instruments using electron impact ionization (EI) (Fenselau and Wang, 1969), field ionization (FI) (Fenselau, Wang, and Brown, 1970), and chemical ionization (CI) (Fales, Khattak, and Wang, private communication). In the latter two cases the largest peak in the molecular ion region is not that of the molecular ion (M), but rather that of a protonated molecular ion ($M+1$). This phenomenon is widely recognized and need not interfere with assignment of the molecular weight. In this particular example the largest M or $M+1$ peak was observed using chemical ionization. In both the FI and CI spectra, the occurrence of fewer peaks reflects the smaller extent to which fragmentation occurs. It should be remembered that some fragmentation is desirable inasmuch as it reveals structural information.

SAMPLE PREPARATION

The preparation of a sample for mass spectral analysis depends on the quantity and purity of the sample, the information desired, and the instrumentation available. Special purification may be necessary. Buffer salts, for example, may not interfere with a bioassay, but their pyrolysis products will be detected in a mass spectrum.

Simple chemical modification may be desirable to increase volatility or to stabilize the molecular ion. Special vessels may be provided in which the sample can be transferred directly into the instrument. Solvents have to be evaporated before analysis. If gas chromatographic introduction into the mass spectrometer is to be used, chromatographic conditions will have to be determined.

IDENTIFICATION OF DRUG METABOLITES

The structural identification of drug metabolites is one of the most straightforward applications of mass spectrometry in terms of interpreting the spectrum. The investigator knows the structure of the drug which was initially administered, has some idea of what kinds of structural changes to expect, and, very often, has a selection of standards or similar compounds available for comparison. Thus, the ideal approach to a drug metabolism problem is to obtain spectra of the parent drug and any similar compounds available and to correlate the fragmentation pattern with the structure. Then when spectra of the metabolites are obtained, comparable fragmentation patterns may be sought, leading by analogy to structural information. A simple example is found in the fragmentation of several human urinary metabolites of the drug L-DOPA used to treat Parkinson's disease. These compounds were treated with bis(trimethylsilyl)trifluoroacetamide and trimethylchlorosilane, and the resultant trimethylsilyl derivatives were purified and analyzed by gas chromatography/mass spectrometry (Peaston and Bianchine, 1971). Peaks of structural significance in the mass spectrum of the parent drug, tris(trimethylsilyl) L-DOPA (Table 2), include the molecular ion peak at m/e 413, $M-15$ peak at m/e 398, the $M-117$ peak at m/e 296 corresponding to loss of the carbotrimethylsiloxy group, and the peak at m/e 267 corresponding to the aromatic nucleus and one methylene group in the side chain. The M^+ and $M-15$ peaks in the spectrum of two human metabolites A and B are indicated in Table 2. As can be seen in the table, the peak at m/e 267 remains strong in the spectrum of metabolite A, but there is no peak at $M-117$. This suggests that the aromatic portion of the molecule has not been changed, but that the metabolite no longer contains a carboxylic acid group. The molecular weight (determined from the M^+ and $M-15$ peaks) is consistent with the structure shown. This structure was confirmed by comparison of the GC retention time and mass spectrum with those of authentic dopamine. The spectrum of metabolite B, on the other hand, contains a peak at $M-117$, confirming a carboxylic acid group in the compound, but no peak at 276. The aromatic nucleus has been changed and is now represented by the major peak at m/e 209. The number of trimethylsilyl groups attached to the benzylic portion of the molecule suggest that one of the phenol groups has been methylated. The loss of 30 mass units (CH_2O) noted in the table is typical of methyl phenyl ethers. The molecular weight and fragmentation pattern is consistent with the structure of the trimethylsilyl derivative of 3-methoxy-4-hydroxy-phenylacetic acid.

The positions of the methoxy and hydroxy substituents shown could not be determined from the mass spectrum alone. However, confirmation of the structure

TABLE 2

Characteristic Peaks in the Spectrum of Trimethylsilyl Derivatives of DOPA and Two Human Metabolites

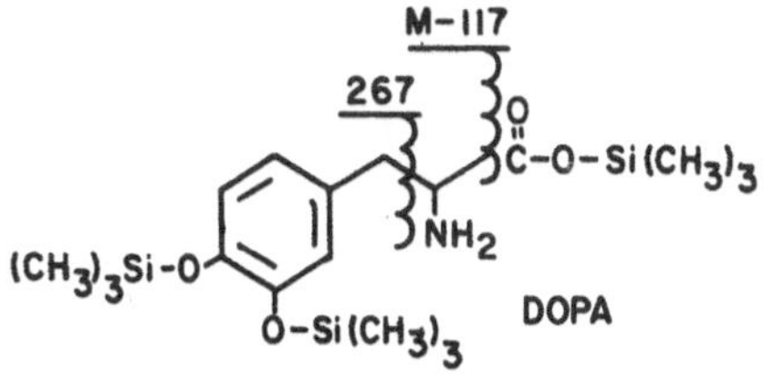

M−117
267
C−O−Si(CH$_3$)$_3$
NH$_2$
(CH$_3$)$_3$Si−O
O−Si(CH$_3$)$_3$ DOPA

M$^+$	413
M−15	398
M−117	296
267	267

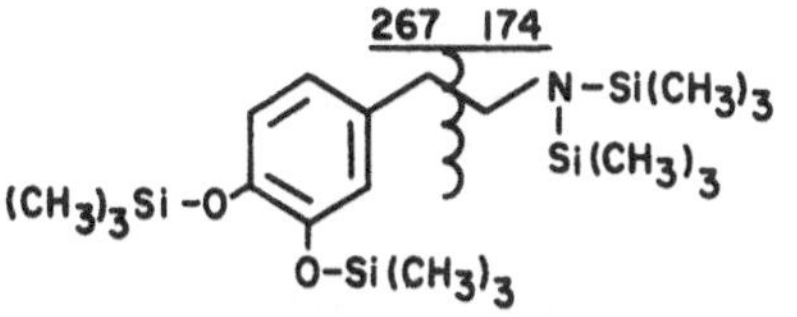

267 174
N−Si(CH$_3$)$_3$
Si(CH$_3$)$_3$
(CH$_3$)$_3$Si−O
O−Si(CH$_3$)$_3$
DOPAMINE

M$^+$	441
M−15	426
M−117	NONE
267	267
M−267	174

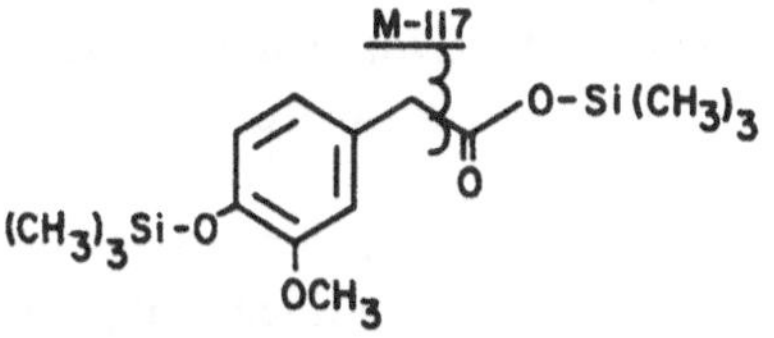

M−117
O−Si(CH$_3$)$_3$
O
(CH$_3$)$_3$Si−O
OCH$_3$
3-METHOXY-4-HYDROXY-PHENYLACETIC ACID

M$^+$	326
M−15	311
M−117	209
267	NONE
M−117−30	179

was obtained by comparison of the spectrum and GC retention time with those of the authentic compound.

A similar approach has been used in the structural analysis of diazepam metabolites in the rat (Bommer and Vane, 1966; Schwartz et al., 1967). The metabolites are reported to have been identified in mixtures where the biggest peak in the metabolite spectrum "was not stronger than a few per cent of the base peak of the entire spectrum" of the mixture (Bommer and Vane, 1966). The use of high resolution measurements (via photoplates) gave the necessary measure of assurance to the assignment of peaks to the metabolites. Rat metabolism includes hydroxylation of the pendent phenyl ring (see Figure 4), and the position of this hydroxyl group could not be determined from the mass spectrum alone. Nuclear magnetic resonance measurements completed this aspect of the identification.

Structural studies of the human urinary metabolites of diazepam have been incorporated into a medical-student experiment at Johns Hopkins (Coulter et al., 1970). The low resolution spectrum of diazepam is shown in Figure 4. The two groups of intense peaks above m/e 250 are critical for elucidation of metabolite structures (Table 3). The doublets arising from the two isotopes of chlorine can be seen. In studies of urine extracts the pairs of peaks resulting from ^{37}Cl and ^{35}Cl (1:3 intensity ratio) can be used to distinguish drug-related ions from impurities.

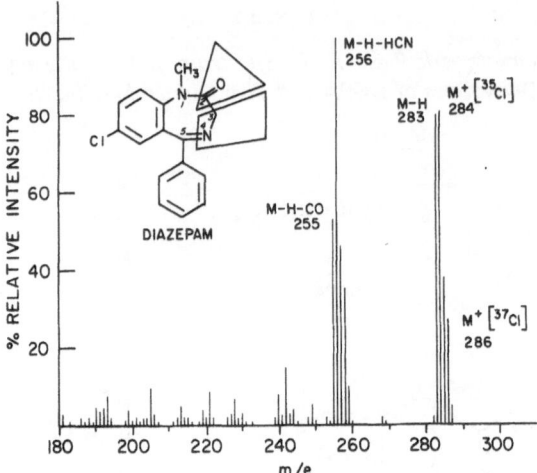

FIG. 4. Low resolution mass spectrum of diazepam.

Earlier studies (Bommer and Vane, 1966) of compounds in this series had indicated that the major primary fragmentation is loss of a hydrogen atom from position 3. This is followed in the decomposition of diazepam by loss of CO and HCN, as blocked out in the structure in Figure 4.

In the student experiment the metabolites are isolated nearly pure by thin-layer chromatography in a single-solvent system, and identified using the tabular approach presented in Table 3. Demethylation and hydroxylation relative to the

TABLE 3

Characteristic Peaks in the Spectra of Human Metabolites of Diazepam

	DIAZEPAM	HUMAN METABOLITES		
		I	II	III
M^+ Composition	$C_{16}H_{13}N_2OCl$	$C_{15}H_{11}N_2OCl$	$C_{16}H_{13}N_2O_2Cl$	$C_{15}H_{11}N_2O_2Cl$
Alteration		$-CH_3$	$+O$	$+O, -CH_3$
M-H,CO	YES	YES	YES	YES
M-H,HCN	YES	YES	NO	NO
M-H,HOCN	NO	NO	YES	YES

parent drug are easily detectable from high resolution measurements of the molecular ion masses. Loss of HCO from all three metabolites confirms that the carbonyl groups are intact. The new hydroxyl group is placed at position 3 when the $M - H_2CN$ peak is replaced by a new $M - H_2OCN$ peak. Other physical measurements support the mass spectral evidence.

Studies of human metabolism employing similar logistics have been reported for a number of different kinds of drugs, including the contraceptive steroids (DeJongh, Perricone, and Gay, 1968; Palmer, Ross, et al., 1969), the sulfonamide derivative probenecid (Perel et al., 1970), the nonsteroid fertility drug bis(p-acetoxyphenyl)cyclohexylidenemethane (Aldercreutz et al., 1967), the cardiac depressant quinidine gluconate (Palmer, Fowler, et al., 1969), methadone (Pohland et al., 1971), the analgesic phenacetin (Burtis, Butts, and Rainey, 1970), a hypnotic benzodiazepine (Schwartz et al., 1968a), perazine (Krauss et al., 1969), and an anthranilate diuretic (Smith and Grostic, 1967). Unmetabolized cytoxan has been identified in blood, sweat, urine, saliva, synovial fluid, and milk in patients receiving the drug in treatment of leukemia and arthritis (Fenselau et al., 1971). Mass spectrometry has also been important in studies of the structures of animal metabolites of drugs, including pentobarbital (Palmer, Fowler, et al., 1969), the tranquilizer chlordiazepoxide (Schwartz et al., 1968b), a pteridine diuretic (Sisenwine and Walkenstein, 1969), the antidepressant thiazesim (Dreyfuss et al., 1968), probenecid (Guarino et al., 1969), and the antitumor agent cyclophosphamide (Hill et al., 1970).

Another group of animal metabolism studies which should be mentioned involves toxic drugs, hallucinogens, and insecticides. Mass spectrometry played a major role in studies identifying metabolites of the active marijuana constituents $\Delta^{1(6)}$- and $\Delta^{1(2)}$-tetrahydrocannabinol from studies in vivo (Burnstein et al., 1970) and in vitro (Foltz et al., 1970; Nilsson et al., 1970; Wall et al., 1970). Metabolites of hallucinogenic indolealkylamines have also been studied (Ahlborg et al., 1968). Pesticides whose animal metabolites have been studied include the chlorinated hydrocarbons aldrin and dieldrin (Weinig et al., 1966; Damico et al., 1968; Matthews and Matsumura, 1969), rotenone (Fukami et al., 1967), terraclor (Kuchar et al., 1969), methyl 1-(butylcarbamoyl)-2-benzimidazolecarbamate (Gardiner et al., 1968), the carbamates carbaryl (Baron et al., 1969) and siduron (Belasco and Reiser, 1969), and the uracil derivatives terbacil (Rhodes et al., 1969) and bromacil (Gardiner et al., 1969).

In a number of papers mass spectra have been reported of metabolites whose chemical structures were already known, usually as a demonstration of the feasibility of an instrumental innovation or the efficacy of some kind of chemical modification. Examples include metabolites of histamine (Tham and Holmstedt, 1965), the catecholamines (Anggard and Sedvall, 1969), and chlorpromazine (Hammar, Holmstedt, and Ryhage, 1968).

The major problem, then, in metabolite identification is not the interpretation of the spectra, but rather the attainment of sufficient amounts of samples of suitable purity. Purification can often be best approached with a combined gas chromatograph/mass spectrometer. However, the forest of peaks obtained on the chromatogram can necessitate continuous scanning, generation of miles of chart paper, and weeks of spectral analysis by the researchers to locate the spectra of the drug metabolites to be studied. Two approaches have been suggested to alleviate this problem. In one (Hites and Biemann, 1970) the data from the continuous scans are stored in a computer. Peaks characteristic of the metabolites being sought are registered and the computer provides a "peakogram" trace of the height of each of these peaks through all the scans stored. If the appropriate peaks are requested, their heights will be maximal in scans of metabolites. When these scans are identified, the complete spectrum of each metabolite can be retrieved from the computer. A more direct approach is to use radioisotope-labeled drugs and a radioactivity detector in a stream-split gas chromatograph/mass spectrometer (Hobbs, 1970). Thus, the total ion monitor of the mass spectrometer provides a complete chromatogram of the mixture, while the radioactivity detector registers peaks only when drug-related material passes through. At these points in the chromatogram the mass spectrometer may be scanned and spectra obtained.

The reader is referred to several reviews (Hammar, Holmstedt, et al., 1969; Fales, 1970); Guarino and Fales, 1970) of the use of mass spectrometry in studying drug metabolism.

STRUCTURE ELUCIDATION OF DRUGS AND TOXINS FROM NATURAL SOURCES

The structure elucidation of a completely unknown sample is a much more difficult undertaking than that of a drug metabolite. In this case any chemical information and other spectroscopic evidence must be considered in conjunction with the mass spectrum. Perhaps the single most valuable piece of information which can be obtained from the mass spectrum is the molecular weight, or empirical formula if a high resolution instrument is used. The empirical formula and considerable information about the structure can be provided by the mass spectrometer from impure, noncrystalline samples, in contrast to combustion analysis and x-ray crystallography.

One of the classical mass-spectral structure proofs in the annals of pharmacology is that of the toxic impurity in the anesthetic halothane, which causes hepatic necrosis. This compound was identified from its mass spectrum as 2,3-dichloro-1,-1,1,4,4,4,-hexafluorobutene-2 (Cohen et al., 1963).

Hallucinogens

An equally interesting structure elucidation was that of the hallucinogen STP (2,5-dimethoxy-4-methylamphetamine), which was successfully achieved in both United States and British government laboratories (Martin and Alexander, 1968; Phillips and Mesley, 1969). These efforts drew on IR, UV, NMR, and TLC information, as well as high resolution mass spectrometry. Mass spectrometry has been employed in structural investigations of the chemical constituents of hashish (Yamauchi et al., 1968; von Spulak et al., 1968; Mechoulam and Ben-Zvi, 1968; Vollner et al., 1969), of a more obscure hallucinogen called HOG (Holmstedt, 1969), and also of some hallucinogens in South American Indian snuffs (Agurell et al., 1969). The extraction and mass-spectral identification of a variety of hallu-cinogenic drugs in commercial formulations have been discussed (Bellman, 1968).

In man a metabolite of ethanol has been identified by the combined techniques of gas chromatography and mass spectrometry (Jaakonmaki et al., 1967).

Toxicological Applications

Toxic substances comprise another group of natural products of pharmaco-logical interest in the elucidation of whose structure, mass spectrometry has played a role. Examples include the necrotoxin from fire ant venom (MacConnell et al., 1970), steroidal alkaloid toxins from the Colombian frog arrow poison (Tokuyama et al., 1969), steroidal alkaloid teratogens from the plant *Veratrum californium* (Keeler, 1969a), fungus metabolites toxic to mammals (Moss et al., 1967; Bamburg et al., 1968; Steyn, 1970), a fish poison from the lower Amazon (Cascon et al., 1965), and the carcinogenic lipid carcinolipin (Hradec and Dolejs, 1968).

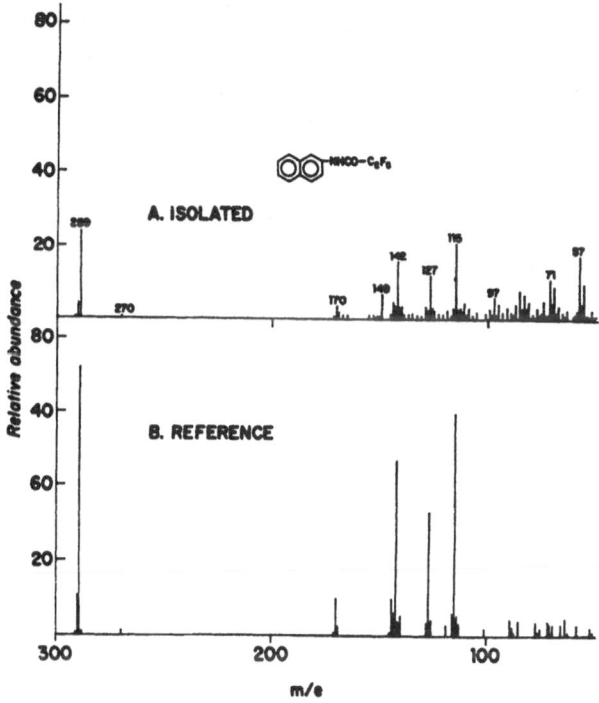

FIG. 5. Mass spectra of 2-naphthylamine pentafluoropropionamide isolated from cigarette smoke and reference 2-naphthylamine pentafluoropropionamide. (From Masuda and Hoffman. 1969. *Anal. Chem.*, 41:650-652.)

Another substance of pharmacological importance whose structure has been identified with the help of mass spectrometry is the bladder carcinogen 2-naphthylamine, isolated from the smoke of 300 cigarettes (Masuda and Hoffmann, 1969; D. Hoffman, Masuda, and Wynder, 1969). Basic material in the smoke was trapped in methanolic hydrogen chloride solution, reacted with pentafluoropropionic anhydride, and analyzed by gas chromatography and mass spectrometry. The spectra of isolated and reference 2-naphthylamine pentafluoropropionamide are shown in Figure 5. These spectra furnish a good example of how actual data often look. The structure assignment was based on comparison of the GC retention times and the mass spectra. The same group has also used mass spectrometry to identify insecticide residues and pyrolysis products in cigarettes (D. Hoffman, Rathkamp, and Wynder, 1969).

Antibiotics

One of the most difficult areas of structure proof is that of new drugs—notably antibiotics and antitumor agents—isolated from natural sources. As mentioned above, the most valuable contribution of a mass spectrum is usually the molecular weight. A good example of this is found in the reports (Rickards et al., 1968; Muxfeldt et al., 1968) of the revised structure of pikromycin, which is based on low and high resolution mass measurements of the molecular ion. The original elemental analysis (Brockmann and Henkel, 1951) shown in Table 4 is consistent with both the original and the revised elemental compositions.

TABLE 4

Analyses for Original and Revised Pikromycin Formulas

	Calculated for Original Formula $C_{25}H_{43}NO_7$	Calculated for Revised Formula $C_{28}H_{47}NO_8$	Observed Analyses
Combustion Analysis	C 63.94 H 9.23 N 2.98	C 63.96 H 9.02 N 2.66	C 63.86 H 9.02 N 2.92
Molecular weight by high resolution mass measurement	469.3028	525.3298	525.3302

Another case where mass spectral analysis caused revision of molecular weight is that of the heptapeptide antibiotic esperin (Thomas and Ito, 1969). Here the terminal N-acyl group was found to be a homologous mixture of β-hydroxy straight chain fatty acids, and the C-terminal amino acid was found to be a 70:30 mixture of leucine and valine (Figure 6).

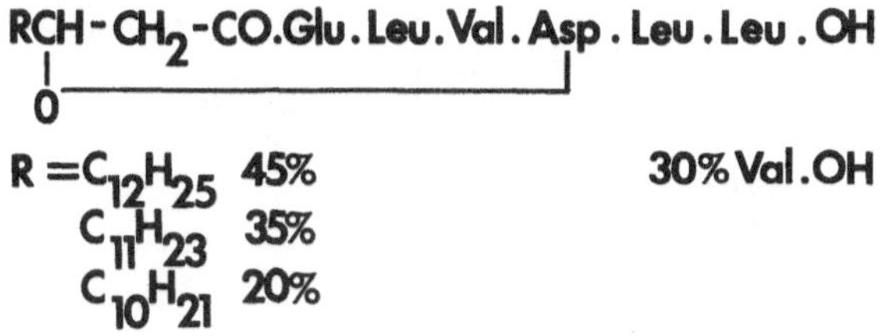

$$RCH-CH_2-CO.Glu.Leu.Val.Asp.Leu.Leu.OH$$

$$\underset{O}{|}$$

$$R = C_{12}H_{25} \quad 45\% \qquad\qquad 30\% \; Val.OH$$
$$ C_{11}H_{23} \quad 35\%$$
$$ C_{10}H_{21} \quad 20\%$$

FIG. 6. Revised structure of the peptide antibiotic esperin.

In this case the compound was converted to an N- and O-permethylated derivative for the analysis, which revealed the sequence of the peptide in addition to the molecular weight of the components of the mixture.

Molar ratios, and thus molecular weights, of the oligomycin antibiotics are important in inhibition studies of oxidative phosphorylation. The difficulty of determining accurate molecular weights for these compounds has been pointed out by three mass spectrometry groups, who have reported a variety of values (Beechey et al., 1967; Chamberlin et al., 1968; Prouty et al., 1969).

A variety of techniques has been used to obtain molecular ions from antibiotics that are too involatile or too unstable to handle routinely. Both chemical ionization (Arsenault et al., 1969) and field ionization (Rinehart and Mathur, 1968) have been used. The spectrum of streptovaricin A was integrated over 10 minutes on a photoplate to obtain a measurable molecular ion peak (Rinehart, 1969). A more extreme approach has also been suggested—analysis of the pyrolysis products of antibiotics that are too labile to be analyzed intact (Brodasky, 1967). Investigators began quite early to use trimethylsilyl ethers as stable volatile derivatives to examine the structures of polyol antibiotics (Golding et al., 1964) and glycoside antibiotics (DeJongh et al., 1967; Tsuji and Robertson, 1969). Even if molecular ions are small, the $M-15$ peak characteristic of trimethylsilyl ethers usually appears unambiguously. The chemical modification worked out for the deoxystreptamine/neomycin class, which includes N-acetylation as well as O-trimethylsilylation, has been used to facilitate mass spectral structure elucidation of four hybrimycins prepared using a mutant bacterium (Shier et al., 1969). The fragmentation pattern of neomycin B and two hybrimycins is indicated in Figure 7. Not only can the structural changes be detected in the molecular weights, which are greater than 1400, but the fragmentation pattern allows their location in the molecule to be determined.

The problems associated with the analysis of a new antibiotic depend to a large extent on the chemical class to which it belongs—peptide, glycoside, alkaloid, macrolide, etc. In a number of cases mass spectrometry has been used to work out a portion of the antibiotic when molecular weight, polarity, or chemical complexity precludes analysis of the entire molecule. Thus the identification of a novel amino acid in the antibiotic peptide edeine A was based in part on high resolution mass measurements (Hettinger and Craig, 1968). The spectrum and structure of the fatty acid portion of amphomycin have been reported (Bodanszky et al., 1969), as

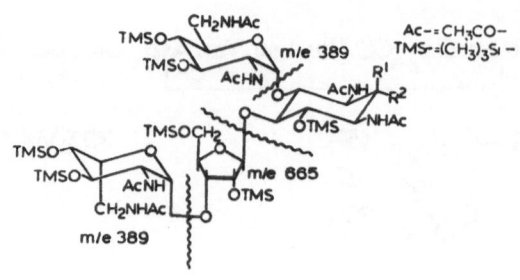

Antibiotic derivatised	R^1	R^2
Neomycin B	H	H
Hybrimycin A1	H	OTMS
Hybrimycin B1	OTMS	H

FIG. 7. Diagnostic fragmentations of *N*-acetyl-*O*-trimethylsilyl antibiotics. (From Shier et al. 1969. *Proc. Nat. Acad. Sci. U.S.A.*, 63:198-204.)

have those of the lipid portion of prasinomycin (Slusarchyk and Weisenborn, 1969). In the case of the polyene macrolide antibiotics, mass spectral analysis of the carbon skeleton has usually been carried out after cleavage of any glycoside bonds and after reduction of the polyene chain. This approach has provided information on the carbon skeleton of fungichromin/lagosin (Cope, Bly, et al., 1962), amphotericin B (Cope, Axen, et al., 1966), and nystatin (Ikeda et al., 1967).

A number of antibiotics, including mitiromycin (Morton et al., 1970), peyocatin/hordenine (Rao, 1970), tryptophol (Lingappa et al., 1969), neoantimycin (Caglioti et al., 1969), beauvericin (Hamill et al., 1969), tetrenolin (Gallo et al., 1969), 1'-demethylclindamycin (Argoudelis, Coats et al., 1969), α_2-rhodomycinon (Brockmann and Niemeyer, 1968), pikromycin (Rickards et al., 1968; Muxfeldt et al., 1968), α-dehydrobiotin (Hanka et al., 1966), and several nucleosides (Hanes et al., 1966; Suhadolnik et al., 1969), have proven amenable to mass spectral analysis without chemical modification or special instrumentation. The biosynthesis of lincomycin from CD_3-methionine has been studied by mass spectral analysis of the unaltered antibiotic (Argoudelis, Eble, et al., 1969). A spectrum of the *N*-acetyl derivative was obtained as part of the elegant structure elucidation of actinobolin (Antosz et al., 1970).

Tumor Inhibitors

The structures of many natural products with antitumor activity have been studied by a variety of techniques, including mass spectrometry (Cote et al., 1969; Kupchan et al., 1970). The structure of the alkaloid vinblastine, used to treat a number of malignancies, including Hodgkin's disease, was confirmed in one of the earliest demonstrations of the usefulness of high-resolution mass spectrometry (Bommer et al., 1964). Alkaloids were early found to be amenable to mass spectral analysis, and a great deal of structure work has been done in this area (Budzikie-wicz et al., 1964).

Vitamins

The vitamins, like the antibiotics, encompass a variety of chemical classes under one functionally derived heading. Work demonstrating the feasibility of mass spectral analysis of ubiquinones and vitamin K-type compounds (Di Mari et al., 1966; Vetter et al., 1967) has been followed by papers (Matschiner and Amelotti, 1968; Campbell and Bentley, 1969) using the technique to demonstrate occurrence of vitamin K_2 from a number of sources as isoprenoid mixtures. Spectra have been obtained of compounds (Figure 8) where $n = 6,7,8,9,10,11,12$. Dihydro-analogs of vitamin K_2 have similarly been found to occur as mixtures (Campbell and Bentley, 1968; Beau et al., 1966). The methyl group on the quinone ring of vitamin K was shown by mass spectral analysis to originate from CD_3-labeled methionine (Jackman et al., 1967). A new epoxide metabolite of vitamin K, whose accumulation in rats is promoted by administration of the anticoagulant warfarin, has been identified by physical methods, including mass spectrometry (Matschiner et al., 1970).

Mass spectrometry has also been used to prove the structures of a dimer of vitamin A (Giannotti et al., 1966), a dimer of vitamin E (Lloyd et al., 1969, Strauch et al., 1969) and biologically active metabolites of vitamin D_3 (Suda et al., 1970). High resolution mass measurements indicated that the first of the D_3 metabolites, isolated from hog blood, weighed 400.3343 atomic mass units (Blunt et al., 1968). This corresponds to an empirical formula of $C_{27}H_{44}O_2$ and reveals that the metabolite contains an additional oxygen atom, compared to vitamin D_3 itself. Loss of the side chain (see Figure 9) led to ions of mass 271.2053 $(C_{19}H_{27}O)$ in the fragmentation of both D_3 and its metabolite, demonstrating that the new hydroxyl group is in the side chain, which is lost. A peak at m/e 59.0492 (C_3H_7O), present in the spectrum of the metabolite and absent in the spectrum of vitamin D_3 (cholecalciferol), suggested that the hydroxyl group was attached to the last three carbon atoms in the side chain. Comparison of the NMR to that of 25-hydroxycholesterol confirmed the metabolite as 25-hydroxycholecalciferol.

Spectra have also been discussed of compounds of known structure in the B_6 (DeJongh, Perricone, and Gay, 1968), B_1 (Hesse et al., 1967), and A (Lin et al., 1970) families.

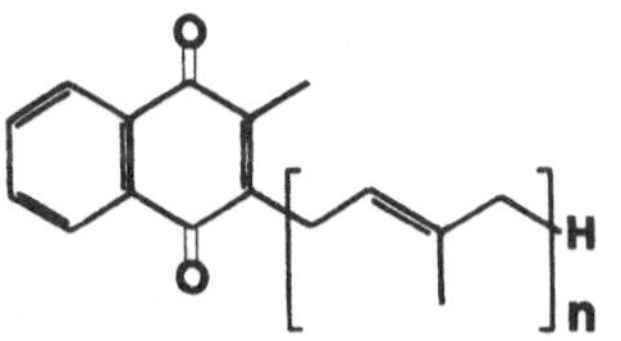

FIG. 8. Vitamin K_2 isoprenoids.

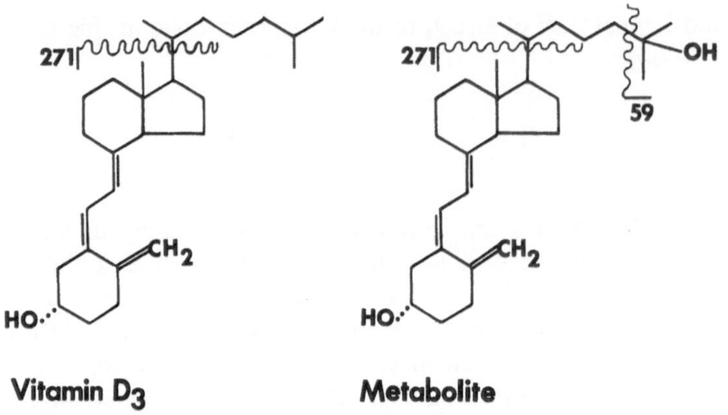

FIG. 9. Diagnostic fragmentation of Vitamin D₃ and its active metabolite.

Prostaglandins

Mass spectrometry has played a major role in the elucidation of structure (Bergstrom et al., 1962, 1963) in the recently delineated prostaglandin family, which appears to have considerable therapeutic potential (Karim and Filshie, 1970; Roth-Brandel et al., 1970). Usually GCMS analyses have been performed on compounds that are esterified with diazomethane or diazoethane (Hamberg and Samuelsson, 1969; Granstrom and Samuelsson, 1969). Trimethylsilylation has also been suggested (Vane and Horning, 1969). Hydroxyl groups may be acetylated, although this is apparently not necessary, and keto groups have been reduced with sodium borodeuteride or converted to *O*-methyloxime derivatives (Green, 1969). Mass spectral analysis has also been important in studies of biosynthesis (Ryhage and Samuelsson, 1965; Samuelsson, 1965; Hamberg and Samuelsson, 1967; Israelsson et al., 1969; Sih et al., 1969). Other reports have dealt with structures of human urinary metabolites (Hamberg and Samuelsson, 1969; Granstrom and Samuelsson, 1969).

Cardiac Glycosides

Mass spectrometry has been used for some time to assist elucidation of the structure of the aglycone portion of cardenolides of the cardiac glycoside type (Lardon et al., 1969; Tschesche and Marwede, 1967). Negative ion spectra have been used in this effort as well as conventional positive ion spectra (S. Hoffmann et al., 1966). A recent report (Brown et al., 1970) suggests that structural information may be obtained from the unmodified intact glucoside carrying up to three sugar units using field ionization. Cleavage occurs between the sugar units, and prominent "sequence peaks" in the spectrum allow the aglycone and component monosaccharides to be characterized and their sequence reconstructed. The stereochemistry of the glycosidic bonds cannot be assigned from the mass spectrum. Electron impact spectra of chemically modified polysaccharide glycosides may also provide structural information (Blessington and Morton, 1970).

Peptides

A great many papers have appeared discussing the use of mass spectrometry to sequence peptides (Jones, 1968; Van Lear and McLafferty, 1969; Das and Lederer, 1970; DeJongh, 1970; Shemyakin et al., 1971). By far the great majority of these papers have reported work with synthetic or commercial peptides of known structures, available in large amounts. In other cases peptides from biological sources, of already known structure, have been analyzed. This work has served to demonstrate that the volatility of peptides is limited by their size, by functional groups in the side chains, and by the polarity of the amide groups themselves. In cases where all the amino acids have nonpolar side chains, chemically modified peptides of 10 to 12 amino acids have been reconstructed from the mass spectrum. Modified arginine has been sequenced in tetrapeptides. Larger peptides, e.g., an octadecapeptide derivative analyzed in 5 mg quantity (Franek et al., 1969), have been introduced into the mass spectrometer, information being obtained for the first 7 to 10 units, but not for the entire molecule.

Some criticism of various kinds of chemical modification has been published (Agarwal et al., 1968; Thomas, 1969; Cheesman, 1970; Lenard and Gallop, 1970). It is probably significant that in most of the work done with larger compounds of unknown structures, modification has included acetylation or trifluoroacetylation of the terminal amino group and permethylation of amide nitrogens, side chain hydroxyl groups, and terminal and side chain carboxylic groups.

One aspect on which most authors agree is that mass spectral sequencing is best done in conjunction with analysis of the hydrolyzed amino acids by ion exchange chromatography (Shemyakin et al., 1970). Thus, any of the amino acids whose side chains require special modification will be recognized. In addition, the interpretation of the spectrum will be easier if all the pieces to be fitted together are known. Comparisons of chemical (Edman's degradation) sequencing with mass-spectral sequencing suggest (Agarwal et al., 1969; Franek et al., 1969) that the latter is faster, but that the former requires less material. Mass spectral analysis of unknown sequences have been reported using 180 nmole (Agarwal et al., 1969) and approximately 300 nmole (Cheesman, 1970). Mass spectrometry offers the advantages that it can distinguish glutamine and asparagine from glutamic acid and aspartic acid, and identify N-terminal pyroglutamyl groups routinely (deHaas et al., 1969).

Of particular interest to pharmacologists are reports of the mass spectral determinations of primary structures of several peptide antibiotics (Hamill et al., 1969; Thomas and Ito, 1969; Terlain and Thomas, 1969; Hiramoto et al., 1970), feline gastrin (Agarwal et al., 1969), gonadotropin-inhibiting peptide from bovine pineal gland (Cheesman, 1970), hypothalamic hypophysiotropic TSH-releasing factor (Burgus et al., 1970), and a chemical code word of memory (Ungar et al., 1970).

DIAGNOSIS

The term "diagnosis" as used here means identifying chemicals from patients with specific disease states. These compounds often occur uniquely with a given syndrome, but whether or not structural or quantitative identification of this sort will permit significant advances in medical treatment remains to be seen.

Gases

At the simplest level of instrumentation are the mass spectrometers with a low mass range, used to monitor respiratory, circulatory, and tissue gases. Either a multiple detector is used with which three to five masses/gases can be monitored at once without scanning, or rapid short-range scanning is used, e.g., six times per minute over the mass range 20 to 50. Both of these approaches allow for calibration of the strip chart in pressure units.

Mass spectrometry has been used to monitor expiratory gas pressure curves for oxygen, argon, and carbon dioxide in determining histamine thresholds in patients with various kinds of asthma (Trendelenburg, 1969). Analysis of expired air has also been related to cardiac output (Bickel et al., 1970). A variety of diffusion membranes have been used for monitoring blood gases (Woldring et al., 1966; Brantigan et al., 1970), and intramuscular (Dardik et al., 1970) and intracerebral (Owens et al., 1969) gas pressures via cannulae connected to mass spectrometers. A review of the field through 1967 has appeared (Fowler, 1969).

A technique for analysis of gaseous metabolites such as ethylene and dimethylsulfide collected from animal tissues has been described (Parker and Ruliffson, 1967), and the analysis of organic compounds in human breath by gas chromatography and mass spectrometry has been reported (Jansson and Larsson, 1969).

Narcotics and Overdoses

Greater challenge is offered to the spectroscopist by several reports of identification of poisons, narcotics, or drugs used in suicidal overdoses extracted from urine (Bohn and Rucker, 1968), stomach contents (Bohn and Rucker, 1968; Fales et al., 1970), or brain and liver tissue (Weinig et al., 1966; De, 1969). Measurement of the spectrum may be preceded by gas phase or thin layer chromatography (Bonn and Rucker, 1968; Alfes and Clasing, 1969), or analysis may be attempted on the extracted mixtures (De and Umberger, 1969; Fales et al., 1970). Obviously this is an area in which the most sophisticated technology can be applied—high resolution measurements, computerized identification procedures,

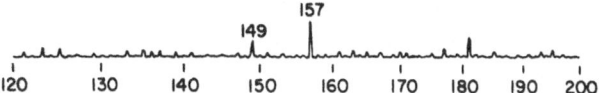

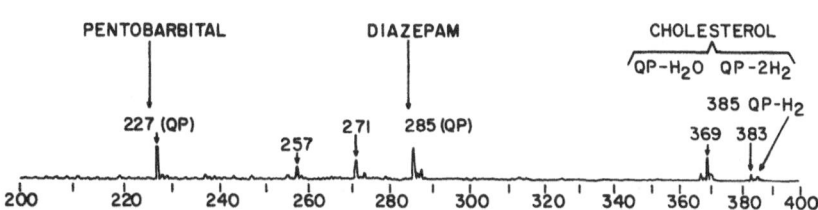

FIG. 10. Partial spectrum of extract from stomach contents. (From H. M. Fales, personal communication.)

specialized ionization techniques. In Figure 10 the middle mass range is reproduced from the mass spectrum of a sample obtained by chloroform extraction of the stomach contents of a comatose overdose victim. This spectrum was obtained using chemical ionization, which has been found (Fales et al., 1970) to give much larger peaks in the molecular ion region of barbiturate spectra than does electron impact (Arnold and Grutzmacher, 1969). A comparable analysis made in Boston has been reported in the popular press (Henahan, 1970).

Urine Analysis

Compounds have been identified from most of the available human body fluids—urine, blood, sweat, amniotic fluid, milk, bile, and stomach contents. Urine has, of course, been the major source. The compounds responsible for the mauve spot test in urine of psychotic patients have been identified (Irvine et al., 1969) as derivatives of kryptopyrrole. On the other hand, mass spectrometry was used in an investigation which demonstrated (Kuehl et al., 1966) that 3,4-dimethoxy-phenylacetic acid was not excreted exclusively by schizophrenic individuals, but occurred at about the same levels in normal and schizophrenic urine. β-Mercaptolactate-cysteine disulfide, a new analog of cystine, was reported present in the urine of a mentally retarded offspring of sibling mating (Crawhall et al., 1968). N-(Phenylacetyl)-L-glutamic acid has been identified as an anomalous and abundant compound in urine of a patient with advanced neuroblastoma (Williams et al., 1969).

Unusual compounds often accumulate in the urine of patients with hereditary enzyme blocks or metabolism disorders. Mass spectrometry has been employed in the identification of N-isovaleryl glycine (Tanaka and Isselbacher, 1967) and

β-hydroxyisovaleric acid (Tanaka et al., 1968) in urine of patients with isovaleryl acidemia and of p-menth-1-ene-8,9-diol (Wade et al., 1966) in urine of a young girl whose hirsutism indicated excessive androgen activity. The unexpected metabolism of allopurinol to oxipurinol by a patient with congenital deficiency of xanthine oxidase was established (Chalmers et al., 1969). Similarly, metabolism of 1,2-^{3}H-20β-dihydrocortisol was studied in a patient with Cushing's Syndrome (Dixon and Pennington, 1968).

In at least one laboratory (Markey et al., 1970) attempts are being made to analyze routinely urine from patients with suspected metabolic lesions at very early stages in the medical diagnosis with integrated gas chromatographic/mass spectrometric-computerized instrumentation. This program has already resolved one ambiguous diagnosis of tyrosinemia where the aromatic compounds detected in urine were found to be, not metabolites of tyrosine, but rather metabolites of heavy doses of anticonvulsants which had been administered to the patient. In the same laboratory α-methyl, β-hydroxybutyric acid as well as methylmalonic acid were identified as trimethylsilyl derivatives in urine of patients with methylmalonic aciduria.

Blood and Sweat

The sensitivity requirements for analysis of compounds in blood are usually greater than for urine analysis because smaller amounts of material are available. In most cases combined GCMS instruments have been used, precluding the need to purify the material completely. Examples include the characterization of 5α-lanost-8,(9)-en-3β-ol in hyperlipemic serum (Gray et al., 1969), the identification of 3α-hydroxyandrost-5-en-17-one in elevated concentrations in the blood, plasma, and bile of patients with uremia (Janne et al., 1969), and characterization of sterol esters from aortal atheroma plaques from patients with advanced aortal lesions (Brooks et al., 1970).

A characteristic odorous substance from the sweat of schizophrenic patients has been identified as trans-3-methyl-2-hexenoic acid by gas chromatography, mass spectrometry, and NMR (K. Smith et al., 1969).

Fluids from Normal Subjects

A great deal of work has been reported on the identification of endogenous compounds from urine, blood, and other fluids of normal humans. This is particularly the case with steroids and fatty acids, which are among the simplest biochemicals to analyze by gas phase procedures. Thus, steroids have been analyzed by GCMS from amniotic fluid (Shackleton and Mitchell, 1967; Siegel et al., 1969), placenta, fetal, and maternal blood (Miettinen and Luukkainen, 1968; Sjovall and Sjovall, 1968; Cronholm et al., 1969), and fatty acids have been identified in human milk (Egge et al., 1969). Steroids in newborn urine and feces (Shackleton et al., 1968; Eneroth and Gustaffson, 1969; Gustafsson et al., 1969) have been related to biosynthetic studies with human fetal liver microsomes (Lisboa and Gustafsson, 1968, 1969).

One program has been described (Horning et al., 1969; Horning, Horning, and Hill, 1969) for routine analysis of urine of all newborns in a large hospital by gas chromatography/mass spectrometry. Besides an array of endogenous compounds, the investigators report that they frequently detect aspirin and occasionally narcotics in newborn urine.

Mass spectrometry is one of the techniques employed in at least one analytical assault on all the compounds in urine (Burtis and Warren, 1968).

Quantitative Analysis

Carefully calibrated mass spectrometers have been used for years to do quantitative analysis of petroleum mixtures introduced through the reservoir-leak inlet system. However, apart from the breath and blood gas analyses described above, the technique has been little used for quantitative work in biochemistry or pharmacology. Mixtures of amino acid esters have been analyzed for internal ratios (Sheehan et al., 1968), and cholines have been analyzed for absolute values in the nanogram range following thermal demethylhalogenation in the reservoir-leak inlet system (Johnston et al., 1968). This paucity of quantitative analyses probably reflects the fact that quantitation is so easily achieved by gas chromatographic techniques. An example of the use of the two techniques in a complementary manner is found in a study of the effect of human pituitary follicle-stimulating hormone on the excretion of a variety of steroids by an amenorrhoeic woman (Luukkainen et al., 1967). Here urinary steroids were identified by mass spectrometry, but quantitative excretion curves were measured by gas chromatography.

Artifacts

Artifacts of isolation and analysis are occasionally identified. Pyroglutamic acid was isolated in high amounts from urine of patients suffering from burns. However, glutamic acid was found to be converted to pyroglutamic acid by the conditions of the separation procedure; and which compound was characteristic of the condition could not be decided (Tham et al., 1968). 3α-Ureido-11β-hydroxy-Δ^4-androsten-17-one was isolable in high amounts from the urine of hypothyroid subjects relative to normal urine. Eventually the ureido steroid was found to be formed during urine incubation at pH 5 from the real metabolite, 11β-hydroxy-Δ^4-androstene-3,17-dione (Fukushima et al., 1966).

The dialkyl phthalate whose characteristic peak is noted at m/e 149 in Figure 10 is probably an artifact derived from plasticizer in clinical tubing or gloves. A variety of phthalate esters are used as plasticizers and also in pump oil, and they show up frequently as artifacts in mass spectra. A liver metabolite of butyl glycolyl

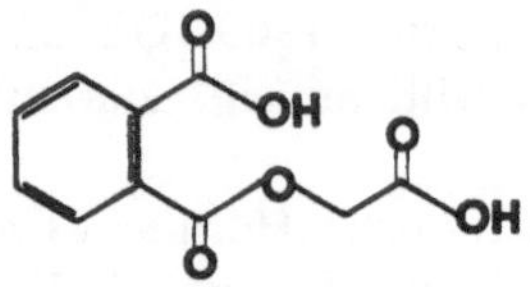

FIG. 11. Liver metabolite of perfusion tubing plasticizer.

butyl phthalate plasticizer leached from tubing in a liver perfusion experiment has been identified using mass spectrometry and other physical methods (Jaeger and Rubin, 1970). The structure is shown in Figure 11.

STABLE ISOTOPE ANALYSIS

One of the earliest contributions of mass spectrometry was the demonstration of the existence of isotopes by the separation of ^{20}Ne and ^{22}Ne (Thomson, 1913). Mass spectrometry is still the most sensitive technique to detect stable isotopes and to measure their occurrence quantitatively. Maximal exploitation of the technique allows the investigator not only to quantitate isotope incorporation, but also to assign the position of the label in the molecule. Use of mass spectral fragmentation to locate isotopic labels obviates multistep chemical degradation. The logistics of such work are quite analogous to those used to locate metabolic alterations in drugs. The fragmentation of the compound must be deciphered before increases in the fragment masses can be used to locate isotopic labels.

Conventional Detection

Enrichments of greater than 10% are normally used to allow quantitation in both molecular and fragment ions with reasonable accuracy with normal scanning, or even on fast scanning GCMS instruments. An example from investigations of the biosynthesis of RNA and DNA demonstrates how information is obtained from the mass spectrum (Caprioli and Rittenberg, 1968a). A sample of D-glucose in which 57% of the molecules carried an ^{18}O-isotope label at C-1 was used as the sole carbon source for growing *Escherichia coli*. Adenosine and deoxyadenosine were isolated and purified and their mass spectra were obtained. The molecular ion of unlabeled adenosine occurs at m/e 267, as indicated in Figure 12. The fragmentation is well understood (McCloskey, in press; Shaw et al., 1970) and the loss of the 5′-oxygen in formation of M-30 ions occurs as indicated in Figure 12. The investigators found that, in the spectrum of their isolated adenosine, 20% of the molecular ions weighed 269, i.e., 20% of the adenosine molecules isolated contained one ^{18}O isotope in place of an atom of ^{16}O. However, virtually all of the M-30 peak occurring at m/e 237 in the spectrum of reference adenosine also appeared at m/e 237 in the spectrum of isolated adenosine, demonstrating that ^{18}O incorporated in the

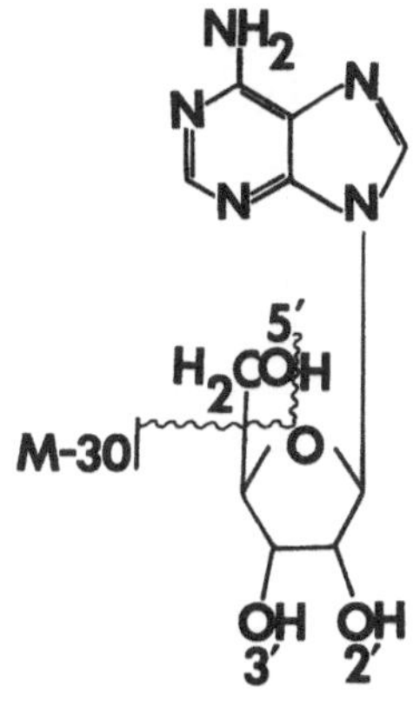

FIG. 12. Diagnostic fragmentation of adenosine.

biosynthesis was located exclusively at the 5'-position. The exclusive incorporation into this position of ^{18}O from the 1-position of glucose confirms the existence of a biosynthetic pathway for conversion of hexose to pentose other than the oxidative removal of terminal C-1. However, the ^{18}O label was not incorporated quantitatively from glucose (57% labeled) to adenosine (20% labeled) in agreement with the hypothesis that several biosynthetic routes operate.

Other investigations of biosynthetic transformations of sugars have been reported (Caprioli and Rittenberg, 1968b; Melo, Elliott, and Glaser, 1968; Sherman et al., 1969) where mass spectrometry has been used to analyze the extent and location of isotope labels. In one case (Melo and Glaser, 1968) results obtained using ^2H-labels were considered more reliable than those obtained using radioactive ^3H-labels because of the larger discrimination against biosynthetic reactions involving tritium atoms.

Water containing ^2H or ^{18}O is one of the most commonly used sources of isotopic labels. The extent and location of incorporation into phytosphingosine synthesized by yeast of ^{18}O from $H_2^{18}O$ was studied with product enrichments of 15 to 20% (Thorpe and Sweeley, 1967). Careful examination of the fragmentation of tetraacetylphytosphinogosine allowed distinction and location of oxygen atoms that were or were not labeled. Mass spectral measurement of heavy atom incorporation from 10%-enriched $H_2^{18}O$ confirmed cleavage of the P-O bond rather than the C-O bond in hydrolysis of 17β-estradiol 3-phosphate by a phosphatase enzyme isolated from human placenta (DiPietro, 1969). Evaluation of heavy atom incorporation from ^2H_2O supported the isomerization of Δ^5-androsten-3,17-dione to Δ^4-androsten-3,17-dione by bovine adrenal steroid isomerase as an intramolecular hydrogen transfer (Murota, Fenselau, and Talalay, 1970).

Gaseous $^{18}O_2$ is another widely used labeled substrate. Oxidative steps in the biosynthesis of steroid hormones (Nakano et al., 1967, 1968), the origin of oxygen incorporated in the biosynthesis of prostaglandins (Ryhage and Samuelsson, 1965; Samuelsson, 1965), and the mammalian hepatic microsomal N-dealkylation reaction (McMahon, Culp, and Occolowitz, 1969) have been studied using $^{18}O_2$

enriched 50 to 98%. The observation (*Ibid.*) that molecular oxygen is the source of oxygen in microsomal *N*-dealkylation reactions supports a mechanism involving direct hydroxylation of the carbon atom rather than preliminary formation of an *N*-oxide.

Studies of biosynthesis of the antibiotic lincomycin (Argoudelis, Eble, et al., 1969) and vitamin K_2 (Jackman et al., 1967) from CD_3-labeled methionine have already been mentioned. Mass spectral aspects of the classical labeling studies of biosynthesis of squalene and steroids have been reviewed (Biemann, 1963; Lederer, 1969).

Studies using higher levels of enrichment of ^{13}C and ^{15}N are less common, presumably because of the hitherto high cost of these isotopes relative to ^2H and ^{18}O. Studies of incorporation of a variety of ^{15}N- and ^{13}C-labeled amino acids into the antibiotic gliotoxin have been reported (Bose, Das, et al., 1968; Bose, Khanchandi, et al., 1968), and a GCMS investigation (Vandenheuval and Cohen, 1970) of amino acids isolated from algae grown in 15% enriched $^{13}CO_2$ suggests that a biosynthetic isotope effect can be detected in the side chains of the amino acids. This conclusion results from examination of fragment ions as well as molecular ions. Studies have also been made of biosynthetic incorporation of ^{15}N from various precursors into the fungal metabolite slaframine (K. L. Rinehart and coworkers, private communication). The masses of the isotope-containing fragment ions were measured with a conventional detector using high resolution to eliminate contributions from other species. Averages were taken of multiple measurements made by switching between two peaks with the peak-matching controls.

Isotope Ratio Detection

Levels of enrichment of less than 1% can be most accurately measured with isotope ratio mass spectrometers. These instruments measure isotope enrichment with double detectors to less than a hundredth of a percent. Most isotope-ratio instruments have a limited mass range and can analyze isotopes in biological material only after conversion to light gases. Such an instrument was used in early investigations of the biosynthesis and metabolism of amino acids by rodents (Rittenberg et al., 1939).

More recently this type of instrument was used to study the extent to which a pool of $^{15}N_2$-urea and $^{14}N_2$-urea is catabolized and regenerated in a patient suffering complete renal failure (Walser et al., 1954; Walser, 1970). Urea was converted unimolecularly to gaseous nitrogen, whose distribution of isotopic species was analyzed. Randomization of the labels, i.e., increase in the amount of $^{15}N^{14}N$ species, reflects metabolic recyclization of urea through ammonium salts and protein, and was found to be extensive when the patient was ingesting only essential amino acids. In another study (D. C. DeJongh and E. B. Hills, private communication), the excretion of labeled nitrogen by dwarf children fed ^{15}N-glycine is being compared to that of normal controls.

If an isotope-ratio detector is used on an instrument with a high enough mass range, biological material can be analyzed without prior conversion to light gases. In this case the investigator can quantitate isotope incorporation at very low levels and also assign the position of the label in the molecule without the necessity of chemical degradation or combustion. In studies of the plant biosynthesis of ricinine, for example (Waller et al., 1966), isotope ratio measurements of molecular (m/e 164) and fragment ions confirmed incorporation of ^{15}N into various parts of the molecule from both ^{15}N-formamide and ^{15}N-aspartate. Levels of incorporation were less than 1%. Quantitatively similar values were obtained by averaging a number of conventional low electron voltage scans.

Metabolic Lesion in Refsum's Disease

A very elegant series of investigations has demonstrated the nature of a metabolic lesion in patients suffering from hereditary Refsum's disease (Steinberg et al., 1967, 1970; Mize et al., 1969). High levels of phytanic acid had been recorded in blood and tissues of these patients, prompting two questions. Does this branched fatty acid derive from exogenous sources or from some unusual biosynthesis? At what point is its metabolism blocked? A very general test for biosynthesis was devised (Steinberg et al., 1967) in which the patient's body fluid was enriched in ^{2}H$_2$O to 0.5% and maintained at this level for four months. Stable isotopes are much safer to use than radioactive labels at this level for this long a time, but their incorporation into phytanic acid and cholesterol (used as an internal standard) is harder to analyze. In order to obtain information on both the location of labels and the extent of incorporation, a technique for averaging multiple scans was used with a conventional instrument.

At the end of four months serum cholesterol was found to be enriched to 91% of theory based on 0.5% body water enrichment. Two hydrogen atoms only were found to be incorporated into phytanic acid, eliminating the possibility of its biosynthesis de novo. Examination of the fragment ion of mass 101 (Figure 13) located these two atoms in the end of the molecule. This suggested that phytanic acid was formed, at least in part, from phytol, which is commonly ingested as a side chain on chlorophyll. This was then confirmed with radioactively labeled phytol.

The second question was also answered by a combination of stable isotope and radioisotope labeling experiments (Mize et al., 1969). The enzymatic block in the catabolism of phytanic acid was shown to be oxidation at the carbon atom α to the carboxylic acid group.

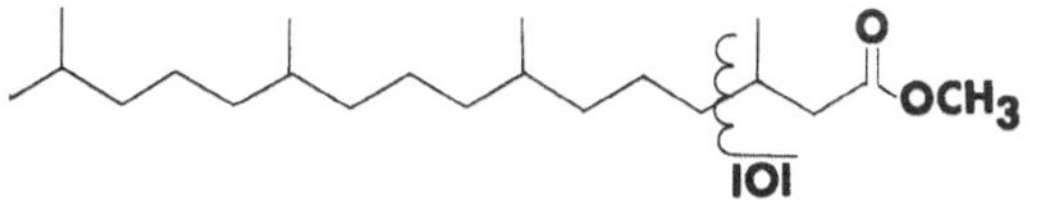

FIG. 13. Diagnostic fragmentation of phytanic acid ester.

Other Investigations

A number of investigations, particularly in nonmammalian systems, in which mass spectrometry was used to evaluate stable isotope enrichment, have not been discussed here. Other reviews of the field (Milne, 1971; Rinehart and Grostic, 1971) should be consulted for other references.

Radioisotope labeling (in metabolism studies, for example) is usually carried out at levels low enough that it does not complicate normal interpretation of conventional mass spectra. If the isotopic enrichment is greater than a few percent, quantitative and positional assignment can be obtained by mass spectrometry by averaging multiple scans (Occolowitz, 1968; McMahon and Occolowitz, 1969) or by autoradiographic reading of the spectrum recorded on a photoplate (Knöppel and Beyrich, 1968).

ENVOI

All the areas of current excitement in pharmacology, medicine, and biochemistry that involve studies with small molecules are areas of potential application of mass spectrometry. Several aspects are discussed below, in which the increased use of mass spectrometry could provide important biochemical and medical information. Most of these applications would be facilitated by increased instrumental sensitivity and by innovations in inlet systems to allow ionization of involatile samples.

Studies in Humans with Stable Isotopes

Investigations of human metabolism and biosynthesis of the type described above with patients with Refsum's disease are very rare in the literature (Cronholm and Sjovall, 1970). There are, however, medical situations where the use of stable isotopes is preferable to radioactive tracers (Pinkus et al., 1971). The lack of radioisotopes of some elements, notably nitrogen, and the possibility of pronounced isotope effects in biosynthetic reactions with tritium, may also necessitate labeling with stable isotopes. Mass spectrometry is the best means available to analyze material containing stable isotopes, since not only the amounts, but also the locations, of labels can be identified. This should be an area of expanded activity.

Sequencing of Biopolymers

Peptide sequencing is another field where technology is available, but reports of applications to biochemical problems are scarce. Mass spectrometry should be useful in the identification of hormones, metabolites, and factors. Sequencing of polynucleotides awaits the development of new inlet systems or efficacious chemical modification (Hunt et al., 1968). Some advances have been reported recently (Duncan et al., 1971) in the analysis of phospholipids. Besides the difficulties of volatility, and chemical modification and interpretation of the spectrum, a problem specific to the elucidation of structures of unknown biochemical samples appears to be the interface energy barrier between biochemist and mass spectroscopist.

Mixtures

In many cases it is attractive to analyze impure material, or material in mixtures, without complete separation and purification (McLafferty et al., 1970; Kaiser et al., 1970; Lovins, 1969; Sharkey et al., 1969). Some mixtures are not suitable for introduction into the mass spectrometer through a gas chromatograph, because they are involatile or unstable. In other instances the time and/or material saved by omitting purification may justify analysis of the more complex data derived from mixtures. This is the case, for example, in the emergency diagnosis shown in Figure 10. The spectrum shown of the mixture extracted from the stomach contents of the overdose victim is a fairly simple example of recognizing individual components in a mixture. Halogen isotope patterns may be used to identify low resolution peaks belonging to a certain compound in a mixture, and high resolution data may allow sorting out of peaks belonging to compounds with unique composition, e.g., phosphorus-containing compounds. Obviously, computerized data analysis can be helpful here. Although mass spectrometry has been used for years to analyze mixtures of petroleum products, there was a movement away from mixture analysis in the decade of the 1960's. In biochemistry and pharmacology, at least, mixture analysis must once again be regarded as desirable, for it may be the most expeditious route to a great deal of information.

Blood-Level Kinetics

The routine use of GCMS to monitor blood levels of drugs and metabolites is a goal whose realization is limited primarily by instrumental sensitivity. The technique of recording only two or three peaks (mass fragmentography or multiple peak detection) may provide increased sensitivity only if enough is known about the structure and fragmentation of metabolites to select three characteristic and intense peaks to monitor.

Forensic Medicine

The routine analysis of narcotics and drugs in urine, blood, and tissue is also limited only by sensitivity of available instrumentation. Mass spectral analysis of this type is very attractive because it is less ambiguous than the color tests and chromatographic procedures now employed.

ACKNOWLEDGMENTS

I wish to thank Drs. Allan H. Fenselau and Paul Talalay for reading and criticizing this chapter for me; Mrs. Christian Sander for technical assistance; and the National Academy of Science of the United States and the American Chemical Society for permission to reproduce figures.

REFERENCES

Agarwal, K. L., R. A. W. Johnstone, G. W. Kenner, D. S. Millington, and R. C. Sheppard. 1968. Mass Spectrometry of N-methylated peptide derivatives. Nature (London), 219:498-499.

———— G. W. Kenner, and R. C. Sheppard. 1969. Feline gastrin. An example of peptide sequence analysis by mass spectrometry. J. Amer. Chem. Soc., 91:3096-3097.

Agurell, S., B. Holmstedt, and J. Lindgren. 1969. Alkaloids in certain species of *Virola* and other South American plants of ethnopharmacologic interest. Acta. Chem. Scand., 23:903-916.

Ahlborg, U., B. Holmstedt, and J. Lindgren. 1968. Fate and metabolism of some hallucinogenic indolealkylamines. Advances Pharmacol., 6B:213-229.

Aldercreutz, H., C. Johansson, and T. Luukkainen. 1967. Gas chromatographic and mass spectrometric studies in the influence of metabolites of bis(*p*-acetoxyphenyl)-cyclohexylidinemethane on the estimation of estrogens in urine. Ann. Med. Exp. Biol. Fenn., 45:269-276.

Alfes, M., and D. Clasing. 1969. Identifizierung geringer mengen Methamphetamins nach Körperpassage durch Kopplung von Dunnschichtchromatographie und Massenspektrometrie. Deutsche Z. Ges. Gerichtl. Med., 64:235-240.

Anggard, E., and G. Sedvall. 1969. Gas chromatography of catecholamine metabolites using electron capture detection and mass spectrometry. Anal. Chem., 41:1250-1256.

Antosz, F. J., D. B. Nelson, D. L. Herald, and M. E. Munk. 1970. The structure and chemistry of actinobolin. J. Amer. Chem. Soc., 92:4933-4942.

Argoudelis, A. D., J. H. Coats, D. J. Mason, and O. K. Sebek. 1969. Conversion of clindamycin to l'-demethylclindamycin and clindamycin sulfoxide by *Streptomyces* species. J. Antibiot. (Tokyo), 22:309-314.

———— T. E. Eble, J. A. Fox, and D. J. Mason. 1969. Studies on the biosynthesis of lincomycin. The origin of methyl groups. Biochemistry (Washington), 8:3408-3409.

Arnold, W., and H. F. Grutzmacher. 1969. Massenspektrometrischer Nachweis von Arzneimittelmetaboliten (Barbiturate, Noludar, Pyramidon) im Rahmen der forensischen Analyse. Z. Anal. Chem., 247:179-188.

Arsenault, G. P., J. R. Althaus, and P. V. Divekar. 1969. Structure of the antibiotic botryodiplodin—use of chemical ionization mass spectrometry in organic structure determination. Chem. Commun., 1414-1415.

———— J. J. Dolhun, and K. Biemann. 1970. Gas chromatography-chemical ionization mass spectrometry. Chem. Commun., 1542-1543.

Bamburg, J. R., N. V. Riggs, and F. M. Strong. 1968. The structures of toxins from two strains of *Fusarium tricinctum*. Tetrahedron, 24:3329-3336.

Baron, R. L., J. A. Sphon, J. T. Chen, E. Lustig, J. D. Doherty, E. A. Hansen, and S. M. Kolbye. 1969. Confirmatory isolation and identification of a metabolite of carbaryl in urine and milk. J. Agr. Food Chem., 17:883-887.

Beau, S., R. Axerad, and E. Lederer. 1966. Isolemen et caracterisation des dihydro-menaquinone des myco- et corgnebacteries. Bull. Soc. Chim. Biol. (Paris), 48:569-581.

Beckey, H. D. 1969. Field desorption mass spectrometry: A technique for the study of thermally unstable substances of low volatility. Int. J. Mass Spectrum. Ion Phys., 2:500-503.

Beechey, R. B., V. Williams, C. T. Holloway, I. G. Knight, and A. M. Robertson. 1967. Estimation of the molecular weights and molecular formulae of oligomycin-A, rutamycin and aurovertin by mass spectrometry. Biochem. Biophys. Res. Commun., 26:339-341.

Belasco, I. J., and R. W. Reiser. 1969. Metabolic fate of siduron in the animal. J. Agr. Food Chem., 17:1000-1003.

Bellman, S. W. 1968. Mass spectral identification of some hallucinogenic drugs. J. Assoc. Off. Anal. Chem., 51:164-175.

Bergstrom, S., R. Ryhage, B. Samuelsson, and J. Sjovall. 1962. The structure of prostaglandin E, F_1 and F_2. Acta Chem. Scand., 16:501-502.

_____ R. Ryhage, B. Samuelsson, and J. Sjovall. 1963. Prostaglandins and related factors. The structures of prostaglandin E, $F_{1\alpha}$ and $F_{1\beta}$. J. Biol. Chem., 238:3555-3564.

Bickel, R. G., C. F. Diener, and H. L. Brammell. 1970. An analog computer program for cardiac output in humans using mass spectrometer analysis of expired air. Aerospace Med., 41:203-207.

Biemann, K. 1962. Mass Spectrometry. New York, McGraw-Hill.

_____ 1963. Mass spectrometry. Ann. Rev. Biochem., 32:755-780.

Biros, F. J. 1970. Enhancement of mass spectral data by means of a time averaging computer. Anal. Chem., 42:537-540.

Blessington, B., and I. M. Morton. 1970. Mass spectrometry in cardenolide chemistry. Org. Mass Spectrom., 3:95-99.

Blunt, J. W., H. F. DeLuca, and H. K. Schnoes. 1968. 25-Hydroxycholecalciferol. A biologically active metabolite of vitamin D_3. Biochemistry (Washington), 7:3317-3322.

Bodanszky, M., N. C. Chaturvedi, and J. A. Scozzie. 1969. The structure of fatty acids from the antibiotic amphomycin. J. Antibiot. (Tokyo), 9:399-408.

Bohn, G., and G. Rucker. 1968. Die Anwendung einer Kombination von Dünnschicht-chromatographie und Massenspektrometrie zum Nachweis von Glutethimid in Organmaterial. Arch. Toxik., 23:221-225.

Bommer, P., W. McMurray, and K. Biemann. 1964. High resolution mass spectra of natural products. Vinblastine and derivatives. J. Amer. Chem. Soc., 86:1439-1440.

_____ and F. Vane. 1966. The use of fragmentation patterns of 1,4 benzodiazepines for the structure determination of their metabolites by high resolution mass spectrometry. Fourteenth Annual Conference on Mass Spectrometry and Allied Topics. May 22-27. Dallas, Texas.

Bose, A. K., K. G. Das, P. T. Funke, I. Kugajevsky, O. P. Shukla, K. S. Khanchandani, and R. J. Suhadolnik. 1968. Biosynthetic studies on gliotoxin using stable isotopes and mass spectral methods. J. Amer. Chem. Soc., 90:1038-1041.

_____ K. S. Khanchandani, R. Tavares, and P. T. Funke. 1968. The mode of incorporation of phenylalanine into gliotoxin. J. Amer. Chem. Soc., 90:3593.

Brantigan, J. W., V. L. Gott, M. L. Vestal, G. J. Fergusson, and W. H. Johnston. 1970. A nonthrombogenic diffusion membrane for continuous in vivo measurement of blood gases by mass spectrometry. J. Appl. Physiol., 28:375-377.

Brockmann, H., and W. Henkel. 1951. Pikromycin, ein bitter schmeckendes Antibioticum aus Actinomyceten. Chem. Ber., 84:284-288.

_____ and J. Niemeyer. 1968. α_2-Rhodomycinon, α-citromycinon, γ-citromycinon. Chem. Ber., 101:1341-1348.

Brodasky, T. F. 1967. Pyrolysis—gas chromatography in the differentiation and characterization of antibiotics. J. Gas Chromatog., 5:311-318.

Brooks, C. J. W., W. A. Harland, G. Steel, and J. D. Gilbert. 1970. Lipids of human atheroma: isolation of hydroxyoctadecadienoic acids from advanced aortal lesions. Biochim. Biophys. Acta, 202:563-566.

Brown, P., F. R. Bruschweiler, G. R. Pettit, and T. Reichstein. 1970. Characterization of cardenolides by field ionization mass spectrometry. J. Amer. Chem. Soc., 92:4470-4472.

Budzikiewicz, H., C. Djerassi, and D. H. Williams. 1964. Structure Elucidation of Natural Products by Mass Spectrometry. Vol. 1, Alkaloids. San Francisco, Holden Day.

Burgus, R., T. F. Dunn, D. Desiderio, D. N. Ward, W. Vale, and R. Guillemin. 1970. Characterization of ovine hypothalamic hypophysiotropic TSH-releasing factor. Nature (London), 226:321-325.

Burnstein, S. H., F. Menezes, and E. Williamson. 1970. Metabolism of $\Delta^{1(6)}$-tetrahydrocannabinol, an active marihuana constituent. Nature (London), 225:87-88.

Burtis, C. A., W. C. Butts and W. T. Rainey, Jr. 1970. Separation of the metabolites of phenacetin in urine by high resolution anion exchange chromatography. Clin. Path., 53:769-777.

_____ and K. S. Warren. 1968. Identification of urinary constituents isolated by anion-exchange chromatography. Clin. Chem., 14:290-301.

Caglioti, L., D. Misiti, R. Mondelli, A. Selva, F. Arcamone, and G. Cassinelli. 1969. The structure of neoantimycin. Tetrahedron, 25:2193-2221.

Campbell, I. M., and R. Bentley. 1968. Inhomogeneity of vitamin K_2 in *Mycobacterium phlei*. Biochemistry (Washington), 7:3323-3327.

_____ and R. Bentley. 1969. Inhomogeneity of vitamin K_2 in *Escherichia coli*. Biochemistry (Washington), 8:4651-4655.

Caprioli, R., and D. Rittenberg, 1968a. Quantitative aspects of the origin of pentose in *Escherichia coli*. Proc. Nat. Acad. Sci. U.S.A., 60:1379-1382.

_____ and D. Rittenberg. 1968b. On the utilization of D-fructose for pentose synthesis in *Escherichia coli*. Proc. Nat. Acad. Sci. U.S.A., 61:1422-1427.

Cascon, S. C., W. B. Mors, B. M. Tursch, R. T. Aplin, and L. J. Durham. 1965. Ichthyothereol and its acetate, the active polyacetylene constituents of *Ichthyothere terminalis* (Spreng.) Malme, a fish poison from the lower Amazon. J. Amer. Chem. Soc., 87:5237-5241.

Chalmers, R. A., R. Parker, H. A. Simmonds, W. Snedden, and R. W. E. Watts. 1969. The conversion of 4-hydroxypyrazolo[3,4-d]pyrimidine (allopurinol) into 4,6-dihydroxypyrazolo[3,4-d]pyrimidine (oxipurinol) in vivo in the absence of xanthine-oxygen oxidoreductase. Biochem. J., 112:527-532.

Chamberlin, J. W., M. Gorman, and A. Agtarap. 1968. Characterization of the oligomycins and related antibiotics. Eighth Interscience Conference on Antimicrobial Agents and Chemotherapy. Oct. 21-23, New York City.

Cheesman, D. W. 1970. Structural elucidation of a gonadotropin-inhibiting substance from the bovine pineal gland. Biochim. Biophys. Acta, 207:247-253.

Cohen, E. N., J. W. Bellville, H. Budzikiewicz, and D. H. Williams. 1963. Impurity in halothane anesthetic. Science, 141:899.

Cooks, R. G., and G. S. Johnson. 1971. Natural products; including oligopeptides, oligonucleotides and oligosaccharides. *In* Williams, D. H., ed., Mass Spectrometry of Organic and Organometallic Compounds. London, Chemical Society, Specialist Reports Series.

Cope, A. C., U. Axen, E. P. Burrows, and J. Weinlich. 1966. Amphotericin B. Carbon skeleton, ring size and partial structure. J. Amer. Chem. Soc., 88:4228.

———— R. K. Bly, E. P. Burrows, O. J. Ceder, E. Ciganek, B. T. Gillis, R. F. Porter, and H. E. Johnson. 1962. Fungichromin: complete structure and absolute configuration at C_{26} and C_{27}. J. Amer. Chem. Soc., 84:2170-2178.

Cote, J. R., E. Bianchi, and E. R. Trumbull. 1969. Antitumor agents from *Bursera microphylla* (Burseraceae) II. Isolation of a new lignan—burseran. J. Pharm. Sci., 58:175-176.

Coulter, A. W., C. Fenselau, P. S. Lietman, and C. H. Robinson, 1970. Unpublished data.

Crawhall, J. C., R. Parker, W. Sneddon, E. P. Young, M. G. Ampola, M. L. Efron, and E. M. Bixby, 1968. Beta mercaptolactate-cysteine disulfide: analog of cystine in the urine of a mentally retarded patient. Science, 160:419-420.

Cronholm, T., and J. Sjovall. 1970. Effect of ethanol metabolism on redox state of steroid sulphates in man. Eur. J. Biochem., 13:124-131.

———— J. Sjovall, and K. Sjovall. 1969. Ethanol induced increase of the ratio between hydroxy- and ketosteroids in human pregnancy plasma. Steroids, 13:671-678.

Damico, J. N., J. T. Chen, C. E. Costello, and E. O. Haenni. 1968. Structure of Klein's metabolites of aldrin and dieldrin. J. Assoc. Off. Anal. Chem., 51:48-55.

Dardik, M., I. Dardik, and H. Laufman. 1970. Paradoxical tissue ischemia with augmentation of collateral flow following arterial occlusion. Ann. Surg., 171:380-384.

Das, B. C., and E. Lederer, 1970. Mass spectrometry of complex natural compounds. *In* Burlingame, A. L., ed., Topics in Organic Mass Spectrometry, 255-326. New York, John Wiley and Sons.

De, P. K., and C. J. Umberger. 1969. Application of mass spectrometry to forensic toxicology. Developments in Applied Spectroscopy, 7A:267-273.

deHaas, G. H., F. Franek, B. Keil, D. W. Thomas, and E. Lederer. 1969. Application of mass spectrometry to the analysis of proteins containing an N-terminal pyroglutamic acid residue. FEBS Lett., 4:25-27.

DeJongh, D. C. 1970. Mass spectrometry. Anal. Chem., 42:169R-205R.

———— J. D. Hribar, S. Hanessian, and P. W. K. Woo. 1967. Mass spectrometric studies on aminocyclitol antibiotics. J. Amer. Chem. Soc., 89:3364-3365.

———— S. D. Hribar, P. Littleton, K. Fotherby, R. W. A. Rees, S. Shrader, T. J. Foell, and H. Smith. 1968. The identification of some human metabolites of norgestrel, a new progestational agent. Steroids, 649-665.

———— S. C. Perricone, and M. L. Gay. 1968. Mass spectrometry of vitamin B_6: different forms of the vitamin, its metabolites, antimetabolites and analogs. Org. Mass Spectrom., 1:151-166 and references therein.

Di Mari, S. J., J. M. Supple, and M. Rapoport. 1966. Mass spectra of naphthoquinones. Vitamin $K_{1(20)}$. J. Amer. Chem. Soc., 88:1226-1232.

DiPietro, D. L. 1969. Mechanism of hydrolysis of estradiol-3-phosphate by placental acid phosphatase III. Biochim. Biophys. Acta, 178:188-190.

Dixon, R., and G. W. Pennington. 1968. In vivo 6β-hydroxylation of 20β-dihydrocortisol. Steroids, 12:423-433.

Dole, M., L. L. Mack, R. L. Hines, R. C. Mobley, L. D. Ferguson, and M. B. Alice. 1968. Molecular beams of macroions. J. Chem. Phys., 49:2240-2249.

Dreyfuss, J., A. I. Cohen, and S. M. Hess. 1968. Metabolism of thiazesim, 5-(2-dimethylaminoethyl)-2,3-dihydro-2-phenyl-1,5-benzothiazepin-4(5H)-one, in the rat in vivo and vitro. J. Pharm. Sci., 57:1505-1511.

Duncan, J. H., W. J. Lennarz, and C. C. Fenselau. 1971. Mass spectral analysis of glycerophospholipids. Biochemistry (Washington), 10:927-932.

Egge, H., U. Murawski, P. Gyorgy, and F. Zilliken. 1969. Minor constituents of human milk. Identification of cyclohexaneundecanoic acid and phytanic acid in human milk fat by a combination gas chromatograph/mass spectrometer. Fed. Eur. Biochem. Soc. Lett., 2:255-258.

Eneroth, P., and J. Gustafsson. 1969. Steroids in newborns and infants. Identification of 20,22-dihydroxycholesterol from the monosulphate and "disulphate" fractions in human meconium. Fed. Eur. Biochem. Soc. Lett., 5:99-103.

─────── J. Gustafsson, and E. Nystrom. 1969. Identification of 24,25-dihydro-$\Delta^{9(11)}$-lanosterol and 4α, 14α-dimethyl substituted sterols among the esterified and free sterols in human meconium. Europ. J. Biochem., 11:456-464.

Fales, H. M. 1971. Ionization techniques other than electron bombardment. In Milne, G. W. A., ed., Mass Spectrometry. New York, John Wiley and Sons.

─────── 1970. Techniques for studying drug biotransformation, isolation and identification procedures—spectral methods. In Way, L., ed., Fundamentals of Drug Metabolism and Disposition. Baltimore, Williams and Wilkins Co.

─────── G. W. A. Milne, and T. Axenrod. 1970. Identification of barbiturates by chemical ionization mass spectrometry. Anal. Chem., 42:1432-1435.

─────── G. W. A. Milne, and M. L. Vestal. 1969. Chemical ionization mass spectrometry of complex molecules. J. Amer. Chem. Soc., 91:3682-3685.

Fenselau, C., and S. Y. Wang. 1969. Mass spectra of some dimeric photoproducts of pyrimidines. Tetrahedron, 25:2853-2863.

─────── J. H. Duncan, and O. M. Colvin. 1971. Unpublished data.

─────── S. Y. Wang, and P. Brown. 1970. Field ionization mass spectra of photopolymers of thymine. Tetrahedron, 26:5923-5927.

Field, F. H., and M. S. B. Munson. 1965. Mass spectrometric studies of methane at pressures to 2 torr. J. Amer. Chem. Soc., 87:3289-3294.

Foltz, R. L., et al. 1970. Metabolite of (-) trans-Δ-tetrahydrocannabinol: identification and synthesis. Science, 168:844-845.

Fowler, K. T. 1969. The respiratory mass spectrometer. Phys. Med. Biol., 14:185-199.

Franek, F., B. Keil, D. W. Thomas, and E. Lederer. 1969. Chemical and mass spectrometric sequence studies of a peptide from the variable part of normal immunoglobulin λ-chains. Fed. Eur. Biochem. Soc. Lett., 2:309-312.

Fukami, J., I. Yamamoto, and J. E. Casida. 1967. Metabolism of rotenone in vitro by tissue homogenates from mammals and insects. Science, 155:713-716.

Fukushima, D. K., S. Noguchi, H. L. Bradlow, B. Zumoff, K. Kozuma, L. Hellman, and T. F. Gallagher. 1966. Isolation, characterization and synthesis of 3α-ureido-11β-hydroxy-Δ^4-androsten-17-one. J. Biol. Chem., 241:5336-5340.

Gallo, G. G., C. Coronelli, A. Vigevani, and G. C. Lancini. 1969. The structure of tetrenolin, a new antibiotic substance. Tetrahedron, 25:5677-5680.

Gardiner, J. A., R. K. Brantley, and H. Sherman. 1968. Isolation and identification of a metabolite of methyl 1-(butylcarbamoyl)-2-benzimidazole carbamate in rat urine. J. Agr. Food Chem., 16:1050-1052.

─────── R. W. Reiser, and H. Sherman. 1969. Identification of the metabolites of bromacil in rat urine. J. Agr. Food Chem., 17:967-973.

Giannotti, C., B. C. Das, and E. Lederer. 1966. Sur la constitution chimique du kitol, dimere de la vitamine A. Bull. Soc. Chim. France, 3299-3303.

Golding, B. T., R. W. Rickards, and M. Barber. 1964. The determination of molecular formulae of polyols by mass spectrometry of their trimethylsilyl ethers; the structure of the macrolide antibiotic filipin. Tetrahedron Lett., 2615-2621.

Granstrom, E., and B. Samuelsson. 1969. The structure of a urinary metabolite of prostaglandin $F_{2α}$ in man. J. Amer. Chem. Soc., 91:3398-3400.

Gray, M. F., A. Morrison, E. Farish, T. D. V. Lawrie, and C. J. W. Brooks. 1969. Characterization of 5α-lanost-8(9)-en-3β-ol in hyperlipaemic serum. Biochim. Biophys. Acta, 187:163-165.

Green, K. 1969. Gas chromatography-mass spectrometry of O-methyloxime derivatives of prostaglandins. Chem. Phys. Lipids, 3:254-272.

Guarino, A. M., W. D. Conway, and H. M. Fales. 1969. Mass spectral identification of probenecid metabolites in rat bile. Europ. J. Pharmacol., 8:244-252.

———— and Fales, H. M. 1970. Isolation and identification of drug metabolites: gas chromatography-mass spectrometry. *In* Brodie, B. B. and J. R. Gillette, eds., Drug Transport and Metabolism. New York, John Wiley and Sons.

Gustafsson, J., C. H. L. Shackelton, and J. Sjovall. 1969. Steroids in newborns and infants. C_{19} and C_{21} steroids in faeces from infants. Europ. J. Biochem., 10:302-311.

Hamberg, M., and B. Samuelsson. 1967. On the mechanism of the biosynthesis of prostaglandins E_1 and $F_{1\alpha}$. J. Biol. Chem., 242:5336-5343.

———— and B. Samuelsson. 1969. The structure of the major urinary metabolite of prostaglandin E_2 in man. J. Amer. Chem. Soc., 91:2177-2178.

Hamill, R. L., C. E. Higgens, H. E. Boaz, and M. Gorman. 1969. The structure of beauvericin, a new depsipeptide antibiotic toxic to *Artemia salina*. Tetrahedron Lett., 4255-4258.

Hammar, C., I. Hanin, B. Holmstedt, R. J. Kitz, D. J. Jenden, and B. Karlen. 1968. Identification of acetylcholine in fresh rat brain by combined gas chromatography-mass spectrometry. Nature (London), 220:915-917.

———— B. Holmstedt, J. Lindgren, and R. Tham. 1969. The combination of gas chromatography and mass spectrometry in the identification of drugs and metabolites. Advances Pharmacol. Chemother., 7:53-89.

———— B. Holmstedt, and R. Ryhage. 1968. Mass fragmentography. Anal. Biochem., 25:532-548.

Hanes, S., D. C. DeJongh, and J. A. McCloskey. 1966. Further evidence on the structure of cordycepin. Biochim. Biophys. Acta, 117:480-482.

Hanka, L. J., M. E. Bergy, and R. B. Kelly. 1966. Naturally occurring antimetabolite antibiotic related to biotin. Science, 154:1667-1668.

Henahan, J. F. 1970. K. Biemann, a renaissance man in mass spectrometry. Chem. Eng. News, July 13, 1970: 50-54.

Hesse, M., N. Bild, and H. Schmid. 1967. Die Massenspektren von Vitamin B_1 und von einigen Modellverbindungen. Helv. Chim. Acta, 50:808-813.

Hettinger, T. P. and L. C. Craig. 1968. The composition of the antibiotic peptide edeine A. Biochemistry (Washington), 7:4147-4153.

Hill, D. C., M. C. Kirk, and R. F. Struck. 1970. Isolation and identification of 4-keto-cyclophosphamide, a possible active form of the antitumor agent cyclophosphamide. J. Amer. Chem. Soc., 92:3207-3208.

Hiramoto, M., K. Okada, and S. Nagai. 1970. The revised structure of viscosin, a peptide antibiotic. Tetrahedron Lett., 1087-1090.

Hites, R. A., and K. Biemann. 1970. Computer evaluation of continuously scanned mass spectra of gas chromatographic effluents. Anal. Chem., 42:855-860.

Hobbs, D. C. 1970. Techniques for mass spectrometry of drug metabolites without extensive purification. Eighteenth Annual Conference on Mass Spectrometry and Allied Topics, June 14-19, San Francisco.

Hoffman, S., E. Weiss, and T. Reichstein. 1966. Adigosid, Struckturbestimmung. Glykoside und Aglykone. Helv. Chim. Acta, 49:1855-1872.

Hoffmann, D., Y. Masuda, and E. L. Wynder. 1969. α-Naphthylamine and β-naphthylamine in cigarette smoke. Nature (London), 221:254-256.

———— G. Rathkamp, and E. L. Wynder. 1969. Chemical studies on tobacco smoke. Quantitative analysis of chlorinated hydrocarbon insecticides. Beitr. Tabakforsch., 5:140-148.

Holmstedt, B. 1969. Gas chromatography-mass spectrometry as a tool to elucidate the structure of unknown psycho-active drugs. *In* Sjoqvist, F., and Tottie, M., eds., Abuse of Central Stimulants, 357-373. New York, Raven Press.

Horning, M. G., E. C. Chambay, C. J. Brooks, A. M. Moss, E. A. Boucher, E. C. Horning, and R. M. Hill. 1969. Characterization and estimation of urinary steroids of the newborn human by gas-phase analytical methods. Anal. Biochem., 31:512-531.

———— E. C. Horning, and R. M. Hill. 1969. Mass spectrometric studies of drugs and drug metabolites in the newborn. Fourth Middle Atlantic Regional Meeting of the American Chemical Society, February 12-15. Washington, D.C.

Hradec, J., and L. Dolejs. 1968. The chemical constitution of carcinolipin. Biochem J., 107:129-133.

Hunt, D. F., C. E. Hignite, and K. Biemann. 1968. Structure elucidation of dinucleotides by mass spectrometry. Biochem. Biophys. Res. Commun., 33:378-383.

Ikeda, M., M. Suzuki, and C. Djerassi. 1967. Nystatin—the structure of the aglycone. Tetrahedron Lett., 3745-3750.

Irvine, D. G., W. Bayne, H. Miyashita, and J. R. Majer. 1969. Identification of kryptopyrrole in human urine and its relation to psychosis. Nature (London), 224:811-813.

Israelsson, U., M. Hamberg, and B. Samuelsson. 1969. Biosynthesis of 19-hydroxy-prostaglandin A_1. Europ. J. Biochem., 11:390-394.

Jaakonmaki, P. I., K. L. Knox, E. C. Horning, and M. G. Horning. 1967. The characterization by gas-liquid chromatography of ethyl β-D-glucosiduronic acid as a metabolite of ethanol in rat and man. Europ. J. Pharmacol., 1:63-70.

Jackman, L. M., I. G. O'Brien, G. B. Cox, and F. Gibson. 1967. Methionine as the source of methyl groups for ubiquinone and vitamin K: a study using nuclear magnetic resonance and mass spectrometry. Biochim. Biophys. Acta, 141:1-7.

Jaeger, R. J., and R. J. Rubin. 1970. Plasticizers from plastic devices. Extraction, metabolism and accumulation by biological systems. Science, 170:460-462.

Janne, O., T. Laatikainen, J. Vainio, and R. Vihko. 1969. Identification of 3α-hydroxyandrost-5-en-17-one in human plasma, urine and bile. Steroids, 13:121-128.

Jansson, B. O., and B. T. Larsson. 1969. Analysis of organic compounds in human breath by gas chromatography-mass spectrometry. J. Lab. Clin. Med., 74:961-966.

Johnston, G. A. R., A. C. K. Triffett, and J. A. Wunderlich. 1968. Identification and estimation of choline derivatives by mass spectrometry. Anal. Chem., 40:1837-1840.

Jones, J. H. 1968. The mass spectra of amino acid and peptide derivatives. Quart. Rev. (London), 22:302-316.

Kaiser, K., H. Obermann, G. Remberg, M. Spiteller-Friedmann, and G. Spiteller. 1970. Möglichkeiten und Grenzender Anwendung einer direkten Kombination Gaschromatographhochauflosendes Massenspektrometer bei der Untersuchung von in biologischen materialien vorkommenden Steroiden. Monatsh., 101:240-263.

Karim, S. M. M., and G. M. Filshie. 1970. Therapeutic abortion using prostaglandin F_2. Lancet, 157-159.

Keeler, R. F. 1969a. Teratogenic compounds of *Veratrum californium* (Durand). The structure of cyclopamine. Phytochem., 8:223-225.

———— 1969b. The structure of the glycosidic alkaloid cycloposine. Steroids, 13:579-588.

Knöppel, H., and W. Beyrich. 1968. A new technique for studying mechanisms of mass spectral reactions using ^{14}C-labelled compounds. Tetrahedron Lett., 291-294.

Krauss, D., W. Otting, and U. Breyer. 1969. Identification of a urinary metabolite of perazine as a piperazine-2,5-dione derivative. J. Pharm. Pharmacol., 21:808-813.

Kuchar, E. J., F. O. Geenty, W. P. Griffith, and R. J. Thomas. 1969. Analytical studies of metabolism of terraclor in beagle dogs, rats and plants. J. Agr. Food Chem., 17:1237-1240.

Kuehl, F. A., R. E. Ormond, and W. J. A. Vandenheuvel. 1966. Occurrence of 3,4-dimethoxyphenylacetic acid in urines of normal and schizophrenic individuals. Nature (London), 211:606-608.

Kupchan, S. M., R. M. Smith, Y. Aynehchi, and M. Maruyama. 1970. Tumor inhibitors. Cucurbitacins O, P, and Q, the cytotoxic principles of *Brandegea bigelovii*. J. Org. Chem., 35:2891-2894.

Lardon, A., K. Stockel, and T. Reichstein. 1969. Gomphogenin-Teilsynthese und Struktur des Calotropagenins. Helv. Chim. Acta, 52:1940-1954.

Lederer, E. 1969. Some problems concerning biological C-alkylation reactions and phytosterol biosynthesis. Chem. Soc. Quart. Rev., 23:453-481.

Lenard, J., and P. M. Gallop. 1970. Sequence analysis of microgram amounts of peptides by mass spectrometry. Anal. Biochem., 34:286-291.

Lin, R. L., G. R. Waller, E. D. Mitchell, K. S. Yang, and E. C. Nelson. 1970. Mass spectra of retinol and related compounds. Anal. Biochem., 35:435-441.

Lingappa, B. T., M. Prasad, Y. Lingappa, D. F. Hunt, and K. Biemann. 1969. Phenethyl alcohol and tryptophol: autoantibiotics produced by the fungus *Candida albicans*. Science, 163:192-194.

Lisboa, B. P., and J. Gustafsson. 1968. Biosynthesis of two new steroids in the human foetal liver. 1β- and 2β-hydroxytestosterone. Europ. J. Biochem., 6:419-424.

_____ and J. Gustafsson. 1969. Biosynthesis of 18-hydroxytestosterone in the human foetal liver. Europ. J. Biochem., 9:402-405.

Lloyd, H. A., E. A. Sokoloski, B. S. Strauch, and H. M. Fales. 1969. The vitamin E dimer, a fluxional system. Chem. Commun., 299-301.

Lovins, R. E. 1969. Identification of pesticides in mixtures by high-resolution mass spectrometry. J. Agr. Food Chem., 17:663-667.

Luukkainen, T., C. A. Gemzell, and M. Adlercreutz. 1967. Effect of human pituitary follicle-stimulating (HP-FSH) hormone on urinary excretion of eight different oestrogens, 11-deoxy-17-ketosteroids and pregnanediol in a patient with polycystic ovaries. Acta Endrocr. (Suppl.), 119:75.

MacConnell, J. G., M. S. Blum, and H. M. Fales, 1970. Alkaloid from fire ant venom: identification and synthesis. Science, 168:840-841.

Markey, S. P., K. B. Hammond, and J. R. Plattner. 1970. Applications of GC-MS to metabolic research problems. Eighteenth Annual Conference on Mass Spectrometry and Allied Topics, June 14-19, San Francisco.

Martin, R. J., and T. G. Alexander. 1968. Analytical procedures used in FDA laboratories for the analysis of hallucinogenic drugs. J. Assoc. Off. Anal. Chem., 51:159-163.

Masuda, Y., and D. Hoffmann. 1969. Quantitative determination of 1-naphthylamine and 2-naphthylamine in cigarette smoke. Anal. Chem., 41:650-652.

Matschiner, J. T., and J. M. Amelotti. 1968. Characterization of vitamin K from bovine liver. J. Lipid Res., 9:176-179.

_____ R. G. Bell, J. M. Amelotti, and T. E. Knauer. 1970. Isolation and characterization of a new metabolite of phylloquinone in the rat. Biochim. Biophys. Acta, 201:309-315.

Matthews, H. B., and F. Matsumura. 1969. Metabolic fate of dieldrin in the rat. J. Agr. Food Chem., 17:845-852.

McCloskey, J. A. (In press.) Mass spectrometry. *In* Ts'o, P. O. P., ed., Basic Principles in Nucleic Acid Chemistry. New York, Academic Press, Inc.

McLafferty, F. W., R. Venkataraghavan, and P. Irving, 1970. Determination of amino acid sequences in peptide mixtures by mass spectrometry. Biochem. Biophys. Res. Commun., 39:274-278.

McMahon, R. E., H. W. Culp, and J. C. Occolowitz. 1969. Studies on the hepatic microsomal N-dealkylation reaction. Molecular oxygen as the source of the oxygen atom. J. Amer. Chem. Soc., 91:3389.

_____ and J. L. Occolowitz. 1969. Nature of compounds uniformly labeled with radiocarbon in a benzene ring. J. Agr. Food Chem., 17:402-403.

Mechoulam, R., and Z. Ben-Zvi. 1968. On the nature of the beam test. Tetrahedron, 24:5615-5624.

Melo, A., W. H. Elliott, and L. Glaser. 1968. The mechanism of 6-deoxyhexose synthesis. Intramolecular hydrogen transfer catalyzed by deoxythymidine diphosphate D-glucose oxidoreductase. J. Biol. Chem., 243:1467-1474.

_____ and L. Glaser. 1968. The mechanism of 6-deoxyhexose synthesis. Conversion of deoxythymidine diphosphate 4-keto-6-deoxy-D-glucose to deoxythymidine diphosphate-L-rhammose. J. Biol. Chem., 243:1475-1478.

Miettinen, T. A., and T. Luukkainen. 1968. Gas-liquid chromatographic and mass spectrometric studies on sterols in *Vernix caseosa,* amniotic fluid and meconium. Acta Chem. Scand., 22:2603-2612.

Milne, G. W. A. 1971. The application of mass spectrometry to problems in medicine and biochemistry. *In* Milne, G. W. A., ed., Mass Spectrometry. New York, John Wiley and Sons.

Milne, T. A. 1969. Proposed use of nozzle-beam sampling of supercritical dense gases in the mass spectrometry of nonvolatile compounds. Int. J. Mass Spectrom. Ion Phys., 3:153-155.

Mize, C. E., J. Avigan, D. Steinberg, R. C. Pittmen, H. M. Fales, and G. W. A. Milne. 1969. A major pathway for the mammalian oxidative degradation of phytanic acid. Biochim. Biophys. Acta, 176:720-739.

Morton, G. O., G. E. Van Lear, and W. Fulmor. 1970. The structure of mitiromycin. J. Amer. Chem Soc., 92:2588-2590.

Moss, M. O., F. V. Robinson, and A. B. Wood. 1967. Observations on the structure of the toxins from *Penicillium rubrum.* Chem. Industr. (Britain), 755-758.

Murota, S., C. Fenselau, and P. Talalay, 1970. Partial purification of a beef adrenal Δ^5-3-ketosteroid isomerase and studies of its mechanism of action. Steroids, 17:25-37.

Muxfeldt, H., S. Shrader, P. Hansen, and H. Brockmann. 1968. The structure of pikromycin. J. Amer. Chem. Soc., 90:4748-4749.

Nakano, H., H. Inano, H. Sato, M. Shikita, and B. Tamaoki. 1967. Side-chain cleavage as related to steroid hormone synthesis. Biochim. Biophys. Acta, 137:335-346.

————— C. Takemoto, H. Sato, and B. Tamaoki. 1968. Location of hydroxy groups introduced to steroid molecules by adrenal and testicular enzymes. Biochim. Biophys. Acta, 152:186-196.

Nilsson, I. M., S. Agurell, J. L. G. Nilsson, A. Ohlsson, F. Sandberg, and M. Wahlqvist. 1970. Δ^1-tetrahydrocannabinol: structure of a major metabolite. Science, 168:1228-1229.

Occolowitz, J. L. 1968. Carbon-14 as a label in mass spectrometry. Chem. Commun., 1226-1227.

Owens, G., L. Belmusto, and S. Woldring. 1969. Experimental intracerebral pO_2 and pCO_2 monitoring by mass spectrography. J. Neurosurg., 30:110-115.

Palmer, K. H., M. S. Fowler, M. E. Wall, L. S. Rhodes, W. J. Waddell, and B. Baggett. 1969. The metabolism of R(+)- and RS-pentobarbital. J. Pharmacol. Exp. Ther., 170:355-363.

————— B. Martin, B. Baggett, and M. E. Wall. 1969. The metabolic fate of orally administered quinidine gluconate in humans. Biochem. Pharmac., 18:1845-1860.

————— F. T. Ross, L. S. Rhodes, B. Baggett, and M. E. Wall. 1969. Metabolism of antifertility steroids. J. Pharmacol. Exp. Ther., 167:207-216.

Parker, D. J., and W. S. Ruliffson. 1967. A mass spectrometric procedure for rapid identification of trace volatile metabolites. Anal. Biochem., 19:418-425.

Peaston, M. J. T., J. R. Bianchine, and C. Fenselau. 1971. Unpublished data.

Perel, J. M., R. F. Cunningham, H. M. Fales, and P. G. Dayton. 1970. Identification and quantitation of probenecid metabolites in man. Life Sciences, 9:1337-1343.

Philips, G. F., and R. J. Mesley. 1969. Examination of the hallucinogen 2,5-dimethoxy-4-methylamphetamine. J. Pharm. Pharmacol., 21:9-17.

Pinkus, J. L., D. Charles, and S. C. Chattoraj. 1971. Deuterium labeled steroids for study in humans. Estrogen production rates in normal pregnancy. J. Biol. Chem., 246:633-636.

Pohland, A., H. E. Boaz, and H. R. Sullivan. 1971. Synthesis and identification of metabolites resulting from the biotransformation of DL-methadone in man and in the rat. J. Med. Chem., 14:194-197.

Prouty, W. F., H. K. Schnoes, and F. M. Strong. 1969. A molecular weight revision for compounds of the oligomycin complex. Biochem. Biophys. Res. Commun., 34:511-516.

Rao, G. S. 1970. Identity of peyocactin, an antibiotic from peyote (*Lophophora williamsii*), and hordenine. J. Pharm. Pharmacol., 22:544-545.

Rhodes, R. C., R. W. Reiser, J. A. Gardiner, and H. Sherman. 1969. Identification of the metabolites of terbacil in dog urine. J. Agr. Food Chem., 17:974-979.

Rickards, R. W., R. M. Smith, and J. Majer. 1968. The structure of the macrolide antibiotic picromycin. Chem. Commun., 1049-1050.

Rinehart, K. L., Jr. 1969. Applications of mass spectrometry in structural and bio-synthetic studies. 158th National Meeting of the American Chemical Society, September 7-12, New York City. Division of Biological Chemistry, paper 8.

————— and M. L. Grostic. 1971. The use of stable isotopes in chemistry and bio-chemistry. *In* Milne, G. W. A., ed., Mass Spectrometry. New York, John Wiley and Sons.

————— and H. M. Mathur. 1968. Chemistry of the streptovaricins. Structure of varicinal A. J. Amer. Chem. Soc., 90:6241.

Rittenberg, D., A. S. Keston, F. Rosebury, and R. Schoenheimer. 1939. Studies in pro-tein metabolism II. The determination of nitrogen isotopes in organic compounds. J. Biol. Chem., 127:291-299.

Roboz, J. 1968. Introduction to Mass Spectrometry. New York, John Wiley and Sons.

Roth-Brandel, U., M. Bygdeman, N. Wigvist, and S. Bergstrom. 1970. Prostaglandins for induction of therapeutic abortion. Lancet, 1:190-191.

Ryhage, R., and B. Samuelsson. 1965. Origin of oxygen incorporated during the bio-synthesis of prostaglandin E_1. Biochem. Biophys. Res. Commun., 19:279-282.

Samuelsson, B. 1965. On the incorporation of oxygen in the conversion of 8,11,14-eicosatrienoic acid to prostaglandin E_1. J. Amer. Chem. Soc., 87:3011-3013.

Schwartz, M. A., P. Bommer, and F. Vane. 1967. Diazepam metabolites in the rat: characterization by high resolution mass spectrometry and nuclear magnetic resonance. Arch. Biochem., 121:508-516.

————— F. M. Vane, and E. Postma. 1968a. Urinary metabolites of 7-chloro-1-(2-diethylaminoethyl)-5-(2-fluorophenyl)-1,3-dihydro-2H-1,4-benzodiazepin-2-one di-hydrochloride. J. Med. Chem., 11:770-774.

————— F. M. Vane, and E. Postma. 1968b. Chlordiazepoxide metabolites in the rat. Characterization by high resolution mass spectrometry. Biochem. Pharmacol., 17:965-974.

Shackleton, C. H. L., R. W. Kelly, P. M. Adhikary, C. J. W. Brooks, R. A. Harkness, P. J. Sykes, and F. L. Mitchell. 1968. The identification and measurement of a new steroid 16β-hydroxydehydroepiandrosterone in infant urine. Steroids, 12:705-716.

————— and F. L. Mitchell. 1967. The measurement of 3β-hydroxy-Δ⁵ steroids in human fetal blood, amniotic fluid, infant urine and adult urine. Steroids, 10:359-385.

Sharkey, A. G., Jr., J. L. Shultz, T. Kessler, and R. A. Friedel. 1969. Determining organic contaminants in air and water. Research/Development, 30-32.

Shaw, S. J., D. M. Desiderio, K. Tsuboyama, and J. A. McCloskey. 1970. Mass spectrometry of nucleic acid components. Analogs of adenosine. J. Amer. Chem. Soc., 92:2510-2522.

Sheehan, J. C., D. Mania, S. Nakamura, J. A. Stock, and K. Maeda. 1968. The struc-ture of telomycin. J. Amer. Chem. Soc., 90:462-470.

Shemyakin, M. M., Y. A. Ovchinnikov, and A. A. Kiryushkin. 1971. Mass spectrometry in peptide chemistry. *In* Milne, G. W. A., ed., Mass Spectrometry. New York, John Wiley and Sons.

————— et al. 1970. The rational use of mass spectrometry for amino acid sequence determination in peptides and extension of the possibilities of the method. FEBS Letters, 7:8-12.

Sherman, W. R., M. A. Stewart, and M. Zinbo. 1969. Mass spectrometric study on the mechanism of D-glucose 6-phosphate-L-myo-inositol-1-phosphate cyclase. J. Biol. Chem., 244:5703-5708.

Shier, W. T., K. L. Rinehart, Jr., and D. Gottlieb. 1969. Preparation of four new antibiotics from a mutant of *Streptomyces fradiae*. Proc. Nat. Acad. Sci. U.S.A., 63:198-204.

Siegel, A. L., H. Aldercreutz, and T. Luukkainen. 1969. Gas chromatographic and mass spectrometric identification of neutral and phenolic steroids in amniotic fluid. Ann. Med. Exp. Fenn., 47:22-32.

Sih, C. J., G. Ambrus, P. Foss, and C. J. Lai. 1969. A general biochemical synthesis of oxygenated prostaglandins E. J. Amer. Chem. Soc., 91:3685-3687.

Sisenwine, S. F., and S. S. Walkenstein. 1969. The metabolic fate of the pteridine diuretic, Wy-5256. J. Pharm. Sci., 58:867-871.

Sjovall, J., and K. Sjovall. 1968. Identification of 5α-pregnane-3α,20α,21-trial in human pregnancy plasma. Steroids, 12:359-366.

Slusarchyk, W. A., and F. L. Weisenborn. 1969. The structure of the lipid portion of the antibiotic prasinomycin. Tetrahedron Lett., 659-662.

Smith, D. L., and M. F. Grostic. 1967. Mass spectrometric identification of the metabolites of methyl N-(o-aminophenyl)-N-(3-dimethylaminopropyl) anthranilate. J. Med. Chem., 10:375-379.

Smith, K., G. F. Thompson, and H. D. Koster. 1969. Sweat of schizophrenic patients: identification of the odorous substance. Science, 166:398-399.

Steinberg, D., C. E. Mize, J. Avigan, H. M. Fales, L. Eldjarn, K. Try, O. Stokke, and S. Refsum. 1967. Studies on the metabolic error in Refsum's disease. J. Clin. Invest., 46:313-322.

_____ C. E. Mize, J. H. Herndon, Jr., H. M. Fales, W. K. Engel, and F. Q. Vroom. 1970. Phytanic acid in patients with Refsum's syndrome and response to dietary treatment. Arch. Intern. Med., 125:75-87.

Steyn, P. S. 1970. The isolation, structure and absolute configuration of secalonic acid D, the toxic metabolite of *Penicillium oxalicum*. Tetrahedron, 26:51-57.

Strauch, B. S., H. M. Fales, R. C. Pittmen, and J. Avigan, 1969. Dimers and trimers of α-tocopherol: metabolic and synthetic studies. J. Nutr., 97:194-202.

Suda, T., H. F. DeLuca, H. K. Schnoes, Y. Tanaka, and M. F. Holick, 1970. 25,26-Dihydroxycholecalciferol, a metabolite of vitamin D_3 with intestinal calcium transport activity. Biochemistry (Washington), 9:4776-4780.

Suhadolnik, R. J., B. M. Chassy, and G. R. Waller. 1969. Isolation, structural elucidation and biological properties of 3′-acetamido-3′-deoxyadenosine from *Helminthosporium* sp. 215. Biochim. Biophys. Acta, 179:258-267.

Tanaka, K., and K. J. Isselbacher. 1967. The isolation and identification of N-isovaleryglycine from urine of patients with isovaleric acidemia. J. Biol. Chem., 242:2966-2972.

_____ J. C. Orr, and K. J. Isselbacher. 1968. Identification of β-hydroxyisovaleric acid in the urine of a patient with isovaleric acidemia. Biochim. Biophys. Acta, 152:638-641.

Terlain, B., and J. Thomas. 1969. The constitution of triselimycin, a polypeptide antibiotic extracted from *Streptomyces* culture. C. R. Acad. Sci. [C] (Paris), 269:1546-1549.

Tham, R., and B. Holmstedt. 1965. Gas chromatographic analysis of histamine metabolites in human urine. J. Chromatogr., 19:286-295.

_____ L. Nystrom, and B. Holmstedt. 1968. Identification by mass spectrometry of pyroglutamic acid as a peak in the gas chromatography of human urine. Biochem. Pharmacol., 17:1735-1738.

Thomas, D. W. 1969. Mass spectrometry of N-permethylated peptide derivatives; artifacts produced by C-methylation. FEBS Lett., 5:53-56.

————— and T. Ito. 1969. The revised structure of the peptide antibiotic esperin, established by mass spectrometry. Tetrahedron, 25:1985-1990.

Thomson, J. J. 1913. Rays of Positive Electricity and Their Application to Chemical Analysis. London, Longmans Green and Co.

Thorpe, S. R., and C. C. Sweeley. 1967. Chemistry and metabolism of sphingolipids. On the biosynthesis of phytosphingosine by yeast. Biochemistry (Washington), 6:887-897.

Tokuyama, T., J. Daly, and B. Witkop. 1969. The structure of batrachotoxin, a steroidol alkaloid from the Colombian arrow poison frog, *Phyllobates aurotaenia*, and partial synthesis of batrachotoxin and its analogs and homologs. J. Amer. Chem. Soc., 91:3931-3938.

Trendelenburg, F. 1969. Mass spectrometric gas analysis and provocation tests in asthma. Respiration, 26, Suppl.: 163-166.

Tschesche, R., and G. Marwede. 1967. Digitanolglykoside zur Konstitution zweier Esteraglykone aus *Caralluma dalzielii*. Tetrahedron Lett., 1359-1363.

Tsuji, K., and J. H. Robertson. 1969. Gas-liquid chromatographic determination of neomycins B and C. Anal. Chem., 41:1332-1335.

Ungar, G., I. K. Ho, L. Galvan, and D. M. Desiderio. 1970. Isolation and identification of a specific behavior-inducing peptide extracted from brain. Proc. West. Pharmacol. Soc., Jan. 30.

Vandenheuvel, W. J. A., and J. S. Cohen. 1970. Gas-liquid chromatography—mass spectrometry of carbon-13 enriched amino acids as trimethylsilyl derivatives. Biochim. Biophys. Acta, 208:251-259.

Vane, F., and M. G. Horning, 1969. Separation and characterization of the prostaglandins by gas chromatography and mass spectrometry. Anal. Lett., 2:357-371.

Van Lear, G. E., and F. W. McLafferty. 1969. Biochemical aspects of high resolution mass spectrometry. Ann. Rev. Biochem., 38:289-321.

Vestal, M. L. 1970. Chemical ionization source for the quadrupole mass spectrometer. Eighteenth Annual Conference on Mass Spectrometry and Allied Topics, June 14-19, San Francisco.

Vetter, W., M. Vecchi, M. Gutmann, R. Ruegg, W. Walther, and P. Meyer. 1967. Gas-chromatographische und massenspectrometrische Untersuchung von Phytylubichinon, Vitamin K₁ und Vitamin K₂. Helv. Chim. Acta, 50:1866-1879.

Vollner, L., D. Bierniek, and F. Korte. 1969. Cannabidivarin, ein neurer Haschisch-Inhaltsstoff. Tetrahedron Lett., 145-147.

Von Spulak, F., U. Claussen, H. Fehlhaber, and F. Korte. 1968. Cannabidiolcarbonsaure-Tetrahydrocannabitriol-Ester, ein neuer Haschisch-Inhaltsstoff. Tetrahedron, 24:5379-5383.

Wade, A. P., G. S. Wilkinson, F. M. Dean, and A. W. Price. 1966. The isolation, characterization and structure of uroterpenol, a monoterpene from human urine. Biochem. J., 101:727-734.

Wall, M. E., D. R. Brine, G. A. Brine, C. G. Pitt, R. I. Freudenthal, and H. D. Christensen. 1970. Isolation, structure and biological activity of several metabolites of O⁹-tetrahydrocannabinol. J. Amer. Chem. Soc., 92:3466-3468.

Waller, G. R., R. Ryhage, and S. Meyerson. 1966. Mass spectrometry of biosynthetically labeled ricinine. Anal. Biochem., 16:277-286.

Walser, M. 1970. Use of isotopic urea to study the distribution and degradation of urea in man. *In* Schmidt-Nielsen, B., ed., Urea and the Kidney, 421-429. Amsterdam, Excerpta Medica Foundation.

————— J. George, and L. J. Bodenlos. 1954. Altered proportions of isotopes of molecular nitrogen as evidence for a monomolecular reaction. J. Chem. Phys., 22:1146.

Watson, J. T. 1969. Gas chromatography and mass spectroscopy. *In* Ettre, L. S., and

W. H. McFadden, eds., Ancillary Techniques for Gas Chromatography. New York, John Wiley and Sons.

Weinig, E., G. Machbert, and P. Zink. 1966. Über den Nachweis des Dieldrins bei einer Dieldrinvergiftung. Arch. Toxik., 22:115-124.

Williams, C. M., A. H. Porter, M. Greer, K. N. Scott, and C. C. Sweeley. 1969. Identification of urinary N-(phenylacetyl)-L-glutamic acid in neuroblastoma. Biochem. Med., 3:164-176.

Woldring, S., G. Owens, and D. C. Woolford. 1966. Blood gases. Continuous in vivo recording of partial pressures by mass spectrography. Science, 153:885-887.

Yamauchi, T., Y. Shoyama, Y. Matsuo, and I. Nishioka. 1968. Cannabigerol monomethyl ether, a new component of hemp. Chem. Pharm. Bull. (Tokyo), 16:1164-1165.

Chapter **13**

Oscillographic Polarography

Raymond J. Gajan

Division of Chemistry and Physics, Food and Drug Administration,
Department of Health, Education, and Welfare, Washington, D.C.

INTRODUCTION

Polarography, a powerful but often neglected technique, is used for the detection, identification, and determination of trace components present in less than microgram amounts. It is equal to and sometimes better than many classical methods for the determination of major components of a sample.

With the advent of newer and more versatile polarographs this technique appears even more promising for the determination of trace amounts of drugs, pesticides, and other foreign organic compounds present in micro and submicro amounts in biological material.

This chapter will be devoted to oscillographic polarography and the ways in which this powerful technique may be utilized in the study of drugs, drug metabolites, and/or their breakdown products. For the purpose of this discussion oscillographic polarography is defined as any process whereby polarographic phenomena are displayed on a cathode ray oscilloscope.

Basic Principles

Professor Jaroslov Heyrovsky of Charles University, Prague, Czechoslovakia, first introduced polarography in 1922. Thirty-seven years later he was awarded the 1959 Nobel prize in chemistry for the discovery and development of this important analytical technique.

Heyrovsky (1956a) defined polarography as the science of studying the processes occurring at the dropping mercury electrode. He limited the term *polar-*

443

ography to capillary mercury electrodes such as the dropping mercury electrode, the streaming mercury electrode, and the hanging drop electrode, because of their unique property of giving exactly reproducible results.

Polarography therefore is that field of electrochemistry which is concerned with interpretations of current-voltage relationships occurring during the electrolysis of a solution between two electrodes, one of which is small and polarizable, and the other large and nonpolarizable. The polarized or polarizable electrode, i.e., a dropping mercury electrode, adapts the potential externally impressed on it with little or no change in current. The depolarized or nonpolarizable electrode retains a constant potential independent of the current and is not altered by the changes in applied potential. Therefore, if only one electrode in a cell is polarizable, its potential will change by the same amount as the change in applied potential.

Polarography consists of gradually applying an increasing potential difference between a polarizable and a nonpolarizable electrode in a solution and measuring the currents produced in microamperes. These currents are caused by the migration of ions to the dropping mercury electrode in the electrical gradient set up around it and the diffusion of ions into a concentration gradient formed by the removal of ions from the solution immediately surrounding the electrode. This latter current is called the *diffusion current* and is the current of interest in polarography.

The current due to migration of ions to the dropping mercury electrode is suppressed by adding a neutral salt to the solution in a concentration of at least 35 times that of the oxidizable or reducible substances. This neutral salt is called the *supporting* or *base* electrolyte and is not itself oxidized or reduced over the potential range being studied. This salt also serves to increase the electrical conductivity of the solution, and in so doing decreases the potential or IR drop through the cell.

If a solution contains an oxidizable or reducible substance, a reaction takes place at the dropping mercury electrode. The potential at which this reaction takes place is a function of the reduction or oxidation potential of the electroactive species and, in a given solution, is characteristic of the substance being oxidized or reduced. The diffusion current produced depends on the concentration of the oxidizable or reducible substance in the solution. A typical current voltage curve is shown in Figure 1.

As the potential increases from *A* to *B*, no reduction takes place at the dropping mercury electrode and we note a small steady increase in current. This is known as the *residual current;* it is independent of any specific ion. The reduction potential of a reducible ion in the solution is reached at *B*, and the current increases sharply to *C*. At this point the effective concentration of the reacting ion at the dropping mercury electrode is zero; the diffusion rate becomes constant and is proportional to the concentration of the reacting ions in the rest of the solution. A state of concentration polarization now exists at the dropping mercury electrode and a steady current flows as indicated, from *C* to *D*. This current is known as the *limiting current*. The difference between the *limiting current* and the *residual current* is known as the *diffusion current;* it is proportional to the concentration of the reacting ion in the solution.

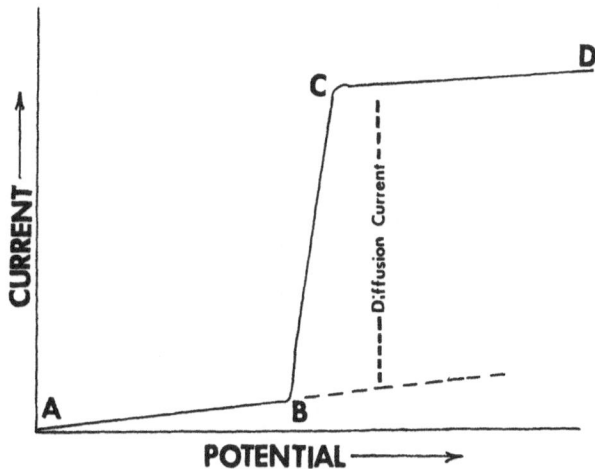

FIG. 1. Typical current voltage curves. (From Gajan. 1965. *J. Assoc. Offic. Anal. Chem.*, 45: 1028-1037.)

Since it is difficult to measure the reduction potential accurately, the potential at which the diffusion current reaches half the value of the limiting current is used. This is a physical constant; it is practically independent of the concentration and is characteristic of the electroactive substance. This potential is called the *half-wave potential* of the electroactive substance, or $E_{1/2}$. Since the half-wave potential of a substance depends on the base electrolyte and the reference electrode used, these parameters should be specified when an $E_{1/2}$ value is cited.

The theoretical aspects of these various polarographic currents have been studied extensively and equations for them have been formulated by Ilkovič (1934) and many others. Detailed accounts of the derivations of these equations may be found in the original papers or in one of the many basic texts on polarography such as those by Milner (1957), Meites (1965), Kolthoff and Lingane (1965), and Heyrovsky and Kuta (1966). An excellent short text for the beginner is that of Heyrovsky and Zuman (1968).

OSCILLOGRAPHIC POLAROGRAPHY

Theory

The cathode ray oscillograph was first used in polarography by Matheson and Nicols (1938). About the same time a similar polarograph was described by Müller and coworkers (1938). The oscilloscope, because of its rapid response, was originally used to shorten the time of a polarographic analysis. However, it was found that the resulting polarotraces differed fundamentally from those of classical polarography and thus increased the potential versatility of the technique.

Among the many investigators who have contributed to the development of both the theory and applications of oscillographic polarography are Heyrovsky and

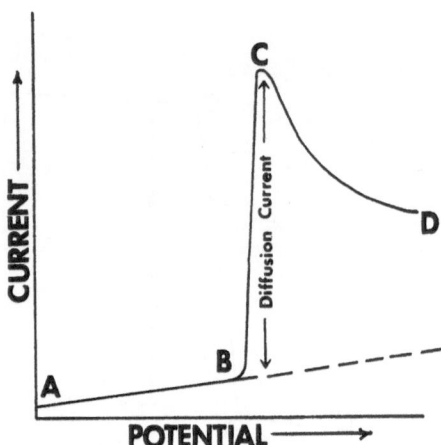

FIG. 2. A typical cathode ray polarotrace. (From Gajan. 1965. *J. Assoc. Offic. Anal. Chem.,* 45: 1028-1037.)

Forejt (1943), Randles (1947), Airey (1947), Ševčik (1948), Delahay (1949), Snowden and Page (1950), and Reynolds and Davis (1953). Loveland and Elving (1952) have written a comprehensive review on oscillographic polarography. Kalvoda (1965) has produced an excellent book on the subject.

Two radically different techniques are used in using the cathode ray oscilloscope in polarography. In the first technique, commonly referred to as the single sweep method, the entire change of potential is effected during the life of a single drop. The resulting curve is observed on a cathode ray oscilloscope. To obtain reproducible results the sweep is synchronized with the dropping rate of the electrode and is confined to the last few seconds of its drop life when its growth rate is smallest. The drop time is usually set at 7 to 10 seconds and the sweep time at about 2 seconds, thus leaving a delay period of 5 to 8 seconds during which time each new drop is forming. The rate of change of cell potential is fixed, usually at 0.3 volt per second. The starting potential may be varied from +4.5 volts to −4.5 volts depending on the instrument used. A typical cathode ray polarotrace is shown in Figure 2.

In the polarotrace shown in Figure 2, the *residual current* is the portion from A to B, the *diffusion current* from B to C, and the *limiting current* C to D. The peak height *BC* is proportional to the concentration of the substance being oxidized or reduced at the dropping mercury electrode, and because of various factors the sensitivity of the technique is greatly increased over that of conventional polarography. The main factor is the elimination of the drop wave, i.e., curves due to the growth and fall of successive drops. The potential at the peak C is known as the *peak potential*; it closely resembles the $E_{1/2}$ of conventional polarography and is usually about 0.05 volt more negative than the conventional half-wave potential. Equations for these waves have been formulated by Delahay (1949) and Randles (1947).

By circuit modifications it is possible to use this type of instrument for derivative polarography in which the rate of change of the direct wave di/dE vs. E is measured instead of C (current) vs. E (volts). The derivative waves occur in the form of peaks on the oscilloscope at a point of inflection analogous to the half-wave potentials of the substance being polarographed. Better resolution but less sensitivity is achieved by using this derivative circuit.

The second method using the cathode ray oscilloscope was developed by Heyrovsky and Forejt (1943) and is referred to as the multisweep method, or oscillographic polarography with alternating current. They devised a polarograph which produced a potential time relationship or its derivatives $\dfrac{dE}{dt}=f(t)$, or dE/dt vs. E. In this technique an alternating current from a 50-Hz source at constant amplitude is regulated to charge the dropping mercury electrode from 0 to -2.0 volts in a hundredth of a second and then back to zero volt in the next hundredth of a second. The frequency of the time sweep is synchronized with the applied alternating current-voltage to produce a stationary potential-time figure on the oscilloscope. Any process resulting in a flow of current at the dropping mercury electrode produces a horizontal inflection on the potential time curve. Thus in this technique the tracings on the oscilloscope indicate depolarization by kinks or lags on the curves. Each depolarizer, that is, the substance which reacts at the dropping mercury electrode, shows one or two kinks, one on the cathodic or upper portion of the polarotrace and, if the reduction is reversible, another on the anodic portion. A typical oscillopolarotrace is shown in Figure 3.

The upper portion of this polarotrace from A to B denotes the cathodic polarization in the potential range scanned, usually from 0 volt to -2.0 volts. The bottom portion of the polarotrace from B to A denotes anodic polarization from -2.0 volts to 0 volts. The horizontal deflections denote the half-wave potential of the depolarizer, that is, the substance being reduced or oxidized at the dropping mercury electrode. The depth of the cut denotes the diffusion current and is proportional to the concentration of the depolarizer. If the depolarizer gives an anodic cut and a cathodic cut at the same potential (cuts a and a' in Figure 3),

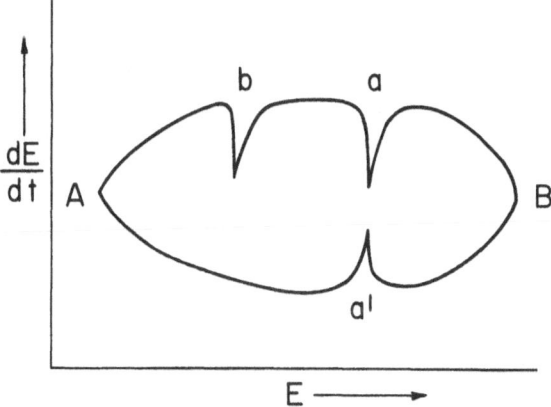

FIG. 3. A typical oscillopolarotrace.

the reaction at the dropping mercury electrode is said to be reversible. If the cuts are at a different potential or one of them is missing, for example, cut *b*, the reaction at the dropping mercury electrode is irreversible.

The multisweep technique is able to detect and measure many reactions at the dropping mercury electrode that cannot be measured by conventional polarography. For example, Heyrovsky (1957) was able to detect and measure *o*-, *p*-, and *m*-nitrophenols in the presence of nitrobenzene.

Another interesting phenomenon specific for this technique is the formation of artifacts. Kalvoda (1965) suggested that the artifacts were due to the formation of new products at the electrode caused by the periodic repetition of the alternating current. For example, Heyrovsky (1965a) reported that, when vapors of carbon disulfide were polarographed, they gave the cut-ins for sulfur anions or hydrogen sulfide. He thought that the carbon disulfide was reduced at negative potentials above -1.5 volts to sulfur anions which formed cut-ins at -0.6 volt. In this case the artifact was the sulfur anion. When the direct current was adjusted so that it did not reach -1.5 volts, the cut-in due to the artifact disappeared.

Oscillographic polarography with alternating current, the multisweep method, is preferred for qualitative analyses and kinetic studies because of its greater resolution and because many more substances can be polarographed by this technique.

The single sweep method is preferred for quantitative analysis because of its greater accuracy and sensitivity, and because it is not subject to errors caused by variation in drop size or by too many sweeps applied to the same drop as in the multisweep method.

Instrumentation

A number of newer and more sophisticated instruments that can be used for oscillographic polarography are now commercially available.

Southern Analytical Ltd. of Surrey, England, has developed a single sweep, differential type of instrument called the Davis Differential Cathode-Ray Polarotrace A1660. This instrument was described by Davis and Rooney (1962) and is designed so that the signal obtained from a reference cell can be subtracted from the signal obtained from a cell containing the sample solution. The dropping mercury electrodes of the two cells are matched to give identical signals from identical solutions. In this single sweep instrument the potential change is rapidly applied and is restricted to the lifetime of a single drop. The trace observed represents the electrode reaction taking place during the last two seconds of drop life when its growth rate is smallest. There is a five-second delay period during which each drop is growing. Thus a complete polarotrace is obtained every seven seconds, the lifetime of each drop. The drop time is automatically synchronized.

The Davis Differential Cathode-Ray Polarotrace may be operated in four distinct modes:

1. The *subtractive mode,* in which one cell contains the sample solution and the other cell contains a sample or reagent blank. Any effects due to reagent impurities are cancelled so that the sensitivity of the instrument is greatly increased.

2. The *comparative mode,* which is used when the approximate composition of the sample is known. One cell contains the sample solution and the other cell contains an accurately known standard of similar composition. The difference in wave height is due to the differences in composition. Measurements can be made with a precision of $\pm 0.1\%$. This mode of operation is most useful in the analysis of major components, i.e., primary standards, alloys, and similar substances.

3. The *twin cell derivative mode,* in which both cells contain the same solution and a small preset difference is maintained between applied potentials. This mode results in a derivative wave form that permits its resolution of waves only 0.04 volt apart. When a parallel resistance capacitance network is introduced into the amplifier system, a second derivative is obtained; this second derivative results in resolution of peaks 0.025 volt apart.

4. The fourth mode of operation is a *single celled instrument.*

The instrument has provision for baseline slope compensation and current zoning controls so that it is possible to measure a very low concentration of the substance in the presence of much higher amounts (1000:1) of a more electropositive or electronegative ion depending on the oxidation or reduction of the substance to be measured.

The instrument may be operated either in a forward or reverse sweep in increments of 0.5 volt from 0 volt to 2.5 volts starting potential. Provisions are made for compensation of the starting current and capacity current. With this instrument, Maienthal and Taylor (1968) were able to determine copper, lead, and zinc in water and acids, in concentrations of less than one part per billion (ppb).

Another dual cell oscillographic polarograph has recently been developed by Chemtrix, Inc., Beaverton, Oregon. This instrument is called the Chemtrix Type SSP-5. With this instrument the display polarotrace can be stored on the face of the cathode ray tube for study and other traces can be added as desired. The scan ranges are 0.5 volt, 1.0 volt, and 2.0 volts, and the scan rates are 0.01, 0.02, 0.05, 0.1, 0.2, and 1 second per division, with the starting potential being adjustable from $+2.0$ to -2.0 volts. The dual dropping mercury assembly is designed for both three-electrode and two-electrode operations. In three-electrode operations the potential applied to the polarographic cell is automatically controlled on a continuous basis to compensate for the effects of electrolyte resistance. In addition to the differential operation, either cell can be used for single cell or cyclic voltammetry. Using the Chemtrix SSP-5, Griffin (1969) determined selenium in a concentration of one ppb.

Several multipurpose electrochemical instruments now available are capable of both single sweep and cyclic voltammetry. These instruments should be a valuable asset to any electrochemical laboratory. In addition to voltammetry, they are designed for potential sweep chronoamperometry, stripping analysis, three-electrode polarography, controlled voltage coulometry, solid electrode voltammetry, controlled voltage electrodeposition and separation, and chronopotentiometry. Instruments now available are the Beckman Electroscan 30, manufactured by Beckman Instruments, Inc., Fullerton, California 92634; the Polarographic Analyzers, Models 170 and 171, manufactured by Princeton Applied Research Corp., Princeton, N.J. 08540; the NIL Electrolabs, manufactured by National Instrument Laboratories, Inc., Rockville, Md. 20852; the MP 1660 console electronic module system, manufactured by McKee-Pedersen Instruments, Danville, California 94526; and the Heath, Malmstadt, Euke controlled potential polarography system manufactured by Heath Co., Benton Harbor, Michigan 49023.

For cyclic or multisweep techniques Kalvoda (1965) recommends the LP600 Polaroscope, manufactured by Labortorui Pristorje, n.p., Prague, Czechoslovakia.

The most common reference electrodes are the standard calomel electrode, the mercury pool electrode, and the silver wire electrode. The silver wire reference electrode (a #20 or #22 silver wire coated with a very thin layer of silver chloride) is generally preferred for trace analysis with the single cell instruments. This electrode is suitable for microanalysis and for routine work because it does not require special cells, does not take up much room, and is easy to clean or replace. Mercury pool electrodes are preferred for dual cell differential polarography since they are more easily reproduced. That is, since each cell has the same reference electrode, it is easier to balance the cells.

There are many different polarographic cells. Zagorski (1962), in his comprehensive review on the various cells and their uses, states: "Because all the phenomena of polarographic electrolysis occur at the surface of the mercury drop the volume and shape of the cell containing the solution has little effect on the reaction." Polarographic analyses have been carried out in large volumes of solution (such as an ocean) on the one hand, and in only a fraction of a milliliter on the other.

Clean mercury is essential for polarographic analysis. Mercury cleaned by the method of Gordon and Wichers (1957) is sufficiently pure for organic analysis. Triple distillation is necessary only when mercury has become contaminated by noble metals. A modification of the Gordon and Wichers method is as follows:

> Transfer mercury to a 1-liter thick-walled filtering flask. Add 250 ml of 20% (v/v) HNO_3 and bubble a strong air current through the solution mixture for 4 to 6 hours. Transfer the mixture to a separatory funnel and draw off the mercury into a clean, dry 1-liter filtering flask. Add 250 ml of distilled H_2O and bubble air through the mixture for about 2 hours. Pour off the H_2O layer and check its pH. Continue washing the mercury with distilled H_2O in this manner until the H_2O is neutral. Transfer the mercury and H_2O to a separatory funnel and draw off the mercury through a filter paper, S & S #589 or equivalent, having a pin hole at the apex. Collect the mercury in a clean, dry

beaker. Repeat the pin-hole filtration twice more and collect the mercury in a clean, dry bottle with a standard taper glass stopper for storage.

GENERAL PROCEDURES

Any compound that contains highly polar or conjugated unsaturated groups can probably be polarographically reduced or oxidized at the dropping mercury electrode. The polarographic reactions of these groups are influenced by the rest of their molecules. Thus the determination of these functional groups affords a means of determining the whole molecule. Moreover, a polarographic reduction or oxidation obtained at a specific peak potential under a definite set of conditions provides a clue to some of the structural characteristics of the substance being polarographed.

In contrast to inorganic polarography, in which most of the reactions are reversible, reactions of most of the organic functional groups that are polarographed are irreversible. Table 1 lists some of the irreversible functional groups.

Many heterocyclic and organometallic compounds also produce irreversible waves. Reversible reactions have been attributed to the quinoidal compounds such as benzoquinone and naphthoquinone. Certain functional groups such as the thiols,

R-SH, and the diethyl dithiocarbamates, $R_2-N-C\overset{\displaystyle S}{\underset{\displaystyle S}{\diagdown}}$, yield insoluble or complex

compounds with mercury, and these compounds give anodic waves. Some nitrogen-containing heterocyclics produce catalytic hydrogen waves. In the presence of ammoniacal cobalt and nickel solutions, other compounds such as cysteine and proteins give catalytic waves. This type of compound usually contains at least one atom of sulfur. This cobalt-catalyzed wave is the basis for the Brdička (1933) protein index reaction for the detection of cancer.

Zuman (1964) divides organic polarographic analysis into two main categories: direct methods and indirect methods. Direct methods are those in which the samples are dissolved, the electrolyte is added, and the resulting solution is polarographed. Indirect methods are used for those compounds which are polarographically unreactive in themselves but can be transformed by a chemical reaction into reaction derivatives. The reactions most commonly used for indirect polarography are nitration, nitrosation, condensation, addition, substitution, oxidation, hydrolysis, and complex formation. Drug metabolites and breakdown products may also fall into this category.

Polarographic methods, like other techniques, require some sort of preliminary separation or cleanup. The techniques most commonly used are extraction, distillation, dialysis, electrophoresis, precipitation, complex formation, and chromatography.

In the development of a polarographic procedure, first the structure of the

TABLE 1

Common Irreversible
Functional Groups

Functional Groups	Examples
Conjugated double or triple	*butadiene*

-C=C-C=C-

-C≡C-C≡C-

```
H   H   H   H
|   |   |   |
C=C  -C=C
|        |
H        H
```

Carbon-halogen   *chloroform*

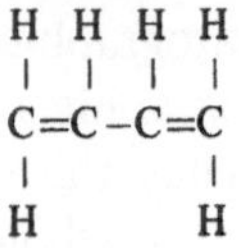

C-X

```
      Cl
      |
  H-C-Cl
      |
      Cl
```

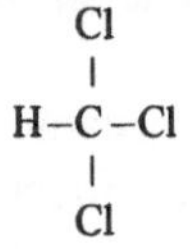

Carbon-oxygen   *formaldehyde*

```
\
 C=O
/
```

```
        O
        ‖
   H-C
        \
         H
```

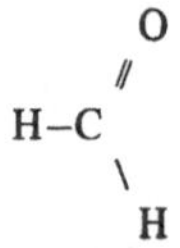

Carbon-nitrogen   *acetamidine*

```
\
 C=N
/
```

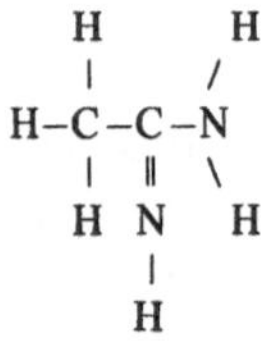

```
   H        H
   |       /
H-C-C-N
   |  ‖   \
   H  N   H
      |
      H
```

Nitrogen-nitrogen   *azobenzene*

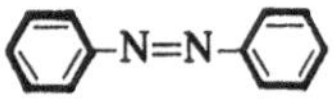

-N=N-

Nitrogen-oxygen   *nitrobenzene*

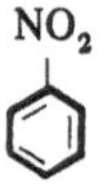

-N=O

Carbon-sulfur   *diphenylsulfone*

-C-S

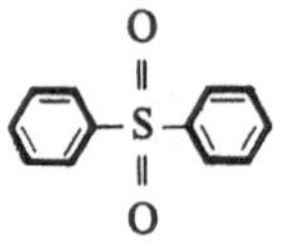

compound under investigation is examined for the presence of a polarographically reactive functional group or for reactions necessary to obtain a derivative possessing such a group. Next, the literature on polarographic procedures is searched for the best way to polarograph these groups. The most helpful sources are "Polarography in Medicine, Biochemistry, and Pharmacy" by Brezina and Zuman (1958) and "Polarography" in two volumes by Kolthoff and Lingane (1965). Of particular interest and assistance to biochemists is a book on electroanalytical methods by Purdy (1965). A very useful text for beginners is "Practical Polarography" by Heyrovsky and Zuman (1968).

The review articles on organic polarography by Wawzonek (1949, 1950, 1952, 1954, 1956, 1958, 1960, and 1962), Wawzonek and Pietrzyk (1964), and Pietrzyk (1966, 1968, and 1970) are also very helpful.

To be polarographed a compound must be in solution and must remain in solution after addition of the base or supporting electrolyte. Because of the low solubility of many organic substances, special solvents are required. Acetone, methanol, and ethanol are most commonly used. Others are acetonitrile, dimethylsulfoxide, dimethylformamide, pyridine, and dioxane. Mixtures of these solvents with less polar solvents such as benzene, hexane, ether, and petroleum ether are also used. Generally, to be usable the solvent system must be miscible with water, although completely nonaqueous systems have been used.

In the selection of a solvent-electrolyte system care must be taken that no interfering substances are present. Substances may interfere either by having similar half-wave potentials or by being present in an amount many times greater than the compound of interest and polarographing before it. Most of the interferences encountered in organic polarography may be traced to impurities, either in the solvent or in the electrolyte solution. Therefore, it is recommended that all solvents be purified and checked frequently for impurities by polarographing a solution containing only the solvent and electrolyte and checking for interfering waves over the potential range of interest. The electrolytes most used are the salts of the alkali metals (potassium, sodium, and lithium), and the salts of the tetraalkylammonium compounds. These salts must also be checked for purity, since they too may contribute interferences to the system.

The choice of solvent and electrolyte are very important; they are to polarography what column packing and carrier gas are to gas-liquid chromatography. The half-wave potential and the ease of oxidation or reduction at the dropping mercury electrode are directly dependent on them. For example, in a mixture containing compounds A and B, A may polarograph before B in one system, and B before A in another. Many interferences may also be eliminated by the proper choice of electrolyte system.

Often when the polarographic behavior of a compound or one of similar composition is reported in the literature, only minor changes, if any, are necessary in adapting these methods for oscillopolarographic analysis. Conversely, because of the difference in electronics and other factors, many of the methods described in the literature based on the conventional type of polarographs are not suitable for oscillopolarography unless some modifications are made, such as increasing the strength of the electrolytes from $0.1N$ to $1.0N$ or from $0.01N$ to $0.1N$. A systematic approach is necessary if the polarographic behavior of the compound of interest is unknown.

A convenient plan is as follows: Prepare standard solutions containing 50 and 100 μg/ml of the compound in various solvents. Next prepare several typical electrolyte solutions such as $0.1N$ HCl, NaOH, NaCl, LiCl, NH$_4$Cl, NH$_4$OH, NaOAc, (CH$_3$)$_4$NBr, and mixtures of these solutions. (The various buffer systems such as those of McIlvaine and Britton-Robinson are also used.) Then add various ratios of sample solutions and electrolyte solution to a polarographic cell. Bubble prepurified nitrogen through the solution for three to five minutes depending on the volatility of the solvent being used, and polarograph over the entire range of the electrolyte used to find a usable polarographic wave. (Nitrogen is bubbled through the solution to remove any oxygen present, which will polarograph and interfere with the polarographs of interest.)

After the best solvent electrolyte system is established, study the effects of pH, temperature, and concentration on the compound being polarographed.

Check the minimum and maximum amounts of compound which can be polarographed, since this varies from compound to compound. (The peak or half-wave potential of many compounds shifts with concentration. However, in the range of concentration usually encountered in trace analysis this phenomenon is rarely, if ever, observed.) Next, determine the type and amount of cleanup necessary for sample analysis. In some instances, a compound can be polarographed after solvent extraction without further cleanup, in which case a slight shift in peak potential may occur due to viscosity and other properties of the uncleaned solutions in the polarographic cells.

The extraction and cleanup procedures used for other trace techniques are usually sufficient for polarographic analysis. Again, all reagents used, especially solvents, should be purified and checked. Occasionally interferences originating in the column packing or drying agents are found. If thin-layer chromatography is used in conjunction with polarography, the adsorbents used on TLC plates should also be checked.

In polarographic analysis the wave height observed from the sample solution is compared to that obtained from polarographing a standard solution at the same time and under the same conditions. This is known as the *comparative method*. Another technique is to add a known amount of a standard to the cell solution and note any increase in wave height. From this increase in wave height the amount of compound in the sample can be calculated after correcting for volume change. This technique, called *standard addition*, is a valuable check on the qualitative determination, since the half-wave potential of the standard added and the compound in the sample should match if they are the same compound.

Polarography, like most other instrumental techniques, is a comparative technique and therefore requires a standard reference material. This standard material must be a well-defined compound whose chemical composition and purity are known and adequately verified by the several techniques available for such purposes.

APPLICATIONS

Determination of the Elements

The single sweep method has been used by a number of investigators to determine trace amounts of elements in various substances, such as bismuth, cadmium, cobalt, copper, manganese, nickel, molybdenum, lead, antimony, tellurium, vanadium, and zinc in plants (Nangnoit, 1964); copper, lead, tin, and zinc in food in the range of 0.1 to 2.5 ppm (Condliffe and Skrimshire, 1961); 0.1 ppm of aluminum, arsenic, cadmium, copper, indium, iodine, iron, lead, tellurium, and zinc in water with a precision of better than 1% (Maienthal and Taylor, 1968); 0.5 ppb arsenic in well water (single sweep dual celled instrument) with a relative accuracy of 5 to 10% of the actual concentration (Whitnack and Brophy, 1969); tin in beer at a level of 0.007 μg/ml (Rooney, 1963); and 0.01 ppm antimony in water (Toren, 1968).

Cernik (1967) compared dry and wet ashing methods for determination of blood level by cathode ray polarography. Within a range of 16 to 200 μg per 100 ml of blood he recovered 82 to 100% by the dry ash technique.

Irving and Watts (1961) developed a polarographic procedure to determine calcium and magnesium in blood serum. Their method compared favorably with the existing chemical procedures.

Fichera and Ferrara (1969) utilized oscillopolarography to determine copper, zinc, molybdenum, and iron in vegetables. The limit of sensitivity of their procedure was 0.03 μg/ml for copper, 0.05 μg/ml for zinc and iron, and 0.01 μg/ml for molybdenum.

In FDA laboratories we have used a single sweep dual cell polarograph to determine copper at 0.02 ppm and tin, lead, zinc, and cadmium at 0.05 ppm. We have also determined sulfur, cyanide, arsenic, and iron in foods.

Organic Compounds

Most of our investigations at FDA have dealt with the determination of pesticides and other residues. Table 2 lists the sensitivity of some of the methods we have developed.

Datta and Gajan (1965) applied the Brdička protein reaction to the study of the effects of aflatoxin-B, a toxic metabolite of the fungus *Aspergillus flavus* Link, on the plasma of ducklings fed the metabolite.

The Brdička protein reaction is based on a catalytic wave observed when a protein solution is added to a buffered ammoniacal solution of cobalt salts. These catalytic waves have also been obtained by polarographing low molecular weight compounds containing sulfur, such as certain amino acids, polypeptides, and proteins. Brdička (1933) found that these polarographic waves revealed dif-

TABLE 2

Sensitivity of Polarographic Residue Analysis[a]

Residue	Pure Electrolyte (μg/ml)	Actual Crop (ppm)	Reference
Parathion	0.004	0.04	Gajan (1963)
Diazinon	0.20	0.20	Gajan (1969)
Malathion	0.20	0.30	Gajan (1969)
Guthion	0.025	0.04	Gajan and Gaither (1968)
Carbaryl	0.02	0.20	Gajan et al. (1965)
Dimethoate	0.025	0.05	Gajan and Gaither (1968)
Systox	0.25	0.25	Gajan (1962)
PCNB	0.02	0.02	Klein and Gajan (1961)
DDT	0.05	0.05	Gajan and Link (1964)
Fumaric Acid	< 1.0	< 1.0	Smith and Gajan (1965)
Aflatoxin B	0.3		Gajan et al. (1964a)
Aflatoxin G	0.3		Gajan et al. (1964a)

[a]From Gajan. 1965. *J. Ass. Offic. Anal. Chem.*, 45:1028-1037.

ferences between plasma taken from cancer patients and that from normal individuals. This is not strange since the presence and the state of these groups in blood and other biological materials reflect the pathological changes in the organisms. The Brdička reaction has been applied not only to clinical diagnosis and prognosis of malignancies and other diseases, but also in biochemical studies of native and denatured proteins. This technique has been applied chiefly in the clinical laboratories of central Europe, where the technique is best understood. Details of the procedure may be found in O. H. Müller's (1963) fine review of the subject.

In an attempt to correlate the results obtained by this procedure, Müller and Davis (1945) suggested that two tests be run under identical conditions and the ratio of the values obtained by these tests used as an index characteristic of the given unknown. This ratio has become known as the Brdička Protein Index.

In one test the oxalated plasma or other biological material is digested with potassium hydroxide, then reacted with ammoniacal cobaltous chloride, and polarographed. In the other test, called the filtrate test, the oxalated plasma is treated with potassium hydroxide followed by a precipitation step using sulfosalicylic acid, and then filtered. The clear filtrate is then reacted with an ammoniacal hexamine cobaltic chloride solution and polarographed. The protein index is obtained from the ratio of the heights of the polarographic waves obtained in the filtrate test, and the digest test is multiplied by an arbitrary constant of 15. In general the values for the digest test tend to decrease and those for the filtrate test tend to increase, with cancer-type infections showing a marked increase in the index value. For hepatitis-type disorders the index shows a decrease in value. In our experiments the ducklings fed aflatoxin-B yielded results significantly higher than those obtained with the controls. These results were correlated with those obtained by histopathological examinations. The protein indexes were relatively quantitative and showed a quantitative relationship between the dosage fed and the abnormality of proteins present in the plasmas of the experimental ducklings. This procedure is probably no more specific than corresponding nonpolarographic clinical tests but it does have the advantage of ease of operation, sensitivity, reproducibility, speed, and widespread application. This technique appears to have promise in monitoring feeding studies in which the test animals can be quickly and easily checked for signs of abnormalities without being sacrificed. Müller (1965) published the results of an extensive study of the clinical significance of this reaction and concluded that it has great value as a general diagnostic test and is useful for following the recovery of a patient during treatment. Seidel (1964) in Germany reported that, on the basis of over 2000 cases studied in a gyneco-logical hospital, the procedure proved useful as a diagnostic test for differentiating between benign and malignant ovarian tumors, recognizing recidivation, and con-trolling therapy. Vorontrov (1967) studied the filtrate reactions and SH groups of serum in 41 children with thrombocytopenic purpura, hemophilia, and capillary toxicosis. With the first two diseases the polarographs were normal in most cases. With capillary toxicosis there were marked shifts in the filtrate reaction and a distinct reduction in the SH group.

Bojanovic et al. (1966) followed the effect of insulin on the sera of schizo-phrenic patients and found a 58% increase in the height of the protein wave after injection of insulin.

Matyus and Scheda (1969) compared 104 mental patients with 24 normal subjects by the original Brdička method and found that, in endogenous psychoses, mostly schizophrenics, the waves were low, indicating a low concentration of sulfur-containing amino acids. In senile psychoses, arteriosclerotic dementias, and acute softenings the curves were high, indicating high concentration of sulfur-containing amino acids. In cerebral tumors and meningitis the curves were high. This was considered due to high protein content. In consolidated schizophrenias and ancient softenings the curves were normal.

Mairanovskaya et al. (1965) studied the polarographic technique for the diagnosis of malignant mediastinal tumors and compared the finding with 52 healthy donors. Sera from 51 patients with tumors were investigated; in 88% of the cases there was correlation between the clinical diagnosis and polarographic data. After successful treatment the polarographic values fell but rose again on recurrences. Obara and coworkers (1963) used the Brdička Index in Japan to study the effect of radiation and storage on meat and fish.

Paleček (1966) studied the oscillographic indentation produced by native and denatured DNA in the anodic part of de/dt vs. E curves and found that they were due to guanine residues in the DNA molecules. He also found that the depth of the indentation of denatured DNA is always greater than that of the native sample and depends on the content of guanine and cytosine in the molecule. A correlation was observed between the depths of the anodic indentation of native DNA's with the same guanine and cytosine content and the genetic relationship of the organism from which the DNA's were isolated. Paleček (1969) has recently reviewed the polarographic behavior of low molecular weight nucleic acid components, polyribonucleotides, native and denatured DNA, and DNA containing single strand breaks.

Lukasova (1968) also studied the influence of single strand breaks in the double helical structure of DNA on the anodic indentations for the oscillogram dE/dt vs. E.

Hawley and coworkers (1967) utilized fast sweep techniques to study the oxidation pathways of catecholamines in vitro. These techniques allowed positive identification of transient intermediates, such as the open chain o-quinones, and the precise determination of the rate of cyclization to the substituted indole and its subsequent aminochrome. They found significant differences in the rate of cyclization of adrenaline and noradrenaline. They also studied 2-methynoradrenaline, dopamine, and isoproterenol.

Dušinský and Antolik (1965) used oscillographic polarography for continuous measurements of the enzymatic inactivation of penicillins by penicillinase in which the penicillinase splits the β-lactam configuration, forming penicilloic acids. They claim that the method is very specific and that it provides fast and direct measurements of enzyme inactivation and thus a determination of the penicillins.

In other applications Khokhol'kova (1963) determined dinitro-orthocresol both quantitatively and qualitatively in the various organs of rats fed the compound, while Jindrichova et al. (1965) utilized polarography to confirm the presence of benzene in the blood, liver, spleen, brain, and bone marrow of a cobbler who died of suspected chronic benzene poisoning due to handling benzene-containing glue in his occupation. Bardodej and Bardodejova (1966) found that rats ingesting α-methylstyrene and persons inhaling the styrene retained approximately 60% of the parent compound and that they excreted a metabolite, atrolactic acid, which was determined polarographically.

Tomana (1966), studying the polarographic behavior of ascorbic acid in tissue homogenates, discovered that the height of the wave was influenced by the amount of glutathione present. He was able to devise a rapid procedure for the determination of ascorbic acid in all types of animal tissue. Valashek et al. (1968) developed an oscillopolarographic procedure for the determination of anhydro-vitamin A in the presence of vitamin A.

Whitnack and Soli (1966) suggested using fast sweep polarography for the characterization and study of bacterial pigments because of its sensitivity and simplicity. They studied the polarography of a red pigment isolated from a culture of marine flagellate. Ruttkay-Nedecky and Anderlova (1967) noted differences in the polarograms of tobacco mosaic virus (TMV) and that of a cucumber virus (CV-4).

In application of polarography to drug analysis, fast sweep polarography was used by Fruedenberg (1967) to analyze trace amounts of a steroid, Δ^4-3-keto A ring steroid, in the presence of large amounts of a similar steroid, $\Delta^{1,4}$-3-keto A steroid, and by Holbrook and Scales (1967) to determine 0.005 μg/g tetramisole in animal tissue.

Oscillographic polarography was used by Skora-Zietek (1967) to determine phentermin (α,α-dimethyl-β-phenylethylamine) in urine and blood; by Arancibia-Mercado (1967) for determining carbamic drugs such as carisoprodol, meprobamate, mebutamate, methocarbamol, and styramate; by Kalab (1960) to study the metabolism of amino acids, purines, pyrimidine, nucleosides, and nucleotides in cultures of *Escherichia coli;* by Oelschlager and Hoffman (1966) in a rapid method for lidocaine content in injections (accuracy of ±1 to 2%); and by Oelschlager et al. (1967) to study the oscillopolarographic properties of chlorodiazepoxide and its synthesis products.

In other studies utilizing oscillographic polarography, Tereshin (1969) found that, among chlortetracycline, oxytetracycline, and streptomycin, streptomycin was the least reactive. The oxy- and chlortetracycline showed sharp and specific oscillopolarographic activity and could be differentiated. Tereshin was able to determine oxytetracycline in an *Escherichia coli* broth at 6 μg/ml. Similarly, Porter (1967) used the technique to determine from 0.5 to 2.0% chlorpromazine sulfoxide in chlorpromazine, and Porter et al. (1967) were able to determine dipicolinic acid in concentrations as low as 2 μg/ml in the presence of bacterial spores and vegetative cells. Their results compared favorably with the time-consuming spore release method of Janssen et al. (1958).

Prasal (1968) used oscillographic polarography to study the electrode processes of ceruloplasmin, which gave a reversible system in an acetate buffer. This system was used to confirm the activation of Fe^{2+} ion of ceruloplasmin for some biologically active compounds.

In an application to pesticides, Westlake et al. (1969) used differential oscillopolarography to determine 0.1 ppm Ciodrin (crotonic acid, 3-hydroxy α-methyl-benzyl ester of dimethyl phosphate) in animal tissues by converting the compound to its acetophenone, which has a reducible carbonyl group.

Polarography is also a valuable tool for investigation of oxygenation changes in biological systems under the influence of chemical and physical factors. Literature references to the use of this type of oxygen determination to monitor metabolic happenings are too numerous to mention. Polarographic probes have been used by Kozam (1968) to study the effect of pilocarpine hydrochloride on the O_2 tension of the submaxillary gland of the rat. Sokalyanskii (1968) has reviewed the clinical applications of polarography to determination of partial pressure of oxygen at increased oxygen pressures.

Mazzela (1967) used oxygenation changes to study the effect of various drugs on myocardial polarographic oxygen determination. Also, Lysina (1968) studied the effect of radiation on 115 individuals having long exposures to radioactive sources by utilizing polarographic oxygenation processes which change due to neurosis dystonia. Pleticha-Lansky (1968), in oscillopolarographic studies of the effect of γ-radiation on adenine, found that a colored product was formed in the presence of oxygen, whereas in anaerobic conditions formamidopyrimidines were the main product. Based on these findings he proposed a mechanism for the radiolysis of adenine in aqueous solutions.

CONCLUSIONS

It has been shown that oscillopolarography is a very rapid, relatively specific, and easily used technique, and that its applicability to the problems encountered in the study of organic compounds, their metabolites, and breakdown products in biological materials is almost limitless.

Successful application of this technique requires certain skills and knowledge, which may be gained only by practical experience coupled with patience. For those who persevere, the rewards will be manifold.

REFERENCES

Airey, L. 1947. The application of the cathode ray oscillograph to polarography: General layout and uses of the cathode-ray polarograph. Analyst, 72:304-307.

Aranciba-Mercado, L. F. 1967. Polarographic and qualitative and quantitative oscillopolarographic studies of some carbamic acids: Carisoprodol, meprobamate, mebutamate, methocarbamol, and styramate. An. Fac. Quim. Farm. Chile, 19:15-17.

Bardodej, Z., and E. Bardodejova. 1966. Atrolactic acid as metabolite of a methyl styrene. Česk. Hyg., 11:302-304 (cited in Chem. Abstr., 65:14319 d).

Bojanovic, J. J., L. M. Sevaljevic, and M. O. Corbic. 1966. Polarographic activity of blood serum protein in schizophrenic patients in deep hypoglycemic coma effected by insulin. Glas. Hem. Drus. Beograd, 28:427-433.

Brezina, M., and P. Zuman. 1958. Polarography in Medicine, Biochemistry, and Pharmacy. New York, Interscience Publishers.

Brdička, R. 1933. Polarographic studies with the dropping mercury electrode. XXXI. New test for proteins in the presence of cobalt salts in ammoniacal salts of ammonium chloride. Collection Czech. Chem. Commun., 5:112-128.

Cernik, A. A. 1967. A dry ashing method for the determination of blood lead using cathode-ray polarography. Comparison with wet ashing technique. Brit. J. Industr. Med., 24:289-293.

Condliffe, W. F., and A. J. H. Skrimshire. 1961. The polarographic determination of copper, lead, tin, and zinc in foodstuffs. J. Polarogr. Soc., 7:10-14.

Datta, P. R., and R. J. Gajan. 1965. Plasma protein index of aflatoxin-fed ducklings. Life Sci., 4:1791-1795.

Davis, H. M., and R. Rooney. 1962. Differential cathode-ray polarography. J. Polarogr. Soc., 8:25-35.

Delahay, P. 1949. An experimental study of the characteristic features of oscillographic polarography. J. Phys. Colloid Chem., 53:1279-1301.

Dušinský, G., and P. Antolik. 1965. Oscillographic polarography as a method for continuous measurements of inactivation of penicillins by pencillinase. Nature (London), 206:196-197.

Fichera, P., and S. Ferrara. 1969. Oscillopolarographic determination of trace elements in vegetables. I. Copper, zinc, molybdenum and iron. Agrochimica, 13:85-90.

Fruedenberg, D. L. 1967. Trace determination of certain 3-keto steroids with the Davis Differential Cathode Ray Polarotrace. Paper #5, Pittsburgh Conference on Analytical Chemistry and Applied Spectroscopy, March 5-10, 1967.

Gajan, R. P. 1962. Applications of oscillographic polarography to the determination of organophosphorus pesticide residues. J. Assoc. Offic. Anal. Chem., 45:401-406.

———— 1963. Applications of oscillopolarography to the determination of organophosphorus pesticides. II. A rapid screening procedure for the determination of parathion in some fruits and vegetables. J. Assoc. Offic. Anal. Chem., 46:216-222.

————— 1965. Analysis of pesticide residues by polarography. J. Assoc. Offic. Anal. Chem., 45:1028-1037.

————— 1969. Collaborative study of confirmative procedures by single sweep oscillographic polarography for the determination of organophosphorus residues in non-fatty foods. J. Assoc. Offic. Anal. Chem., 52:811-817.

————— W. Benson, and J. Finochiarro. Determination of carbaryl in plants by oscillographic polarography. J. Assoc. Offic. Anal. Chem., 48:958-962.

————— and R. Gaither. 1968. Polarographic procedures for pesticide residues. *In* Pesticide Analytical Manual, vol. I, par. 641.01, U.S. Food and Drug Administration, Washington, D.C.

————— and J. Link. 1964. An investigation of the oscillopolarography of DDT and certain analogs. J. Assoc. Offic. Anal. Chem., 47:1119-1124.

—————S. Nesheim, and A. D. Campbell. 1964. Note on identification of aflatoxins by oscillographic polarography. J. Assoc. Offic. Anal. Chem., 47:27-28.

Gordon, C. L., and E. Wichers. 1957. Purification of mercury and its physical properties. Ann. N.Y. Acad. Sci., 65:369-387.

Griffin, D. J. 1969. Optimization of parameter for single sweep polarographic analysis of selenium diamidobenzidine complex. Anal. Chem., 41:462-466.

Hawley, M. D., S. V. Talawawdi, S. Piekarski, and R. N. Adams. 1967. Electrochemical studies of the oxidation of catecholamines. J. Amer. Chem. Soc., 89:447-450.

Heyrovsky, J. 1956a. Trends in polarographic analysis. Chem. Age, 74:1449.

————— 1956b. The development of polarographic analysis. Analyst, 81:189-192.

————— 1957. Anwendung des Kathodenstrahloscillographie in der Polarographie mit Wechselstrom. Chem. Tech., 9:257.

————— and J. Forejt. 1943. Oscillographische polarographie. Z. Phys. Chem., 193:77-96.

————— and J. Kuta. 1966. Principles of Polarography. New York, Academic Press.

————— and P. Zuman. 1968. Practical Polarography. New York, Academic Press.

Holbrook, A., and B. Scales. 1967. Polarographic determination of tetramisole hydrochloride in extracts of animal tissues. Anal. Biochem., 18:46-53.

Ilkovič, D. 1934. The dropping mercury electrode. XLIV. Dependence of the limiting currents on the diffusion constant, on the rate of dropping and on the size of drops. Collection Czech. Chem. Commun., 6:498-513.

Irvin, E. A., and P. S. Watts. 1961. Estimate of calcium and magnesium in blood serum by cathode ray polarograph. Biochem. J., 79:429-432.

Janssen, F. W., A. S. Lund, and L. E. Andersen. 1958. Colorimetric assay for dipicolinic acid in bacterial spores. Science, 127:26.

Jindrichova, J., V. Vortel, A. Fingerland, K. Juidrak, and L. Chroback. 1965. Fatal panmyelophthisis connecting to subacute myelosis caused by benzene. Vnitrni Lek., 11:995 (cited in Chem. Abstr., 65:8837 [1966]).

Kalab, V. 1960. Application of oscillographic polarography in microbiology. Chem. Zvesti, 14:823-828.

Kalvoda, R. 1965. Techniques of Oscillographic Polarography, 2nd ed. New York, Elsevier Publishing Co.

Khokhol'kova, G. A. 1963. Polaroraphic determination of dinitro-orthocresol in biological media. Gigiena i Fiziol. Truda Proizv. Toksikol., Klinika, Profzabolevanii, 2:343 (cited in Chem. Abstr., 63:11981d [1965]).

Klein, A. K., and R. J. Gajan. 1961. Determination of pentachloronitrobenzene in vegetables. J. Assoc. Offic. Anal. Chem., 44:712-719.

Kolthoff, I. M., and J. J. Lingane. 1965. Polarography, 3rd ed. New York, Wiley/ Interscience Publishers.

Kozam, G. 1968. Effect of pilocarpine on the oxygen tension of rat submaxillary gland. J. Dent. Res. 47:370-373.

Loveland, J. W., and P. J. Elving. 1952. Cathode ray oscilloscopic investigation of phenomena at polarisable mercury electrodes. Chem. Rev., 51:67-117.

Lukasova, E. 1968. The relationship between irregularities in the double helical structure of *Bacillus subtilis* and *Bacillus orevis* DNA's and their oscillopolarographic behavior. Biophysik, 5:183-191.

Lysina, G. G. 1968. Oxygenation of the organism in those working for a prolonged period with sources of ionizing radiation. Vrach. Delo, 6:100-103.

Maienthal, J., and J. K. Taylor. 1968. Polarographic methods for the determination of trace inorganics in water. Advances Chem. Series, 73:172-182.

Mairanovskaya, E. F., A. S. Mamontov, V. V. Garoditova, and N. D. Garin. 1965. The utilization of polarographic methods in the diagnostics of malignant mediastinal tumors. Grudn. Khir., 3:89-93.

Matheson, L. A., and N. Nicols. 1938. The cathode ray oscillograph applied to the dropping mercury electrode. Trans. Electrochem. Soc., 73:193-208.

Matyus, L., and V. Scheda. 1969. Polarographic study of cerebrospinal fluid (Brdička reaction). Ideggvogy. Szemle, 22:410-416.

Mazzela, H. 1967. Effects of several compounds on the dog's myocardial oxygen as determined by polarography. Arq. Brasil. Cardiol., 20:215-220.

Meites, L. 1965. Polarographic Techniques, 2nd ed. New York, Wiley/Interscience Publishers.

Milner, G. W. C. 1957. The Principles and Application of Polarography. London, Longmans, Green and Company.

Müller, O. H. 1963. Polarographic analysis of proteins, amino acids, and other compounds by means of the Brdička Reaction. Meth. Bioch. Anal., 11:329-403.

_____ 1965. Polarographic reaction of plasma proteins and their clinical significance. Clin. Chem., 11, Suppl. 2:270-289.

_____ and J. S. Davis. 1945. Polarographic studies of proteins and their degradation products. J. Biol. Chem., 159:667-679.

Müller, R. H., R. H. Garmor, M. E. Droz, and J. Peters. 1938. The cathode-ray polarograph. Ind. Eng. Chem., Anal. Ed., 10:339.

Nangnoit, P. 1964. Le dosage oscillopolarographique des oléoéléments metalliques dans les végétaux. J. Electrochem., 7:50-59.

Obara, T., and Y. Ogasawara. 1963. Polarographic studies on storage of meats. XII. Influence of proteolytic enzymes on the polarographic wave of beef protein solution. J. Food Sci., 28:8-14.

Oelschlager, H., and H. Hoffman. 1966. Polarographic determination of lidocaine in injection solutions. Arch. Pharm. (Weinheim), 299:1025-1030.

_____ J. Volke, H. Hoffman, and E. Kurek. 1967. Mechanisms of polarographic reduction of chlordiazepoxides. Arch. Pharm. (Weinheim), 300:250-257.

Paleček, E. 1966. Oscillopolarographic polarography of guanine residues of deoxyribonucleic acid. Collection Czech. Chem. Commun., 31:2360-2372.

_____ 1969. Polarographic techniques in nucleic acid research. Progr. Nucl. Acid Res., 9:31-73.

Pietrzyk, D. J. 1966. Organic polarography. Anal. Chem., 38:278R-296R.

_____ 1968. Organic polarography. Anal. Chem., 40:194R-223R.

_____ 1970. Organic polarography. Anal. Chem., 42:139R-152R.

Pleticha-Lansky, R. 1968. Oscillopolarographic studies of the effects of gamma radiation on adenine in aqueous solutions. Int. J. Radiat. Biol., 14:331-339.

Porter, G. S. 1967. A polarographic limit test for sulphoxide in chlorpromazine. J. Pharm. Pharmacol., 19:176-179.

_____ M. W. Brown, and M. R. W. Brown. 1967. Polarographic determination of dipicolinic acid in the presence of bacterial spores and vegetative cells. Biochem. J., 102:19c-20c.

Prasal, Z. 1968. A study of the oxido-reductive properties of caeruloplasmin by oscillographic polarography. Acta Biochim. [Pol.], 15:235-239.

Purdy, W. C. 1965. Electroanalytical Methods in Biochemistry. New York, McGraw-Hill Book Co.

Randles, J. E. P. 1947. The application of the cathode ray oscillography to polarography: Underlying principles. Analyst, 72:301-304.

Reynolds, G. F., and H. M. Davis. 1953. An improved Randles type cathode ray polarograph. Analyst, 78:314-319.

Rooney, R. C. 1963. The determination of tin in beer. Analyst, 88:959-962.

Ruttkay-Nedecky, G., and A. Anderlova. 1967. Polarography of proteins containing cysteine. Nature (London), 213:564-565.

Seidel, K. H. 1964. The Brdička reaction in a gynecological hospital. Abh. Deut. Akad. Wiss. Berlin, Kl. Chem. Geol. Biol., 1:261-266 (cited in Chem. Abstr., 62:6921b).

Ševčik, A. 1948. Oscillographic polarography using periodical triangular voltage. Collection Czech. Chem. Commun., 13:349-377.

Skora-Zietek, M. 1967. A method for the polarographic determination of phentermin in urine and blood. Mikrochim. Acta, 3:528-534.

Smith, H., and R. J. Gajan. 1965. Detection and determination of fumaric acid in foods. J. Assoc. Offic. Anal. Chem., 48:699-700.

Snowden, F. C., and H. T. Page. 1950. A cathode ray polarograph. Anal. Chem., 22:969-981.

Sokalyanskii, I. F. 1968. Use of a polarographic method to determine partial pressure of oxygen at increased oxygen pressures. Polyarogr. Opred. Kisloroda Biol. Ob'ektakh., pp. 199-202. (cited in Chem. Abstr., 72:51591n, 1970).

Tereshin, I. M. 1969. Oscillopolarographic studies on certain antibiotics. Lab. Delo, 1:44-46.

Tomana, M. 1966. Contribution to the problem of polarographic determination of ascorbic acid in animal tissues. Collection Czech. Chem. Commun., 31:4728-4734.

Toren, P. E. 1968. Determination of traces of antimony by single sweep polarography. Anal. Chem., 40:1152-1154.

Valashek, I. E., V. G. Mairanovskii, M. K. Shakhova, and G. I. Samokhvalov. 1968. Polarographic determination of vitamin A acetate in the presence of anhydrovitamin A. Khim.-Farm. Zh., 2:51-54.

Vorontrov, I. M. 1967. Blood serum proteins in children suffering from hemorrhagic diathesis (polarographic study). Pediatriia, 46:45-48.

Wawzonek, S. 1949. Organic polarography. Anal. Chem., 21:61-66.

———— 1950. Organic polarography. Anal. Chem., 22:30-33.

———— 1952. Organic polarography. Anal. Chem., 24:32-40.

———— 1954. Organic polarography. Anal. Chem., 26:65-77.

———— 1956. Organic polarography. Anal. Chem., 28:638-649.

———— 1958. Organic polarography. Anal. Chem., 30:661-674.

———— 1960. Organic polarography. Anal. Chem., 32:144R-161R.

———— 1962. Organic polarography. Anal. Chem., 34:182R-200R.

———— and D. J. Pietrzyk. 1964. Organic polarography. Anal. Chem., 36:220R-239R.

Westlake, A., F. E. Hearth, F. A. Gunther, and W. E. Westlake. 1969. Determination of Ciodrin from fortified animal tissue by oscillopolarography of the conversion product, acetophenone. J. Agr. Food Chem., 17:1160-1163.

Whitnack, G. C., and R. G. Brophy. 1969. A rapid and highly sensitive single sweep polarographic method of analysis for arsenic (III) in drinking water. Anal. Chim. Acta, 48:123-127.

———— and G. Soli. 1966. Characterization of bacterial pigments by single sweep polarography. J. Electroanal. Chem., 12:60-63.

Zagorski, Z. P. 1962. Cells for polarographic electrolysis. In Zuman, P., and I. M. Kolthoff, eds., Progress in Polarography, vol. 2:549-568. New York, Interscience Publishers.

Zuman, P. 1964. Organic Polarographic Analysis. New York, The Macmillan Company.

Chapter **14**

Heatburst Microcalorimetry

Colin F. Chignell

*Laboratory of Chemical Pharmacology, National Heart and Lung Institute,
National Institutes of Health, Bethesda, Maryland*

and

Theodor H. Benzinger

National Bureau of Standards, Gaithersburg, Maryland

Part 1   C. F. Chignell and T. H. Benzinger

INTRODUCTION

Although it is now more than a century since Hess first discovered the equivalence between chemical transformations and their heats of reaction, calorimetry has yet to establish itself in the laboratory as a standard procedure. One of the main difficulties has been that classical calorimetry normally measures only very large amounts of heat. For example, in the measurement of heats of combustion, 10,000 gram-calories are normally required, while for conventional reaction-calorimetry, about 200 gram-calories are usually considered necessary. In contrast, many biologically important reactions liberate only a few thousandths of a gram-calorie of heat. In order to measure such extremely small amounts of heat, it has been necessary to develop special microcalorimetric techniques. One such ultra-sensitive technique, pulse or heatburst microcalorimetry, is the subject of this chapter.

In this chapter the heatburst principle will be briefly discussed followed by a description of the construction and operation of the heatburst microcalorimeter. In the next section, it will be shown how heat can not only be used as an indicator for chemical or biochemical change but can also be used to derive thermodynamic data for the system under study. In a third section, some further possible applications of heatburst microcalorimetry to current problems in molecular biology and pharmacology will be suggested. In Part 2 of this article, the classical determination of the laws of chemical equilibrium and the driving energies of chemical change will be re-examined, and a new determination, more suited to the objects of molecular biology and pharmacology, will be derived.

INSTRUMENTATION

The Heatburst Principle of Microcalorimetry

The difficulties which have held back the development of heat measurements can be traced to one main source: unlike material particles, heat cannot be confined in a test tube. It leaks freely through any boundary or barrier, including empty spaces, which it traverses by electromagnetic radiation. The goal of defeating this ever-present and inevitable dissipation of heat has been approached from two opposite avenues: through the adiabatic principle of classical calorimetry, which prevents the flow of heat by building almost insurmountable "adiabatic" barriers; and through the heat pulse or heatburst principle (Benzinger and Kitzinger, 1954, 1963), which makes no attempt to keep the heat confined or trapped.

The objective of the heatburst approach is to discharge the heat at maximum attainable velocity into a blank or heat sink, and to measure it on its path by converting the energy of the heat flow into an electric potential. The total energy available for measurement can produce either a relatively weak (and long-lasting) or a relatively strong (and short-lasting) electric signal depending on the velocity of heat flow. The second type of response is desirable for two reasons: (1) the intensity of the signal determines the sensitivity of the instrument to small amounts of heat, and (2) shortening the flow duration minimizes disturbances and errors from environmental changes of temperature and flows of heat. At infinite speed of response such errors would disappear. Therefore, the heatburst or pulse principle calls for the highest attainable acceleration and intensity of heat flow, and it will be seen from the next section how this is achieved.

The Heatburst Microcalorimeter

In this section the construction and operation of two commercial heatburst microcalorimeters are described. The Beckman Model 190B is similar to the heatburst microcalorimeter originally designed by Benzinger and Kitzinger (1954, 1963), while the LKB 10700-2 Batch Microcalorimeter was first described by Wadsö (1968).

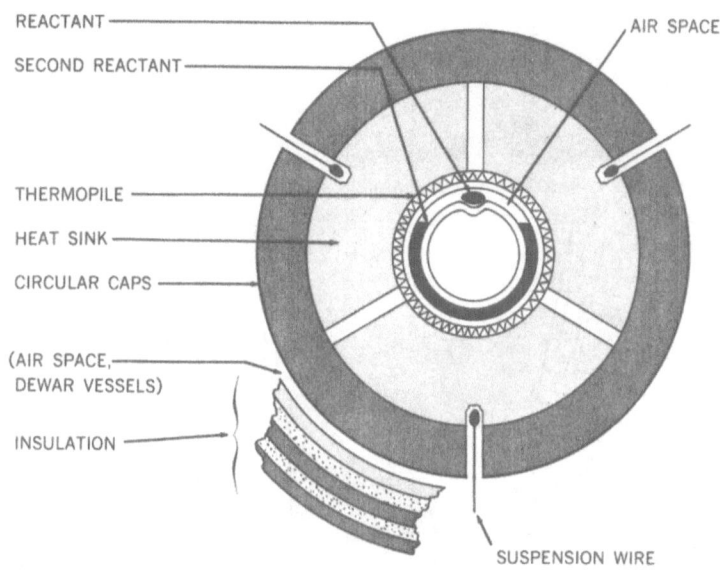

FIG. 1. A transverse section through the Beckman 190B microcalorimeter. (From Benzinger. 1965. *Fractions*, No. 2:1-10. Courtesy of Beckman Instruments, Inc.)

THE REACTION VESSEL.   In the Beckman 190B, the reaction vessel is essentially a double-walled tube sealed at each end with an annular space between the walls for the reactants (Figures 1 and 2). The vessel is bicompartmented to keep the reactants separated until they are mixed when the heat sink is tumbled. The reaction vessel of the LKB 10700-2 consists of a narrow rectangular can divided by a partition wall into two compartments (Figures 3, 4). Although the reaction vessels are normally made of glass, for special applications they can also be made of stainless steel or gold.

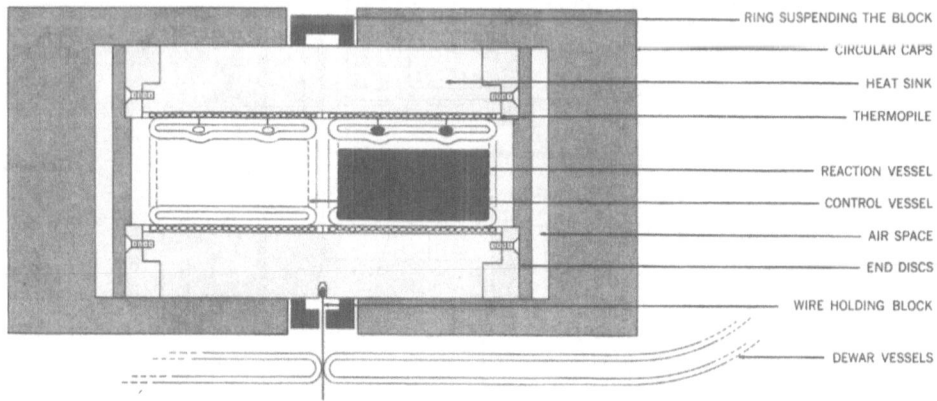

FIG. 2. A longitudinal section through the Beckman 190B Microcalorimeter. (From Benzinger. 1965. *Fractions*, No. 2:1-10. Courtesy of Beckman Instruments, Inc.)

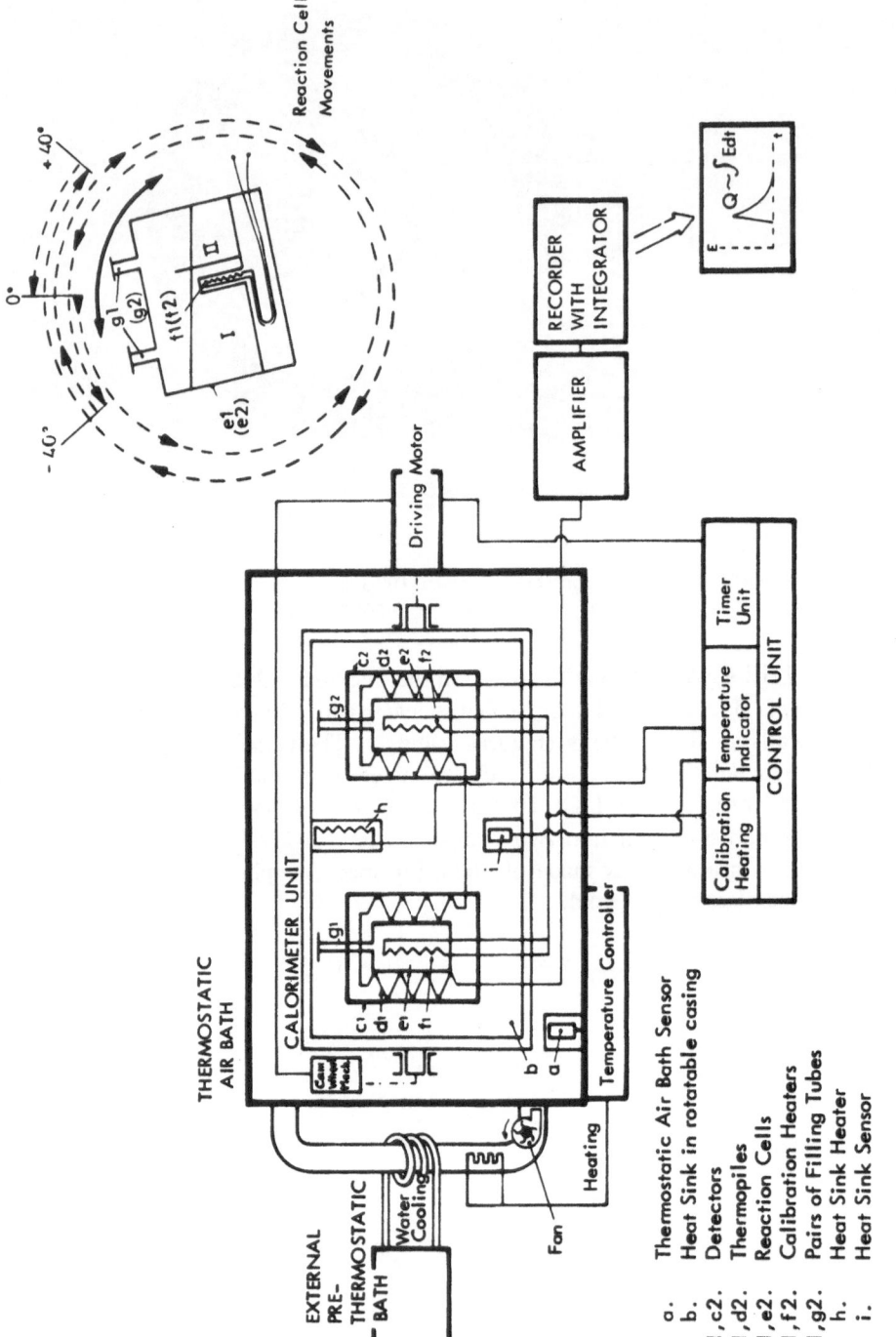

FIG. 3. The LKB 10700-2 batch microcalorimeter. (Photo courtesy of LKB Instruments, Inc.)

a.   Thermostatic Air Bath Sensor
b.   Heat Sink in rotatable casing
c1,c2.   Detectors
d1,d2.   Thermopiles
e1,e2.   Reaction Cells
f1,f2.   Calibration Heaters
g1,g2.   Pairs of Filling Tubes
h.   Heat Sink Heater
i.   Heat Sink Sensor

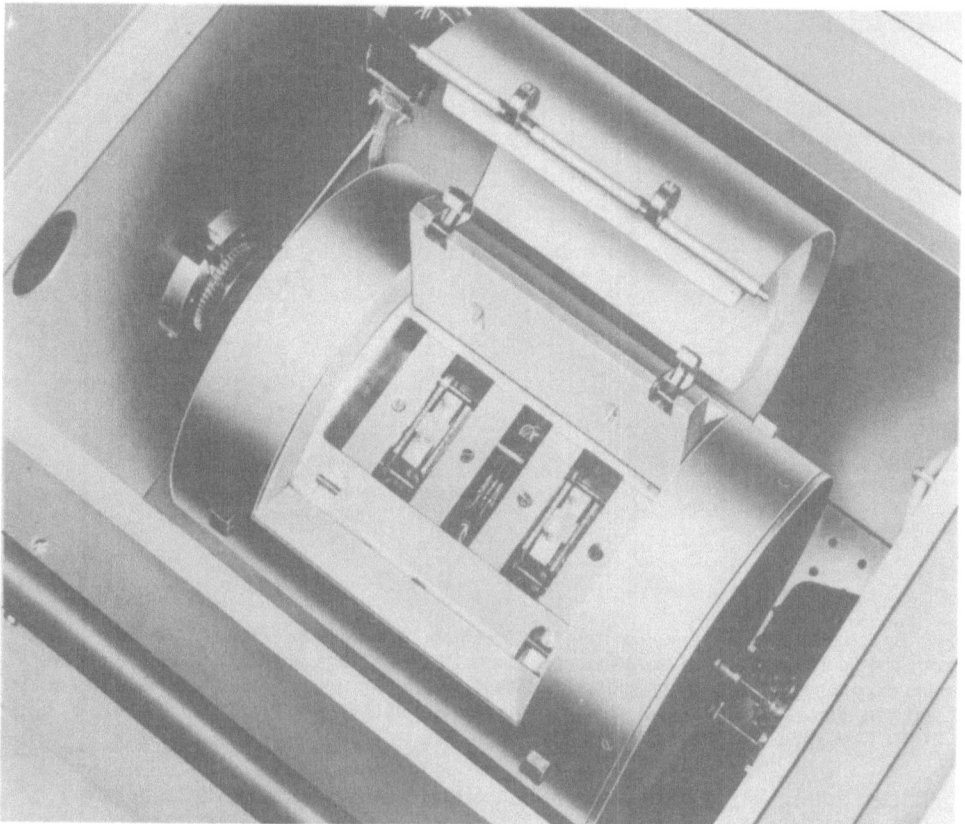

FIG. 4. The LKB 10700-2 batch microcalorimeter with the inner lid of the rotatable unit open showing the reaction cells. (Photo courtesy of LKB Instruments, Inc.)

THE THERMOPILE.   The heat that is generated in the reaction vessel is converted into an electric potential by a thermopile. The Beckman 190B thermopile contains approximately 10,000 junctions. However, since soldering, individually, 10,000 straight conductors in the narrow space between the vessel and the sink would be a tedious task, the "coiled helix" design is employed (Benzinger and Kitzinger, 1963). This gives alternating semicircular conductors of constantan and copper-plated constantan, which are made as follows. First, a helix is made by winding enameled constantan wire of 0.15 mm o.d. on flexible TFE tubing of 3 mm o.d. Then the enamel is removed from one half (180°) of the coil so that two straight rows of thermoelectric junctions are formed when the unenameled half is electroplated with copper. Electroplated thermocouples were first obtained by Hamilton Wilson in 1920. The helix is then coiled upon a thin-wall tubing of aluminum on which a thin electrical insulating deposit has been formed by anodic oxidation. In coiling the helix, twisting is carefully avoided, and the helix is kept oriented so that all the "hot junctions" face, and touch tangentially, the

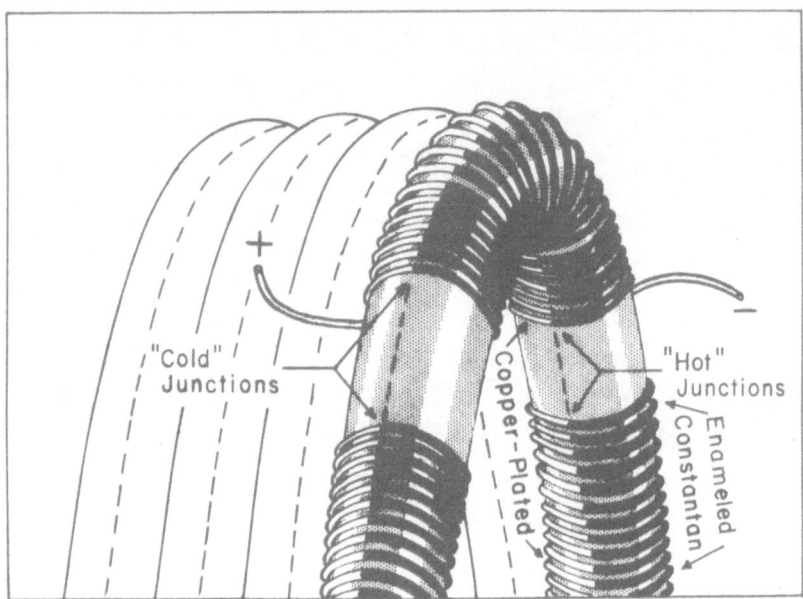

FIG. 5. The coiled helix thermopile from the Beckman 190B Microcalorimeter. The coil is made from constantan wire which is half copper plated. Hot-junctions envelop the reaction-vessels while cold-junctions touch the hollow heat-sink. (From Benzinger. 1969b. *In* Alexander and Lundgren, eds., *A Laboratory Manual of Analytical Methods of Protein Chemistry*, Vol. 5, pp. 95-149. Courtesy of Pergamon Press, Inc.)

anodized tubing on the side which holds the reaction vessel. The other row of junctions faces outward for thermal contact with the heat sink (Fig. 5).

The LKB 10700-2 thermopiles are made from a semiconducting material whose low resistance facilitates amplification of the voltage signal. Each cell has two such thermopiles in the form of rectangular plates, which are placed in close contact with the walls of the reaction vessel (Fig. 3).

THE HEATSINK. Both the Beckman 190B and the LKB 10700-2 have aluminum heatsinks (Figs. 1 to 3), since this metal combines the features of high thermal conductivity and low weight. In the Beckman 190B, the heatsink is split radially into three parts, at 120° angles, so that the three sectors can be forced on the coiled helix with considerable pressure and close tolerance (Fig. 1). Due to the resilience of the coils a uniform thermal contact is obtained between the heat sink, the thermocouples, and the aluminum tubing on which the helix is coiled. End-discs hold the three sectors together. Circular caps fit on both ends of the longitudinal sectors, and the sectors in turn serve as a thermal bridge to connect the two caps (Fig. 2). Thermal coherence and integrity of the sink are thereby achieved. The heatsink is surrounded and enclosed by two Dewar vessels, which in turn are contained in twin heat shields (Fig. 1).

In the LKB 10700-2, the main heatsink is an aluminum cylinder of two parts (diameter 150 mm, length 140 mm) having a 75-mm central bore and 5-mm end walls. In the bore are the two calorimetric units (Figs. 3 and 4). The upper and smaller part of the block is used as a lid and can be fastened to the main part by locking clips. The aluminum cylinder is suspended by horizontal steel shafts between ball bearings positioned on the inner walls of the surrounding thermostated air bath. The shafts are connected to each end of the cylinder through vertical aluminum discs, which are joined to the end-walls of the cylinder by 4 mm steel pins. The metal block is covered with a 20-mm layer of styrofoam (Fig. 4). The temperature difference between the metal block and the air bath is indicated by a 200-junction copper-constantan thermopile (made by electroplating an 0.8 mm constantan wire wound on a mica strip). A 20-ohm electrical heater winding is also attached to the metal block. Electrical windings from the calorimetric units and from the block are taken out through the end walls and several turns are wound on the shafts before being taken to contacts on the inner wall of the air bath (Fig. 3). The thermostated air bath consists of a 50-liter aluminum box, which is insulated on the outside by a 50-mm layer of styrofoam. Fifty-millimeter PVC tubes are used to circulate air between the bath and another air container. The temperature is regulated by a LKB proportional controller 7602-A connected to a thermistor in the thermostated bath and a heater of bare resistance wires is positioned close to a fan in the outside air container. Cooling water is circulated through a copper spiral also positioned in the container.

THE TWIN PRINCIPLE. Heat flows through the ultrasensitive thermoelectric pile not only when it is generated or absorbed in a chemical reaction, but also when liquids inside the reaction vessel are stirred and tiny gradients of temperature are thereby inverted, when friction-heat is generated in the vessels, and when the temperature of the sink changes as a result of external changes in temperature. In order to minimize the effects of such heat flows, the principle of twin-calorimetry is employed. Two reaction vessels (Figs. 2 to 4), one filled with reactants and the other with nonreacting liquid, are placed symmetrically tandem-fashion within the one heat sink. The two cells each have their own thermopile, which is wired in opposition to the other so that electrical responses to all kinds of heat flow tend to cancel—except for the heat of reaction, which is generated in only one of the two vessels.

CALIBRATION. Heat flows through a thermopile when a temperature difference exists between its junctions and ceases to flow as soon as this difference equals zero. This may be expressed as follows:

$$W = K_1 \Delta t \tag{1}$$

where W = heat effect (calories per second), K_1 = heat leakage constant, and Δt = temperature difference. The temperature is in turn proportional to E, the thermopile voltage, so that the amount of heat (Q) transported during the total reaction time is given by

$$Q = K_2 \int E dt \tag{2}$$

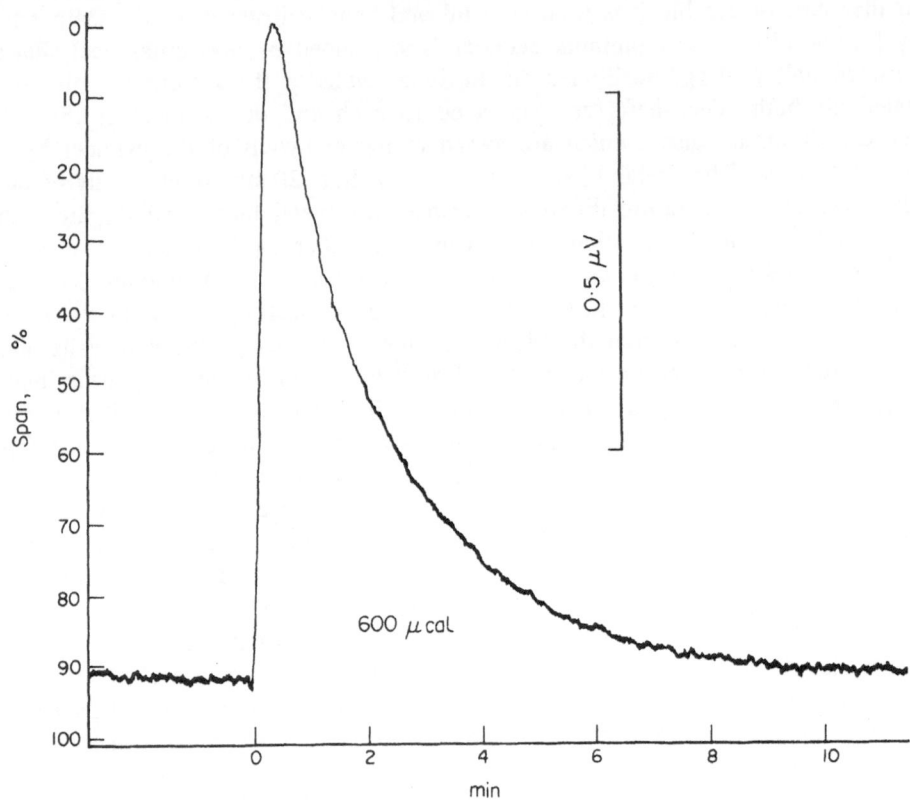

FIG. 6. Electric calibration with a heat pulse of 600 microcalories, total. (From Benzinger. 1969b. *In* Alexander and Lundgren, eds., *A Laboratory Manual of Analytical Methods of Protein Chemistry*, Vol. 5, pp. 95-149. Courtesy of Pergamon Press, Inc.)

where K_2 is a constant. In heatburst microcalorimetry the thermopile voltage is measured during the mixing of the reactants until such time as no more heat is evolved.

In order to evaluate K_2, it is necessary to calibrate the heatburst microcalorimeter. This may be done either chemically or electrically. For chemical calibration, the protonation of tris(hydroxymethyl)aminomethane may be employed. Electrical calibration may be achieved either by a pulse of current or by steady inputs of current. The LKB 10700-2 has an electrical heater built into the cell for calibration purposes (Fig. 3). The Beckman 190B is calibrated by means of a special cell, which contains a heating wire. The appearance of an electrical calibration pulse of just 600 microcalories total is shown in Fig. 6. The area under the curve represents the integral in equation (2) and is therefore directly proportional to the amount of heat (Q) evolved during the experiment.

SOME APPLICATIONS OF HEATBURST MICROCALORIMETRY

Analytical Applications

With the instrumental capabilities described above, calorimetry can now take its place with other standard analytical methods in the modern molecular laboratory. It can be extended to rare or precious substances, to perishable compounds, to molecules of enormous weight, and to poorly soluble materials. Applications may range from physiochemical processes such as solution, dilution, or solid-liquid interactions at surfaces, to the most complex systems of molecular biology and pharmacology. They may extend to systems of which literally nothing is known, except the purity and molecular weight of one reaction partner.

The strength of calorimetry lies in the ubiquity of the phenomenon of heat and the total nonspecificity of the procedure. When there is no otherwise measureable sign of interaction, heat is still available. So not only the presence but also, with rare exceptions where $\Delta H = 0$, the absence of chemical interaction can be demonstrated by microcalorimetry.

ENZYMES AND SUBSTRATES. In a mixture of any number of enzymes, for example, the presence and activity of one enzyme attacking one substrate can be identified by addition of the substrate to the unknown enzyme preparation in the microcalorimeter; heat will detect the interaction (Fig. 7). Similarly, in a mixture of any number of substrates, one substrate can be identified by addition of a pure enzyme preparation. Thus, the determination of purity

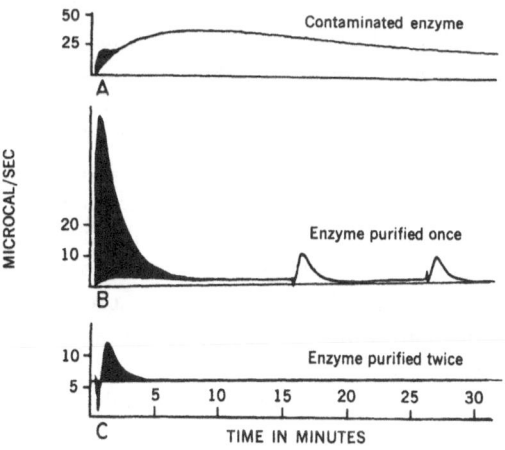

FIG. 7. The purification of glutaminase contaminated with carboxylase: (A) Contaminated enzyme. (B) Enzyme purified once. (C) Enzyme purified twice. The shaded areas represent the heat evolved by the action of the glutaminase. (From Benzinger. 1965. *Fractions*, No. 2:1-10. Courtesy of Beckman Instruments, Inc.)

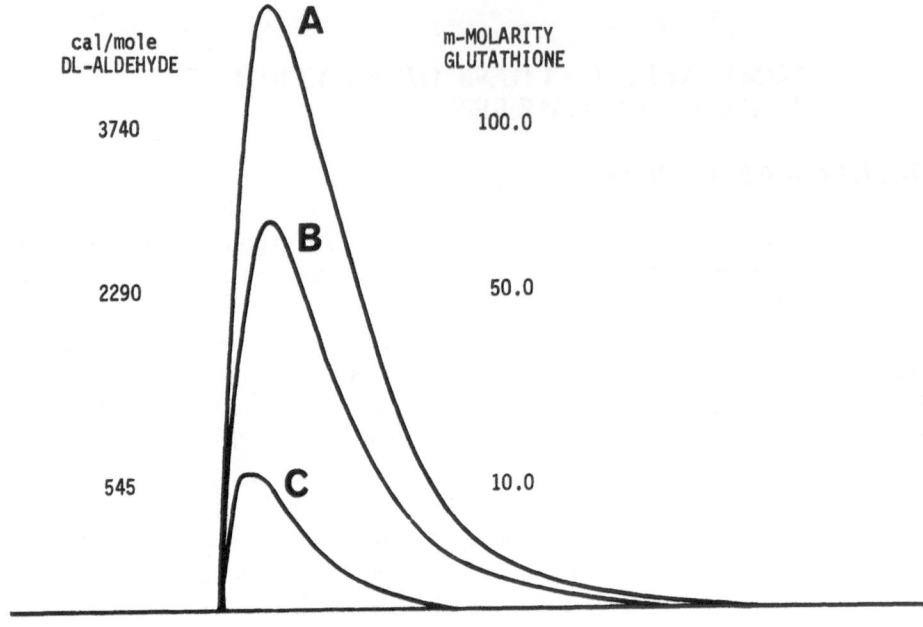

m—MOLARITY GLYCERALDEHYDE: 0.27

FIG. 8. An unknown reaction between D,L-glyceraldehyde and glutathione and its reversibility demonstrated by microcalorimetry. (From Benzinger. 1965. *Fractions*, No. 2:1-10. Courtesy of Beckman Instruments, Inc.)

and the assay of any number of different systems of enzymes could be performed with one technique and instrument.

UNKNOWN INTERACTIONS.   Calorimetry can be used to detect interactions where no other method for separation, identification, or detection of a product exists. For example, L. Kiesow (Benzinger, personal communication) suspected that glutathione with its SH-groups would interact with glyceraldehyde in a model reaction comparable to the interaction of SH-dehydrogenases with their substrates. Calorimetry demonstrated not only the existence of such an interaction (Fig. 8) but also its reversibility. For this reaction, it would be possible in principle to find the heat, free energy and entropy changes without using any other method of chemical analysis except calorimetry. The procedure can be applied to interactions of proteins with many kinds of agents including drug molecules or to the interactions of nucleic acids.

ANTIGEN-ANTIBODY   INTERACTION. Steiner   and   Kitzinger (1956) measured the heat of an antigen-antibody interaction directly (Fig. 9) and were able to identify immunological reactions that do not form insoluble complexes. Insolubility, as a criterion, may be absent in many immunological reactions, and calorimetry might be applied as a probing tool in this field. The authors were able to demonstrate beyond doubt that the heat change was exclu-

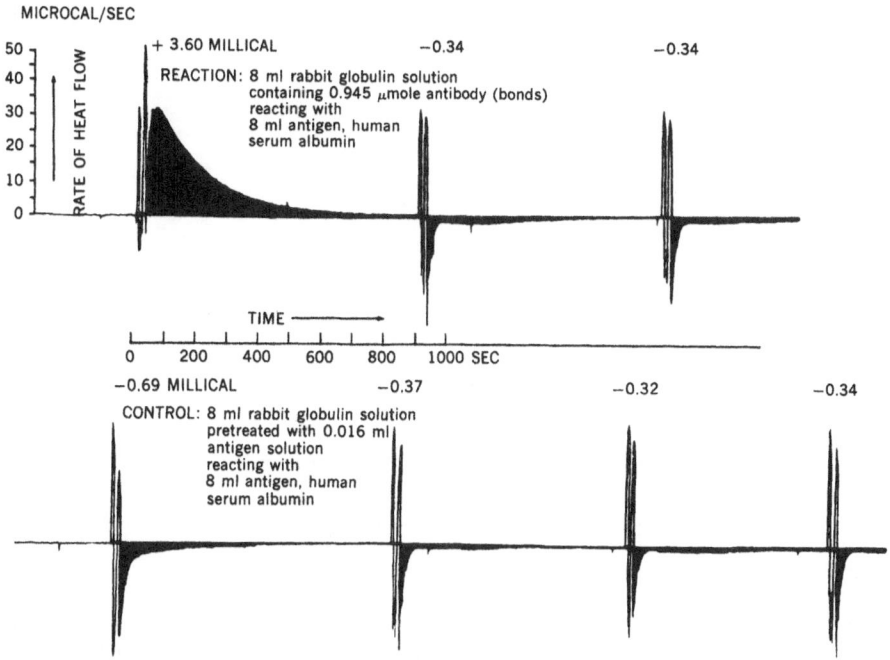

FIG. 9. The demonstration of a specific antigen-antibody reaction. The top curve is before and the bottom curve after the removal of the antibody by preinteraction with a small amount of antigen. (From Benzinger. 1965. *Fractions*, No. 2:1-10. Courtesy of Beckman Instruments, Inc.)

sively associated with the species-specific immunological reaction. Moreover, previous equilibrium studies had permitted a determination of free energy. The data combined with the direct measurements enabled the authors to find the entropy change of the antigen-antibody interaction—between globulins of a rabbit immunized with human serum and human serum albumin as the antigen. For reactions of still unknown mechanisms, estimates of the degree of change of molecular order or disorder are especially valuable.

POLYNUCLEIC ACIDS. With increasing yields of the pure compounds involved it becomes possible to employ microcalorimetry in the study of nucleic acids and their implications in chemical genetics, protein synthesis, virology, tumors, and molecular diseases. In a pioneering study by Steiner and Kitzinger (1962), the heat of formation of double helices from random coils of polyriboadenylic and polyribouridylic acids was measured (Fig. 10). Fortunately, transitions of this kind are reversible and therefore lend themselves (at elevated temperatures, even if not at room temperature) to studies of free energy and entropy changes by calorimetry.

An indication of the potential of calorimetry in the field of nucleic acids was given with the finding of different heats of helix formation at different ionic strengths. When electrical charges on the single strands are neutralized by high ionic strength, the total heat evolved is smaller because the coiled chain molecules must

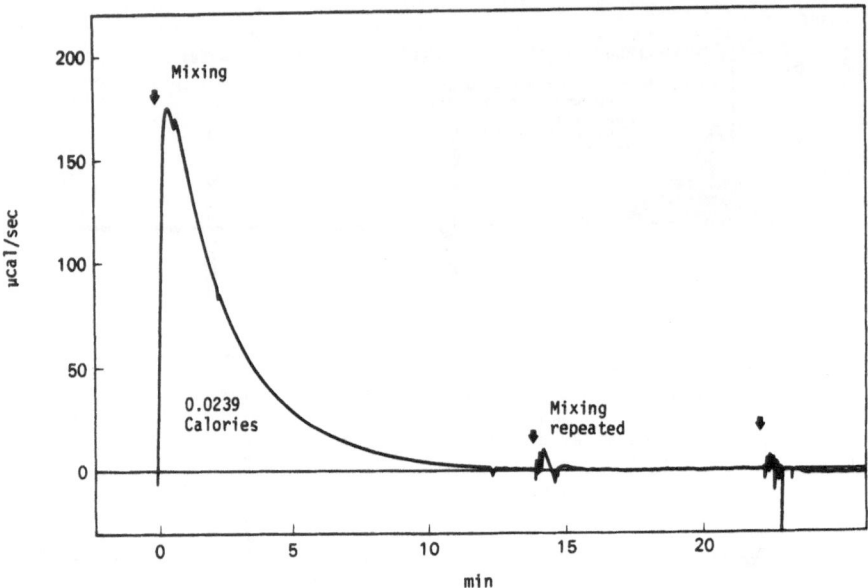

FIG. 10. Heat of formation of polynucleotide helix. Heat of formation of double helices from single-stranded molecules of polyribouridylic and polyriboadenylic acids. The amount of Poly-U was 4.78 μmoles. Poly-A was present in excess. The heat evolved was 23.9 mcal. Note the "zero-spikes" and the reproducibility of the zero baseline in this range. (From Benzinger. 1969b. *In* Alexander and Lundgren, eds., *A Laboratory Manual of Analytical Methods of Protein Chemistry*, Vol. 5, pp. 95-149. Courtesy of Pergamon Press, Inc.).

first be stretched before they form an elongated helix. The absorption of heat in this change is 800 cal/mole. Cooperative structures of this kind are difficult but interesting subjects. Reliable measurements of reaction heats and equilibria could be a basis for further development of the theory of polynucleic acid interactions. It is important to know the forces that drive the combination or separation or recombination of the material on which the transmission of genetic information and the replicating of living matter depend.

ADENOSINE TRIPHOSPHATE HYDROLYSIS. Turning from the high organizational level of proteins and nucleic acids to the less complicated substrate level where decisive transformations of energy for the life process are taking place, we find two crucial steps indicated: oxidation-reduction of the NAD-NADH systems, and the hydrolysis or synthesis of ATP. Fortunately, electrical measurements gave an insight into NAD-thermodynamics at an early stage. For ATP hydrolysis these became known much later.

With the heat pulse microcalorimeter, reliable thermodynamic data on ATP hydrolysis were obtained in 1955 (Kitzinger and Benzinger, 1955) (Fig. 11), and free energy was determined in 1956 (Benzinger and Hems, 1956). While the heat had previously been estimated at −12,000 cal/mole, these measurements revealed that it was −4,800 cal/mole. The standard free energy is considerably higher, −7,000 cal/mole (in the presence of magnesium at pH 7.0 and 36°C). From these standard values free energies can be readily estimated for other

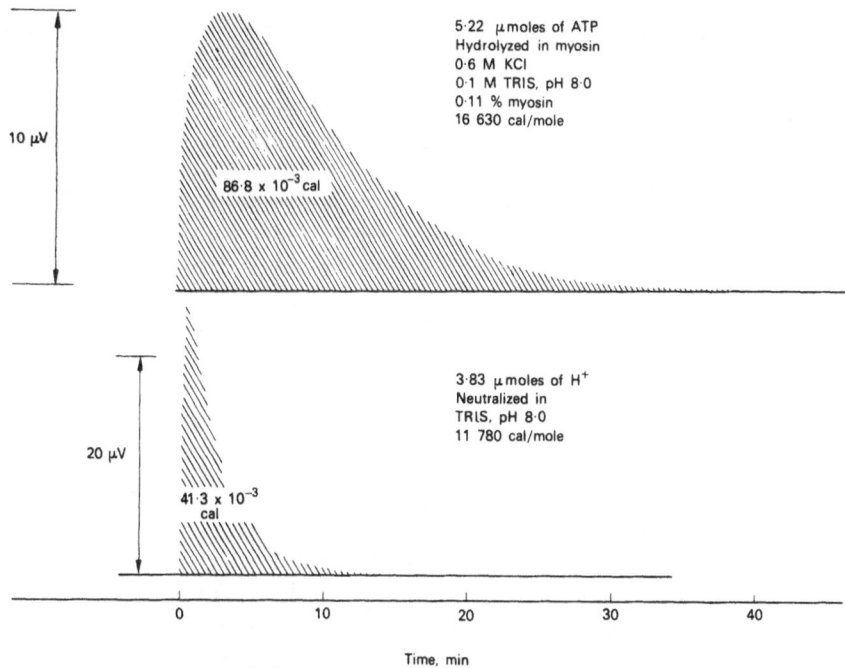

FIG. 11. Adenosinetriphosphate hydrolysis and proton neutralization. Enzymatic hydrolysis of ATP by myosin in the calorimeter (upper recording). The heat of ATP hydrolysis includes the heat of neutralization of one proton in the buffer. The heat of ionization of tris (hydroxymethyl) ammomethane was separately determined (lower recording) and subtracted. The difference, $-4,800$ cal/mole, is the heat of ATP hydrolysis proper. (From Benzinger. 1969b. *In* Alexander and Lundgren, eds., *A Laboratory Manual of Analytical Methods of Protein Chemistry*, Vol. 5, pp. 95-149. Courtesy of Pergamon Press, Inc.)

temperatures, pH values, and concentrations of reactants. Dilution favors the hydrolysis of ATP and makes the free energy more negative. The useful energy properties of ATP are based to a considerable extent on the disappearance of protons, one product of the reaction, in a buffer where the proton concentration is fixed at 10^{-7} M or even lower. That the heat of reaction is not higher in ATP hydrolysis than in the splitting of a phospho-ester bond suggests that use of the "high energy phosphate bond" description should be discontinued.

Thermodynamics and Ultrasensitive Calorimetry

Although calorimetry complements other methods as a tool of chemical analysis, it is in a class of its own as a tool of chemical thermodynamics. Heat (enthalpy) is a quantity as unchangeable as the atomic or molecular weights of the participants. When one more quantity, the entropy change, ΔS, is known, the thermodynamic analysis of a reaction and knowledge of its driving forces are complete in the classical tradition. For discussion of the application of classical thermodynamic principles to biological systems the reader is referred to an excellent monograph by Klotz (1967). However, an extension of these classical concepts is required for a full understanding of the driving energies of chemical change, particularly with respect to the systems studied in molecular biology. This will be dealt with in Part 2 of this article.

Thermodynamic knowledge is significant to both the chemist and the biochemist. For the chemist who seeks control over a process that he makes proceed according to his wishes, thermodynamics reveals the conditions to select—the optimal concentrations or pressures of the participants and the optimal temperature of reaction. For the biochemist, thermodynamics is a vital key to the understanding of the complex world of living matter. The world of life unfolds on our planet in a narrow temperature range and at atmospheric pressure. Yet, under these conditions, the living world produces a perplexing wealth of compounds with astonishing properties for replication, motility, enzymic catalysis, immunological defense, membrane-transport, message-transmission, energy-transformation, and many other functions—all with only one design at its disposal: reaction coupling. And the key to reaction-coupling is thermodynamics.

The particular importance of ultrasensitive calorimetry to chemical thermodynamics was demonstrated by a new approach to determination of entropy and free energy changes (Benzinger, 1956). For the first time heats of reaction—instead of the laborious techniques of low temperature physics—permitted the classical thermodynamic analysis of important systems such as that which hydrolyzes adenosinetriphosphate.

With modern microcalorimetry, quantities of heat and substances required for thermodynamic studies are now smaller by at least six orders of magnitude than those required for classical combustion calorimetry. The significance of this change is evident when, for example, one considers an antigen and an antibody and the complex which they form in a reversible reaction. Combustion calorimetry could not reveal the minute heat change associated with the interaction of a pair of molecules of such size, with secondary and tertiary structures of such importance. And it is unthinkable that substances like these could have been treated with the methods of low-temperature physics (using the third law of thermodynamics to obtain measurements of their entropies). Ultrasensitive calorimetry permits the study of these and similar systems, since heat of reaction of microquantities is the first and direct objective.

All individual steps of chemical reactions are considered to be reversible, at least in concept. However, if a reaction that is irreversible in practice—$A + B \rightleftarrows C + D$—proceeds from left to right with liberation of reaction-heat to near completion, ultrasensitive calorimetry can discover the tiny amount of heat that is absorbed when products C and D interact. Once the reversibility of a reaction has been demonstrated in this way, minute amounts of reactants are added to a highly concentrated solution of products. Interaction of these partners absorbs less heat, or indeed produces heat, when the components are mixed or when a catalyst or enzyme is added. Among these various combinations there is one that neither produces nor absorbs any heat at all. It is found by interpolation between two actual experiments. It represents the state of chemical equilibrium, which is

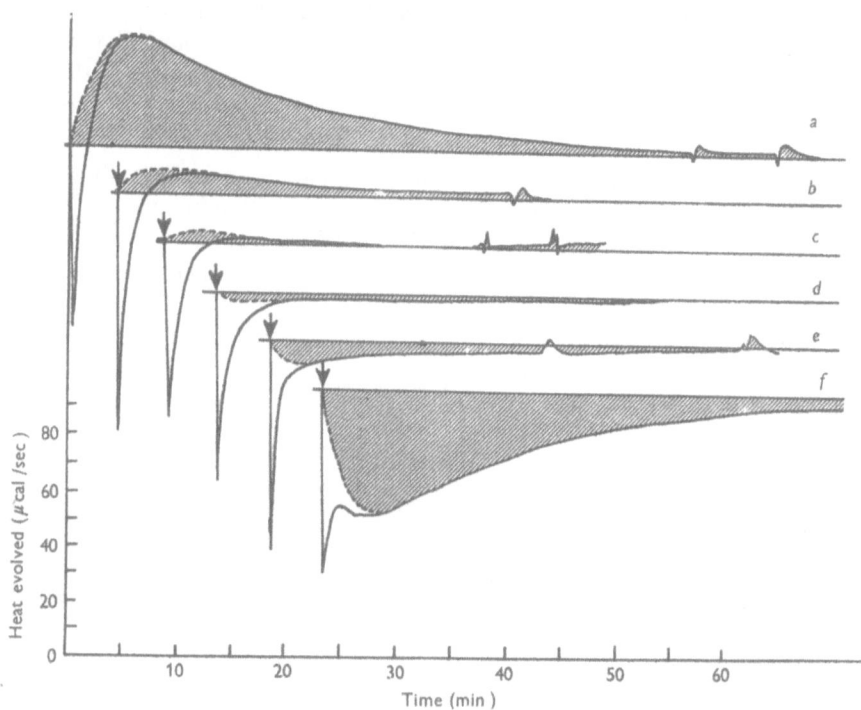

FIG. 12. Tracings of calorimeter recordings. The continuous line is the rate of heat flow recorded after mixing 0.16 ml of glutaminase with 16 ml of glutamine solution in 0.884 *M*-ammonium glutamate at 25°C. The broken line is the heat flow of the enzymic reaction after correcting for the initial mixing heat; the shaded areas represent the amount of the corresponding heat change. (Above the horizontal line heat was evolved, below the line heat was absorbed.) The initial concentration of glutamine in the 16.16 ml of solution immediately after mixing was (m*M*): *a*, 1.57; *b*, 0.923; *c*, 0.876; *d*, 0.785; *e*, 0.672; *f*, zero. Successive tracings have been displaced in the time axis. Arrows indicate time of addition of enzyme, in each experiment. (From Benzinger et al. 1959. *Biochem. J.*, 71:400-407.)

by no means a state of chemical inactivity. Instead, it is a state in which the reaction proceeds with identical speed from left to right and simultaneously from right to left. Any disturbance by addition of reactants or products would cause the reaction to proceed immediately from left to right, or vice versa, depending on liberation or absorption of heat. Knowing the initial composition of the mixture one can, with two experiments, find the heat of reaction ΔH, the equilibrium constant K, the free energy change ΔF, and the entropy change $T\Delta S$.

This procedure is shown in Fig. 12 for a reaction that is practically irreversible—the hydrolysis of glutamine. In the experiment of the lowest curve, pure products (glutamic acid and ammonia) were added to an enzyme solution in the microcalorimeter, and an absorption of heat appeared. The products were transformed into reactants at an initial rate of $\sim 10^{-8}$ mole/second. This rate could be expected not to change, since the high concentration of reacting products remains practically unchanged during such an extremely slow and limited transformation.

Nevertheless, the rate of heat absorption soon declined and became zero. The reason is that the reactant which was formed, glutamine, began immediately to react forward, reforming products from reactants. Later, when glutamine had accumulated to such an extent that the rate of this forword reaction became equal to the rate of the reverse reaction as initially observed, chemical equilibrium was attained.

This one experiment does not reveal the quantity of net chemical change required for the attainment of equilibrium, since ΔH is unknown. In a second experiment a known amount of glutamine is added to the same solution of glutamic acid and ammonia, after which the microcalorimetric experiment is repeated.

Where Q_1 and Q_2 are the heats produced or liberated in the two experiments and M_1 and M_2 are the quantities of glutamine added (zero in the case of the lowest curve), the heat of reaction ΔH is

$$\frac{Q_1 - Q_2}{M_1 - M_2} \tag{3}$$

The apparent equilibrium constant K is readily found by interpolation between two measured points in a plot of heats against reactant concentrations (Fig. 13).

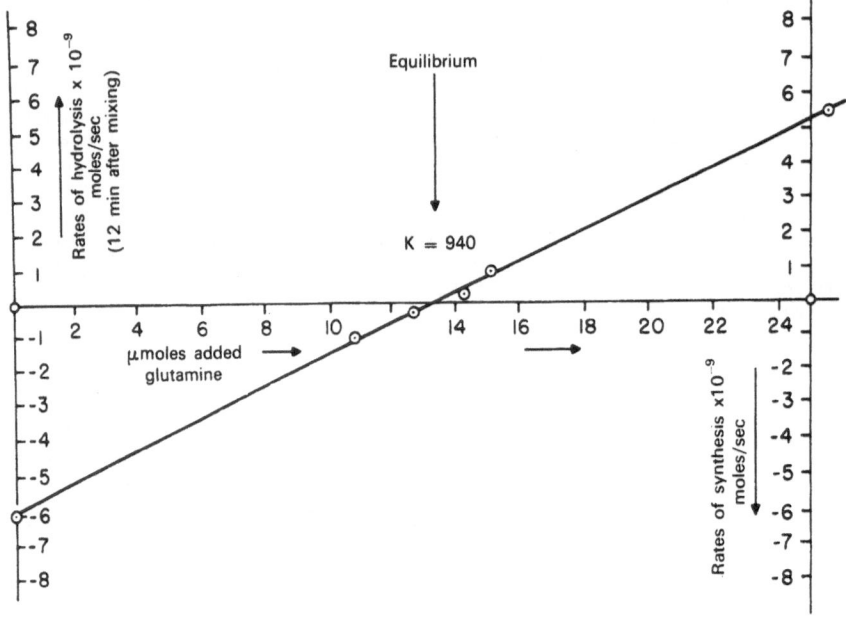

FIG. 13. Equilibrium-constant by interpolation. Net reaction rates (or total heats measured) in the experiments of Figure 12 permit the finding of the point of equilibrium by interpolation. Linearity is caused by linear relation between hydrolysis-rate and glutamine-concentration. A constant rate of glutamine synthesis causes the displacement of the intersect from 0 to −6 ×10⁻⁹ moles/sec. (From Benzinger. 1969b. *In* Alexander and Lundgren, eds., *A Laboratory Manual of Analytical Methods of Protein Chemistry*, Vol. 5, pp. 95-149. Courtesy of Pergamon Press, Inc.).

Corrected for activity coefficients, the constant K reveals the thermodynamic equilibrium and the free energy change, ΔF. From ΔF and ΔH follows $T\Delta S$, the entropy term.

O'Reilly and coworkers (1969) have recently employed heatburst microcalorimetry to study the thermodynamics of warfarin binding to human plasma albumin. They found that the average enthalpy for the reaction by direct calorimetry was -3.14 kcal per mole of warfarin. This value was very close to the -3.48 kcal per mole calculated indirectly from the temperature dependence of the equilibrium constant (Klotz, 1967). Since their equilibrium studies gave a value of -7.37 kcal per mole of warfarin as the free energy change of the reaction, they were able to calculate an entropy change of $+14.2$ cal per mole-degree. They suggested that the negative enthalpy and positive entropy resulted from hydrogen and hydrophobic bonding between the drug and the protein (O'Reilly et al., 1969).

PROGNOSIS

The principle and instrumentation of heatburst microcalorimetry have been described in this chapter to introduce this versatile technique to the pharmacologist. A few examples have been described in order to illustrate what can be done with this type of instrumentation. At the present time, there are few instances where heatburst microcalorimetry has been applied to pharmacology. Nevertheless, since heat is a universal indicator of chemical change, the potential of this technique is almost unlimited. One of the main problems in molecular pharmacology has often been to find a technique that will detect the interaction of a drug with a given biological system. If such an interaction involves the generation or uptake of heat, then microcalorimetry can be used to monitor the reaction. Thus, under the appropriate conditions, it may be possible by means of heatburst microcalorimetry to detect complex formation between a drug and that elusive tissue element, the drug receptor.

Part 2   Theodor H. Benzinger

A NEW CONCEPT IN THERMODYNAMICS AND ITS IMPLICATION IN MOLECULAR BIOLOGY AND PHARMACOLOGY

Introduction

In the previous examples, it has been shown how the classical principles of chemical thermodynamics have been applied to molecular biology and pharmacology. The microcalorimeter method was used to obtain heat of reaction (enthalpy), Clausius entropy, and Gibbs' free energy data. These data satisfy the classical determination of chemical equilibrium. In the following section, it will be shown that an extended statement and determination are required for the thermodynamic objectives of molecular biology and pharmacology. This article is reproduced with minor changes from *Nature* (London), 229:100–102 (1970), with the permission of Macmillan (Journals) Ltd.

The laws of chemical equilibrium are conventionally determined in terms of the heat of reaction term ΔH_T^0 and the Clausius entropy term $T\Delta S_T^0$. Indeed, these two quantities provide the thermodynamic foundations of the chemical and life sciences, and the statement

$$-RT \ln K = \Delta H_T^0 - T\Delta S_T^0 \qquad (4)$$

is as infallible as the laws of thermodynamics. (Here $-RT \ln K$ is a numerical expression for collective or mass action, not individual thermodynamic properties of products and reactants.) Any number of equally infallible statements can, however, be obtained by simultaneously adding to or subtracting from the enthalpy and entropy terms in equation (4) some quantity—let it be called $\Delta\Gamma_T^0$:

$$-RT \ln K = (\Delta H_T^0 - \Delta\Gamma_T^0) - (T\Delta S_T^0 - \Delta\Gamma_T^0) \qquad (5)$$

Although this simple operation does not affect the infallibility of equation (4) for thermodynamic accounting, it completely changes the physical interpretation of the two terms on the right hand side. Most of the possible choices for the magnitude of $\Delta\Gamma_T^0$ would no doubt produce physically nonsensical quantities in a new equation. Thus the question arises whether or not the choice of ΔH_T^0 and $T\Delta S_T^0$ is the only meaningful one and, if not, whether it is the best choice that could have been made.

Thermodynamic Concepts

Early in the development of chemical thermodynamics ΔH_T^0 was chosen (and $T\Delta S_T^0$ followed inevitably from the definition of entropy $dS = dq/dT$). (Even earlier the conceptual uniqueness of ΔH_T^0 had been overrated in Berthelot's view of the work obtainable from chemical reactions.) Although ΔH_T^0 is certainly the logical choice for a direct thermodynamic measurement with chemical reactions, the ease and precision of such measurements do not necessarily mean that ΔH_T^0 is also the best choice for a fundamental statement such as equation (4). Suitable criteria must be adopted to investigate other possibilities from a viewpoint of conceptual clarity and power. When chemical thermodynamics is used for common-sense purposes and extended by molecular interpretations beyond purist formalism, it is supposed to describe the transformations of energy that are inseparably linked with transformations of matter. Our criteria will therefore be the direct relations of the thermodynamic quantities selected, to the formation or breaking of chemical bonds between atoms, the only processes by which chemical product matter can be formed from chemical reactant matter.

Two Contributions

It is difficult to show a direct relation between chemical bonding or bond breaking and the classical ΔH_T^0 and $T\Delta S_T^0$ terms. It can be shown that ΔH_T^0 is a composite, not a uniform quantity, and that the two contributions of which it is composed are of fundamentally different origin. They may be present in any conceivable known or unknown proportion and in the molecular view only one of the two contributions has a direct relation to chemical bonding.

Proof of this contention may be found by allowing reactants and products to be taken separately from temperature T down to $0°K$ or from $0°K$ up to T, while heat capacity differences ΔC_p are measured for every infinitesimal step to find the integral $\int_0^T \Delta C_p dT$. Whenever this integral is not zero, an amount of heat $\int_0^T \Delta C_p dT$ must be liberated or absorbed during the reaction, in addition to other heat changes that arise from the formation or undoing of chemical bonds between atoms. In our low temperature experiment the reaction did not take place and the chemical bonds, which the reaction equation describes, were not formed. In these low-temperature experiments, we have, however, measured $\int_0^T \Delta C_p dT$, one contribution to the heat of reaction ΔH_T^0. The other contribution obtained by subtraction, $\Delta H_T^0 - \int_0^T \Delta C_p dT$, is chemical-bonding energy. It can be observed only when the reaction takes place, and even then it is in most cases obscured by the contribution $\int_0^T \Delta C_p dT$.

Integrals and Chemical Bonds

Because $\int_0^T \Delta C_p dT$ is obviously unrelated to the formation or breaking of chemical bonds between atoms, our concept proposes that $\int_0^T \Delta C_p dT$ be subtracted out of equation (4) for a determination of the laws of chemical equilibrium, extended to cases where $\int_0^T \Delta C_p dT$ is finite or large (Benzinger, 1969a).

One obtains from equation (5)

$$-RT \ln K = \left(\Delta H_T^0 - \int_0^T \Delta C_p dT\right) - \left(T\Delta S_T^0 - \int_0^T \Delta C_p dT\right)$$

This may be written

$$-RT \ln K = \Delta H_0^0 - \Delta W_T^0 \tag{6}$$

where

$$\Delta W_T^0 = [T \int_0^T \frac{\Delta C_p}{T} dT - \int_0^T \Delta C_p dT]$$

In equation (6) ΔH_0^0 represents the amount of heat (or, when the reaction is properly harnessed, energy of any kind: chemical, osmotic, mechanical, electrical, or other) obtainable from the energy of formation of chemical bonds between atoms. At 0°K, ΔH_0^0 is defined as the heat of reaction; at other temperatures, ΔH_0^0 is a virtual quantity, invariant with temperature unless bond stretching as a result of thermal agitation leads to a slight reduction of the amount of work required to separate bond partners. (Such variations with temperature, if they exist, are subject to experimental proof by measurements of $\int_0^T \Delta C_p dT$ and ΔH_T^0 over the range under consideration. If the states concerned are inaccessible experimentally, they are reached in a mental process comparable with the concept of infinite dilution in solution theory.)

The term ΔW_T^0 of equation (6) represents "thermal free energy" or the work obtainable by conversion of "thermal" heat contained in chemical compounds and expendable in the performance of separating chemically bonded atoms in the compounds concerned. Equation (6) is consistent with the pertinent statement of statistical mechanics: $-RT \ln K = \Delta E_0 - RT \ln (Q_B/Q_A)$ regardless of the interpretation of the terms. The classical statement (4) presents a different view of the forces competing for chemical equilibrium.

Our equation (6) uses for determination of the laws of chemical equilibrium two quantities with dimensions (calorie mol^{-1}). No quantity with the dimensions of entropy (calorie mol^{-1} K^{-1}) is involved and this may be considered a simplification.

Links with Planck

In an effort to relate the contents of equation (6) more closely to the classical statement (4) and, particularly, to one of three characteristic functions developed by Planck (1945, pp. 120-122), we have previously (Benzinger, 1969a) given the formulation

$$-RT \ln K = \Delta H_0^0 - T \Delta \Phi_T^0 \tag{7}$$

The term $T\Delta\Phi_T^0$ may be regarded as an entropy term, which is free and not bound and is not compensated in a simultaneous exchange of heat and entropy $\times T$ in equivalent amounts in the same direction between the reactant system and the surroundings, which would make the net change in free energy zero. Φ_T^0 represents standard "free entropy."

The symbol Φ was chosen because of the identity of our expression for free entropy with one of the three characteristic functions already discussed, which was designated Ψ, or Φ in earlier editions of Planck's treatise. Φ_T^0 is also identical with the free energy functions $([F-H_0^0]/T)$, tabulated in numerous standard works and textbooks. Planck's only important mention of chemical change in connection with Ψ or Φ reads:

"The additive constant of integration still has to be considered. This could depend on p, and, besides, on the chemical composition of the system. The dependence on p is given by the first equation of (79b) by a measurement of the volume, V. The dependence on the chemical composition can be concluded from the measurement of such processes as are accompanied by chemical changes of state."

At that point Planck left the issue as it stood. At the time of his writing, the man-made macromolecules of the modern chemist and the coded giant molecules of biological systems were of no concern to the physicist. The thermodynamics of most of the chemical reactions then known could be described satisfactorily with the terms of equation (4), as $\int_0^T \Delta C_p dT$ is often close to zero in these cases.

Near the end of the *Treatise*, however, Planck made a far-seeing statement and prediction, important to modern macromolecular chemistry and to molecular biology: "Accordingly, the determination of the laws of chemical equilibrium is

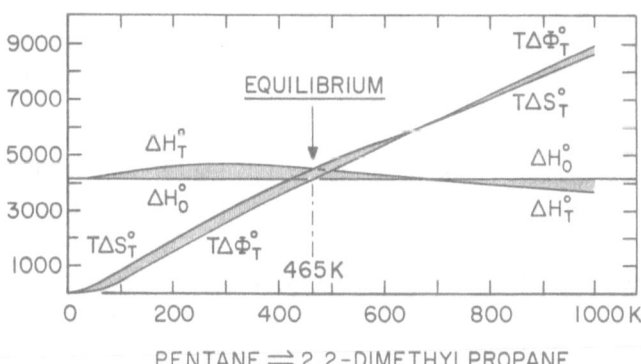

FIG. 14. Isomerization of a 5-carbon compound. Thermodynamic data from 0°K to 1,000°K, (a) in classical form (ΔH_T^0 and $T\Delta S_T^0$) and (b) in accordance with the free entropy concept by ΔH_T^0 and $T\Delta\Phi_T^0 = T\int_0^T \frac{\Delta C_p}{T}dT - \int_0^T \Delta C_p dT$. At the equilibrium point, 465°K, the difference between the two presentations is 10%. (From Benzinger. 1971. *Nature* [London], 229:100-102. Courtesy of Macmillan [Journals] Ltd.)

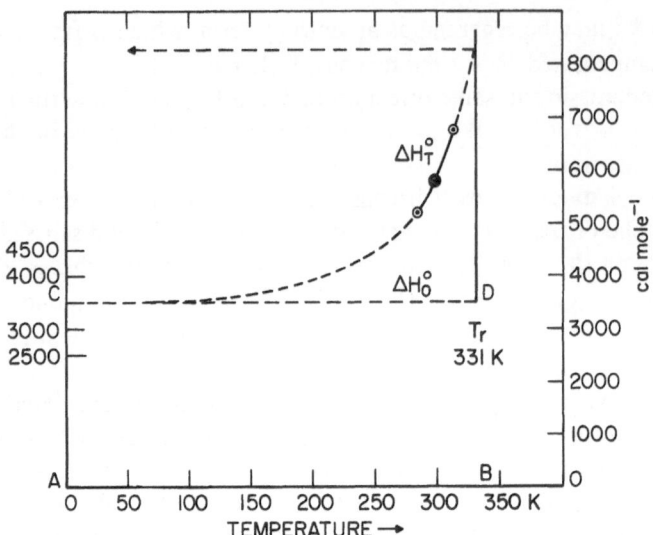

FIG. 15. Thermodynamics of unwinding the poly-A:poly-U double helix. Heats of reaction, one measured by Kitzinger et al. (1962) and three by Rawitscher et al. (1963), are plotted against the temperature axis *AB*. The plot is tentatively extrapolated to $\Delta H_0^0 = (\Delta H_T^0 - \int_0^T \Delta C_p dT)$ with zero slope at 0°K (on third law considerations). This gives a tentative value for ΔH_0^0 (chemical bond energy for two hydrogen bonds per base pair) between 2,500 and 4,500 calorie mole^{-1} or possibly less, compared with more than 8,000 measured as heat of reaction. (The curve cannot be sensibly extrapolated for zero slope at 0°K to 8,000 calorie mole^{-1} (uppermost broken line), taking heat of reaction for chemical bond energy in classical manner (see Pauling, 1960). The plot represents $\Delta\Gamma_T = \int_0^T \Delta C_p dT$ with the temperature axis *CD*. (From Benzinger. 1971. *Nature* [London], 229:100-102. Courtesy of Macmillan [Journals] Ltd.)

made to depend on measurements of heat capacity and heat of reaction . . . to be sure, the experimental results available are not sufficiently extensive to test completely this far reaching conclusion from the theory."

In contrast to Planck's postulate the experimental determination of ΔH_T^0 and $T\Delta S_T^0$ in the classical equation (4) does not depend on measurements of heat capacity, either at room temperature or at any temperature between T and 0°K. Values of ΔH_T^0 and $T\Delta S_T^0$ follow simply from one measurement of heat and one chemical determination of K at room temperature, or even from two measurements of heat at room temperature without chemical analysis (Benzinger, 1956).

If Planck was right in postulating that measurements of heat capacity are indispensable for a determination of the laws of chemical equilibrium, and if our extension of equation (4) into equation (7) has carried out Planck's mandate correctly, then the experimental art of chemical thermodynamics with macromolecules is faced with a necessity for time consuming efforts. Only the first of the two integrals

$$\int_0^T \frac{\Delta C_p}{T} dT = \Delta S_T^0 \quad \text{and} \quad \int_0^T \Delta C_p dT = \Delta\Gamma_T^0$$

is easily obtained from ΔH_T^o and K or even from two measurements of heat at room temperature (Benzinger, 1956). The second integral looks less complex than the first, but cannot be determined by any shortcut procedure. It is only possible to obtain it by measurements of ΔC_p at all temperatures between 0°K and T.

The treatment of $\int_0^T \Delta C_p dT$ as a negligible quantity is not a serious omission in ideal gas reactions, electron transport or other interactions of the smallest chemical entities. The contribution which our concept can make to the thermodynamic understanding of various kinds of chemical change is measured in differences between ΔH_T^o and ΔH_0^o and between $T\Delta S_T^o$ and $T\Delta \Phi_T$.

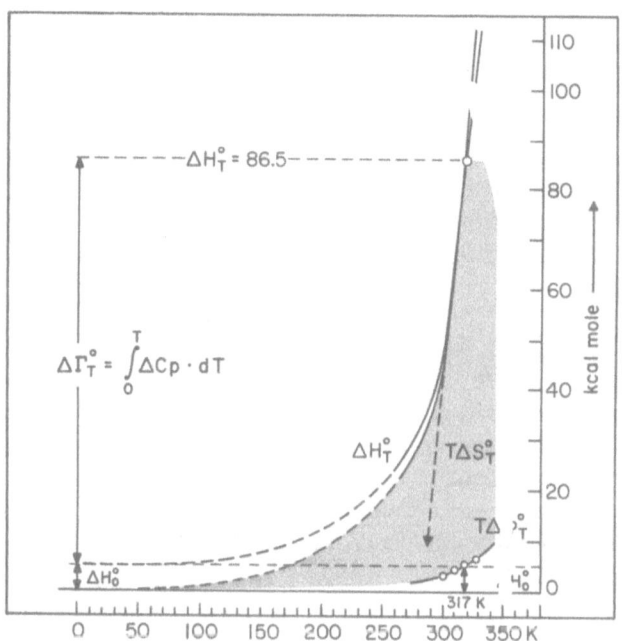

FIG. 16. Thermodynamics of protein unfolding (ribonuclease) using data measured by Danforth et al. (1967). Midpoint of unfolding, 317°K; heat of unfolding, 86,500 calorie mole^{-1} and "slope" of ΔH_T^o against temperature $\Delta_{p317}^o = 2,300$ calorie mole^{-1} K^{-1}. Tentative plots of ΔH_T^o or $\Delta \Gamma_T^o$ $= \int_0^T \Delta C_p dT$, $T\Delta S_T^o$ and $T\Delta \Phi_T^o = [T\int_0^T \frac{\Delta C_p}{T} dT - \int_0^T \Delta C_p dT]$ were obtained by extrapolation to zero slopes at 0°K as required by the third law. A tentative value of ~5,000 calorie mole^{-1} is found for ΔH_0^o, the energy of those few bonds that hold the chain of amino acids in its peculiar, biologically active, conformation. The experimental plot of ΔH_T^o with the given slope at 317°K cannot be sensibly extrapolated to zero slope at 0°K with 86,500 calorie mole^{-1} (broken straight line) as would be required if heat of reaction were taken for bond energy in classical fashion (see Pauling, 1960). The graph of $T\Delta \Phi_T^o$ (circles) is based on $\Delta \Gamma_T^o$ values from optically determined, reactant and product concentrations (Danforth et al., 1967). The slopes are experimental. The magnitude of ΔH_0^o is tentative and subject to revision in the light of low temperature measurements of heat capacity differences. (From Benzinger. 1971. Nature [London], 229:100-102. Courtesy of Macmillan [Journals] Ltd.)

Numerical Differences

In the formation of water vapor from the elements in the gas state, for example, this difference is about 1%. The difference is, however, of order 10% for isomerization of an organic molecule of only five carbon chain length shown in Figure 14, and for the formation of the double helix from single stranded polynucleotides shown in Figure 15 the preliminary estimate of the difference is 100% or more. An even higher difference can be predicted from available data for the unfolding of a protein after breakage of only a few bonds that hold the chain in its peculiar conformation (Figure 16).

Our thermodynamic concept thus offers an explanation for heats of reaction of more than 8,000 calorie mol^{-1} per base pair in Figure 15; estimates for two hydrogen bonds per base pair would be much lower. The concept offers an explanation for the dramatic dependence of ΔH_T^0 on temperature observed in recent years in molecular biology. It is our conclusion that indirect or direct determinations of heat capacities ΔC_p down to the lowest attainable temperatures or determination of chemical-bond energies from atomic data (Sanderson, 1971) are indispensable for a future understanding of the thermodynamics of macromolecular change.

ACKNOWLEDGMENTS

The authors wish to express their gratitude to the Spinco Division of Beckman Instruments Inc. for permission to reprint parts of an article appearing in their publication *Fractions* (Benzinger, 1965) and to Macmillan (Journals) Ltd. for permission to reproduce an article appearing in *Nature* (Benzinger, 1971). The authors are also grateful to Mr. Paul Mills of LKB Instruments Inc. for reading the manuscript.

REFERENCES

Benzinger, T. H. 1956. Equations to obtain for equilibrium reactions free energy, heat and entropy changes from two calorimetric measurements. Proc. Nat. Acad. Sci. U.S.A., 42:109-113.

———— 1965. Heatburst microcalorimetry. Fractions, No. 2:1-10. Palo Alto, California, Spinco Division, Beckman Instruments, Inc.

———— 1969a. Thermodynamic basis of life and growth: The driving forces of chemical change. In Heald, F. P., ed., Adolescent Nutrition and Growth. New York, Appleton-Century-Crofts.

———— 1969b. Ultrasensitive reaction calorimetry. In Alexander, P., and H. P. Lundgren, eds., A Laboratory Manual of Analytical Methods of Protein Chemistry, Vol. 5, pp. 95-149. Oxford and New York, Pergamon Press.

———— 1971. Thermodynamics, chemical reactions and molecular biology. Nature (London), 229:100-102.

———— and R. Hems. 1956. Reversibility and equilibrium of the glutaminase reaction observed calorimetrically to find the free energy of adenosine triphosphate hydrolysis. Proc. Nat. Acad. Sci. U.S.A., 42:896-900.

———— and C. Kitzinger. 1954. Microcalorimetry of simple biochemical systems. Fed. Proc., 13:11.

———— and C. Kitzinger. 1963. Microcalorimetry, new methods and objectives. *In* Hardy, J. D., ed., Temperature—Its Measurement and Control in Science and Industry, Vol. 3, 43-60. New York, Reinhold Press.

———— C. Kitzinger, R. Hems, and K. Burton. 1959. Free energy changes of the glutaminase reaction and the hydrolysis of the terminal pyrophosphate bond of adenosinetriphosphate. Biochem. J., 71:400-407.

Danforth, R., H. Krakauer, and J. Sturtevant. 1967. Differential calorimetry of thermally induced processes in solution. Rev. Sci. Instrum., 38:484-487.

Kitzinger, C., and T. H. Benzinger. 1955. Wärmetönung der Adenosintri-phosphorsäure-Spaltung. Z. Naturforsch., 10B:375-382.

———— and T. H. Benzinger. 1960. Principle and method of heatburst microcalorimetry and the determination of free energy, enthalpy, and entropy changes. Meth. Biochem. Anal., 8:309-360.

———— R. F. Steiner, and T. H. Benzinger. 1962. Proc. Int. Union Physiol. Sci., 2:547.

Klotz, I. 1967. Energy Changes in Biochemical Reactions. New York, Academic Press.

O'Reilly, R. A., J. I. Ohms, and C. H. Motley. 1969. Studies on coumarin anticoagulant drugs. Heat of interaction of sodium warfarin and human plasma albumin by heatburst microcalorimetry. J. Biol. Chem., 244:1303-1305.

Pauling, L. 1960. The Nature of the Chemical Bond. Ithaca, New York, Cornell University Press.

Planck, M. 1945. Treatise on Thermodynamics, 3rd ed. New York, Dover Press.

Rawitscher, M. A., P. D. Ross, and J. Sturtevant. 1963. The heat of the reaction between polyriboadenylic acid and polyribouridylic acid. J. Amer. Chem. Soc., 85:1915-1918.

Sanderson, R. T. 1971. Chemical Bonds and Bond Energy. New York, Academic Press.

Steiner, R. F., and C. Kitzinger 1956. A calorimetric determination of the heat of an antigen-antibody reaction. J. Biol. Chem., 222:271-284.

———— and C. Kitzinger. 1962. Heat of reaction of polyriboadenylic acid and polyribouridylic acid. Nature (London), 194:1172-1173.

Wadsö, I. 1968. Design and testing of a microcalorimeter. Acta Chem. Scand., 22:927-937.

INDEX